The Cardiomyopathic Heart

The Cardiomyopathic Heart

Editors

Makoto Nagano, M.D.

Professor and Director
Department of Internal Medicine
Jikei University School of Medicine
Tokyo, Japan

Nobuakira Takeda, M.D.

Department of Internal Medicine
Jikei University School of Medicine
Tokyo, Japan

Naranjan S. Dhalla, Ph.D.

Distinguished Professor and Head
Division of Cardiovascular Sciences
St. Boniface General Hospital Research Centre
University of Manitoba
Winnipeg, Canada

Raven Press **New York**

Raven Press, Ltd., 1185 Avenue of the Americas, New York, New York 10036

Made in the United States of America

Library of Congress Cataloging-in-Publication Data

The cardiomyopathic heart / editors, Makoto Nagano, Nobuakira Takeda,
  Naranjan S. Dhalla.
       p.   cm.
    Includes bibliographical references and index.
    ISBN 0–7817–0092–2 (hardcover)
    1. Myocardium—Pathophysiology—Congresses.   2. Hamsters as
laboratory animals—Congresses.   I. Nagano, Makoto, 1928–
II. Takeda, Nobuakira.   III. Dhalla, Naranjan S.
    [DNLM: 1. Myocardial Diseases—congresses.   2. Heart Failure,
Congestive—congresses.   3. Disease Models, Animal—congresses.
4. Hamsters—congresses.   WG 280 C26665 1993]
RC685.M9C354   1994
616.1′24—dc20
DNLM/DLC
for Library of Congress   93–4656
                                                        CIP

9   8   7   6   5   4   3   2   1

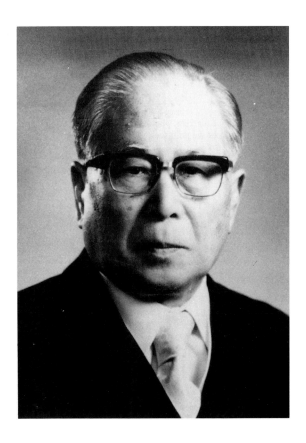

Contents

I. Hamster Cardiomyopathy and Congestive Heart Failure

Cellular and Subcellular Basis of Contractile Dysfunction

II. Hypertrophic, Congestive, and Metabolic Cardiomyopathies

Mechanisms of Heart Dysfunction in Cardiomyopathies

Contributors

Naohiko Akiyama

Department of Internal Medicine
Faculty of Medicine
University of Nagoya
Tsuruma
Showa-ku
Nagoya 466, Japan

Nikolai Aldag

Zentrum der Inneren Medizin
Abteilung für Kardiologie
Johann Wolfgang Goethe-Universität
Theodor-Stern-Kai 7
D-6000 Frankfurt am Main, Germany

Tsutomu Araki

The Second Department of Internal
*   Medicine*
Kanazawa University School of Medicine
Takara-machi 13-1
Kanazawa 920, Japan

Xiuqi Bai

Institute of Preclinical Sciences
N. Bethune University of Medical Sciences
National Key Laboratory of Enzyme
*   Engineering*
Jilin University
Xinmin Street 6
Chang Chun, Jilin, China

Rong Bang Hong

The Third Department of Internal
*   Medicine*
Hamamatsu University School of Medicine
3600 Handa-cho
Hamamatsu 431-31, Japan

Robert E. Beamish

Division of Cardiovascular Sciences
St. Boniface General Hospital Research
*   Centre*
351 Tache Avenue
Winnipeg, Manitoba R2H 2A6, Canada

Marcel Borgers

Department of Physiology
Life Sciences
Janssen Research Foundation
Turnhoutseweg 30
B-2340 Beerse Belgium

Lesley A. Brown

Department of Cardiac Medicine
National Heart and Lung Institute
Dovehouse Street
London SW3 6LY, United Kingdom

Martin Büchler

Medizinische Klinik III
Kardiologie
Universität Freiburg
Hugstetter Str. 55
7800 Freiburg, Germany

René Cardinal

Centre de Recherche
Hôpital Sacré-Coeur
Montréal H4J 1C5, Canada

Gonghe Dai

Institute of Preclinical Sciences
N. Bethune University of Medical Sciences
National Key Laboratory of Enzyme
*   Engineering*
Jilin University
Xinmin Street 6
Chang Chun, Jilin, China

Barbara A. Danowski
Department of Anatomy
Pennsylvania Muscle Institute
School of Medicine
University of Pennsylvania
Philadelphia, Pennsylvania 19104

Federica del Monte
Department of Cardiac Medicine
National Heart and Lung Institute
Dovehouse Street
London SW3 6LY, United Kingdom

Ken S. Dhalla
Division of Cardiovascular Sciences
St. Boniface General Hospital Research
 Centre
351 Tache Avenue
Winnipeg, Manitoba R2H 2A6, Canada

Naranjan S. Dhalla
Division of Cardiovascular Sciences
St. Boniface General Hospital Research
 Centre
351 Tache Avenue
Winnipeg, Manitoba R2H 2A6, Canada

Hitoshi Ebata
Department of Cardiology
Jichi Medical School
Minamikawachi-Machi
Tochigi 329-04, Japan

Vijayan Elimban
Division of Cardiovascular Sciences
St. Boniface General Hospital Research
 Centre
351 Tache Avenue
Winnipeg, Manitoba R2H 2A6, Canada

Terumoto Fukuchi
The Third Department of Internal
 Medicine
Hamamatsu University School of Medicine
3600 Handa-cho
Hamamatsu 431-31, Japan

Hugo Geerts
Department of Physiology
Life Sciences
Janssen Research Foundation
Turnhoutseweg 30
B-2340 Beerse, Belgium

Yoshihio Hanaki
Department of Internal Medicine
Faculty of Medicine
University of Nagoya
Tsuruma
Showa-ku
Nagoya 466, Japan

Haruo Hanawa
The First Department of Internal Medicine
Niigata University School of Medicine
Niigata 951, Japan

Sian E. Harding
Department of Cardiac Medicine
National Heart and Lung Institute
Dovehouse Street
London SW3 6LY, United Kingdom

Gerd Hasenfuss
Medizinische Klinik III
Kardiologie, Universität Freiburg
Hugstetter Str. 55
7800 Freiburg, Germany

Hidekazu Hashimoto
The Second Department of Internal
 Medicine
Nagoya University School of Medicine
65 Tsuruma-cho
Showa-ku
Nagoya 466, Japan

Kazuki Hattori
Department of Internal Medicine II
Faculty of Medicine
University of Nagoya
Tsuruma
Showa-ku
Nagoya 466, Japan

Jitsuo Higaki
Department of Geriatric Medicine
Osaka University Medical School
1-1-50 Fukushima
Fukushima-ku
Osaka 553, Japan

Yuji Hiraoka
The Second Department of Internal
Medicine
Faculty of Medicine
Toyama Medical and Pharmaceutical
University
2630 Sugitani
Toyama 930-01, Japan

Yoshiyuki Hirota
Department of Internal Medicine
Aoto Hospital
Jikei University School of Medicine
Aoto 6-41-2
Katsushika-ku
Tokyo 125, Japan

Yukihiro Hojo
Department of Cardiology
Jichi Medical School
Minamikawachi-Machi
Tochigi 329-04, Japan

Christian Holubarsch
Medizinische Klinik III
Kardiologie, Universität Freiburg
Hugstetter Str. 55
7800 Freiburg, Germany

Hiroyuki Hosono
The First Department of Internal Medicine
Niigata University School of Medicine
Niigata 951, Japan

Lizhong Hou
Institute of Preclinical Sciences
N. Bethune University of Medical Sciences
National Key Laboratory of Enzyme
Engineering
Jilin University
Xinmin Street 6
Chang Chun, Jilin, China

Uichi Ikeda
Department of Cardiology
Jichi Medical School
Minamikawachi-Machi
Tochigi 329-04, Japan

Takayoshi Ikegaya
The Third Department of Internal
Medicine
Hamamatsu University School of Medicine
3600 Handa-cho
Hamamatsu 431-31, Japan

Susumu Imai
The Second Department of Internal
Medicine
Gunma University School of Medicine
3-39-15, Showa-machi
Maebashi-city
Gunma 371, Japan

Issei Imanaga
Department of Physiology
School of Medicine
Fukuoka University
Fukuoka 814-01, Japan

Kyoko Imanaka-Yoshida
The First Department of Internal Medicine
Mie University School of Medicine
Tsu, Mie 514, Japan

Hidekazu Ino
The Second Department of Internal
Medicine
Kanazawa University School of Medicine
Takara-machi 13-1
Kanazawa 920, Japan

Takayuki Ito
The Second Department of Internal
Medicine
Nagoya University School of Medicine
65 Tsuruma-cho
Showa-ku
Nagoya 466, Japan

Takaaki Iwai
Department of Internal Medicine
Aoto Hospital
Jikei University School of Medicine
Aoto 6-41-2
Katsushika-ku
Tokyo 125, Japan

Yoshio Iwama
The Second Department of Internal
  Medicine
Nagoya University School of Medicine
65 Tsuruma-cho
Showa-ku
Nagoya 466, Japan

Tutomu Iwasaki
The Second Department of Internal
  Medicine
Gunma University School of Medicine
3-39-15, Showa-machi
Maebashi-city
Gunma 371, Japan

Tohru Izumi
The First Department of Internal Medicine
Niigata University School of Medicine
Niigata 951, Japan

Gaëtan Jasmin
Département de Pathologie, Faculté de
  Médecine
Université de Montréal
C.P. 6128
Succursale A
Montréal, Québec H3C 3J7, Canada

Hanjörg Just
Medizinische Klinik III
Kardiologie, Universität Freiburg
Hugstetter Str. 55
7800 Freiburg, Germany

Martin Kaltenbach
Zentrum der Inneren Medizin
Abteilung für Kardiologie
Johann Wolfgang Goethe-Universität
Theodor-Stern-Kai 7
D-6000 Frankfurt am Main, Germany

Yojiro Kamegawa
Department of Physiology
School of Medicine
Fukuoka University
Fukuoka 814-01, Japan

Toshiko Kanbe
Department of Cardiology
Jichi Medical School
Minamikawachi-Machi
Tochigi 329-04, Japan

Masanori Kaneko
The Third Department of Internal
  Medicine
Hamamatsu University School of Medicine
3600 Handa-cho
Hamamatsu 431-31, Japan

Valery I. Kapelko
Cardiology Research Center
15A Cherepkovskaya St.
125252 Moscow, Russia

Mitsutoshi Kato
Department of Internal Medicine
Aoto Hospital
Jikei University School of Medicine
Aoto 6-41-2
Katsushika-ku
Tokyo 125, Japan

Tomoko Kato
Department of Biomedical Chemistry
Faculty of Medicine
University of Nagoya
Tsuruma
Showa-ku
Nagoya 466, Japan

Nalini Kaul
Division of Cardiovascular Sciences
St. Boniface General Hospital Research
  Centre and Department of Physiology
Faculty of Medicine
University of Manitoba
351 Tache Avenue
Winnipeg, Manitoba R2H 2A6, Canada

Hideaki Kawaguchi
Department of Cardiovascular Medicine
Hokkaido University School of Medicine
Sapporo 060, Japan

Naomasa Kawaguchi
Department of Pathology
College of Biomedical Technology
Osaka University
Toyonaka, Japan

Shoji Kawazu
The Second Department of Internal
  Medicine
Gunma University School of Medicine
3-39-15, Showa-machi
Maebashi-city
Gunma 371, Japan

Zaza A. Khuchua
Cardiology Research Center
15A Cherepkovskaya St.
125252 Moscow, Russia

Chiharu Kishimoto
The Second Department of Internal
  Medicine
Faculty of Medicine
Toyama Medical and Pharmaceutical
  University
2630 Sugitani
Toyama 930-01, Japan

Akira Kitabatake
Department of Cardiovascular Medicine
Hokkaido University School of Medicine
Sapporo 060, Japan

Junzoh Kitoh
Institute for Laboratory Animal Research
Nagoya University School of Medicine
65 Tsuruma-cho
Showa-ku
Nagoya 466, Japan

Akira Kobayashi
The Third Department of Internal
  Medicine
Hamamatsu University School of Medicine
3600 Handa-cho
Hamamatsu 431-31, Japan

Ryuichi Kobayashi
Department of Geriatric Medicine
Osaka University Medical School
1-1-50 Fukushima
Fukushima-ku
Osaka 553, Japan

Makoto Kodama
The First Department of Internal Medicine
Niigata University School of Medicine
Niigata 951, Japan

Department of Medical Technology
The College of Biomedical Technology of
  Niigata University
Niigata 951, Japan

Sen Koyama
Tachikawa Hospital
Nagaoka, Japan

Kazimierz Krupinski
Zentrum der Inneren Medizin
Abteilung für Kardiologie
Johann Wolfgang Goethe-Universität
Theodor-Stern-Kai 7
D-6000 Frankfurt am Main, Germany

Toshiyuki Kudo
Department of Cardiovascular Medicine
Hokkaido University School of Medicine
Sapporo 060, Japan

Atushi Kuroda
The First Department of Internal Medicine
Kagoshima University Medical School
Kagoshima, Japan

Masahiko Kurokawa
Department of Virology
Faculty of Medicine
Toyama Medical and Pharmaceutical
*   University*
2630 Sugitani
Toyama 930-01, Japan

Shue-L. Lee
Division of Cardiovascular Sciences
St. Boniface General Hospital Research
*   Centre*
351 Tache Avenue
Winnipeg, Manitoba R2H 2A6, Canada

Fen Li
Département de Pathologie, Faculté de
*   Médecine*
Université de Montréal
C.P. 6128
Succursale A
Montréal, Québec H3C 3J7, Canada

Guang-qu Li
Institute of Preclinical Sciences
N. Bethune University of Medical Sciences
National Key Laboratory of Enzyme
*   Engineering*
Jilin University
Xinmin Street 6
Chang Chun, Jilin, China

Shaowei Li
Institute of Preclinical Sciences
N. Bethune University of Medical Sciences
National Key Laboratory of Enzyme
*   Engineering*
Jilin University
Xinmin Street 6
Chang Chun, Jilin, China

Naoki Makino
Department of Bioclimatology and
*   Medicine*
Medical Institute of Bioregulation
Kyushu University
Beppu 874, Japan

Ashwani Malhotra
Division of Cardiology
Department of Medicine
Montefiore Medical Center
111 East 210th Street
Bronx, NY 10467

Toru Maruyama
Department of Bioclimatology and
*   Medicine*
Medical Institute of Bioregulation
Kyushu University
Beppu 874, Japan

Fumiaki Masani
Division of Cardiology
Niigata Kuwana Hospital
Niigata 951, Japan

Hisamichi Masuda
The Third Department of Internal
*   Medicine*
Hamamatsu University School of Medicine
3600 Handa-cho
Hamamatsu 431-31, Japan

Kazuhiro Masutomo
Department of Bioclimatology and
*   Medicine*
Medical Institute of Bioregulation
Kyushu University
Beppu 874, Japan

Felix Z. Meerson
Institute of General Pathology and
*   Pathophysiology*
Baltijskaya 8
Moscow 125315, Russia

Hiroshi Mikami
Department of Geriatric Medicine
Osaka University Medical School
1-1-50 Fukushima
Fukushima-ku
Osaka 553, Japan

Yutaka Miyazaki
The Second Department of Internal
Medicine
Nagoya University School of Medicine
65 Tsuruma-cho
Showa-ku
Nagoya 466, Japan

Shin-ichi Momomura
The Second Department of Internal
Medicine
University of Tokyo
Hongo 7-3-1, Bunkyo-ku
Tokyo 113, Japan

Ursula Müller
Department of Medicine I
Klinikum Grosshadern
University of München
München, Germany

Kazuhiko Murata
The Second Department of Internal
Medicine
Gunma University School of Medicine
3-39-15, Showa-machi
Maebashi-city
Gunma 371, Japan

Ernst Mutschler
Pharmakologisches Institut für
Naturwissenschaftler
Johann Wolfgang Goethe-Univerisität
Theodor-Stern-Kai 7
D-6000 Frankfurt am Main, Germany

Makoto Nagai
Department of Internal Medicine
Aoto Hospital
Jikei University School of Medicine
Aoto 6-41-2
Katsushika-ku
Tokyo 125, Japan

Makoto Nagano
Department of Internal Medicine
Aoto Hospital
Jikei University School of Medicine
Aoto 6-41-2
Katsushika-ku
Tokyo 125, Japan

Masahiro Nagano
Department of Geriatric Medicine
Osaka University Medical School
1-1-50 Fukushima
Fukushima-ku
Osaka 553, Japan

Fumiaki Nakamura
Department of Geriatric Medicine
Osaka University Medical School
1-1-50 Fukushima
Fukushima-ku
Osaka 553, Japan

Masayuki Nishimura
Department of Clinical Genetics
Medical Institute of Bioregulation
Kyushu University
Beppu 874, Japan

Toshihiro Obayashi
Department of Internal Medicine II
Faculty of Medicine
University of Nagoya
Tsuruma
Showa-ku
Nagoya 466, Japan

Hiroshi Ochiai
Department of Virology
Faculty of Medicine
Toyama Medical and Pharmaceutical
University
2630 Sugitani
Toyama 930-01, Japan

Peter O'Gara
Department of Cardiac Medicine
National Heart and Lung Institute
Dovehouse Street
London SW3 6LY, United Kingdom

Toshio Ogihara
Department of Geriatric Medicine
Osaka University Medical School
1-1-50 Fukushima
Fukushima-ku
Osaka 553, Japan

Tadanari Ohkubo
Department of Internal Medicine
Aoto Hospital
Jikei University School of Medicine
Aoto 6-41-2
Katsushika-ku
Tokyo 125, Japan

Naoki Ohta
The Second Department of Internal
* Medicine*
Gunma University School of Medicine
3-39-15, Showa-machi
Maebashi-city
Gunma 371, Japan

Toshiko Ohta
Department of Microbiology
Tsukuba University School of Medicine
Ibaragi, Japan

Hiroshi Okada
Department of Cardiovascular Medicine
Hokkaido University School of Medicine
Sapporo 060, Japan

Yoshiya Oku
The First Department of Internal Medicine
Kagoshima University Medical School
Kagoshima, Japan

Kenji Okumura
The Second Department of Internal
* Medicine*
Nagoya University School of Medicine
65 Tsuruma-cho
Showa-ku
Nagoya 466, Japan

Ko Okumura
Department of Immunology
School of Medicine
Juntendo University
Tokyo, Japan

Hans-Georg Olbrich
Zentrum der Inneren Medizin
Abteilung für Kardiologie
Johann Wolfgang Goethe-Universität
Theodor-Stern-Kai 7
D-6000 Frankfurt am Main, Germany

Shunzo Onishi
Department of Pathology
College of Biomedical Technology
Osaka University
Toyonaka, Japan

Bohuslav Ošťádal
Institute of Physiology
Academy of Sciences of the Czech
* Republic*
Vídeňská 1083
142 20 Prague 4, Czech Republic

Ivana Ošťádalová
Institute of Physiology
Academy of Sciences of the Czech
* Republic*
Vídeňská 1083
142 20 Prague 4, Czech Republic

Yibing Ouyang
Institute of Preclinical Sciences
N. Bethune University of Medical Sciences
National Key Laboratory of Enzyme
* Engineering*
Jilin University
Xinmin Street 6
Chang Chun, Jilin, China

Takayuki Ozawa
Department of Biomedical Chemistry
Faculty of Medicine
University of Nagoya
Tsuruma
Showa-ku
Nagoya 466, Japan

Vincenzo Panagia
Division of Cardiovascular Sciences
St. Boniface General Hospital Research
* Centre*
351 Tache Avenue
Winnipeg, Manitoba R2H 2A6, Canada

Bukert Pieske
Medizinische Klinik III
Kardiologie, Universität Freiburg
Hugstetter Str. 55
7800 Freiburg, Germany

Philip A. Poole-Wilson
Department of Cardiac Medicine
National Heart and Lung Institute
Dovehouse Street
London SW3 6LY, United Kingdom

Mikhail I. Popovich
Institute of Prophylactic and Clinical
  Medicine
20 Kubinskoi Revolutsii St.
Kishinev, Moldova

Herbert Posival
Klinik für Thorax- und
  Kardiovaskularchirurgie
Herzzentrum
Nordrhein-Westfalen
Bad Oeynhausen, Germany

Libuse Proschek
Département de Pathologie
Faculté de Médecine
Université de Montréal
C.P. 6128
Succursale A
Montréal, Québec H3C 3J7, Canada

Arvinder Randhawa
Division of Cardiovascular Sciences
St. Boniface General Hospital Research
  Centre and Department of Physiology
Faculty of Medicine
University of Manitoba
351 Tache Avenue
Winnipeg, Manitoba R2H 2A6, Canada

Tatiana Ravingerová
Institute for Heart Research
Slovak Academy of Sciences
Dubravska cesta 9
842 33 Bratislava, Czech and Slovak
  Federative Republic

Heinz Rupp
Institute of Physiology II
University of Tübingen
Gmelinstrasse 5
D-7400 Tübingen 1, Germany

Zdeněk Rychter
Institute of Physiology
Academy of Sciences of the Czech
  Republic
Vídeňská 1083
142 20 Prague 4, Czech Republic

Makihiko Saeki
The First Department of Internal Medicine
Niigata University School of Medicine
Niigata 951, Japan

Kazuto Saito
Health Service Center
National Institute of Fitness & Sports
Shiromizu-1
Kanoya City 8911-23, Japan

Valdur A. Saks
Cardiology Research Center
15A Cherepkovskaya St.
125252 Moscow, Russia

Jean M. Sanger
Department of Anatomy
Pennsylvania Muscle Institute
School of Medicine
University of Pennsylvania
Philadelphia, Pennsylvania 19104

Joseph W. Sanger
Department of Anatomy
Pennsylvania Muscle Institute
School of Medicine
University of Pennsylvania
Philadelphia, Pennsylvania 19104

Hitoshi Sano
Department of Cardiovascular Medicine
Hokkaido University School of Medicine
Sapporo 060, Japan

Shigetake Sasayama
The Second Department of Internal
  Medicine
Faculty of Medicine
Toyama Medical and Pharmaceutical
  University
2630 Sugitani
Toyama 930-01, Japan

Markward Schneider
Zentrum der Pathologie
Johann Wolfgang Goethe-Universität
Theodor-Stern-Kai 7
D-6000 Frankfurt am Main, Germany

Yoshitane Seino
Department of Cardiology
Jichi Medical School
Minamikawachi-Machi
Tochigi 329-04, Japan

Yoshinori Seko
The Third Department of Internal
  Medicine
Faculty of Medicine
University of Tokyo
Tokyo, Japan

Takashi Serizawa
The Second Department of Internal
  Medicine
University of Tokyo
Hongo 7-3-1
Bunkyo-ku
Tokyo 113, Japan

Rajat Sethi
Division of Cardiovascular Sciences
St. Boniface General Hospital Research
  Centre
351 Tache Avenue
Winnipeg, Manitoba R2H 2A6, Canada

Kanu R. Shah
Division of Cardiovascular Sciences
St. Boniface General Hospital Research
  Centre
351 Tache Avenue
Winnipeg, Manitoba R2H 2A6, Canada

Akira Shibata
The First Department of Internal Medicine
Niigata University School of Medicine
Niigata 951, Japan

Kazuyuki Shimada
Department of Cardiology
Jichi Medical School
Minamikawachi-Machi
Tochigi 329-04, Japan

Masami Shimizu
The Second Department of Internal
  Medicine
Kanazawa University School of Medicine
Takara-machi 13-1
Kanazawa 920, Japan

Yoichi Shinkai
Department of Immunology
School of Medicine
Juntendo University
Tokyo, Japan

Kimiyasu Shiraki
Department of Virology
Faculty of Medicine
Toyama Medical and Pharmaceutical
  University
2630 Sugitani
Toyama 930-01, Japan

Pawan K. Singal
Division of Cardiovascular Sciences
St. Boniface General Hospital Research
  Centre and Department of Physiology
Faculty of Medicine
University of Manitoba
351 Tache Avenue
Winnipeg, Manitoba R2H 2A6, Canada

Natasa Siveski-Iliskovic
Division of Cardiovascular Sciences
St. Boniface General Hospital Research
  Centre and Department of Physiology
Faculty of Medicine
University of Manitoba
351 Tache Avenue
Winnipeg, Manitoba R2H 2A6, Canada

Jan Slezak
Institute for Heart Research
Slovak Academy of Sciences
Dubravska cesta 9
842 33 Bratislava, Czech and Slovak
  Federative Republic

Tetsuro Suetugu
The First Department of Internal Medicine
Kagoshima University Medical School
Kagoshima, Japan

Norihiko Sugihara
The Second Department of Internal Medicine
Kanazawa University School of Medicine
Takara-machi 13-1
Kanazawa 920, Japan

Seiryo Sugiura
The Second Department of Internal Medicine
University of Tokyo
Hongo 7-3-1
Bunkyo-ku
Tokyo 113, Japan

Satoru Sugiyama
Department of Biomedical Chemistry
Faculty of Medicine
University of Nagoya
Tsuruma
Showa-ku
Nagoya 466, Japan

Shingo Suzuki
Division of Cardiovascular Sciences
St. Boniface General Hospital Research Centre
351 Tache Avenue
Winnipeg, Manitoba R2H 2A6, Canada

Tadashi Suzuki
College of Medical Care and Technology
Gunma University
Showa-machi
Maebashi-city
Gunma 371, Japan

László Szekeres
Institute of Pharmacology
Albert Szent-Györgyi Medical University
H-6720, Szeged, Hungary

Hitoshi Takada
The Second Department of Internal Medicine
Faculty of Medicine
Toyama Medical and Pharmaceutical University
2630 Sugitani
Toyama 930-01, Japan

Atsushi Takeda
Department of Internal Medicine
Aoto Hospital
Jikei University School of Medicine
Aoto 6-41-2
Katsushika-ku
Tokyo 125, Japan

Nobuakira Takeda
Department of Internal Medicine
Aoto Hospital
Jikei University School of Medicine
Aoto 6-41-2
Katsushika-ku
Tokyo 125, Japan

Ryoyu Takeda
The Second Department of Internal Medicine
Kanazawa University School of Medicine
Takara-machi 13-1
Kanazawa 920, Japan

Yutaka Takino
The Second Department of Internal Medicine
Gunma University School of Medicine
3-39-15, Showa-machi
Maebashi-city
Gunma 371, Japan

Hiromitsu Tanaka
The First Department of Internal Medicine
Kagoshima University Medical School
Kagoshima, Japan

Masashi Tanaka
Biomedical Chemistry
Faculty of Medicine
University of Nagoya
Tsuruma
Showa-ku
Nagoya 466, Japan

Akira Tanamura
Department of Internal Medicine
Aoto Hospital
Jikei University School of Medicine
Aoto 6-41-2
Katsushika-ku
Tokyo 125, Japan

Thomas P. Thomas
Division of Cadiovascular Sciences
St. Boniface General Hospital Research
*   Centre and Department of Physiology*
Faculty of Medicine
University of Manitoba
351 Tache Avenue
Winnipeg, Manitoba R2H 2A6, Canada

Yukio Toki
The Second Department of Internal
*   Medicine*
Nagoya University School of Medicine
65 Tsuruma-cho
Showa-ku
Nagoya 466, Japan

Shoichi Tomono
The Second Department of Internal
*   Medicine*
Gunma University School of Medicine
3-39-15, Showa-machi
Maebashi-city
Gunma 371, Japan

Narcisa Tribulová
Institute for Heart Research
Slovak Academy of Sciences
Dubravska cesta 9
842 33 Bratislava, Czech and Slovak
*   Federative Republic*

Yoshio Tsuruya
Department of Cardiology
Jichi Medical School
Minamikawachi-Machi
Tochigi 329-04, Japan

Vladimir I. Veksler
Cardiology Research Center
15A Cherepkovskaya St.
125252 Moscow, Russia

Renee Ventura-Clapier
Université Paris-Sud
Orsay, France

Luc ver Donck
Department of Physiology
Life Sciences
Janssen Research Foundation
Turnhoutseweg 30
B-2340 Beerse Belgium

Greet Verellen
Department of Physiology
Life Sciences
Janssen Research Foundation
Turnhoutseweg 30
B-2340 Beerse Belgium

Michel Vermeulen
Centre de Recherche
Hôpital Sacré-Coeur
Montréal H4J 1C5, Canada

Jingxin Wang
Institute of Preclinical Sciences
N. Bethune University of Medical Sciences
National Key Laboratory of Enzyme
*   Engineering*
Jilin University
Xinmin Street 6
Chang Chun, Jilin, China

Ken-ichi Watanabe
Division of Cardiology
Niigata Kuwana Hospital
Niigata 951, Japan

Karl Werdan
Department of Medicine I
Klinikum Grosshadern
University of München
München, Germany

Hans-Joachim Woltersdorf
Zentrum der Inneren Medizin
Abteilung für Kardiologie
Johann Wolfgang Goethe-Universität
Theodor-Stern-Kai 7
D-6000 Frankfurt am Main, Germany

Dylan G. Wynne
Department of Cardiac Medicine
National Heart and Lung Institute
Dovehouse Street
London SW3 6LY, United Kingdom

Hideo Yagita
Department of Immunology
School of Medicine
Juntendo University
Tokyo, Japan

Keiji Yamamoto
Department of Cardiology
Jichi Medical School
Minamikawachi-Machi
Tochigi 329-04, Japan

Hiroshi Yamashita
The Second Department of Internal
  Medicine
University of Tokyo
Hongo 7-3-1
Bunkyo-ku
Tokyo 113, Japan

Noboru Yamazaki
The Third Department of Internal
  Medicine
Hamamatsu University School of Medicine
3600 Handa-cho
Hamamatsu 431-31, Japan

Takashi Yanaga
Department of Bioclimatology and
  Medicine
Medical Institute of Bioregulation
Kyushu University
Beppu 874, Japan

Jie Yang
Biochemistry Department
China-Japan Friendship Hospital
Beijing, China

Tongshu Yang
Institute of Preclinical Sciences
N. Bethune University of Medical Sciences
National Key Laboratory of Enzyme
  Engineering
Jilin University
Xinmin Street 6
Chang Chun, Jilin, China

Yoshio Yazaki
The Third Department of Internal
  Medicine
Faculty of Medicine
University of Tokyo
Tokyo, Japan

Mitsuhiko Yoshino
The Second Department of Internal
  Medicine
Nagoya University School of Medicine
65 Tsuruma-cho
Showa-ku
Nagoya 466, Japan

Hiroyuki Yoshio
The Second Department of Internal
  Medicine
Kanazawa University School of Medicine
Takara-machi 13-1
Kanazawa 920, Japan

Shaosong Zhang
The First Department of Internal Medicine
Niigata University School of Medicine
Niigata 951, Japan

Ping Zhu
Institute of Preclinical Sciences
N. Bethune University of Medical Sciences
National Key Laboratory of Enzyme
  Engineering
Jilin University
Xinmin Street 6
Chang Chun, Jilin, China

Attila Ziegelhoeffer
Institute for Heart Research
Slovak Academy of Sciences
Dubravska cesta 9
842 33 Bratislava, Czech and Slovak
  Federative Republic

Heinz-Gerd Zimmer
Department of Physiology
University of Munich
Pettenkoferstr. 12
8000 München 2, Germany

Ladislav Zlatos
Institute of Pathophysiology
Medical Faculty
Comenius University
Bratislava, Czech and Slovak
  Federative Republic

Preface

Since the coinage of the term *cardiomyopathy* by Brigden in 1957, investigative cardiologists and pathologists have been classifying all sorts of cardiac diseases in this category, with the exception of coronary artery disease caused by obstruction of coronary vessels. In spite of the confusion regarding the usage of terminology, cardiomyopathies are generally divided into two types—primary cardiomyopathies and secondary cardiomyopathies. Primary cardiomyopathies include diseases affecting the myocardium alone by a process of unknown etiology; secondary cardiomyopathies include diseases of unusual pathogenesis in which the heart is involved in a generalized process underlying the disease. The large number of diseases associated with cardiomyopathy is impressive, so perhaps it is appropriate to use this terminology in a broad sense of the definition. Some of the commonly used terms in this area include congestive cardiomyopathy, hypertrophic cardiomyopathy, dilated cardiomyopathy, genetic cardiomyopathy, ischemic cardiomyopathy, alcoholic cardiomyopathy, diabetic cardiomyopathy, metabolic cardiomyopathy, infective cardiomyopathy, viral cardiomyopathy, catecholamine cardiomyopathy, and adriamycin cardiomyopathy. Regardless of the pathogenetic factors leading to the development of cardiomyopathy, it is becoming clear that a derangement of cardiac structure and metabolism occurs in cardiomyopathy, and this is usually associated with impaired heart function. Furthermore, hypertrophy of the myocardium is frequently associated with the process of cardiomyopathy. Because of the difficulties in assessing the cellular, metabolic, and molecular mechanisms involved in dysfunction of cardiomyopathic hearts in humans, a wide variety of experimental animal models have been developed. The exact mechanisms leading to the development of heart dysfunction in any experimental model of cardiomyopathys are not clear; however, imbalance of hormonal pattern has been commonly observed. The occurrence of intracellular Ca^{2+} overload is routinely suggested to explain the development of cellular damage and contractile failure in cardiomyopathic hearts.

Over the past 30 years much has been written on subcellular and metabolic alterations in different types of cardiomyopathic hearts. It is now timely to examine the literature closely if we are to improve our knowledge concerning the pathophysiology of heart dysfunction in cardiomyopathies.

The symposium "Cellular Abnormalities Associated with Cardiomyopathies in Animals," held in Tokyo in May 1992, organized by the Aoto Hospital of the Jikei University under the direction of Professor Makoto Nagano, provided an excellent forum for a meeting of experimental cardiologists and basic scientists to discuss problems related to heart dysfunction in cardiomyopathies.

Since cardiomyopathic hamsters have been widely used as an experimental model of heart disease, Part I of this book is devoted to hamster cardiomyopathy. The second part of the book examines hypertrophic, congestive, and metabolic cardio-myopathies in different experimental models. Together, the contributions provide a comprehensive synthesis of recent advances in the physiology, pharmacology, and biochemistry of the cardiomyopathic heart.

We believe that this book will provide a unified framework for a multidisciplin-ary approach to further studies in this highly complex field of cardiomyopathies. Because cardiomyopathies have been identified in all parts of the world, this book will be of interest to all practicing, clinical, and investigative cardiologists. It should serve as a valuable reference for basic scientists and postgraduate students, as well.

Makoto Nagano
Nobuakira Takeda
Naranjan S. Dhalla

Acknowledgments

We would like to thank the Eisai Co., Ltd., Mrs. T. Kikuchi, and several Japanese pharmaceutical companies for their generous financial support for the organization of the symposium as well as for the publication of the book. We also thank the Japanese Section of the International Society for Heart Research, the Research Committee for Etiology of Idiopathic Cardiomyopathy of the Ministry of Health and Welfare of Japan, and the Japan Heart Foundation for help in recruiting the outstanding investigators who contributed to the conference and this book. We express our deep appreciation to the members of the Department of Internal Medicine, Aoto Hospital, for their untiring efforts to make this symposium a success. Our cordial thanks go to the Council of Cardiac Metabolism of the International Society and Federation of Cardiology for the sponsorship of this symposium. The help of Mary Brown for the preparation of this book is highly appreciated. Special thanks are due to Ms. Lisa S. Berger and her editorial staff at Raven Press for their patience, interest, and hard work in assembling this volume.

The Cardiomyopathic Heart, edited by Makoto
Nagano, Nobuakira Takeda, and Naranjan S.
Dhalla. Raven Press, Ltd., New York © 1994.

1

Behavior of Subcellular Organelles during the Development of Congestive Heart Failure in Cardiomyopathic Hamsters (UM-X7.1)

*Naranjan S. Dhalla, Shue-L. Lee, Kanu R. Shah,
Vijayan Elimban, Shingo Suzuki, and †Gaetan Jasmin

*Division of Cardiovascular Sciences, St. Boniface General Hospital Research Centre,
Faculty of Medicine, University of Manitoba, Winnipeg; and †Department of Pathology,
Faculty of Medicine, University of Montreal, Montreal, Canada*

INTRODUCTION

By virtue of their contractile properties and ability to utilize energy, myofibrils are directly involved in generating contractile force. Mitochondria, the major sites of energy production, are considered to determine the status of heart function (1–4). On the basis of their properties to raise and lower the concentration of intracellular Ca^{2+}, both sarcoplasmic reticulum and sarcolemma primarily and mitochondria to some extent are involved in the regulation of heart function and metabolism (3,5–8). According to a current concept, excitation of myocardium is considered to open Ca^{2+} channels in the sarcolemmal membrane to permit the entry of a small amount of Ca^{2+} into the cell; some Ca^{2+} is also believed to enter via the sarcolemmal Na^+-Ca^{2+} exchange system upon depolarization. The source of this Ca^{2+} is primarily the sarcolemmal Ca^{2+} storage sites located on the exterior of the myocardial cell, which are in equilibrium with the extracellular Ca^{2+}. The exact mechanisms for opening Ca^{2+} channels are not clear, but these channels appear to be gated where the hydrolysis of ATP by a low-affinity Ca^{2+} ATPase may be required for proper opening under physiologic situations (9,10). The Ca^{2+} entering the cell is not sufficient to cause contraction per se but is considered to release an additional amount of Ca^{2+} from the intracellular Ca^{2+} storage sites such as those present in the sarcoplasmic reticulum; this Ca^{2+} release channel has now been identified. The increased level of cytoplasmic free Ca^{2+} promotes the binding of Ca^{2+} with troponin, relieves the inhibitory effect of the troponin-tropomyosin complex on actin and myosin, and results in the sliding of thin and thick filaments for the generation of contractile force. The Ca^{2+} pump present in the sarcoplasmic reticulum and both

1

the Ca^{2+} pump and the Na^+-Ca^{2+} exchange system in the sarcolemmal membrane (the latter to a lesser extent) lower the cytoplasmic level of free Ca^{2+} and allow the troponin-tropomyosin complex to exert an inhibitory effect on actin and myosin, producing relaxation of the myofibrils. Although mitochondria have the ability to accumulate Ca^{2+}, their participation in lowering the cytoplasmic level of free Ca^{2+} under physiologic conditions is less certain. Nonetheless, mitochondria are considered to regulate the intracellular concentration of Ca^{2+} under pathophysiologic conditions. Thus, it is evident that the functional integrity of myofibrils, mitochondria, sarcoplasmic reticulum, and sarcolemma is crucial for proper functioning of the heart, and any change in the behavior of these organelles is associated with the development of heart dysfunction under pathologic conditions. We will review the existing information on subcellular alterations during the development of heart dysfunction in cardiomyopathic hamsters in general and in the UM-X7.1 strain of cardiomyopathic hamsters with congestive heart failure in particular.

PATHOPHYSIOLOGY OF HEART DYSFUNCTION IN CARDIOMYOPATHIC HAMSTERS

A wide variety of alterations in subcellular organelles have been reported in various types of heart disease, including cardiomyopathy such as that seen in cardiomyopathic hamsters (1,3,6,8). A study concerning the pathologic course of heart disease in different strains of cardiomyopathic hamsters (11–16) has revealed that myocardial necrosis in these animals begins to appear at 30 to 45 days of age and reaches its maximum at 60 to 75 days. This necrotizing phase is followed by cardiac hypertrophy at 90 to 120 days of age, and thereafter varying degrees of congestive heart failure are seen in these cardiomyopathic hamsters. The contractile force development and work performance are markedly depressed in the cardiomyopathic failing heart (17–20). Dramatic alterations of myocardial metabolism in cardiomyopathic hamsters have also been reported (21–24). These changes in heart function, structure, and metabolism are considered to be the consequence of energy depletion (21,22), carnitine deficiency (25,26), increased sympathetic activity (27–30), decreased oxidation of long-chain fatty acids (31), microangiopathy (32,33), and intracellular Ca^{2+} overload (34,35). The hypothesis that the occurrence of intracellular Ca^{2+} overload may be of crucial importance in the genesis of cardiomyopathy and contractile failure in cardiomyopathic hamsters was substantiated by the finding that verapamil, a Ca^{2+} antagonist, prevented cardiac necrosis, contractile dysfunction, microangiopathy, electrical abnormality, and metabolic changes in these hamsters (33,36–41). However, the exact mechanisms for the occurrence of intracellular Ca^{2+} overload and its relationships to alterations in the functions of different organelles in the cardiomyopathic heart are poorly understood.

Although some investigators have reported a slight increase in myofibrillar ATPase activities (1,42), others have observed a depression in the actomyosin or myosin ATPase activities in cardiomyopathic hamster hearts (43,44). Both increase and decrease in myofibrillar ATPase activities were found to depend upon the stage of cardiomyopathy (45), and in fact these conflicting results were explained on the basis of alterations in both contractile and regulating proteins (46,47). A careful analysis of the data reveals that Ca^{2+} sensitivity of myofibrils is altered in relatively older cardiomyopathic hamsters, and this may contribute to cardiac dysfunction at late stages of cardiomyopathy. Likewise, defects in mitochondrial membranes related to the electron transport system for the generation of energy and for binding Ca^{2+} (1,16,48–53) appear to be the consequence of the cardiomyopathic process in which the occurrence of intracellular Ca^{2+} overload induces the observed mitochondrial changes in cardiomyopathic hamsters. On the other hand, abnormalities in the ability of sarcoplasmic reticulum to handle Ca^{2+} are considered to be associated with diastolic problems in the hearts of cardiomyopathic hamsters (52–56). It should also be pointed out that defects in Ca^{2+} binding, Ca^{2+} pump, Na^+-Ca^{2+} exchange, and Ca^{2+} channel density in the sarcolemmal membrane have been identified in the cardiomyopathic hamster heart (57–60). Varying degrees of changes in sarcolemmal Na^+-K^+ ATPase and Ca^{2+}/Mg^{2+} ATPase activities, depending upon the stage of disease, have also been reported in the cardiomyopathic hamster heart (61–64). Although all these studies suggest impaired function of the sarcolemma, sarcoplasmic reticulum, mitochondria, and myofibrils, the sequence of changes in these subcellular organelles during the development of congestive heart failure in this experimental model has not been clearly established. It was therefore considered of interest to examine the time course of alterations in subcellular organelles in cardiomyopathic hamsters to gain information regarding their cause-effect relationship with the degree of congestive heart failure.

Subcellular Changes During the Development of Congestive Heart Failure

In order to investigate the status of various subcellular organelles during the development of congestive heart failure, we employed the UM-X7.1 strain of cardiomyopathic hamsters as an experimental model. From the data in Table 1, it is evident that these animals showed a progressive increase in the amount of abdominal fluid accumulation with age. In comparison to the control groups, lung weight, liver weight, and heart/body weight ratio also showed a progressive increase with respect to age in the cardiomyopathic animals. On the basis of these and other general characteristics, the cardiomyopathic hamsters at the ages of 90 to 100 days were considered at prefailure stage, whereas those 120 to 160 days old, 160 to 200 days old, and 200 to 280 days old were grouped as being at early, moderate, and severe stages of congestive heart failure, respectively (53). The energy levels of the hearts from these cardiomyopathic animals and control hamsters were determined by measuring creatine phosphate and ATP contents according to the method used earlier (22), and the results are shown in Fig. 1. Whereas cardiomyopathic animals at moderate and severe stages of heart failure showed marked reductions in both cre-

TABLE 1. *Changes in general characteristics of cardiomyopathic hamsters (UM-X7.1) compared with age-matched control animals[a]*

Age groups	Ascites (ml)	Lung weight	Liver weight	Heart/body weight
		(% Increase)		
90 to 100 days (Prefailure)	ND	0.5 ± 0.34	1.3 ± 0.69	$8.9 \pm 0.4^*$
120 to 160 days (Early failure)	$1.3 \pm 0.42^*$	$5.4 \pm 0.49^*$	1.2 ± 0.58	$15.6 \pm 0.8^*$
160 to 200 days (Moderate failure)	$2.9 \pm 0.31^*$	$26.2 \pm 1.7^*$	$14.5 \pm 0.86^*$	$22.5 \pm 1.7^*$
200 to 280 days (Severe failure)	$7.8 \pm 0.84^*$	$35.2 \pm 1.9^*$	$41.2 \pm 2.13^*$	$24.6 \pm 1.5^*$

[a]Alterations in lung, liver, and heart weights were calculated on the basis of fresh tissue weights. Changes in lung weight, liver weight, and heart/body weight ratio are expressed as a percentage of the control values from healthy animals of the same age group.
$^*p < 0.05$.
ND, not detectable.

atine phosphate and ATP contents, animals at the early stage exhibited a significant decrease in creatine phosphate content only. No significant changes in energy levels were seen in hearts from cardiomyopathic animals at prefailure stages. These results indicate that depletion in the energy status of the myocardium may not initiate congestive heart failure in cardiomyopathic hamsters; however, the fall in the cardiac energy level appears to be closely associated with the development of heart failure in this experimental model.

For the isolation of different subcellular organelles, the hearts from six to ten cardiomyopathic animals in each group were pooled; control hamsters of the same age group were used for comparison. Purified myofibrillar, mitochondrial, sarcoplasmic reticular, and sarcolemmal fractions were isolated from each batch according to the methods described elsewhere (65–68). The myofibrillar Mg^{2+} ATPase and Ca^{2+}-stimulated ATPase activities were determined as before (69), whereas methods for the measurement of mitochondrial oxidative phosphorylation, Ca^{2+} uptake, and ATPase activities were the same as described earlier (53). The sarcoplasmic reticular ATP-dependent Ca^{2+} uptake and Mg^{2+} ATPase and Ca^{2+}-stimulated ATPase activities were determined according to the methods of Alto and Dhalla (70). All techniques for measuring sarcolemmal Mg^{2+} ATPase, Na^+-K^+ ATPase, ATP-independent Ca^{2+}, binding, and low-affinity Ca^{2+} ATPase activities were the same as those described earlier (68,71,72). The results were analyzed statistically and presented as means $\pm$ SE (standard error), and the difference between control and experimental preparations was considered significant when $p < 0.05$.

The results shown in Table 2 indicate no changes in the myofibrillar Mg^{2+} ATPase and Ca^{2+}-stimulated ATPase activities in cardiomyopathic hearts at different stages of failure. Likewise, no changes in mitochondrial ATPase and Ca^{2+} uptake activities were seen in cardiomyopathic hearts, except that the Ca^{2+} uptake activity

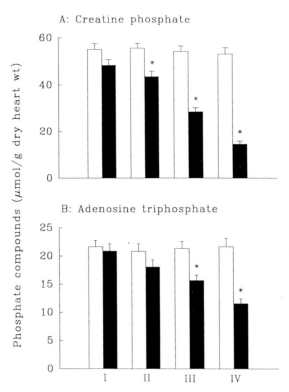

FIG. 1. Myocardial creatine phosphate **(A)** and adenosine triphosphate **(B)** in cardiomyopathic hamsters (UM-X7.1) at prefailure (I), early failure (II), moderate failure (III), and severe failure (IV) stages. The control (□) and cardiomyopathic (■) hamsters were 90 to 100 days old (I), 120 to 160 days old (II), 160 to 200 days old (III), and 200 to 280 days old (IV). Each value is a mean ± SE of six hearts. *$p<0.05$.

TABLE 2. *Myofibrillar ATPase activities in cardiomyopathic hamsters (UM-X7.1) at different stages of congestive heart failure[a]*

| | ATPase activity (μmol Pi/mg/min) | | | |
| | Mg^{2+} ATPase | | Ca^{2+}-stimulated ATPase | |
	Control	Failing	Control	Failing
Prefailure	0.15 ± 0.03	0.19 ± 0.03	0.27 ± 0.04	0.31 ± 0.03
Early failure	0.14 ± 0.02	0.17 ± 0.02	0.29 ± 0.02	0.33 ± 0.04
Moderate failure	0.15 ± 0.04	0.17 ± 0.03	0.29 ± 0.02	0.35 ± 0.03
Severe failure	0.15 ± 0.03	0.18 ± 0.02	0.30 ± 0.03	0.34 ± 0.05

[a]Each value is a mean ± SE of four to six experiments. Different groups of cardiomyopathic hamsters were selected on the basis of their age, as described in Table 1. Age-matched control hamsters were used for each group.
ATPase, adenosine triphosphatase.

TABLE 3. *Mitochondrial Ca^{2+} uptake and ATPase activities in cardiomyopathic hamsters (UM-X7.1) at different stages of congestive heart failure[a]*

	Ca^{2+} uptake (nmol Ca^{2+}/mg/5 min)		ATPase activity (μmol Pi/mg/min)	
	Control	Failing	Control	Failing
Prefailure	190 ± 18	181 ± 21	0.87 ± 0.13	0.88 ± 0.11
Early failure	187 ± 15	174 ± 19	0.95 ± 0.12	0.91 ± 0.07
Moderate failure	160 ± 17	145 ± 16	0.91 ± 0.08	0.95 ± 0.09
Severe failure	148 ± 12	$95 \pm 13^*$	0.95 ± 0.06	1.00 ± 0.11

[a]Each value is a mean $\pm$ SE of four to six experiments. Different groups of cardiomyopathic hamsters were selected on the basis of their age, as described in Table 1. Age-matched control hamsters were used for each group.
$^*p < 0.05$.

was depressed significantly at the severe stages of congestive heart failure (Table 3). Furthermore, the mitochondrial oxidative phosphorylation activities in the cardiomyopathic hearts, as assessed by adenosine diphosphate or ADP:0 ratio and phosphorylation rate, were not different from their respective control values; except that the phosphorylation rate was slightly but significantly depressed at the severe stages of heart failure (Table 4). These results suggest that no major changes in the myofibrillar or mitochondrial membrane occur during the development of congestive heart failure in the UM-X7.1 strain of cardiomyopathic hamsters. In this regard, it should be pointed out that the medium employed for the isolation of mitochondria contained ethylenediaminetetra-acetic acid (EDTA), and thus the mitochondrial Ca^{2+} content (10 μmol/mg protein) in cardiomyopathic hearts was not different from that of the controls. However, when mitochondria were isolated in the absence of EDTA or ethylene glycol tetra-acetic acid (EGTA), the mitochondrial Ca^{2+} content in cardiomyopathic hearts was five to seven times higher

TABLE 4. *Oxidative phosphorylation by heart mitochondria in cardiomyopathic hamsters (UM-X7.1) at different stages of congestive heart failure*

	ADP:0 ratio		Phosphorylation rate (μmol ADP phosphorylated/ min/g protein)	
	Control	Failing	Control	Failing
Prefailure	2.8 ± 0.07	2.9 ± 0.05	477 ± 25	484 ± 21
Early failure	2.8 ± 0.09	3.0 ± 0.08	482 ± 29	495 ± 23
Moderate failure	2.9 ± 0.07	2.9 ± 0.08	522 ± 66	482 ± 62
Severe failure	2.3 ± 0.05	2.4 ± 0.11	390 ± 9.2	$350 \pm 5.8^*$

Each value is a mean $\pm$ SE of four to six experiments. The substrate employed was 1.5 mM pyruvate plus 0.3 mM malate. Different groups of cardiomyopathic hamsters were selected on the basis of their age, as described in Table 1. Age-matched control hamsters were used for each group.
$^*p < 0.05$.
ADP, adenosine diphosphate.

than that seen in the control preparations. Furthermore, the mitochondrial oxidative phosphorylation activity was markedly depressed at early, moderate, and severe stages of congestive heart failure. Thus, it appears that the depletion of high-energy phosphate stores in the cardiomyopathic heart may partly be caused by the depressed ability of mitochondria to generate energy as a consequence of Ca^{2+} overload. Although myofibrillar ATPase activity was not altered when myofibrils were isolated, this does not rule out participation in depleting the levels of cardiac energy owing to excessive activation of Ca^{2+}-stimulated ATPase by high levels of the intracellular concentration of free Ca^{2+} in cardiomyopathic failing hearts.

Adenosine triphosphate–dependent Ca^{2+} uptake in the sarcoplasmic reticular vesicles was determined in the absence or presence of a permeant anion, oxalate, and the results are shown in Fig. 2. Although Ca^{2+} uptake in the presence of oxalate was not altered, Ca^{2+} accumulation in the sarcoplasmic reticulum in the absence of

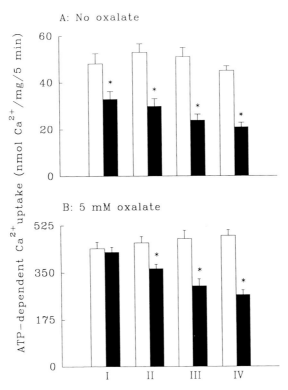

FIG. 2. Adenosine triphosphate–dependent Ca^{2+} uptake activities of cardiac sarcoplasmic reticulum in the absence of **(A)** or presence **(B)** of 5 mM potassium oxalate in cardiomyopathic hamsters (UM-X7.1) at prefailure (I), early failure (II), moderate failure (III), and severe failure (IV) stages. The control (□) and cardiomyopathic (■) hamsters in each of the four groups were of the same age as those described in Fig. 1. Each value is a mean ± SE of four experiments. $^*p < 0.05$.

TABLE 5. *Sarcoplasmic reticular Mg^{2+} ATPase and Ca^{2+}-stimulated ATPase activities in cardiomyopathic hamsters (UM-X7.1) at different stages of congestive heart failure[a]*

| | ATPase activity (μmol Pi/mg/min) | | | |
| | Mg^{2+} ATPase | | Ca^{2+}-stimulated ATPase | |
	Control	Failing	Control	Failing
Prefailure	1.18 ± 0.17	1.27 ± 0.13	0.94 ± 0.07	0.89 ± 0.14
Early failure	1.31 ± 0.15	1.29 ± 0.17	0.89 ± 0.04	0.93 ± 0.08
Moderate failure	1.29 ± 0.14	1.32 ± 0.18	0.85 ± 0.11	0.91 ± 0.09
Severe failure	1.36 ± 0.19	1.43 ± 0.21	0.94 ± 0.10	0.90 ± 0.14

[a]Each value is a mean $\pm$ SE of six experiments. Different groups of cardiomyopathic hamsters were selected on the basis of their age, as described in Table 1. Age-matched control hamsters were used for each group.

oxalate was significantly depressed in cardiomyopathic hearts at prefailure stage. The Ca^{2+} uptake activity of the sarcoplasmic reticulum in the absence or presence of oxalate was decreased at early, moderate, and severe stages of heart failure. However, no changes in sarcoplasmic reticular Mg^{2+} ATPase and Ca^{2+}-stimulated ATPase activities were seen in cardiomyopathic hearts (Table 5). These results suggest an uncoupling of the Ca^{2+} pump present in the sarcoplasmic reticulum from the cardiomyopathic heart. They also appear to indicate some membrane abnormality at the level of the sarcoplasmic reticulum. Nonetheless, the observed defect in sarcoplasmic reticular Ca^{2+} uptake can be seen to explain the impaired relaxation of the cardiomyopathic heart at early, moderate, and severe stages of heart failure. The depressed ability of the sarcoplasmic reticulum to handle Ca^{2+} also favors the availability of an excessive amount of Ca^{2+} for mitochondrial accumulation, which may result in the occurrence of mitochondrial Ca^{2+} overload in the cardiomyopathic heart.

The data in Fig. 3 show sarcolemmal Mg^{2+} ATPase and Na^{+}-K^{+} ATPase activities in cardiomyopathic hearts at different stages of congestive heart failure. It is interesting to observe that although the sarcolemmal Na^{+}-K^{+} ATPase was depressed at all stages, sarcolemmal Mg^{2+} ATPase activity was decreased only at the severe stage of heart failure. The depressed sarcolemmal Na^{+}-K^{+} ATPase would result in an increase in the intracellular concentration of Na^{+}, thus promoting the occurrence of intracellular Ca^{2+} overload through the participation of the Na^{+}-Ca^{2+} exchange system. On the other hand, sarcolemmal Ca^{2+} ATPase having a low affinity for Ca^{2+} was decreased at moderate and severe stages of congestive heart failure only (Table 6). Since the low-affinity sarcolemmal Ca^{2+} ATPase is considered to serve as a gating mechanism for the entry of Ca^{2+}, the observed depression in the activity of this enzyme at moderate and severe stages of heart failure may serve as an adaptive change for reducing the entry of Ca^{2+} into the myocardium. Furthermore, it was noted that the low-affinity sarcolemmal ATP-independent Ca^{2+} binding (measured at 1.25 mM Ca^{2+}), which is considered to represent the superficial stores of Ca^{2+} in the sarcolemmal membrane, was de-

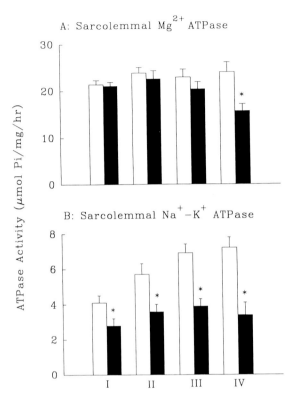

FIG. 3. Sarcolemmal Mg^{2+} ATPase **(A)** and Na^+-K^+ ATPase **(B)** activities in hearts from cardiomyopathic hamsters (UM-X7.1) at prefailure (I), early failure (II), moderate failure (III), and severe failure (IV) stages. The control ($\square$) and cardiomyopathic ($\blacksquare$) hamsters in each of the four groups were of the same age as that described in Fig. 1. Each value is a mean $\pm$ SE of four experiments. *$p<0.05$.

TABLE 6. *Sarcolemmal Ca^{2+} ATPase activity at millimolar concentrations of Ca^{2+} in cardiomyopathic hamsters (UM-X7.1) at different stages of congestive heart failure[a]*

| | Ca^{2+} ATPase activity (μmol Pi/mg/min) | | | |
| | 1.25 mM Ca^{2+} | | 4 mM Ca^{2+} | |
	Control	Failing	Control	Failing
Prefailure	15.0 ± 1.3	14.3 ± 1.4	24.2 ± 2.1	23.6 ± 2.2
Early failure	15.6 ± 1.2	16.1 ± 1.1	25.8 ± 2.7	24.1 ± 1.8
Moderate failure	17.3 ± 1.5	$12.2 \pm 0.8^*$	28.3 ± 2.5	$17.6 \pm 1.1^*$
Severe failure	17.2 ± 1.2	$10.4 \pm 0.6^*$	28.0 ± 2.3	$16.4 \pm 1.0^*$

[a]Heavy sarcolemmal preparations were employed. Each value is a mean $\pm$ SE of six experiments. Different groups of cardiomyopathic hamsters were selected on the basis of their age, as described in Table 1. Age-matched control hamsters were used for each group.
*$p<0.05$.

pressed at all stages of heart failure (Fig. 4). This change in the low-affinity ATP-independent Ca^{2+} binding was specific because the high-affinity ATP-independent Ca^{2+} binding (measured at 50 μM Ca^{2+}) was depressed only at the severe stage of heart failure (Fig. 4). The reduction in the superficial store of Ca^{2+} in the sarcolemmal membrane would favor a decrease in the entry of Ca^{2+} into the cardiac cell and thus could explain the development of depressed contractile force in the cardiomyopathic heart. This mechanism can also be considered to play an adaptive role in preventing the occurrence of intracellular Ca^{2+} overload in the cardiomyopathic heart.

From the results presented here, it is evident that the sarcolemmal and sarcoplasmic reticulum membranes are altered at the prefailure stages in cardiomyopathic hamsters. Depressed sarcolemmal Na^+-K^+ ATPase activity as well as impaired Ca^{2+} handling ability of the sarcoplasmic reticulum would promote the occurrence of intracellular Ca^{2+} overload, and this may result in heart failure. Although some

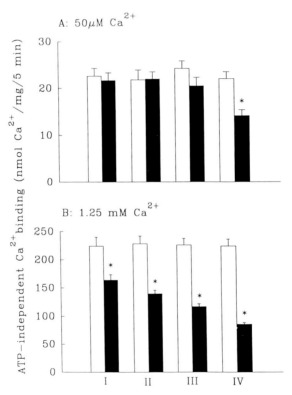

FIG. 4. Sarcolemmal ATP-independent Ca^{2+} binding at 50 μM Ca^{2+} **(A)** and 1.25 mM Ca^{2+} **(B)** in hearts from cardiomyopathic hamsters (UM-X7.1) at prefailure (I), early failure (II), moderate failure (III), and severe failure (IV) stages. The control (□) and cardiomyopathic (■) hamsters in each of the four groups were of the same age as those described in Fig. 1. Each value is a mean ± SE of four experiments. *$p < 0.05$.

defect in the mitochondrial membrane was seen in the cardiomyopathic heart, this change was found only at severe stages of heart failure and can be viewed as the consequence of such failure. On the other hand, no apparent alteration in myofibrils was identified in the cardiomyopathic hamsters. Nevertheless, excessive stimulation of myofibrillar ATPase owing to the occurrence of intracellular Ca^{2+} overload as well as mitochondrial Ca^{2+} overloading and associated impairment in the process of energy production may contribute to depleting the high-energy phosphate stores in the cardiomyopathic heart. The reduction in the sarcolemmal superficial stores of Ca^{2+}, which are available for Ca^{2+} influx, as well as depressed activity of the low-affinity Ca^{2+} ATPase, which is considered to serve as a Ca^{2+} gating mechanism in the sarcolemmal membrane, would point to a decreased amount of Ca^{2+} entering the cell. These Ca^{2+}-related mechanisms in the sarcolemmal membrane may represent an adaptive system and can be considered to explain the reduced ability of the cardiomyopathic heart to generate contractile force.

ACKNOWLEDGMENT

The work reported in this article was supported by a grant from the Heart and Stroke Foundation of Manitoba.

SUMMARY

By examining the UM-X7.1 strain of cardiomyopathic hamsters at different stages of congestive heart failure, we have observed the sequence of subcellular alterations in the failing myocardium. The prefailure stage of heart failure in this experimental model was associated with depressed activities of sarcolemmal Na^+-K^+ adenosine triphosphatase (ATPase) and adenosine triphosphate (ATP)-independent low-affinity Ca^{2+} binding and of sarcoplasmic reticular ATP-dependent Ca^{2+} uptake in the absence of oxalate. Early, moderate, and severe stages of congestive heart failure were associated with decreased sarcoplasmic reticular ATP-dependent Ca^{2+} uptake in the presence of oxalate as well as decreased sarcolemmal Na^+-K^+ ATPase and ATP-independent Ca^{2+} binding activities. Sarcolemmal low-affinity Ca^{2+} ATPase was depressed at moderate and severe stages of heart failure, whereas no changes were seen in the sarcoplasmic reticular Ca^{2+}-stimulated ATPase in cardiomyopathic hearts. Although some subtle changes in mitochondrial membrane were seen at severe stages of heart failure, no apparent change in myofibrillar ATPase was identified. The impaired Ca^{2+} handling by the sarcoplasmic reticulum and the depressed sarcolemmal Na^+-K^+ ATPase activity was seen to result in the occurrence of intracellular Ca^{2+} overload, mitochondrial Ca^{2+} overload, energy depletion, and contractile failure. On the other hand, the sarcolemmal ATP-independent Ca^{2+} binding and Ca^{2+} ATPase are considered to serve as adaptive changes because they can be seen to decrease the entry of Ca^{2+}, thereby reducing the extent of intracellular Ca^{2+} overload in the cardiac cells of cardiomyopathic hamsters. Thus, it appears that a remodeling of heart membranes such as sarcolemma and sarcoplasmic reticulum occurs, and alterations in the function of these membranes may lead to the development of congestive heart failure in the UM-X7.1 strain of cardiomyopathic hamsters.

REFERENCES

1. Dhalla NS, Sulakhe PV, Fedelesova M, Yates JC. Molecular abnormalities in cardiomyopathy. *Adv Cardiol* 1974;13:282–300.
2. Tomlinson CW, Lee SL, Dhalla NS. Abnormalities in heart membranes and myofibrils during bacterial infective cardiomyopathy in rabbits. *Circ Res* 1976;39:82–92.
3. Dhalla NS, Das PK, Sharma GP. Subcellular basis of cardiac contractile failure. *J Mol Cell Cardiol* 1978;10,363–85.
4. Lindenmayer GE, Sordahl LA, Harigaya S, Allen JC, Besch JR Jr, Schwartz A. Some biochemical studies on subcellular systems isolated from fresh recipient human cardiac tissue obtained during transplantation. *Am J Cardiol* 1971;27:277–83.
5. Carafoli E. Mitochondria, Ca^{2+} transport and the regulation of heart function and metabolism. *J Mol Cell Cardiol* 1975;7:83–9.
6. Dhalla NS, Pierce GN, Panagia V, Singal PK, Beamish RE. Calcium movements in relation to heart function. *Basic Res Cardiol* 1982;77:117–39.
7. Lehninger AL. Mitochondria and calcium transport in heat. *Biochem J* 1970;119:129–38.
8. Dhalla NS, Dixon IMC, Beamish RE. Biochemical basis of heart function and contractile failure. *J Appl Cardiol* 1991;6:7–30.
9. Dhalla NS, Zhao D. Cell membrane Ca^{2+}/Mg^{2+} ATPase. *Prog Biophys Mol Biol* 1988;52:1–37.
10. Dhalla NS, Zhao D. Possible role of sarcolemmal Ca^{2+}/Mg^{2+} ATPase in heart function. *Magnesium Res* 1989;2:161–72.
11. Bajusz E, Baker J, Nixon CW, Hamburger F. Spontaneous hereditary myocardial degeneration and congestive heart failure in a strain of Syrian hamsters. *Ann NY Acad Sci* 1969;156:105–29.
12. Gertz EW. Cardiomyopathic Syrian hamster: a possible model of human disease. *Prog Exp Tumor Res* 1972;16:242–60.
13. Paterson RA, Layberry RA, Nadkarni BB. Cardiac failure in the hamster. A biochemical and electron microscopic study. *Lab Invest* 1972;26:755–66.
14. Colgan JA, Lazarus ML, Sachs HG. Post-natal development of the normal and cardiomyopathic Syrian hamster heart: a quantitative electron microscopic study. *J Mol Cell Cardiol* 1978;10:43–54.
15. Jasmin G, Proschak L. Hereditary polymyopathy and cardiomyopathy in the Syrian hamster I. Progression of heart and skeletal muscle lesions in the UM- X7.1 line. *Muscle Nerve* 1982;5:20–5.
16. Proschek L, Jasmin G. Hereditary polymyopathy and cardiomyopathy in the Syrian hamster II. Development of heart necrotic changes in relation to defective mitochondrial function. *Muscle Nerve* 1982;5:26–32.
17. Brink AJ, Lochner A. Contractility and tension development of the myopathic hamster (B10 14.6) heart. *Cardiovasc Res* 1969;3:453–8.
18. Mass-Schwartz A, Weinstock RS, Wagner RL, Abelman WH. Right and left ventricular compliance in the hereditary cardiomyopathy of the Syrian hamster. *Cardiovasc Res* 1977;11:367–74.
19. Brink AJ, Lockner A. Work performance of the isolated perfused beating heart in the hereditary myocardiopathy of the Syrian hamster. *Circ Res* 1967;21:391–401.
20. Kumar AE, Plenge R, Gamble WJ, Monasek FJ, Monroe RG. Ventricular performance, coronary flow, and MVO_2 in hamster cardiomyopathy with failure. *Am J Physiol* 1971;221:684–9.
21. Lochner A, Brink AJ, Van Der Walt JJ. The significance of biochemical and structural changes in the development of the myocardiopathy of the Syrian hamster. *J Mol Cell Cardiol* 1970;1:47–64.
22. Fedelesova M, Dhalla NS. High energy phosphate stores in the hearts of genetically dystrophic hamsters. *J Mol Cell Cardiol* 1971;3:93–102.
23. Witmer JT. Energy metabolism and mechanical function in perfused hearts of Syrian hamsters with dilated or hypertrophic cardiomyopathy. *J Mol Cell Cardiol* 1986;18:307–17.
24. Sievers R, Parmley HW, Tames T, Wikman-Coffelt J. Energy levels at systole vs diastole in normal hamster hearts vs myopathic hamster hearts. *Circ Res* 1983;53:759–66.

25. Hoppel CL, Tandler B, Parland W, Turkaly JS, Albers LD. Hamster cardiomyopathy: a defect in oxidative phosphorylation in the cardiac interfibrillar mitochondria. *J Biol Chem* 1982;257:1540–8.
26. York CM, Cantrell CR, Borum PR. Cardiac carnitine deficiency and altered carnitine transport in cardiomyopathic hamsters. *Arch Biochem Biophys* 1983;221:533–56.
27. Angelakos ET, King MP, Carballo L. Cardiac adrenergic innervation in hamsters with hereditary myocardiopathy: chemical and histochemical studies. *Rec Adv Stud Card Struc Met* 1973;2:519–31.
28. Angelakos ET, Carbello LC, Daniels JB, King MP, Bajusz E. Adrenergic neurohumorous in the heart of hamsters with hereditary myopathy during cardiac hypertrophy and failure. *Rec Adv Stud Card Struc Met* 1972;1:262–78.
29. Sole MJ, Lo C-M, Laird CW, Sonnenblick EH, Wurtman RJ. Norepinephrine turnover in the heart and spleen of the cardiomyopathic Syrian hamster. *Circ Res* 1975;41:855–62.
30. Sole MJ, Kamble AB, Hussain MN. A possible change in the rate-limiting step for cardiac norepinephrine synthesis in the cardiomyopathic Syrian hamster. *Circ Res* 1977;41:814–17.
31. Kelly TF. Altered lipoprotein lipase and lipid metabolism in the myocardium of B10 14.6 myopathic hamsters. *Trans NY Acad Sci* 1968;30:960–1.
32. Factor S, Sonnenblick EH. Microvascular spasm as a cause of cardiomyopathies. *Cardiovasc Rev Rep* 1983;4:1177–82.
33. Factor SM, Minase T, Cho S, Dominita R, Sonnenblick EH. Microvascular spasm in cardiomyopathic Syrian hamster: a preventable cause of focal myocardial necrosis. *Circulation* 1982; 66:342–5.
34. Lossnitzer K, Bajusz E. Water and electrolyte alterations during the life course of the B10 14.6 Syrian golden hamster. A disease model of a hereditary cardiomyopathy. *J Mol Cell Cardiol* 1974;6:163–77.
35. Jasmin G, Proschek L. Calcium and myocardial cell injury. An appraisal in the cardiomyopathic hamster. *Can J Physiol Pharmacol* 1984;62:891–8.
36. Jasmin G, Solymoss B. Prevention of hereditary cardiomyopathy in the hamster by verapamil and other agents. *Proc Soc Exp Biol Med* 1975;149:193–8.
37. Wikman-Coffelt J, Sievers R, Parmley WW, Jasmin G. Verapamil preserves adenine nucleotide pool in cardiomyopathic Syrian hamster. *Am J Physiol* 1986;250:H22–8.
38. Rouleu J-L, Chuck LHS, Hollosi G, et al. Verapamil preserves myocardial contractility in the hereditary cardiomyopathy of the Syrian hamster. *Circ Res* 1982;50:405–12.
39. Kobayashi A, Yamashita T, Kaneko M, Nishiyama T, Hayashi H, Yamazaki N. Effects of verapamil on experimental cardiomyopathy in the B10 14.6 Syrian hamster. *J Am Coll Cardiol* 1987;10:1128–34.
40. Yamashita T, Kobayashi A, Yamazaki N, Miura T, Shirasawa H. Effects of L-carnitine and verapamil on myocardial carnitine concentration and histopathology of Syrian hamster B10 14.6. *Cardiovasc Res* 1986;20:614–20.
41. Capasso JM, Sonnenblick EH, Anversa P. Chronic calcium blockade prevents the progression of myocardial contractile and electrical dysfunction in the cardiomyopathic Syrian hamster. *Circ Res* 1990;67:1381–93.
42. Wada A, Yoneda H, Shibata N, Invie Y, Onishi S. Morphological and biochemical studies on the heart of cardiomyopathic Syrian hamster. *Rec Adv Stud Card Struc Met* 1975;6:275–82.
43. Bhan A, Malhotra A, Hatcher VB, Sonnenblick EH, Scheuer J. Depressed myosin ATPase activity in hearts of myopathic hamsters: dissociation from neutral protease activity. *J Mol Cell Cardiol* 1978;10:769–77.
44. Malhotra A, Karell M, Scheuer J. Multiple cardiac contractile protein abnormalities in myopathic Syrian hamsters (B10 53.58). *J Mol Cell Cardiol* 1985;17:95–107.
45. Pang DC, Weglicki WB. Alterations of myofibrillar ATPase activities in hearts of cardiomyopathic hamsters (B10 53.58). *J Mol Cell Cardiol* 1980;12:445–56.
46. Malhotra A. Regulatory proteins in hamster cardiomyopathy. *Circ Res* 1990;66:1309–15.
47. Malhotra A, Scheuer J. Troponin-tropomyosin abnormalities in hamster cardiomyopathy. *J Clin Invest* 1990;86:286–92.
48. Lindenmayer GE, Harigaya S, Bajusz E, Schwartz A. Oxidative phosphorylation and calcium transport of mitochondria isolated from cardiomyopathic hamster hearts. *J Mol Cell Cardiol* 1970;1:249–59.
49. Lochner A, Opie LH, Brink AJ, Bosman AR. Defective oxidative phosphorylation in hereditary myocardiopathy in the Syrian hamster. *Cardiovasc Res* 1968;3:297–307.
50. Wrogeman K, Blanchaer MC, Jacobson BE. Oxidative phosphorylation in cardiomyopathic hamsters. *Am J Physiol* 1972;222:1453–7.

51. Wrogeman K, Nylan EG. Mitochondrial calcium overloading in cardiomyopathic hamsters. *J Mol Cell Cardiol* 1978;10:185–95.
52. Sulakhe PV, Dhalla NS. Excitation-contraction coupling in heart VII. Calcium accumulation in subcellular particles in congestive heart failure. *J Clin Invest* 1971;50:1019–29.
53. Panagia V, Lee SL, Singh A, Pierce GN, Jasmin G, Dhalla NS. Impairment of mitochondrial and sarcoplasmic reticular functions during the development of heart failure in cardiomyopathic (UM-X7.1) hamsters. *Can J Cardiol* 1986;2:236–47.
54. Gertz EW, Stam AC Jr, Sonnenblick EH. A quantitative and qualitative defect in the sarcoplasmic reticulum in the hereditary cardiac myopathy of the Syrian hamster. *Biochem Biophys Res Commun* 1970;40:746–53.
55. McCollum WB, Crow C, Harigaya S, Bajusz E, Schwartz A. Calcium binding by cardiac relaxing system isolated from myopathic Syrian hamsters (strains) 14.6, 82.62 and 40.54). *J Mol Cell Cardiol* 1970;1:445–57.
56. Sulakhe PV, Dhalla NS. Excitation-contraction coupling in heart X. Further studies on the energy-linked calcium transport by subcellular particles in the failing heart of myopathic hamsters. *Biochem Med* 1973;8:18–27.
57. Matts, Baker JC, Bailey LE. Excitation-contraction coupling in normal and myopathic hamster hearts III: functional deficiencies in interstitial glycoproteins. *Cardiovasc Res* 1979;13:568–77.
58. Panagia V, Singh JN, Anand-Srivastava MB, Pierce GN, Jasmin G, Dhalla NS. Sarcolemmal alterations during the development of genetically determined cardiomyopathy. *Cardiovasc Res* 1984; 18:567–72.
59. Makino N, Jasmin G, Beamish RE, Dhalla NS. Sarcolemmal Na^+-Ca^{2+} exchange during the development of genetically determined cardiomyopathy. *Biochem Biophys Res Commun* 1985;133:491–7.
60. Wagner JA, Weisman HF, Snowman AM, Reynolds IJ, Weisfeldt ML, Snyder SH. Alterations in calcium antagonist receptors and sodium-calcium exchange in cardiomyopathic hamster tissues. *Circ Res* 1989;65:205–14.
61. Singh JN, Dhalla NS, McNamara DB, Bajusz E, Jasmin G. Membrane alterations in failing hearts of cardiomyopathic hamsters. *Rec Adv Stud Card Struc Met* 1975;6:259–68.
62. Dhalla NS, Tomlinson CW, Singh JN, et al. Role of sarcolemmal changes in cardiac pathophysiology. *Rec Adv Stud Card Struc Met* 1976;9:377–94.
63. Dhalla NS, Singh JN, Bajusz E, Jasmin G. Comparison of heart sarcolemmal enzyme activities in normal and cardiomyopathic (UM-X7.1) hamsters. *Clin Sci Mol Med* 1976;57:233–42.
64. Sulakhe PV, Dhalla NS. Alterations in the activity of cardiac Na^+-K^+ stimulated ATPase in congestive heart failure. *Exp Mol Pathol* 1973;18:100–11.
65. Solaro RJ, Pang DC, Briggs FN. The purification of cardiac myofibrils with Triton X-100. *Biochim Biophys Acta* 1971;245:259–62.
66. Sordahl LA, Johnson C, Blailock ZR, Schwartz A. The mitochondrion. In: Schwartz A, ed. *Methods in pharmacology.* New York: Appleton-Century-Crofts; vol 1, 1971;247–86.
67. Harigaya S, Schwartz A. Rate of calcium binding and uptake in normal animals and failing human cardiac muscle membrane vesicles (relaxing system) and mitochondria. *Circ Res* 1969;25:781–94.
68. Dhalla NS, Anand-Srivastava MB, Tuana BS, Khandelwal RL. Solubilization of calcium-dependent adenosine triphosphate from rat heart sarcolemma. *J Mol Cell Cardiol* 481;13:413–23.
69. Pierce GN, Dhalla NS. Cardiac myofibrillar ATPase activity in diabetic rats. *J Mol Cell Cardiol* 1981;13:1063–9.
70. Alto LE, Dhalla NS. Role of change in microsomal calcium uptake in the effects of reperfusion of Ca^{2+}-deprived rat hearts. *Circ Res* 1981;48:17–24.
71. Pierce GN, Dhalla NS. Sarcolemmal Na^+-K^+ ATPase activity in diabetic rat heart. *Am J Physiol* 1983;245:C241–7.
72. Pierce GN, Kutryk MJB, Dhalla NS. Alterations in calcium binding and composition of the cardiac sarcolemmal membrane in chronic diabetes. *Proc Natl Acad Sci USA* 1983;80:5412–16.

The Cardiomyopathic Heart, edited by Makoto Nagano, Nobuakira Takeda, and Naranjan S. Dhalla. Raven Press, Ltd., New York © 1994.

2

Na, K ATPase Gene Expression in the Cardiomyopathic Heart

Yoshio Tsuruya, Uichi Ikeda, *Toshiko Ohta, Keiji Yamamoto, Yoshitane Seino, Hitoshi Ebata, Yukihiro Hojo, Toshiko Kanbe, Kazuyuki Shimada

*Department of Cardiology, Jichi Medical School, Tochigi 329-04, Japan; *Department of Microbiology, Tsukuba University School of Medicine, Ibaragi, Japan*

INTRODUCTION

Na, K-ATPase or the Na, K pump plays an important role in myocardial function. Thus, active transport of Na^+ and K^+ across the cell membrane by the Na, K pump is essential for the occurrence of myocardial excitability and contractility. The re-uptake by the Na, K pump of K^+ that is lost from the cell during the action potential prevents a possible arrhythmogenic rise of interstitial K^+. By maintaining the Na^+ gradient across the cell membrane and associated Na^+-Ca^{2+} exchange, the Na, K pump plays a significant role in cellular Ca^{2+} clearance.

Na, K ATPase is composed of two subunits: a catalytic α subunit ($Mr = 110,000$) and a glycosylated β subunit ($Mr = 35,000$). It is generally agreed that nonvectorial functions of Na, K ATPase, such as ATPase activity and cardiac glycoside binding, are localized to the α subunit. The role of the β subunit is unknown, but full reconstitution of the vectorial function of Na, K ATPase requires both α and β subunits in a 1:1 stoichiometry. At least three subunit isoforms, α1, α2, and α3, have been characterized in rats (1) and humans (2). Among the three α isoforms, α1 isoform is the major isoform expressed through all developmental stages in rat hearts (3).

The cardiomyopathic Syrian hamster of the inbred strain Bio 14.6 is an animal model of human idiopathic cardiomyopathy that shows susceptibility to the development of myocardial necrosis, fibrosis, and calcification at 35 to 40 days of life, followed by cardiac hypertrophy and congestive heart failure (4,5). A decrease in Na, K ATPase activity in the cardiac plasma membrane has been shown to be one of the earliest abnormalities in the course of hereditary cardiomyopathy (6), and it might be of importance in the associated intracellular calcium accumulation, mitochondrial calcification, and cell necrosis. However, it is still unknown whether the abnormality in Na, K ATPase activity is the primary defect or a result of cardiac damage. To answer this question, we investigated Na, K ATPase α1 isoform gene expression in the cardiomyopathic Syrian hamster heart.

MATERIALS AND METHODS

Animals

Three- and thirty-week-old male Bio 14.6 Syrian hamsters and sex and age-matched, healthy F1β hamsters (Charles River, MA) were used for experiments. Standard laboratory feed was given to the animals until the day before the experiment.

Northern Blot Analysis

For Northern blot analysis, equal amounts of total RNA (15 μg) from control and cardiomyopathic hearts were used. Total RNA was isolated from hamster ventricles by the guanidine isothiocyanate–cesium chloride (GITC-CsCl) method, size-fractionated by electrophoresis on denaturing 1.0% agarose/formaldehyde gels, and transferred to nylon membranes (Hybond N$^+$, Amersham, UK) (7). Membranes were hybridized with a rat Na, K ATPase α1 isoform-specific complementary DNA probe labeled with ^{32}P-dCTP (Amersham, UK), using a multiprime DNA labeling kit (Amersham, UK). The rat α1 complementary DNA probe consisted of a 2.2 kb *Nco*I-*Bgl*II fragment (1). After hybridizations, filters were washed once in 2 × SSPE (IxSSPE contains 150 mmol/L NaCl, 10 mmol/L NaH$_2$PO$_4$, and 1 mmol/L ethylenediaminetetra-acetic acid [EDTA] with 1% sodium dodecyl sulfate (SDS) at room temperature for 15 minutes and then once in 0.1 × SSPE with 1% SDS at 65°C for 10 minutes. Filters were exposed to Kodak XAR-5 film at −80°C for 1 to 2 days with one intensifying screen and quantitated by densitometric scanning (Immunomedica, Image Analyzer TIF-64, Japan) (8).

Measurement of Na, K ATPase Activity

Na, K ATPase activity was measured in membrane fractions from 3-week-old Bio 14.6 and F1β hamster ventricles with the method previously described (9).

Southern Blot Analysis of Genomic DNA

Genomic DNA was taken from 3-week-old Bio 14.6 and F1β hamster livers. Ten micrograms of genomic DNA were digested with 50 units of various restriction endonucleases (*Eco*RI, *Hind*III, *Bgl*II, *Kpn*I, *Pvu*II) (BRL, MD) under conditions recommended by the manufacturer, size-fractionated on 1.0% agarose gels, and transferred to nylon membranes. Hybridizations were performed with a rat Na, K ATPase α1 isoform complementary DNA probe labeled with ^{32}P-dCTP. Washing was performed as described in the Northern blot analysis.

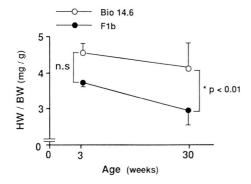

FIG. 1. Heart weight (HW) to body weight (BW) ratio of 3- and 30-week-old Bio 14.6 and F1b hamsters. Data are the mean ± SE of eight samples.

Statistical Analysis

All data are expressed as the mean ± SE; a *p* value of less than 0.05 was considered statistically significant.

RESULTS

The average heart weight to body weight ratio of Bio 14.6 hamsters was almost equal to that of F1β hamsters at the age of 3 weeks (4.68 ± 0.25 mg/g and 3.90 ± 0.65 mg/g, respectively, $n = 6$, $p > 0.05$) (Fig. 1). However, at the age of 30 weeks, the ratio became significantly higher in Bio 14.6 hamsters than in F1β hamsters, with a ratio of 4.30 ± 0.11 mg/g and 3.13 ± 0.41 mg/g, respectively ($n = 6$, $p < 0.01$), indicating moderate cardiac hypertrophy in Bio 14.6 hamsters at this age.

In Northern blot analysis, the Na, K ATPase α1 mRNA signal was detected as a single band with an approximate size of 3.7 kb in both Bio 14.6 and F1β hamsters (Fig. 2). The α1 mRNA level was quantitated by densitometric scanning. As shown in Fig. 3, the cardiac α1 mRNA level in Bio 14.6 hamsters was significantly lower

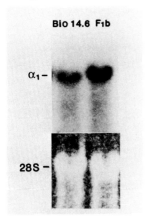

FIG. 2. Northern blot analysis of Na, K ATPase α1 mRNA expression in 3-week-old Bio 14.6 and F1b hamster hearts. Total RNA was isolated from Bio 14.6 and F1b hamster ventricles by the GITC-CsCl method. Equal amounts of total RNA (15 μg) were size-fractionated on 1.0% agarose-formaldehyde gels and transferred to nylon membranes. Hybridizations were performed with a ^{32}P-labeled rat Na, K ATPase α1 subunit complementary DNA probe. Autoradiography was performed at −80°C for 1 to 2 days with one intensifying screen.

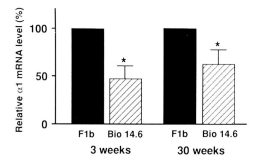

FIG. 3. Relative Na, K ATPase α1 mRNA level in 3- and 30-week-old Bio 14.6 and F1b hamster hearts. Autoradiography was quantitated by laser densitometer. *$p < 0.05$ in Bio 14.6 compared with F1b hamsters. Data are the mean ± SE of four samples.

than that in F1β hamsters at the age of both 3 and 30 weeks ($48 \pm 13\%$ and $62 \pm 14\%$, respectively, $n = 4$, $p < 0.05$) (Fig. 3).

To ascertain whether the decreased cardiac α1 mRNA expression in Bio 14.6 hamsters was accompanied by a decrease in Na, K ATPase activity, we measured its activity in membrane fractions of Bio 14.6 and F1β hamster ventricles. As shown in Fig. 4, Na, K ATPase activity was approximately 20% lower in 3-week-old Bio 14.6 hamsters than in F1β hamsters of the same age (5.9 versus 7.0 μmol Pi/h/mg protein, respectively).

We next investigated restriction fragment length polymorphisms (RFLPs) of the α1 isoform gene between the two strains. A 2.9-kb *Sac*I fragment of rat Na, K ATPase α1 complementary DNA was tested for its ability to detect RFLPs between Bio 14.6 and F1β hamster genomic DNA that had been digested with a panel of restriction endonucleases. However, RFLPs were not detected by these enzymes (data not shown).

To determine Na, K ATPase gene expression in other types of cardiac hypertrophy, we studied the α1 mRNA expression in spontaneous hypertensive rats and normotensive Wistar Kyoto (WKY) rat ventricles. At both 8 weeks (early hypertrophic) and 16 weeks (established hypertrophic) of age, the cardiac α1 mRNA level in spontaneous hypertensive rats was almost equal to that in WKY rats of the same age. (Fig. 5).

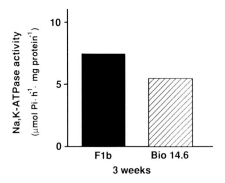

FIG. 4. Na, K ATPase activity of 3-week-old Bio 14.6 and F1b hamster hearts. Na, K ATPase activity was measured in membrane fractions from Bio 14.6 and F1b hamster ventricles. The inorganic phosphate released from their ATPase reaction was estimated by the methods of the Fiske and Subbarow assay. Data are the mean of two separate samples.

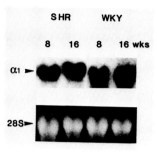

FIG. 5. Northern blot analysis of Na, K ATPase α1 mRNA expression in spontaneous hypertensive rat and WKY rat hearts. Total RNA was isolated from 8- and 16-week-old spontaneous hypertensive and WKY rat ventricles by the GITC-CsCl method. Equal amounts of total RNA (15 μg) were loaded and size-fractionated on 1.0% agarose-formaldehyde gels and transferred to nylon membranes (Hybond N$^+$, Amersham, UK). Hybridizations were performed with a ^{32}P-labeled rat Na, K ATPase α1 subunit complementary DNA probe. Autoradiography was performed at $-80°C$ for 1 to 2 days with one intensifying screen.

DISCUSSION

The results of the present study demonstrate a significant decrease in Na, K ATPase gene expression and Na, K ATPase activity in ventricular myocardium from Bio 14.6 hamsters. The possibility that the alterations observed in Na K ATPase gene expression were not specific to cardiomyopathy but were related to the development of cardiac hypertrophy in the experimental animals must be considered. In this regard, it should be noted that no alteration in cardiac Na, K ATPase gene expression was found in spontaneous hypertensive rats with cardiac hypertrophy compared with WKY rats without cardiac hypertrophy. Thus, myocardial hypertrophy of the left ventricle cannot be considered an explanation of the observed alteration of Na, K ATPase gene expression in Bio 14.6 hamsters.

Na, K ATPase creates and maintains the concentration gradients for Na$^+$ and K$^+$ across the cell membrane (10). Na$^+$ that has been actively transported out of the cell can be exchanged with intracellular Ca^{2+} (11) and H$^+$ (12). Thus, Na, K ATPase in the myocardial sarcolemma contributes to the cellular clearance of Ca^{2+} and H$^+$. A decreased Na$^+$ gradient across the cell membrane may lead to intracellular acidosis and Ca^{2+} accumulation, which in turn may activate Ca^{2+}-sensitive protein-splitting enzymes. Several studies have disclosed certain cardiac sarcolemmal abnormalities that are important in regulating trans-sarcolemmal flux and cytoplasmic levels of calcium in relatively young cardiomyopathic hamsters (13,14). Earlier studies have revealed a decrease in Na, K ATPase activity in hearts from the Bio 14.6 strain of cardiomyopathic hamsters (6); however, Sulakhe and Dhalla (15) described increased Na, K ATPase activity in Bio 14.6 hamster hearts. In this study, we observed decreased Na, K ATPase mRNA expression in Bio 14.6 hamster hearts in both the prehypertrophic and hypertrophic stages. The suppression of Na, K ATPase gene expression associated with decreased Na, K ATPase activity may be of importance to the increase in intracellular calcium observed in the myocardium of cardiomyopathic hamsters. In humans, Norgaard et al (16) also reported a reduction in Na, K ATPase pump numbers in endomyocardial biopsy specimens taken from patients with dilated cardiomyopathy; these findings are compatible with our results in the cardiomyopathic hamster hearts.

It is important to clarify whether the observed abnormality in Na, K ATPase gene expression is a primary defect or a result of cardiac damage. In the cardiomyopathic hamsters, a decrease in Na, K ATPase activity occurs before the ensuing myocardial necrosis and ventricular failure. The cardiac pathology becomes most apparent after 35 to 40 days of age (4,5), and cardiac abnormality is minimal in 3-week-old cardiomyopathic hamsters. Therefore, our findings that the α1 mRNA expression was depressed in the cardiomyopathic hamsters at the age of 3 weeks suggest that the abnormality of Na, K ATPase α1 mRNA expression in the cardiomyopathic hamsters might be a primary defect.

To further support our premise that there is a genetic abnormality in the regulatory systems of the α1 mRNA expression in Bio 14.6 hamsters, we investigated RFLPs between the genomes of Bio 14.6 and F1β hamsters when their DNAs were digested with various endonucleases. However, we could not detect any RFLPs between Bio 14.6 and F1β hamsters, although further investigations using different lengths of complementary DNA probes and other restriction enzymes are needed to reach any meaningful conclusions.

ACKNOWLEDGMENTS

We thank K. Kawakami (Jichi Medical School) for donating rat Na, K ATPase α1 cDNA probe. This study was supported by the Ministry of Education, Culture and Science (#2670407, #5670632), the Japan Foundation for Health Science, and the Takeda Medical Research Foundation.

SUMMARY

In order to investigate the mechanisms of depressed Na, K adenosine triphosphatase (ATPase) activity in cardiomyopathic hearts, Na K ATPase gene expression was observed in 3- and 30-week-old Bio 14.6 strains of cardiomyopathic hamsters. The results indicate that cardiomyopathy in the hamster was associated with a decrease in cardiac Na, K ATPase gene expression and Na, K ATPase activity. This study supports the view that a genetic defect in Na, K ATPase may contribute to the pathogenesis of cardiomyopathy in this animal model.

REFERENCES

1. Shull GE, Greeb J, Lingrel JB. Molecular cloning of three distinct forms of the Na,K-ATPase α subunit from rat brain. *Biochemistry* 1986;25:8125–32.
2. Shull MM, Lingrel JB. Multiple genes encode the human Na,K-ATPase catalytic subunit. *Proc Natl Acad Sci USA* 1987;84:4039–43.
3. Orlowski J, Lingrel JB. Tissue-specific and developmental regulation of Na,K-ATPase catalytic α isoforms and β subunit mRNAs. *J Biol Chem* 1989;263:104–36.
4. Homberger F, Bajusz E. New models of human disease in Syrian hamsters. *JAMA* 1970;212:604–10.

5. Jasmin G, Proschek L. Hereditary polymyopathy and cardiomyopathy in the Syrian hamster. *Muscle Nerve* 1982;5:20–5.
6. Makino N, Jasmin G, Reamish RE, Dhalla NS. Sarcolemmal Na^+-Ca^{2+} exchange during the development of genetically determined cardiomyopathy. *Biochem Biophys Res Commun* 1985;133:491–7.
7. Ikeda U, Hyman R, Smith TW, Medford RM. Aldosterone-mediated regulation of Na,K-ATPase gene expression in adult and neonatal rat cardiocytes. *J Biol Chem* 1991;266:12058–66.
8. Tsuruya Y, Ikeda U, Kawakami K, et al. Augmented Na,K-ATPase gene expression in spontaneously hypertensive rat hearts. *Clin Exp Hypertens [A]* 1991;13:1213–22.
9. Ohta T, Kishi K, Nojima H, Nagano K, Sokabe H. Purification and characterization of Na,K-ATPase from the kidney of spontaneously hypertensive and Wistar Kyoto rats. *Biomed Res* 1984; 5:521–5.
10. Skou JC. Enzymatic basis for active transport of Na^+ and K^+ across cell membrane. *Physiol Rev* 1965;45:596–617.
11. Philipson KD. Sodium-calcium exchange in plasma membrane vesicles. *Annu Rev Physiol* 1985; 47:561–71.
12. Lazdunski M, Frelin C, Vigne P. The sodium/hydrogen exchange system in cardiac cells: its biochemical and pharmacological properties and its role in regulating internal concentrations of sodium and external H. *J Mol Cell Cardiol* 1985;17:1029–42.
13. Angewlakos ET, King MP, Carballo L. Cardiac adrenergic innervation in hamsters with hereditary myocardiopathy. *In*: Bajusz E, Rona G, eds. *Recent advances in studies on cardiac structure and metabolism*. Baltimore: University Park Press, 1973;519–31.
14. Limas CJ, Limas C. Decreased siaryltransferase activity in the hearts of cardiomyopathic hamsters. *Biochim Biophys Acta* 1978;540:543–46.
15. Sulakhe PV, Dhalla NS. Alterations in the activity of cardiac Na^+-K^+-stimulated ATPase in congestive failure. *Exp Mol Pathol* 1973;18:100–11.
16. Norgaard A, Bagger JP, Bjerregaard P, Baandrup U, Kjeldsen K, Thomsen PEB. Relation of left ventricular function and Na,K-pump concentration in suspected idiopathic dilated cardiomyopathy. *Am J Cardiol* 1987;61:1312–15.

The Cardiomyopathic Heart, edited by Makoto
Nagano, Nobuakira Takeda, and Naranjan S.
Dhalla. Raven Press, Ltd., New York © 1994.

3

Alterations of Myocardial Contractility in Cardiomyopathic J-2-N Hamsters

Nobuakira Takeda, Jie Yang, Takaaki Iwai, Akira Tanamura,
Atsushi Takeda, Mitsutoshi Kato, Tadanari Ohkubo,
Makoto Nagano

*Department of Internal Medicine, Aoto Hospital, Jikei University School of Medicine,
Aoto 6-41-2, Katsushika-ku, Tokyo 125, Japan*

INTRODUCTION

Cardiomyopathic hamsters have been used to investigate the pathophysiology of idiopathic cardiomyopathy, and various alterations of the myocardial organelles such as changes in contractile proteins and calcium transport by cardiac sarcoplasmic reticulum have been reported (1–3). In the present study, we investigated myocardial contractility and ventricular myosin isoenzymes in the cardiomyopathic J-2-N hamster, which was developed in our laboratory from the cardiomyopathic Bio 14.6 hamster. Cardiomyopathic J-2-N hamsters are characterized by their large size and ease of propagation. The process by which their hearts become dilated is slow but is similar to what occurs in human idiopathic cardiomyopathy, especially dilated cardiomyopathy.

MATERIALS AND METHODS

Male J-2-N hamsters aged 52 weeks to 54 weeks were separated into two groups (groups A and B) on the basis of their electrocardiographic findings. In group A, the electrocardiogram showed no pathologic findings, whereas those in group B showed left axis deviation. Other male J-2-N hamsters aged 37 weeks to 39 weeks were also separated into two groups (groups I and II) on the basis of electrocardiographic findings. Group I showed no pathologic changes in the electrocardiogram, whereas group II showed a QS pattern in leads II, III, and aVF plus the precordial leads in addition to left axis deviation (Table 1).

Isometric contraction of isolated left ventricular papillary muscle was measured at a stimulation frequency of 0.2 Hz while the muscles were suspended in an organ

TABLE 1. *Age and electrocardiographic findings in the J-2-N hamster*

	Age (weeks)	Electrocardiogram
Group A	52–54	WNL
Group B	52–54	LAD
Group I	37–39	WNL
Group II	37–39	LAD, QS pattern (V_1, V_2, V_3)

WNL, within normal limit; LAD, left axis deviation.

bath perfused with Tyrode's solution (millimolar composition: glucose, 25.0; NaCl, 130.0; $NaHCO_3$, 20.0; NaH_2PO_4, 1.2; KCl, 4.1; $CaCl_2$, 2.2; $MgCl_2$, 1.5; pH 7.4 and 32°C) bubbled with 95% O_2 and 5% CO_2. After a steady state was obtained at L_{max}, both developed tension (T) and $\pm dT/dt_{max}$ were measured.

The left ventricular myosin isoenzyme pattern was determined by pyrophosphate gel electrophoresis (4–6). The gel contained 3.88% acrylamide and 0.12% N,N'-methylene-*bis* acrylamide, while the electrophoresis buffer was 20 mM $Na_4P_2O_7$ (pH 8.8) with 10% glycerol. Native left ventricular myosin was extracted with a solution of 100 mM $Na_4P_2O_7$ (pH 8.8), 5 mM dithiothreitol, 5 mM ethylene glycol tetra-acetic acid (EGTA), and 5 μg/ml leupeptin. Electrophoresis was performed for 30 hours at 3°C with a voltage gradient of 13.3 V/cm.

The left ventricular free wall was observed by light microscopic examination after Masson's staining. Statistical comparisons were carried out using Student's t-test.

RESULTS

Nine rats in group A, five in group B, five in group I, and four in group II were examined. Figure 1 shows that there were no significant differences in ventricular weight between groups A and B, whereas the ventricular-to-body-weight ratio was significantly lower in group B because of the greater body weight in this group (group A versus group B, body weight: 87 ± 8 versus 104 ± 4 g, $p < 0.01$; ventricular weight: 307 ± 33 versus 304 ± 10 mg, not significant; ventricular weight to body weight: 3.52 ± 0.17 versus 2.92 ± 0.12 mg/g, $p < 0.01$). There were no significant differences in body weight between groups I and II, but ventricular weight was significantly greater in group II than in group I (group I versus group II, body weight: 116 ± 14 versus 109 ± 15 g, not significant; ventricular weight: 324 ± 39 versus 398 ± 40 mg, $p < 0.05$; ventricular weight to body weight: 2.80 ± 0.04 versus 3.71 ± 0.61 mg/g, not significant, $p < 0.10$).

There were no significant differences in papillary muscle size between groups A and B or between groups I and II (group A versus group B, length: 3.8 ± 0.2 versus 3.6 ± 0.4 mm, not significant; cross-sectional area: 0.8 ± 0.2 versus 0.9 ± 0.4 mm^2, not significant; group I versus group II, length: 3.8 ± 0.8 versus 4.2 ± 0.4 mm, not significant; cross-sectional area: 0.9 ± 0.3 versus 1.1 ± 0.3 mm^2, not significant).

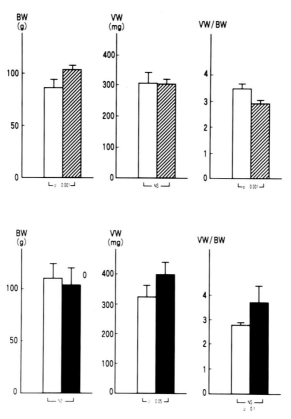

FIG. 1. Comparison of body weight and ventricular weight in the four groups. BW, body weight; VW, ventricular weight; ns, not significant.

Active and resting tension as well as $\pm dT/dt_{max}$ at L_{max} showed no significant differences between groups A and B (group A versus group B, active tension: 0.9 ± 0.4 versus 1.0 ± 0.6 g/mm^2, not significant; resting tension, 0.6 ± 0.2 versus 0.5 ± 0.2 g/mm^2, not significant; $+ dT/dt_{max}$: 12.8 ± 6.9 versus 13.6 ± 8.0 g/mm^2·s, not significant; $- dT/dt_{max}$: 9.4 ± 4.9 versus 10.5 ± 6.3 g/mm^2·s, not significant). Figure 2 shows a comparison of the mechanical parameters between groups I and II. Active tension tended to be lower in group II compared with group I (group I versus group II: 0.8 ± 0.3 versus 0.4 ± 0.1 g/mm^2·s, $p<0.10$). There was no significant difference in resting tension between the two groups (group I versus group II: 0.5 ± 0.2 versus 0.5 ± 0.2 g/mm^2). The value of $+ dT/dt_{max}$ was significantly lower in group II than in group I, and $- dT/dt_{max}$ also showed a tendency to be lower in group II (group I versus group II, $+ dT/dt_{dax}$: 11.6 ± 4.0 versus 6.5 ± 1.5 g/mm^2·s, $p<0.05$; $- dT/dt_{max}$: 8.1 ± 3.4 versus 5.0 ± 1.3 g/mm^2·s, $p<0.10$).

The ventricular myosin isoenzyme pattern was shifted toward VM-3 in group B compared with that in group A (group A versus group B, VM-1: 56.3 ± 7.8 versus

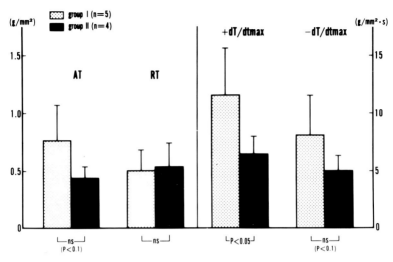

FIG. 2. Comparison of myocardial mechanical parameters between groups I and II. AT, active tension; RT, resting tension; ns, not significant.

$47.8 \pm 7.2\%$, $p < 0.10$; VM-3: 16.0 ± 4.3 versus $22.3 \pm 3.5\%$, $p < 0.05$). This phenomenon was found to be even more marked in the comparison between groups I and II (group I versus group II, VM-1: 67.1 ± 3.9 versus $35.0 \pm 9.6\%$, $p < 0.01$; VM-3: 10.1 ± 1.7 versus $32.8 \pm 6.6\%$, $p < 0.01$) (Fig. 3).

Light microscopic examination revealed fibrosis in the left ventricular free wall in group II (Fig. 4).

DISCUSSION

Many reports have demonstrated a reduction in contractility in cardiomyopathic hamsters (7,8). The morphologic, physiologic, and biochemical alterations of the myocardium that have been reported by other authors in cardiomyopathic hamsters may provide a basis for such changes in cardiac contractility. These changes include a shortened action potential duration (9), abnormalities of the voltage-dependent calcium channels (10,11), other sarcolemmal abnormalities (12,13), a functional defect in the α-subunit of G_s (14), altered G-protein messenger RNA levels (15), abnormalities of regulatory proteins (16,17), and a decrease in the volume or number of calcium transport sites in the sarcoplasmic reticulum (3). The electrocardiographic findings of group II, which showed a QS pattern in leads II, III, and aVF and the precordial levels, reflected morphologic changes in the ventricle. The tendency for a decrease in isometric developed tension in the isolated left ventricular papillary muscles from group II was probably partly attributable to these morphologic changes, i.e., the necrosis of myocardial cells and interstitial fibrosis. Although they were not examined in this study, the biochemical alterations in car-

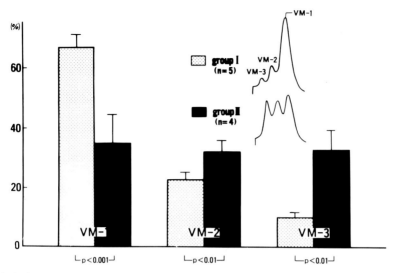

FIG. 3. Left ventricular myosin isoenzymes in J-2-N hamsters. The curves show representative densitometric profiles.

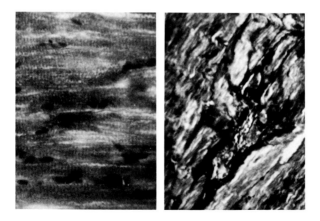

FIG. 4. Histologic comparison of the left ventricular free wall by light microscopic examination. Masson's stain was used (×600). The left panel shows ventricular tissue from group I; the right panel shows tissue from group II.

diomyopathic hamsters mentioned above could also partly explain our mechanical data, despite the fact that J-2-N hamsters must have genetic differences from other cardiomyopathic hamsters.

The alterations in the ventricular myosin isoenzyme pattern that we noted were consistent with previous reports (1,2). In the pressure-overloaded hypertrophied myocardium, a shift of the ventricular myosin isoenzyme pattern toward VM-3 can occur as an adaptation to maintain myocardial developed tension with a low energy utilization (18–21). In diabetic rats, the ventricular myosin isoenzyme pattern also shifts toward VM-3, and this change can be considered an adaptation to disorders of cardiac metabolism (21,22). Thus, the shift in ventricular myosin isoenzymes toward VM-3 in cardiomyopathic J-2-N hamsters may be partly the result of abnormal energy metabolism in the myocardial cells (23).

SUMMARY

Myocardial contractility and energetics were investigated in cardiomyopathic J-2-N hamsters developed at our laboratory. Hamsters were classified into groups on the basis of electrocardiographic findings. Myocardial contractility was assessed by measuring the isometric developed tension in isolated left ventricular papillary muscles perfused with Tyrode's solution (32°C, pH 7.4, stimulation frequency, 0.2 Hz). Ventricular myosin isoenzymes were separated by pyrophosphate gel electrophoresis, and the isoenzyme pattern was determined by densitometry. In the hamsters with electrocardiograms that showed a QS pattern in the precordial leads, isometric maximum developed tension tended to decrease and the maximum rate of increase in tension was significantly less than that in hamsters with normal electrocardiograms. The ventricular myosin isoenzyme pattern was shifted toward VM-3, and myocardial histologic changes were more severe in the group with a QS pattern. These results suggested that myocardial contractility and energetics were altered in cardiomyopathic J-2-N hamsters.

REFERENCES

1. Wiegand V, Stroh E, Hennings A, Lossnitzer K, Kreuzer H. Altered distribution of myosin isoenzymes in the cardiomyopathic Syrian hamster (Bio 8.262). *Basic Res Cardiol* 1983;78:665–70.
2. Malhotra A, Karell M, Scheuer J. Multiple cardiac contractile protein abnormalities in myopathic Syrian hamsters (Bio 53.58). *J Mol Cell Cardiol* 1985;17:95–107.
3. Whitmer JT, Kumar P, Solaro J. Calcium transport properties of cardiac sarcoplasmic reticulum from cardiomyopathic Syrian hamsters (Bio 53.58 and 14.6): evidence for a quantitative defect in dilated myopathic hearts. *Circ Res* 1988;62:81–5.
4. Hoh JY, McGrath PA, Hale PT. Electrophoretic analysis of multiple forms of rat cardiac myosin: effects of hypophysectomy and thyroxin replacement. *J Mol Cell Cardiol* 1978;10:1053–76.
5. d'Albis A, Pantolani C, Becher JJ. An electrophoretic study of native myosin isoenzymes and of their subunit content. *Eur J Biochem* 1979;99:261–72.
6. Rupp H, Jacob R. Response of blood pressure and cardiac myosin polymorphism to swimming training in the spontaneously hypertensive rat. *Can J Physiol Pharmacol* 1982;60:1098–1103.

7. Capasso JM, Olivetti G, Anversa P. Mechanical and electrical properties of cardiomyopathic hearts of Syrian hamsters. *Am J Physiol* 1989;257:H1836–42.
8. Sen L, O'Neill M, Marsh JD, Smith TW. Myosite structure, function, and calcium kinetics in the cardiomyopathic hamster heart. *Am J Physiol* 1990;259:H1533–43.
9. Wiederhold K-F, Nilius B. Increased sensitivity of ventricular myocardium to intracellular calcium–overload in Syrian cardiomyopathic hamster. *Biomed Biochim Acta* 1986;45:1333–7.
10. Wagner JA, Weisman HF, Snowman AM, Reynolds IJ, Weisfeldt ML, Snyder SH. Alterations in calcium antagonist receptors and sodium-calcium exchange in cardiomyopathic hamster tissues. *Circ Res* 989;65:205–14.
11. Rossner KL. Calcium current in congestive heart failure of hamster cardiomyopathy. *Am J Physiol* 1991;260:H1179–86.
12. Makino N, Jasmin G, Beamish RE, Dhalla NS. Sarcolemmal Na^+-Ca^{2+} exchange during the development of genetically determined cardiomyopathy. *Biochem Biophys Res Commun* 1985;133:491–7.
13. Kuo TH, Tsang W, Wiener J. Defective Ca^{2+}-pumping ATPase of heart sarcolemma from cardiomyopathic hamster. *Biochim Biophys Acta* 1987;900:10–16.
14. Kessler PD, Cates AE, Van Dop C, Feldman AM. Decreased bioactivity of the guanine nucleotide-binding protein that stimulates adenylate cyclase in hearts from cardiomyopathic Syrian hamsters. *J Clin Invest* 1989;84:244–52.
15. Katoh Y, Komuro I, Takaku F, Yamaguchi H, Yazaki Y. Messenger RNA levels of guanine nucleotide-binding proteins are reduced in the ventricle of cardiomyopathic hamsters. *Circ Res* 1990;67:235–9.
16. Malhotra A. Regulatory proteins in hamster cardiomyopathy. *Circ Res* 990;66:1302–9.
17. Malhotra A, Scheuer J. Troponin-tropomyosin abnormalities in hamster cardiomyopathy. *J Clin Invest* 1990;86:286–92.
18. Alpert NR, Mulieri LA. Increased myothermal economy of isometric force generation in compensated cardiac hypertrophy induced by pulmonary artery constriction in the rabbit. *Circ Res* 1982;50:491–500.
19. Kissling G, Rupp H, Malloy L, Jacob R. Alterations in cardiac oxygen consumption under chronic pressure overload. Significance of the isoenzyme pattern of myosin. *Basic Res Cardiol* 1982;77:255–69.
20. Jacob R, Kissling G, Ebrecht G, Holubarsch Ch, Medugorac I, Rupp H. Adaptive and pathological alterations in experimental cardiac hypertrophy. In: Chazov E, Saks V, Rona G, eds. *Advances in myocardiology*. New York: Plenum Press, 1983;55–77.
21. Holubarsch Ch, Litten RZ, Mulieri LA, Alpert NR. Energetic changes of myocardium as an adaptation to chronic hemodynamic overload and thyroid gland activity. *Basic Res Cardiol* 1985;80:582–93.
22. Takeda N, Nakamura I, Hatanaka T, Ohkubo T, Nagano M. Myocardial mechanical and myosin isoenzyme alterations in streptozotocin-diabetic rats. *Jpn Heart J* 1988;29:455–63.
23. Takeda N, Ohkubo T, Tanamura A, et al. Myocardial mechanics and myosin isoenzymes in streptozotocin-induced diabetic rats. In: Nagano M, Dhall NS, eds. *The diabetic heart*. New York: Raven Press, 1991;291–9.

The Cardiomyopathic Heart, edited by Makoto
Nagano, Nobuakira Takeda, and Naranjan S.
Dhalla. Raven Press, Ltd., New York © 1994.

4

Contractile and Regulatory Proteins in Hamster Cardiomyopathy

Ashwani Malhotra

*Division of Cardiology, Department of Medicine, Montefiore Medical Center,
111 East 210th Street, Bronx, New York 10467*

INTRODUCTION

Primary congestive cardiomyopathy represents a poorly understood group of clinical disorders. The Syrian hamster with a genetic cardiomyopathy is a reproducible, gradually progressive animal model of cardiac hypertrophy, cardiac dilation, and congestive heart failure resembling cardiomyopathy in humans (1–4). The terminal phase of the disease is characterized by progressive cardiac dilation and decompensation, ultimately leading to congestive heart failure and death at 10 to 12 months of age compared with 20 to 24 months for normal hamsters. Cardiomyopathy in the genetically myopathic Syrian hamster is associated with depressed contractile performance and a variety of ultrastructural alterations in the myocardium (5,6). Biochemical abnormalities have been reported by us and others in the contractile proteins, sarcolemma, sarcoplasmic reticulum, mitochondria, and lysosomes (7–16). Recently, Capasso and coworkers (17) reported that the early stages of cardiomyopathy in the Syrian hamster consist of alterations in the mechanical properties of the myocardium and electrical characteristics of the cell membrane. These may have important implications in the evolution of the dilated congestive form of myocardial disease in this animal model. Little is known about the role of contractile proteins and the regulatory protein(s) system in this model of cardiomyopathy.

Because of the central role contractile proteins may play in the mechanical properties of the cardiac muscle, we conducted studies in cardiac myosin and regulated actomyosin ATPase from myopathic hamsters to elucidate the role of cardiac myosin and regulatory complex, Troponin-Tropomyosin (TnTm) in hamster cardiomyopathy.

ANIMAL MODEL AND METHODS

Male or female random bred (RB) and Bio 53.58 or TO2 (myopathics) at 1 to 10 months of age were used in this study. Bio TO2s, formerly known as Bio 53.58

31

(strain 14.6), are an inbred strain with a hereditary abnormality in skeletal and cardiac muscle (atrial and ventricular hypertrophy), which results in subsequent development of congestive heart failure (17–21). The onset of disease is identical to that in Bio 53.58 and 14.6 hamsters from which this strain was developed. Animals younger than 40 to 50 days of age display little gross or light microscopic evidence of heart disease. At this time they enter the "necrotic phase" of the disease, developing multiple focal areas of myocytolytic necrosis in the heart and skeletal muscle. After 3 to 4 months, the lesions begin to decrease as the heart gradually undergoes hypertrophy, and they are replaced in the heart by fibrous calcified deposits.

Genetically myopathic Syrian hamsters (TO2) were obtained from Bio Breeders Inc. (Watertown, MA). For controls, RB animals of the same age were used. The animals were anesthetized with ether and their hearts removed. The atria and the connecting vessels were removed, and the ventricular portions were homogenized with a Tekmar homogenizer for the isolation and purification of different contractile proteins and the regulatory protein(s) complex, as described earlier (8,9,22,23).

RESULTS AND DISCUSSION

SDS-PAGE and Myosin ATPase Activity

Sodium dodecyl sulfate (SDS) gel electrophoresis of cardiac myosin from control and myopathic animals showed two light chains (LC_1 and LC_2) in the myosin from control hamsters with molecular weights of approximately 28,000 and 18,000 daltons. Myosin from myopathic animals showed a loss of the 18,000 dalton component with the appearance of two to three additional low molecular weight bands (9). However, SDS gel electrophoresis of triton- X–washed myofibrils from control and myopathic hearts demonstrated that the light chain-2 (LC_2) was present in the myofibrils from myopathic hearts. Thus, it appears that the loss of LC_2 had occurred during the purification of myosin (9).

The Ca^{2+} ATPase activity of myosin in both low and high potassium chloride was significantly depressed in the myopathic animals at 7 to 8 months of age. However, the K^+ ethylenediaminetetra-acetic acid (EDTA) ATPase activity of myosin did not show any differences in the myopathic and control animals. There was no significant difference in the Ca^{2+} ATPase levels in the hearts of the male and female myopathic animals.

Proteolytic Activity in Myopathic Hamsters

To determine the mechanism of the degradation of the light chain, proteolytic activity was determined in the myofibrils from control and myopathic hearts measured at different pH values, using ^{2}[H]-acetyl casein as the substrate. There was an overall increase in the proteolytic activity of myofibrils in the myopathic hearts. The increase was highest at pH 7 and above (9). The protease activity copurifies with the myosin, with an apparent increase in the specific activity from myofibrils to myosin preparation in the case of myopathic hearts. We purified this protease, and in vitro studies demonstrated that the protease can specifically degrade the LC_2 of cardiac myosin and other thin filamental proteins (24). These studies indicated that actomyosin and myosin ATPase activities are depressed in myopathic hearts. The myosin prepared from the myopathic hearts showed a consistent loss of LC_2, which was an artifact of preparation owing to a high level of neutral protease activity in these hearts. The depressed ATPase activity may have contributed to the decreased contractile performance observed in these hearts.

Myofibrillar Proteins and Myosin Isoenzymes

The next study was undertaken to determine (a) at which stage during the course of cardiomyopathy the ATPase activity of myofibrillar proteins becomes altered, (b) whether changes in the distribution of myosin isoenzymes occur as cardiomyopathy develops, and (c) how the changes in myofibrillar proteins relate to changes in myosin ATPase activity during the course of cardiomyopathy. To address these questions, the effects of graded calcium on the myofibrillar ATPase activity in the hearts of 1-month-old, 4-month-old, and 7-month-old control (C) and myopathic (M) hamsters were analyzed. The basal Mg^{2+} and Ca^{2+} stimulated Mg^{2+} ATPase activity of myofibrils at different free Ca^{2+} ions was significantly higher in myopathics than in control hearts at 4 and 7 months. This study suggested that ATPase regulation by Ca^{2+} was altered in the myopathic animals (8). To study the time course, we determined the Ca^{2+} ATPase activity of cardiac myosin from C and M animals in three different age groups (1 month, 4 to 5 months, and 7 months). No changes in activity were seen at 1 month. There were significant decreases in cardiac Ca^{2+} myosin ATPase activities at 4 and 7 months in M animals compared to those in C groups (8).

Figure 1 shows isoenzyme (V1, V2 and V3) profiles as seen on the pyrophos-

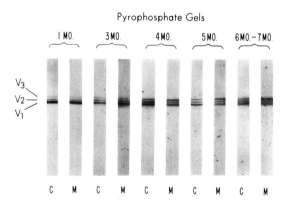

FIG. 1. Pyrophosphate gel electrophoresis of cardiac myosin isoenzymes (V_1,V_2,V_3) at various stages (1 month to 7 months old) in developing normal (C) and cardiomyopathic (M) hamster hearts.

phate gels in samples obtained from hearts of control and myopathic animals at 1 month to 7 months of age. V1 isomyosin predominated in 1- to 3-month-old animals in C and M groups. However, in M and 4- to 7-month-old controls, there was a gradual shift to predominance of V3 isoenzyme. The actin-activated Mg^{2+} myosin ATPase paralleled the proportion of cardiac myosin isoenzyme (V1 or V3%) content in C and M groups at 1, 4, and 7 months, respectively (see Fig. 6 in ref. 8).

Reversal of Myofibrillar ATPase and Isoenzyme Content with Verapamil Therapy

Contractile protein and myosin isoenzymes were analyzed in four groups of hamsters (control, untreated, discontinuously treated, and continuously treated with verapamil therapy, 1 g verapamil/1 L of H_2O) at 50 days of age (25). The basal Mg^{2+} ATPase (ethylene glycol tetra-acetic acid [EGTA] ATPase) and Ca^{2+}-stimulated Mg^{2+} ATPase activity of myofibrils was significantly higher in myocardium from untreated animals, whereas treatment with verapamil normalized the differences in net ATPase activation (Ca^{2+}-Mg^{2+} activity minus basal EGTA ATPase) in control and myopathic groups. Distribution of myosin isoenzymes demonstrated a predominance of the V1 band in the control adult group, with a decrease of 28% V1 content in untreated hamsters. The inverse pattern was seen with the V3 isoenzyme. A partial correction was attained with discontinuous verapamil therapy, and a complete reversal of the control pattern was attained with continuous treatment (25). Thus, the study suggests that the biochemical indices of cardiomyopathy in this genetic model parallel the morphologic index in their sensitivity to and normalization by long-term verapamil therapy.

These data demonstrate that cardiac myofibrils ATPase regulation by calcium is altered in genetic myopathic hamsters, and there are shifts in myosin isoenzyme distribution (V1→V3) suggesting abnormalities in multiple components of the contractile apparatus.

The regulatory proteins TnTm constitute a key protein complex involved in the control of muscular contraction in vertebrate striated muscle. The role of TnTm in physiologic and pathologic states of skeletal and cardiac muscle has been explored in a limited way. To further elaborate on the contributory role of TnTm in the cardiomyopathic hamsters, we studied alteration in the regulatory proteins based on the enzymatic analysis of reconstituted actomyosin system. TnTm complex isolated from the skeletal muscle of control and myopathic hamsters was subjected to SDS-PAGE. Co-electrophoresis and scans of the TnTm complex, with individually purified skeletal Tn subunits and Tm, demonstrated a reduction in the TnI and TnC subunits. SDS-PAGE and densitometric scans of cardiac TnTm complex showed small visible changes in the regions of TnI and TnC in the cardiac TnTm complex (22).

Figure 2 shows the Ca^{2+}-dependent skeletal and cardiac actomyosin ATPase activity using control myosin in the presence of control or myopathic skeletal and

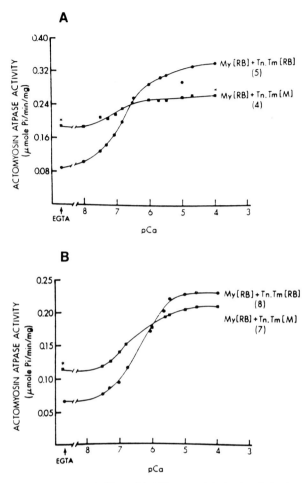

FIG. 2. A: Regulated actomyosin Ca^{2+}-Mg^{2+} ATPase activity in the skeletal muscle of control (random bred [RB]) and myopathic (M) hamsters. ●——●, RB control skeletal myosin (My[RB]) plus actin plus TnTm from control hamster skeletal muscle (Tn.Tm[RB]); ■——■, RB control skeletal myosin (My[RB]) plus actin plus TnTm from M hamster skeletal muscle (Tn.Tm[M]). **B:** Cardiac actomyosin Ca^{2+}-Mg^{2+} ATPase activity in the hearts of control (random-bred [RB]) and myopathic (M) hamsters. ●——●, RB cardiac myosin (My[RB]) plus actin plus TnTm from control hamster cardiac tissue (Tn.Tm[RB]; ■——■, RB cardiac hamster myosin (My[RB]) plus actin plus TnTm from M hamster hearts (Tn.Tm[M]). Numbers in parentheses indicate the number of studies. *$p<0.05$ when RB was compared with M at 10^{-4} M Ca^{2+} or in the presence of EGTA. (Reprinted by permission of the American Heart Association. *Circulation* 1990;66:1302–09.)

cardiac regulatory complex. The basal Mg^{2+} ATPase (EGTA ATPase) of skeletal actomyosin (Fig. 2A) was significantly elevated with myopathic relaxing factor, but the overall activation by free calcium in the range of 1 μM to 0.1 mM was slightly decreased when control myosin was reconstituted with myopathic relaxing factor. On the lower panel (Fig. 2B), the data demonstrate that as with skeletal proteins, cardiac regulatory proteins exhibited a basal EGTA ATPase significantly higher in myopathic samples than in control samples. The overall activation of cardiac actomyosin ATPase activity using myopathic cardiac TnTm complex was minimally depressed in the range of free Ca^{2+} ion concentration (1 μM to 0.1 mM).

In summary, our data show that the regulatory proteins (TnTm) from skeletal and cardiac muscle of myopathic hamsters have decreased inhibitory action on Mg^{2+} actomyosin ATPase activity. Actomyosin studies paralleled the myofibrillar Mg^{2+} ATPase activity, as shown in Fig. 3. The graph on the top (Fig. 3A) shows the Ca^{2+} dependent activity of cardiac myofibrillar ATPase activity with increasing free Ca^{2+} concentrations (10^{-8}M to 10^{-4}M). The basal Mg^{2+} ATPase (EGTA ATPase) and Ca^{2+}-stimulated Mg^{2+} ATPase activity of myofibrils at different free Ca^{2+} concentrations were significantly higher in myopathic (M) than control (C) hearts. The free Ca^{2+} dose-response curve and regulated ATPase activity of reconstituted myosin plus actin with TnTm from control or myopathic hearts is shown on the lower side (Fig. 3B). The basal EGTA ATPase in myopathics also exhibited a significantly higher activity than controls as shown in myopathic myofibrils (Fig. 3A).

To explore the role of the cardiac TnTm complex in the regulation of cardiac myofibrillar regulation in the hearts of cardiomyopathic hamsters, cross-hybridization experiments were conducted by mixing cardiac myofibrils from control and myopathic hamsters with myopathic and control TnTm and vice versa (23). Preparations from control, myopathic, and myopathic plus control TnTm on SDS-PAGE showed similar patterns, thus ruling out any additional or missing subunits in the three different preparations. Dose-response curves of cardiac Ca^{2+}-Mg^{2+}–activated myofibrillar ATPase versus free calcium ion concentration in myofibrils from control, myopathic, control myofibrils (MF) mixed with control TnTm complex and myopathic myofibrils plus control TnTm, demonstrated that cardiac TnTm had no effect on ATPase activity when mixed with control myofibrils. However, in the case of myopathic myofibrils plus control TnTm, the curve reverted to normal in both the absence and presence of free Ca^{2+} ion (23).

To confirm the binding of the control regulatory complex in the myofibrils from the myopathic group, hybridization studies were conducted combining ^{125}I-[TnTm] with myofibrillar preparations from control and myopathic hamster hearts and vice versa. The data were calculated and plotted as a percentage of EGTA inhibitory ATPase in cardiac myofibrils and reconstituted actomyosin with cold and ^{125}I-[TnTm]. Loss in Ca^{2+} sensitivity, as shown by the percentage of EGTA ATPase inhibition in myopathic myofibrils, could be reversed by the addition of cold control (TnTm) or ^{125}I-control [TnTm] complex (23). These data further suggest that TnTm from myopathics has less inhibitory effect than TnTm from controls, diminishing the degree of calcium control of myofibrillar ATPase in cardiomyopathic hamster hearts. The loss in calcium sensitivity in myopathic myofibrils could be reversed by exchanging or binding of cardiac control TnTm complex myofibrils from dystrophic hamsters (23).

In summary, the data on cardiac contractile proteins in the genetic model of hamster cardiomyopathy suggest the following: (a) shifts in myosin isoenzymes

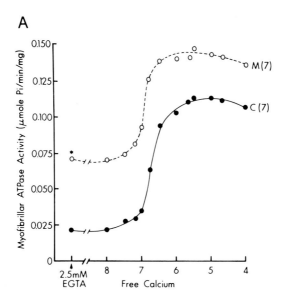

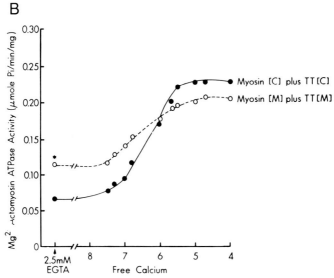

FIG. 3. **A:** Effect of graded calcium on the myofibrillar ATPase activity in the hearts of control (●) and myopathic (○) 7-month-old hamsters. *$p < 0.05$. **B:** Cardiac Mg^{2+} ATPase activity of reconstituted actomyosin versus free Ca^{2+} in control (C) and myopathic (M) hamsters. TT, troponin-tropomyosin. *$p < 0.05$. (Reprinted by permission of Academic Press, Inc. (London) Ltd. J Mol Cell Cardiol 1985;17:95–107.)

(V1→V3); (b) diminished myosin ATPase activity; (c) abnormalities in myofibrillar dose-response curves, as shown by Mg^{2+} and Ca^{2+}-Mg^{2+} ATPase; (d) reversal of myofibrillar ATPase and isoenzyme content with verapamil therapy; and (e) myofibrillar ATPase could be normalized with the addition of TnTm from control hearts.

CONCLUSIONS

Multiple abnormalities are demonstrated in the contractile protein machinery in the skeletal as well as cardiac muscles of myopathic hamsters. In addition to the shifts in myosin isoenzymes and ATPase, changes in the TnTm alter myofibrillar dose response, which may result in altered contractile function in hamster cardiomyopathy.

ACKNOWLEDGMENTS

This chapter is dedicated to the late Dr. Ashok Bhan, who was instrumental in carrying out some of the earlier studies on contractile proteins. I wish to thank Dr. James Scheuer, Chairman, Department of Medicine, for his encouragement and advice during the course of these studies. I would also like to acknowledge the helpful suggestions of Dr. David Geenen during the preparation of this manuscript. Sincere thanks are due to Ms. Cecilia Lopez, Mr. Kirit Patel, and Mr. Antonio Nakouzi for their excellent technical assistance. Secretarial help by Ms. Janice Brewton is deeply appreciated. This work was supported by U.S. Public Health Service Grants HL-15498 and HL-37412.

SUMMARY

Primary congestive cardiomyopathy is poorly understood as a clinical disorder. The Syrian hamster with a genetic cardiomyopathy is a reproducible model of cardiac hypertrophy, cardiac dilation, and congestive heart failure resembling cardiomyopathy in humans. Cardiomyopathy in the genetically myopathic Syrian hamster (Bio 14.6 or Bio 53.58) is associated with altered contractile performance and a variety of ultrastructural changes in the myocardium. Not much is known about the role of the contractile proteins and the regulatory proteins (troponin-tropomyosin) in this genetic model. Because of the central role the contractile proteins may play in the mechanical properties of the striated muscle, the studies on cardiac and skeletal actomyosin and its regulation by troponin-tropomyosin (TnTm) are reported here. Our studies demonstrate multiple abnormalities in the contractile protein machinery in the skeletal as well as cardiac muscle of myopathic hamsters. In addition to the shifts in myosin isoenzymes and myosin adenosine triphosphatase (ATPase), changes in the TnTm alter myofibrillar dose response, which may result in altered contractile function in hamster cardiomyopathy.

REFERENCES

1. Bajusz E, Homberger F, Baker JR, Opie LH. The heart muscle in muscular dystrophy with special reference to involvement of the cardiovascular system in the hereditary myopathy of the hamster. *Ann NY Acad Sci*, 1966;138:213–29.
2. Gertz EW. Cardiomyopathic Syrian hamster: a possible model of human disease. *Prog Exp Tumor Res*, 1972;16:242–60.
3. Bishop S, Sole MJ, Tilley LP. In: Andrews EJ, Ward BC, Altman NH, eds. *Cardiomyopathies, spontaneous animal model of human disease*. New York: Academic Press, 1979;59–64.
4. Jasmin G, Proshek L. Hereditary polymyopathy and cardiomyopathy in the Syrian hamster: I. Progression of heart and skeletal muscle lesions in the UM-X7.1 line. *Muscle Nerve* 1982;5:20–5.
5. Abelmann WH, Jeffrey, FE, Wagner R. In: Bajusz E, Rona G, eds. *Recent advances in studies on cardiac structure and metabolism*, vol. 1, *Myocardiology*. Baltimore: University Park Press, 1972; 225–34.
6. Paterson, RA, Layberry RA, Nadkarni BB. *Lab Invest* 1972;26:755–66.
7. Dhalla NS, Sulakhe PV, Fedelesova M, Yates JC. Molecular abnormalities in cardiomyopathy; comparative pathology of the hearts. *Adv Cardiol* 1974;13:282–300.
8. Malhotra A, Karell M, Scheuer J. Multiple cardiac contractile protein abnormalities in myopathic Syrian hamsters (Bio 53:58). *J Mol Cell Cardiol* 1985;17:95–107.
9. Bhan A, Malhotra A, Hatcher VB, Sonnenblick EH, Scheuer J. Depressed myosin ATPase activity in hearts of myopathic hamsters: dissociation from neutral protease activity. *J Mol Cell Cardiol* 1978;10:769–77.
10. Sulakhe PV, Dhalla NS. Alterations in the activity of cardiac Na^+-K^+ stimulated ATPase in congestive heart failure. *Exp Mol Pathol* 1973;18:100–11.
11. Gertz EW, Stam AC, Jr, Sonnenblick EH. A quantitative and qualitative defect in the sarcoplasmic reticulum in the hereditary cardiac myopathy of the Syrian hamster. *Biochem Biophys Res Commun* 1970;40:746–53.
12. Lindenmayer, GE, Harigaya S, Bajusz E, Schwartz A. Oxidative phosphorylation and calcium transport of mitochondria isolated from cardiomyopathic hamster hearts. *J Mol Cell Cardiol* 1970; 1:249–59.
13. Sole MJ, Kamble AB, Hussain MN. A possible change in the rate-limiting step for cardiac norepinephrine synthesis in the cardiomyopathic Syrian hamster. *Circ Res* 1977;41:814–17.
14. Jasmin G, Proschek L. Calcium and myocardial injury: an appraisal in the cardiomyopathic hamster. *Can J Physiol Pharmacol* 1984;62:891–98.
15. Factor SM, Minase T, Cho S, Domintz R, Sonnenblick EH. Microvascular spasm in the cardiomyopathic Syrian hamster: a preventable cause of focal myocardial necrosis. *Circulation* 1982; 66:342–54.
16. Kato M, Nagano M. The animal model of cardiomyopathy. *Jpn J Clin Med* 1991;49:239–45.
17. Capasso JM, Sonnenblick EH, Anversa P. Chronic calcium channel blockade prevents the progression of myocardial contractile and electrical dysfunction in the cardiomyopathic Syrian hamster. *Circ Res* 1990;67:1381–93.
18. Jasmin G, Bajusz E. In: Fleckenstein A, Rona G, eds. *Recent advances in the study of cardiac structure and metabolism*. Baltimore: University Park Press, 1975;6:219–29.
19. Singh JN, Dhalla NS, McNamara DB, Bajusz E, Jasmin G. In: Fleckenstein A, Rona G, eds. *Recent advances in the study of cardiac structure and metabolism*. Baltimore: University Park Press, 1975; 6:259–68.
20. Sole MJ, Factor SM. Hamster cardiomyopathy: a genetically transmitted sympathetic dystrophy. In: Beamish RE, Panagia V, Dhalla NS, eds. *Pathogenesis of stress-induced heart disease*. Boston: Martinus Nijhoff, 1985:34–43.
21. Rouleau JL, Chuck LHS, Hollosi G, et al. Verapamil preserves myocardial contractility in the hereditary cardiomyopathy of the Syrian hamster. *Circ Res* 1982;50:405–12.
22. Malhotra A. Regulatory proteins in hamster cardiomyopathy. *Circ Res* 1990;66:1302–09.
23. Malhotra A, Scheuer J. Troponin-tropomyosin abnormalities in hamster cardiomyopathy. *J Clin Invest* 1990;86:286–92.
24. Kuo TH, Giacomelli F, Kithier K, Malhotra A. Biochemical characterization and cellular localization of serine protease in myopathic hamster. *J Mol Cell Cardiol* 1981;13:1035–49.
25. Factor SM, Cho S, Scheuer I, Sonnenblick EH, Malhotra A. Prevention of hereditary cardiomyopathy in the Syrian hamster with chronic verapamil therapy. *J Am Coll Cardiol* 1988;12:1599–1604.

The Cardiomyopathic Heart, edited by Makoto
Nagano, Nobuakira Takeda, and Naranjan S.
Dhalla. Raven Press, Ltd., New York © 1994.

5

Sliding Velocity of Cardiomyopathic Hamster Cardiac Myosin on *Nitellopsis* Actin Cables: A Study Using an In Vitro Motility Assay

Seiryo Sugiura, Hiroshi Yamashita, Shin-ichi Momomura,
Takashi Serizawa

*The Second Department of Internal Medicine, School of Medicine, University of Tokyo,
Hongo 7-3-1, Bunkyo-ku, Tokyo 113, Japan*

INTRODUCTION

Syrian hamsters have been used as useful models for studying the pathophysiology of human idiopathic dilated cardiomyopathy. In particular, the contractile dysfunction that develops at a later stage of their lives has been the focus of research for many years. To understand this problem, various approaches have been undertaken and multiple abnormalities have been identified. These abnormalities are metabolic changes such as inhibition of glycolysis resulting in a disturbance in Ca^{2+} buffering (1), diminished response to β-adrenergic receptor stimulation associated with a functional abnormality of the G protein (2), functional changes in regulatory proteins (3,4), and shifts in myosin isozyme distribution (5). Of these, myosin isozyme redistribution is of importance because of the central role played by myosin molecules in muscle contraction. Myosin of myopathic hamsters consists of three isozymes: V1 (homodimer of α-myosin heavy chains), V2 (heterodimer of α- and β-myosin heavy chains), and V3 (homodimer of β-myosin heavy chains). In normal or young (1- to 3-month-old) myopathic hamsters, V1 is the predominant isozyme. However, as the myopathic hamsters grow older and disease stage progresses, V3 content increases and dominates the distribution (5).

The relationship between isozyme distribution and the unloaded shortening velocity of muscle has been reported using rat or rabbit papillary muscles (6,7). In addition, isozyme distribution has a significant influence on the energetics of muscle contraction (8). However, these findings must be interpreted cautiously, because, as pointed out earlier, multiple structural changes take place simultaneously and contribute to the pathogenesis of contractile dysfunction observed in myopathic hamsters. In other words, identification of a direct relationship between myosin isozyme redistribution and contractile dysfunction is difficult in intact muscle preparations that maintain complex cell structure. A novel approach to overcome this problem is the in vitro motility assay system in which we can observe the sliding of isolated myosin and actin molecules under a photomicroscope. In one of these assays developed independently by Sheetz and Spudich (9) and Shimmen and Yano (10), actin cables in an internodal cell of an alga *Nitellopsis obtusa* were used as the substratum of myosin sliding. Using this assay system, we have already shown that the sliding velocity of cardiac myosin obtained from rabbit and rat ventricle correlated with the Ca^{2+}-activated adenosine triphosphatase (ATPase) activity and the myosin isozyme content (11,12). The advantage of this study is that the mechanical property of myosin molecule can be studied under completely controlled conditions without any influence being exerted by the regulatory systems in cardiac muscle. Our preliminary data on the mechanical property of cardiac myosin obtained from myopathic hamsters are presented here. We believe that this line of investigation will help us understand the pathogenesis of cardiac dysfunction in cardiomyopathic hamsters.

METHOD

Myosin Preparation

Forty-week-old cardiomyopathic hamsters (Bio 14.6: B)(n = 4) and age-matched control animals (golden hamster: C)(n = 4) were studied. Animals were anesthetized with an intravenous injection of sodium pentobarbital (40 mg/kg body weight), and their hearts were excised quickly. Because the hamster hearts were small, they were pooled for each group. Cardiac myosin was prepared from left ventricular muscle according to the method described by Katz et al. (13) with some modifications. All the procedures were carried out at 4° C, with 5 mM dithiothreitol and 5 μg/ml leupeptin added to the solution. The final centrifugation was performed for 3 hours at 100,000 g to remove the actin.

Determination of Adenosine Triphosphatase Activity

We determined calcium (Ca^{2+})-activated ATPase activity of myosin according to the method described by Yazaki et al. (14) with minor modifications. The reaction was run for 5 minutes in a solution containing 50 mM tris(hydroxymethy) aminomethane (TRIS), 1 mM adenosine triphosphate (ATP), 10 mM $CaCl_2$, pH 7.5 at 25°C. Inorganic phosphate liberated in ATP hydrolysis was measured according to the method by Youngberg and Youngberg (15). Specific activity was obtained using the myosin concentration determined by the Lowry method (16).

Myosin Isozyme Analysis

Myosin isozyme distribution was analyzed by pyrophosphate polyacrylamide gel electrophoresis described by Pagani et al. (7). The gel was scanned by a densitometer, and the areas under the peaks of V1, V2, and V3 were measured to determine the relative amount of each isozyme. The percentage of α-myosin heavy chain (% α-MHC) was determined by the following formula: % α-MHC = %V1 + %V2/2.

In Vitro Motility Assay

We used the in vitro motility assay technique (Fig. 1) developed by Shimmen and Yano (10). Briefly, this method is composed of three procedures:

Myosin-Coated Bead Preparation

Latex beads (2 μm in diameter) were incubated in poly-L-lysine solution. These poly-L-lysine coated beads were mixed with purified myosin in a high ionic strength buffer (400 mM KCl, 10 mM imidazole HCl, pH 7.0). After reduction of the ionic strength of the buffer solution, filamentous myosin attached to the bead surface. After unbound myosin was removed by centrifugation, the myosin-coated beads were suspended in an Mg-ATP solution containing 1 mM ATP, 6 mM MgCl₂,

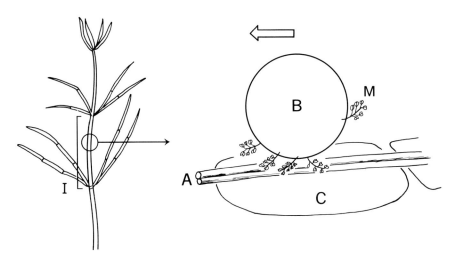

FIG. 1. Schematic presentation of in vitro motility assay. **Left panel,** *Nitellopsis obtusa.* I, internodal cell. **Right panel,** Sliding movement of a myosin-coated bead on *Nitellopsis* actin cables. B, latex bead; M, filamentous myosin; C, chloroplast rows; A, actin cables. **Arrow** indicates the direction of movement.

70 mM KOH, 5 mM ethylene glycol-bis(β-aminoethyl ether)-*N,N,N',N'*-tetra-acetic acid (EGTA), 30 mM piperazine-*N,N'*-bis(2-ethanesulfonic acid) (PIPES), and 200 mM sorbitol (pH 7.0) for the in vitro motility assay.

Preparation of Actin Donor Cells

Actin cables in the internodal cell of a green alga, *Nitellopsis obtusa*, were used as the substratum for the myosin sliding. Under natural conditions, these actin cables interact with the myosin of this plant and generate motive force for the cytoplasmic streaming. *Nitellopsis* was cultured in a plastic bucket filled with tap water and mold at the bottom. This plant consists of long, internodal cells connected in a series, and each cell has well-organized rows of chloroplasts on its inner surface. Because long, straight actin cables run on these chloroplast rows, the direction of myosin sliding is always straight, and thus a steady state is maintained for many seconds. Before each experiment an internodal cell was isolated, trimmed free of branches, and stored in artificial pond water (0.1 mM each of KCl, NaCl, and $CaCl_2$, pH 5.6). Then both ends of an internodal cell were cut open, and the cell was perfused with the Mg-ATP medium and left in a moist chamber to keep from drying out. After 20 minutes, the cell was perfused again with a solution containing 5 mM ethylenediaminetetra-acetic acid (EDTA), 1 mM ATP, 71 mM KOH, 30 mM PIPES, and 200 mM sorbitol (pH 7.0). By means of these procedures the membrane system inside the cell was disintegrated and the cell content was washed out, whereas the actin cables remained intact. The cell was placed in the moist chamber again for 1 minute and perfused with the Mg-ATP medium. The actin donor (actin cables exposed) cell thus prepared was used for the motility assay.

Introduction of Myosin-Coated Beads into the Actin Donor Cell

Myosin-coated beads suspended in the Mg-ATP solution were introduced into the actin donor cell by intracellular perfusion. Both ends of the cell were ligated with polyester thread to avoid passive movement of intracellular fluid, and the cell was placed on the glass slide in a solution containing 0.1 mM K_2SO_4, 1 mM NaCl, 0.1 mM $CaCl_2$, and 150 mM sorbitol. The movement of the beads was observed using a photomicroscope and recorded on videotapes. The measurement of the sliding velocity was performed on the replay of the videotapes. All the experiments were carried out at 21° C to 23° C.

RESULTS

Myosin Isozyme Distribution

Densitometric scan patterns of pyrophosphate gel electrophoresis for native myosin obtained from control and myopathic hamsters are shown in Fig. 2. In control

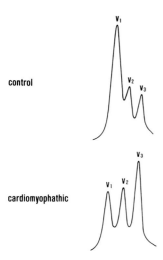

control

cardiomyophathic

FIG. 2. Densitometric scans of pyrophosphate gel of cardiac myosin from control and cardiomyopathic hamsters.

animals, cardiac myosin showed V1 predominance, whereas in the myopathic hamster myosin V3 isozyme predominated.

Adenosine Triphosphatase Activity

Ca^{2+} activated ATPase activity of cardiac myosin was decreased in myopathic hamsters compared with that of controls (0.486 versus 0.579 μM P_1/mg/min). In Fig. 3, the relationship between Ca^{2+}-activated ATPase activity and % α-MHC

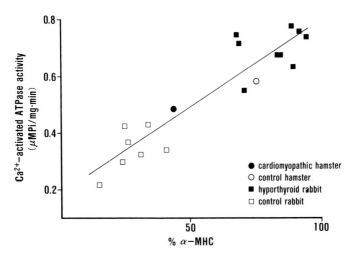

FIG. 3. Relationship between myosin Ca^{2+}-activated ATPase activity and relative content of α-myosin heavy chain. Data from hamsters and rabbit were plotted on same graph for comparison.

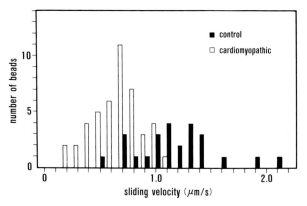

FIG. 4. Histogram showing the velocity distribution for cardiac myosin from cardiomyopathic and control hamsters.

was plotted for both hamster myosin and rabbit cardiac myosin. The data obtained from different species seemed to fall on the same relation.

In Vitro Motility Assay

The sliding movement of the beads coated with hamster myosin was similar in nature to that of beads coated with rabbit skeletal or rabbit cardiac myosin (9–12). When the myosin-coated beads were introduced into the actin donor cell, the myosin on the bead began to interact with the actin and to drag the beads. The beads in the core portion of the cell (not attached to the actin layer) showed only brownian movement. The direction of bead movement was determined by the polarity of the actin cables, as was the direction of cytoplasmic streaming. Figure 4 shows the velocity distribution of beads coated with myosin from both control and myopathic hamsters. Apparently, the distribution for myopathic hamsters shifted left, indicating the reduction in sliding velocity (average 0.71 versus 1.14 μm/sec).

DISCUSSION

Hereditary cardiomyopathic hamsters were studied as animal models of dilated cardiomyopathy, and various biochemical abnormalities were identified. Although these multiple factors contribute to the pathogenesis of impaired contractile function observed in these animals at various stages, we focused on the myosin isozyme redistribution and its functional significance.

In myopathic hamster myosin, relative content of α-myosin heavy chain decreases during the course of the disease. The change in myosin isozyme distribution is associated with a decrease in Ca^{2+}-activated ATPase and actin-activated ATPase activities. These changes have been shown to correlate with the maximal shortening velocity studied with papillary muscle (17). Interestingly, however, myofibrillar

ATPase activity increases in myopathic animals, suggesting a change in the regulatory proteins (5).

To circumvent this problem, we used an in vitro motility assay system and found that the structure and catalytic activity of myosin correlate with the velocity of actin-myosin sliding at the molecular level. Because no regulatory proteins are included, only the property of myosin can be studied in this assay system. However, there are some limitations when applying the present result to cardiac dysfunction in myopathic animals. First, in this assay myosin molecules are randomly arranged so that they may not all be able to work very efficiently. Second, actin-myosin sliding was observed under only unloaded conditions. Because muscle contracts against some load under physiologic conditions, we need information on the mechanical property of myosin molecules under loaded conditions. Finally, as stated previously, changes in contractile protein are not the entire explanation for the cardiac dysfunction of myopathic hamsters.

In summary, we applied the in vitro motility assay technique and studied the mechanical property of cardiac myosin obtained from myopathic hamsters. Compared to normal hamster myosin, myopathic hamster myosin showed low sliding velocity that parallels the Ca^{2+}-activated ATPase activity and relative content of α-myosin heavy chain. This technique can be a useful tool to establish a direct relationship between biochemical and mechanical properties.

SUMMARY

Relative content of myosin isozyme is known to change in cardiomyopathic hamster cardiac muscle. To clarify the effect of isozyme redistribution on cardiac function, we examined both biochemical (isozyme content by pyrophosphate gel electrophoresis and Ca^{2+}-activated adenosine triphosphatase [ATPase] activity) and mechanical (sliding velocity of myosin on actin cables) properties of isolated cardiac myosin. Cardiac myosin was obtained from 3- to 18-month-old cardiomyopathic (Bio 14.6) and control hamsters. Long well-organized actin cables of an alga *Nitellopsis* were used for motility assay. Small latex beads were coated with cardiac myosin and made to slide on algal actin cables in the presence of Mg adenosine triphosphate (ATP). Active movement of bead on the actin cables was observed under the photomicroscope, and the velocity was measured. The sliding velocity was lower in cardiomyopathic myosin, and there was a positive correlation between the velocity and both α-myosin heavy chain content and myosin Ca^{2+}-activated ATPase activity. These results suggest that myosin isozyme redistribution may play a role in the genesis of cardiac dysfunction in cardiomyopathic hamsters.

REFERENCES

1. Wikman-Coffelt J, Stefenelli T, Wu ST, et al. [Ca^{2+}]$_i$ transient in the cardiomyopathic hamster heart. *Circ Res* 1991;68:45–51.
2. Feldman AM, Tena RG, Kessler PD, et al. Diminished β-adrenergic receptor responsiveness and

cardiac dilation in hearts of myopathic Syrian hamsters (Bio 53.58) are associated with a functional abnormality of the G stimulatory protein. *Circulation* 1990;81:1341–52.

3. Malhotra A. Regulatory proteins in hamster cardiomyopathy. *Circ Res* 1990;66:1302–09.
4. Malhotra A, Scheuer J. Troponin-tropomyosin abnormalities in hamster cardiomyopathy. *J Clin Invest* 1990;86:286–92.
5. Malhotra A, Karell M, Scheuer J. Multiple cardiac contractile protein abnormalities in myopathic Syrian hamsters (Bio 53;58). *J Mol Cell Cardiol* 1985;17:95–107.
6. Ebrecht G, Rupp H, Jacob R. Alterations of mechanical parameters in chemically skinned preparations of rat myocardium as a function of isoenzyme pattern of myosin. *Basic Res Cardiol* 1982; 77:220–34.
7. Pagani ED, Julian FJ. Rabbit papillary muscle myosin isozymes and the velocity of muscle shortening. *Circ Res* 1984;54:586–94.
8. Alpert NR, Mulieri LA. Heat, mechanics, and myosin ATPase in normal and hypertrophied heart muscle. *Fed Proc* 1982;41:192–98.
9. Sheetz MPR, Spudich JA. ATP-dependent movement of myosin in vitro: characterization of a quantitative assay. *J Cell Biol* 1984;99:1867–71.
10. Shimmem T, Yano M. Active sliding movement of latex beads coated with skeletal muscle myosin on *Chara* actin bundles. *Protoplasma* 1984;121:132–37.
11. Sugiura S, Yamashita H, Serizawa T, Iizuka M, Shimmen T, Sugimoto T. Active movement of cardiac myosin on *Characeae* actin cables. *Pflügers Arch* 1992; in press.
12. Yamashita H, Sugiura S, Serizawa T, et al. Sliding velocity of isolated rabbit cardiac myosin correlates with isozyme distribution. *Am J Physiol* 1992; in press.
13. Katz AM, Repke DI, Rubin BB. Adenosinetriphosphatase activity of cardiac myosin. Comparison of the enzymatic activities and activation by actin of dog cardiac, rabbit cardiac, rabbit white skeletal and rabbit red skeletal muscle myosins. *Circ Res* 1966;19:611–21.
14. Yazaki Y, Raben MS. Effects of the thyroid state on the enzymatic characteristics of cardiac myosin. *Circ Res* 1975;36:208–15.
15. Youngberg GE, Youngberg MV. Phosphorous metabolism: a system of blood phosphorous analysis. *J Lab Clin Med* 1930;16:158–66.
16. Lowry OH, Rosenbrough NJ, Farr AL, Randall RJ. Protein measurement with the folin phenol reagent. *J Biol Chem* 1951;193:265–75.
17. Rouleau JL, Chuck LHS, et al. Verapamil preserves myocardial contractility in the hereditary cardiomyopathy of the Syrian hamster. *Circ Res* 1982;50:405–12.

The Cardiomyopathic Heart, edited by Makoto
Nagano, Nobuakira Takeda, and Naranjan S.
Dhalla. Raven Press, Ltd., New York © 1994.

6

Altered Contractile Behavior of Cardiomyocytes from Cardiomyopathic Hamsters

Luc Ver Donck, Greet Verellen, Hugo Geerts,
*Hans-Georg Olbrich, †Ernst Mutschler, and Marcel Borgers

*Department of Physiology, Life Sciences, Janssen Research Foundation,
Turnhoutseweg 30, B-2340 Beerse, Belgium; *Zentrum der Inneren Medizin,
Abteilung Kardiologie; and †Pharmakologisches Institut für Naturwissenschaftler,
JW Goethe University Frankfurt, Theodor-Stern-Kai 7, D-6000 Frankfurt/Main, Germany*

INTRODUCTION

The genetically inbred cardiomyopathic Syrian hamster has been shown to provide an elegant animal model of cardiomyopathy and congestive heart failure (1). These animals develop focal necrotic lesions in the heart after the first month of life, followed by cardiac hypertrophy during later months. Finally, death as a consequence of congestive heart failure is usually observed within 1 year (2–4). A variety of characteristic pathologic features that develop during progression of the disease have been described (for review, see elsewhere in this volume): vascular spasms leading to focal ischemic damage (5), elevated catecholamine tonus and sensitivity (6), and failure of cellular ion–regulating mechanisms leading to a disturbed calcium homeostasis (4,7–9). Whether these characteristics are causally related or merely represent epiphenomena remains unclear.

Many authors have identified alterations in the intracellular calcium homeostasis as an important property of cardiomyopathic hamster heart cells. In fact, abnormal intracellular calcium regulation is claimed to represent a major cause of cardiac dysfunction in the failing heart (10). In view of this, we investigated the cellular calcium handling capacity of "calcium-stressed" isolated cardiomyocytes by evaluation of their contractile behavior in the absence of systemic influences. Single cells from necrotic (45 days of age) and hypertrophic (75 and 105 days old) cardiomyopathic hamster hearts were used.

METHODS AND MATERIALS

Isolation of Cardiomyocytes

Calcium-tolerant cardiomyocytes were enzymically isolated from the hearts of 45-, 75-, and 105-day-old cardiomyopathic hamsters (Bio 82.62) and age-matched controls by an enzymatic digestion procedure, as previously described for rat heart (11). Hearts were isolated and retrogradely perfused (3.5 ml/min, 37°C) with calcium-free salt solution (KRH [mM]: NaCl [125.0], KCl [2.6], KH_2PO_4 [1.2], $Mg(SO_4).7H_2O$ [1.2], HEPES [10.0], and glucose [5.5]; pH 7.4 [NaOH]). After 5 minutes, collagenase (0.06%, Wako), bovine serum albumin (0.1%, Serva), and $CaCl_2$ (25 μM) were added to the perfusate for 25 minutes. Then the heart was minced and disaggregated by gentle agitation in the collagenase solution. The cell suspension was washed, the calcium concentration was gradually augmented to 1 mM, and cells were seeded in plastic Petri dishes (60 mm, Falcon). Cells attached to the dishes within 15 minutes, the remaining unattached cells (nonviable) were rinsed off, and the dishes were stored in an oxygen chamber (100% O_2) at room temperature. The yield of rod-shaped isolated cardiomyocytes was similar in both animals, and cells were used in the experiments within 5 hours after isolation.

Evaluation of Contractile Behavior

Electrical Stimulation

Two 4-cm-long platinum electrodes were placed in parallel on to the bottom of a Petri dish at a fixed distance of 3.5 cm. Cardiomyocytes could then be paced at various frequencies by a home-built electrical stimulator generating rectangular, bipolar 10 msec pulses of 100 mA.

Experiments

Cardiomyocytes in Petri dishes were incubated in phosphate-free KRH containing either 0.25, 1, 4, 6, 10, or 16 mM $CaCl_2$ (pH 7.4). Pacing was induced at 2 Hz, and the fraction of synchronously contracting cells was determined after 30 seconds using a light microscope (40 ×, Laborlux, Leitz). At least 100 cardiomyocytes were evaluated in each condition. Cells were scored as "responding" when synchronous twitch contractions could be observed in phase with the pacing rhythm, as indicated by an auditory signal from the stimulator. Cells not displaying a visible response to pacing or those contracting out of phase with the pacing rhythm were scored as "nonresponding." In the same dish, the percentage of cells remaining rod-shaped after 5 minutes of pacing was determined (11,12). In a separate set of experiments, cells were incubated in KRH + 1 mM $CaCl_2$, pH 7.4, and electrically stimulated at increasing pacing rates (2–4 Hz). The percentage of responding cells was determined as described above. All experiments were performed at room temperature.

Statistical Analysis

Data are presented as mean ± standard error of the mean of n independent experiments. Statistical significance was tested by analysis of variance of individual data. Probabilities of less than .05 were considered significant.

RESULTS

Effect of Extracellular Calcium on Response to Field Stimulation

Isolated cardiomyocytes from normal and cardiomyopathic hamster hearts are mechanically silent (quiescent) in the presence of a physiologic calcium concentration but respond to electrical field stimulation by displaying a synchronous twitch contraction. Extracellular calcium affects the number of cardiomyocytes from control hearts responding to pacing in a bell-shaped way: the fraction of responding cells increases at 0.25 to 1 mM $CaCl_2$, is maximal at 1 to 4 mM $CaCl_2$, and then declines again with a further rise in calcium (Fig. 1). This response is similar in cells from 45- and 75-day-old control hearts, whereas a slight reduction is observed at 1 to 6 mM $CaCl_2$ in 105-day-old controls. The percentage of contracting cells tends to be lower in cardiomyopathic cells than in controls at 0.25 to 1 mM $CaCl_2$ in necrotic and early hypertrophic animals (45 and 75 days old), whereas in the hypertrophic phase (105 days), more cells from cardiomyopathic hearts respond to pacing at 4 to 16 mM $CaCl_2$. This is evidenced by a rightward shift of the curve (see Fig. 1). Cells from 105-day-old cardiomyopathic hearts do not display the reduction in responding cells shown in younger animals, as was observed in controls.

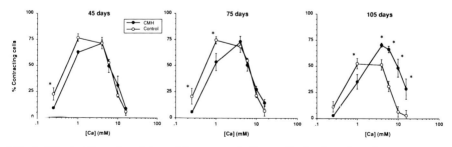

FIG. 1. Effect of the extracellular calcium concentration on the fraction of cardiomyocytes responding to electrical field stimulation. CMH, cardiomyopathic heart; electrical pacing, 100 mA, 2 Hz; *$p<.05$ by analysis of variance, n = 3–5 (45 days); n = 3–4 (75 days); n = 5–8 (105 days).

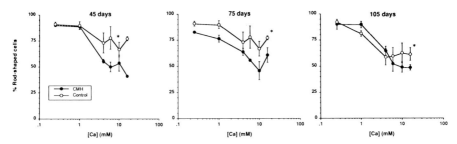

FIG. 2. Effect of the extracellular calcium concentration on the fraction of cardiomyocytes remaining rod-shaped after exposure to electrical field stimulation for 5 minutes. CMH, cardiomyopathic heart; electrical pacing, 100 mA, 2 Hz; $*p<.05$ by analysis of variance; n = 3–5 (45 days), n = 3–4 (75 days), n = 5–8 (105 days).

Effect of Extracellular Calcium on Cell Morphology

The percentage of cells that remains rod-shaped after pacing slightly decreases with increasing calcium concentrations (>1 mM $CaCl_2$) in cells from both cardiomyopathic hamster and control hearts, independent of age (Fig. 2). Cells from cardiomyopathic hearts tend to be more susceptible to increasing calcium than do those from controls. However, this difference reached significance only at 16 mM $CaCl_2$.

Effect of Pacing Frequency on Response to Field Stimulation

The response to elevated pacing rates (3 and 4 Hz, 1 mM $CaCl_2$) is significantly impaired in cells from 45- and 75-day-old cardiomyopathic hearts, as compared with the response in control hearts. However, the response to higher pacing rates is equally depressed in cells from hypertrophic hamsters (105 days old) and those from age-matched controls (Fig. 3).

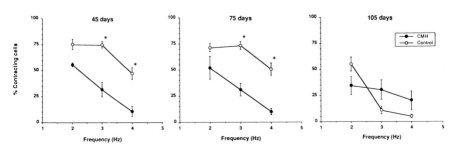

FIG. 3. Effect of the pacing frequency on the fraction of cardiomyocytes responding to electrical field stimulation. CMH, cardiomyopathic heart; electrical pacing, 100 mA, 2–4 Hz in medium + 1 mM $CaCl_2$; $*p<.05$ by analysis of variance; n = 3–4 (45 days), n = 2–3 (75 days), n = 5–8 (105 days).

DISCUSSION

The present experiments demonstrate a bell-shaped response of cardiomyocytes to an increase in the extracellular calcium concentration that shifted to higher calcium in cells from 105-day-old cardiomyopathic hamster hearts. Cardiomyopathic myocytes also tend to be less resistant to increased calcium load and showed fewer responders to increased pacing rate. These findings suggest age-related alterations in the calcium handling capacity of cells from the cardiomyopathic hamster. Comparable findings were reported earlier (13,14).

At present, there is no clear-cut indication of the factors possibly underlying the impaired calcium handling capacity of cardiomyocytes from cardiomyopathic hamsters. Earlier reports demonstrated age-related changes in the calcium-regulating systems of the cell: loss of sarcolemmal calcium-binding capacity (30 to 60 days) (9), depressed myofilament calcium responsiveness (60–120 days) (7), depression of sarcolemmal Na^+/K^+–adenosine triphosphatase (ATPase) activity (30–280 days) (15–17), Ca^{2+}-ATPase activity and Na^+/Ca^{2+}-exchange (120–280 days) (15,16), and decreased myofilament Ca^{2+}-ATPase activity (200 days) (7). On the other hand, calcium current, resting membrane potentials, and action potentials of cardiomyopathic hamster cells in the necrotic or hypertrophic phase have been reported to display normal characteristics (18, 19).

These data suggest the onset of abnormalities in the intracellular calcium-regulating capacity of cardiomyopathic hamsters from a young age onward, which is compatible with the observations on shifts in the contractile behavior of cardiac cells. The rightward shift of the cells' response to elevated calcium upon pacing in 105-day-old cardiomyopathic hearts may be related to reduced myofilament calcium responsiveness as well as reduced Ca^{2+}-ATPase activity and Na^+/Ca^{2+} exchange at this age. The latter two factors may further increase the intracellular calcium level when extracellular calcium rises, such that responsiveness of myofilaments is enhanced. Shape changes of cardiomyocytes from rod-shaped to hypercontracted cells, a relevant measure of loss of cellular tolerance to calcium (12,20), were observed at all ages tested, as was the reduced response to elevated pacing rate. These observations may therefore be related to depressed Na^+/K^+–ATPase activity leading to elevated cellular calcium load. Reduced calcium extrusion capacity (15–17) may also be involved in cells of 105-day-old animals.

In conclusion, these data suggest that cardiomyocytes from cardiomyopathic hamster hearts in the necrotic and hypertrophic stage display impaired cellular calcium handling. This may play a significant role in the future development of congestive heart failure in these animals.

SUMMARY

The cardiomyopathic Syrian hamster displays cardiac cell necrosis as a consequence of calcium overload from 30 days of age onward, followed by hypertrophy at 60 to 200 days of age. We investigated the calcium handling capacity of cardio-myocytes isolated from necrotic and hypertrophic cardiomyopathic hamster hearts. Cardiomyocytes were obtained from the hearts of 45-, 75- and 105-day-old Bio 82.62 hamsters and age-matched healthy controls. The percentage of cells contracting synchronously and remaining rod-shaped upon electrical field stimulation (2 Hz) at increasing extracellular $CaCl_2$ (0.25–16 mM) was evaluated. In cells from control animals, the percent of responders was maximal at 1 to 4 mM $CaCl_2$ and decreased at higher extracellular calcium (6–16 mM) at all ages studied. The percent of responding cardiomyocytes from 45- and 75-day-old cardiomyopathic hamsters was slightly depressed versus those of controls at 0.25 to 1 mM $CaCl_2$ ($p <$ .05), whereas the response to higher extracellular calcium was significantly increased in 105-day-old cardiomyopathic hamsters ($p < .05$). The percent of cardiomyocytes remaining rod-shaped after pacing tended to decrease with increasing extracellular calcium. This was more pronounced in cells from cardiomyopathic hamster hearts but reached significance only at 16 mM $CaCl_2$. At higher pacing frequencies (3–4 Hz; 1 mM $CaCl_2$), the percent of decrease of responders was more pronounced in cardiomyopathic hamsters than in controls. The data suggest altered intracellular calcium handling during the contraction-relaxation cycle in hypertrophic cardiomyopathic hamsters.

REFERENCES

1. Homburger F, Bajusz E. New models of human disease in Syrian hamsters. *JAMA* 1970;212:604–10.
2. Bajusz E, Baker JR, Nixon CW, Homburger F. Spontaneous, hereditary myocardial degeneration and congestive heart failure in a strain of Syrian hamsters. *Ann NY Acad Sci* 1969;156:105–29.
3. Bajusz E, Homburger F, Baker JR, Bogdonoff P. Dissociation of factors influencing myocardial degeneration and generalized cardiocirculatory failure. *Ann NY Acad Sci* 1969;156:396–420.
4. Jasmin G, Procheck L. Calcium and myocardial cell injury. An appraisal in the cardiomyopathic hamster. *Can J Physiol Pharmacol* 1984;62:891–8.
5. Factor SM, Minase T, Cho S, Dominitz R, Sonnenblick EH. Microvascular spasm in the cardiomyopathic Syrian hamster: a preventable cause of focal myocardial necrosis. *Circulation* 1982;66:342–54.
6. Sole MJ, Factor SM. Hamster cardiomyopathy. A genetically transmitted sympathetic dystrophy? In: Beamisch RE, Panagia V, Dhalla NS, eds. *Pathogenesis of stress-induced heart disease.* Boston: Martinus Nijhoff, 1984;34–43.
7. Strobeck JE, Factor SM, Bhan A, et al. Hereditary and acquired cardiomyopathies in experimental animals: mechanical, biochemical and structural features. *Ann NY Acad Sci* 1979;317:59–88.
8. Panagia V, Singh JN, Anand-Srivastava MB, Pierce GN, Jasmin G, Dhalla NS. Sarcolemmal alterations during the development of genetically determined cardiomyopathy. *Cardiovasc Res* 1984;18:262–70.
9. Olbrich HG, Borgers M, Thoné F, et al. Ultrastructural localization of calcium in the myocardium of cardiomyopathic Syrian hamsters. *J Mol Cell Cardiol* 1988;20:753–62.
10. Morgan JP. Abnormal intracellular modulation of calcium as a major cause of cardiac dysfunction. *N Engl J Med* 1991;325:625–32.
11. Ver Donck L, Pauwels PJ, Vandeplassche G, Borgers M. Isolated rat cardiac myocytes as an experimental model to study calcium overload: the effect of calcium-entry blockers. *Life Sci* 1986;38:765–72.
12. Borgers M, Ver Donck L, Vandeplassche G. Pathophysiology of cardiomyocytes. *Ann NY Acad Sci* 1988;522:433–53.

13. Sen L, Donghee K, O'Neill M, Thomas W. Contractile state and Ca flux in isolated adult cardiomyocytes of normal and cardiomyopathic hamsters. *Circulation* 1987;76[Suppl IV]:340.
14. Nag AC, Cheng M. Isolation, long-term culture and ultrastructural characterization of adult cardiomyopathic cardiac muscle cells. *In Vitro Cell Dev Biol* 1987;23:261–66.
15. Makino N, Jasmin G, Beamisch RE, Dhalla NS. Sarcolemmal Na^+/Ca^{2+}-exchange during development of genetically determined cardiomyopathy. *Biochem Biophys Res Commun* 1985;133:491–7.
16. Kuo TH, Tsang W, Wiener J. Defective Ca^{2+}-pumping ATPase of heart sarcolemma from cardiomyopathic hamster. *Biochim Biophys Acta* 1987;900:10–16.
17. Rossner KL, Maskarenhas DAN. The effect of ouabain on hearts of cardiomyopathic hamsters: potentiation by isoproterenol. *J Mol Cell Cardiol* 1987;19:627–32.
18. Hunter EG. Adult ventricular myocytes isolated from CHF146 and CHF147 cardiomyopathic hamsters. *Can J Physiol Pharmacol* 1985;64:1503–6.
19. Howlett SE, Gordon T. Calcium channels in normal and dystrophic hamster cardiac muscle: [^{3}H]nitrendipine binding studies. *Biochem Pharmacol* 1987;36:2653–9.
20. Geerts H, Nuydens R, Nuyens R, Ver Donck L. The effect of flunarizine on intracellular calcium in isolated rat cardiomyocytes. A digital image processing study. *Cardiovasc Res* 1989;23:797–806.

The Cardiomyopathic Heart, edited by Makoto
Nagano, Nobuakira Takeda, and Naranjan S.
Dhalla. Raven Press, Ltd., New York © 1994.

7

Cardiac Collagen Expression in the Development of Two Types of Cardiomyopathic Hamsters (Bio 14.6 and Bio 53.58)

Naoki Makino, Kazuhiro Masutomo, *Masayuki Nishimura,
Toru Maruyama, and Takashi Yanaga

*Departments of Bioclimatology and Medicine and *Clinical Genetics,
Medical Institute of Bioregulation, Kyushu University, Beppu, Japan*

INTRODUCTION

The cardiomyopathic hamsters form an excellent genetically determined model to study the pathophysiology of events during the course of cardiomyopathy and congestive heart failure (1). The pathogenesis of the disease state is not fully understood, but as early as 30 days of age, focal necrosis is apparent and continues up to 4 months, resulting in extensive replacement of viable myocardial fibrotic connective tissue (2). It is now accepted that the myocardium contains a collagen matrix, consisting primarily of type I and type III collagen (3); this matrix is a major determinant of myocardial architecture, structural integrity, and mechanical properties (4). However, alterations in collagen content and collagen gene expression in the cardiomyopathic hamster have not been studied. Our study deals with alterations of collagen concentration and the expression from mRNA of collagen type I and type III in the cardiomyopathic hamster. This arrangement of collagen components is thought to play an important role in the function of the heart, including the compliance of the heart wall (5), proper alignment of the cardiac cells (6), and myofibrillogenesis (7).

In our study we used two strains of hamsters, one that develops a hypertrophic cardiomyopathy (Bio 14.6) and another more recently introduced strain that develops a dilated cardiomyopathy (Bio 53.58). Most studies on myopathic hearts have been carried out in hamster models using either the Bio 14.6 strain introduced by Bajusz et al. (8) or the UM-X7.1 strain introduced by Bajusz and Jasmin (9). These strains develop a hypertrophic form of cardiomyopathy resulting in a thick ened ventricular wall and septum, similar to the cardiomyopathy often seen in the animal model with catecholamine-induced myopathy (10). A more recently available hamster strain (Bio 53.58) develops a dilated, i.e., congestive form of cardiomyopathy characterized by a thin ventricular wall and dilated chambers. This dilated form is morphologically more typical of that seen in forms of cardiomyopathy caused by certain cardiotoxins such as alcohol and some anticancer agents (11). Both the hypertrophic and dilated cardiomyopathies result in a disease that progresses to the same end-point of congestive heart failure. We have examined which stage of cardiomyopathy is associated with altered arrangement of the extracellular matrix, especially interstitial collagen subtypes. To address this question, we attempted to examine alterations of protein concentration and mRNA expression for type I and type III collagen in cardiomyopathic hamsters. In addition, we observed the histologic distribution of the immunohistochemistry of these collagen subtypes and compared it with that in F1-β control hamsters.

METHODS

Animals

Bio 14.6 and Bio 53.58 (Bio-Breeders Inc., Fitchburg, MA) strains of cardiomyopathic hamsters were selected for study. The first group consisted of animals 30 to 40 days old that did not have cardiomegaly. This group is defined as the prehypertrophic stage. The second group consisted of animals between 100 and 110 days old that were in the initial stage of cardiac hypertrophy. The third group consisted of animals between 150 and 160 days old that had significant cardiac hypertrophy without peripheral signs of heart failure. This group is defined as the hypertrophic stage. The fourth group contained animals that were 280 to 300 days old and had marked cardiomegaly and moderate peripheral signs of heart failure. This group is defined as the early stage of heart failure. Animals in these four stages were compared with age-matched normal golden F1-β hamsters.

RNA Isolation and Northern Blot-Analyses

Total cellular RNA was isolated by the methods outlined by Chirgwin et al. (12). RNA was quantitated by absorbance at 260 nm and 310 nm. Quantitation was confirmed by size determination of ribosomal bands that had been fractionated on agarose-formaldehyde gels stained with ethidium bromide. RNA (10 μg) was electrophoresed on a 1% agarose, 6% formaldehyde gel and transferred to a nitrocellulose filter. The filter was prehybridized for 4 to 24 hours at 42°C. Hybridization was performed using 0.5 to 1.0×10^6 cpm per lane of labeled probe (specific activity, 4 to 1.0×10^8 cpm/μg). The complementary DNA probes used in these experiments were α2(type I) collagen and α1(type III) collagen (kindly provided by Dr. de Crombrugghe) and a β-actin probe. After hybridization, the nitrocellulose filter was washed according to methods described by Thomas (13). The filter was autoradiographed onto x-ray film for 1 to 2 days. Densitometric analysis was performed with a Vide-Densitometer (Model 620) (Bio-Rad).

Determination of Hydroxyproline

Hydroxyproline was determined by the method of Bergman and Loxley (14). Myocardial tissue was homogenized, and hydrolysis of the sample solution was done with 6 N HCl at 100°C for 24 hours. The hydrolyzed samples were dried using a flash evaporator. A hydroxyproline standard solution of 2, 4, 6, 8, and 10 μg/ml was made. A reagent blank was included in the procedure by substituting water for the hydroxyproline solution; 0.5 ml of hydroxyproline standard solutions of different strengths and homogenates of heart samples were taken in glass tubes, and 1 ml of isopropanol was added to each. The tubes were then vortexed. To this solution, 0.5 ml of oxidant (0.35 g chloramine-T + 5 ml water + 20 ml citrate buffer) was added, and all elements were vortexed and allowed to stand for 4 minutes. Subsequently, 3.25 ml of Ehrlich reagent (3 ml Ehrlich + 16 ml isopropanol) was added. After the tubes were kept at 25°C for 18 hours, the intensity of red coloration was measured at a wavelength of 558 nm using a model DU50 spectrophotometer (Hitachi, Inc., Japan). The amount of hydroxyproline in the unknown samples was calculated using the standard curve. The collagen content was estimated by multiplying the hydroxyproline content by a factor of 8.2.

Immunofluorescence Studies

Immediately after decapitation of the animals, the hearts were removed from experimental and control hamsters, washed with phosphate-buffered saline, and then snap-frozen in liquid nitrogen. Frozen sections of 8 to 10 μm-thick were cut in a cryostat. The procedures for indirect immunostaining are basically the same as those described previously (15). The following antibodies were used at 1:20 to 1:80 dilutions: rabbit polyclonal antisera to anti–rat type I collagen and those to anti–rat type III collagen (Chemicon Intern., Inc., Temecula, CA) for the primary antibodies and fluorescein-conjugated goat affinity purified antibodies to rabbit IgG (Organon Teknika Corp., Durham, NC) for the second antibodies. As a negative control, parallel sections were incubated with rabbit preimmune serum but not with the primary antibody. Specimens were examined with a fluorescence microscope, BH-II (Olympus Inc, Tokyo, Japan) and both the distribution and the intensity of the specific immunostaining were evaluated. Findings were documented photographically using Kodak Extachrome 400 daylight film (Eastman Kodak Co, Rochester, NY).

RESULTS

Northern blot analysis was performed on total RNA in hearts obtained from 30 to 280 day old control (F1-β) and cardiomyopathic hamsters (Bio 14.6 and Bio

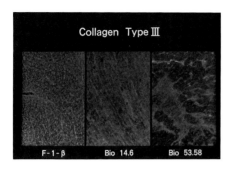

FIG. 1. Northern blot analysis with complementary DNA-specific 2(I) and 1(III) collagen mRNA from hearts of control and experimental hamsters at 280 days old.

53.58). Steady-state mRNA levels for cardiac type III (α1) collagen were higher in hearts of both the Bio 14.6 and Bio 53.58 hamsters than in the hearts of F1-β hamsters at 30 days old. However, there was no difference in type I collagen α2) among F1-β, Bio 14.6, and Bio 53.58 hamsters (data not shown). Enhanced expression of mRNA for type III (α1) collagen was seen in the hearts of Bio 53.58 hamsters at 280 days old, at which stage cardiomyopathic hamsters have progressive heart failure; this expression observed in the hearts of Bio 14.6 hamster was less than that detected in Bio 53.58 hamster hearts at the same age (Fig. 1). In addition, this type of collagen expression was noticeably undetected in F1-β hamsters at 280 days old (Fig. 1). Type I (α2) collagen was not different in 280-day-old Bio strain hamsters from that in 30-day-old animals.

Myocardial collagen concentration, defined by the amount of collagen in milligrams per gram of heart tissue and estimated from the quantification of hydroxyprolines, increased in hearts of cardiomyopathic hamsters (Bio 14.6 and Bio 53.58) at 100 days old (Table 1). However, the collagen concentration in the heart tissue of the F1-β hamster as a normal control animal did not change at 30 or 100 days old (Table 1). The relative ratio of type III (α1) to type I (α2) collagen expression in control and experimental hamsters at four different stages of the development is shown in Table 2. These ratios for two types of cardiomyopathic hamsters (Bio 14.6 and Bio 53.58) were higher than that for the F1-β hamster from 100 to 280 days old. However, a significant increase of this ratio had continued even at 280 days old compared with that in Bio 14.6 hamsters.

TABLE 1. *Collagen contents estimated by hydroxyproline in Syrian hamsters at 30 and 100 days of age[a]*

Days	30~40	100~110
F1-β	0.89 ± 0.04	1.1 ± 0.04
Bio 14.6	0.91 ± 0.03	1.58 ± 0.05[*]
Bio 53.58	0.90 ± 0.03	2.28 ± 0.09[*][+]

[a]Values are the mean $\pm$ SE of four experiments.
[*]$p < 0.05$ compared with F1-β hamster.
[+]$p < 0.05$ compared with Bio 14.6 hamster at the same age.

TABLE 2. *Relative ratio of type III/type I collagen expression in Syrian hamsters*[a]

Days	30	100	150	280
F1-β	0.94	1.56	2.50	1.84
Bio 14.6	1.6	2.0*	10.3*	4.3*
Bio 53.58	1.4	2.7*	10.8*	8.9*[+]

[a]Values represent the mean of four experiments.
*$p < 0.05$ compared with F1-β hamster.
[+]$p < 0.05$ compared with Bio 14.6 hamster at the same age.

Immunofluorescence studies showed an increased expression of type III collagen in Bio 14.6 and Bio 53.58 hamsters compared with control hamster F1-β. Although interstitial immunostaining with anti–type III collagen was seen in every experimental group when compared with the control F1-β hamster, more intense and diffuse staining with anti–type III collagen was seen in Bio 14.6 and Bio 53.58 hamsters (see Fig. 2). On the other hand, there was no significant difference in the intensity or distribution of the immunostaining with anti–type I collagen among Bio 14.6, Bio 53.58, and F1-β control hamsters (data not shown).

DISCUSSION

The study examined collagen expression in hearts from normal controls and two clinically and morphologically different types of cardiomyopathy using the Syrian hamster model. Age comparisons were made between these hamsters from 30 to 280 days old. It was of interest to study the dilated cardiomyopathic strain, i.e., Bio 53.58, since it represents a more prevalent form of the disease seen in the clinical setting. Also, the rapid development of a myocardial collagen network that sur-

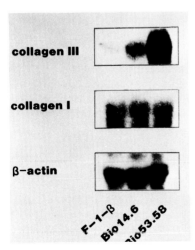

FIG. 2. Immunostaining of type III collagen in sections of heart from F1-β, Bio 14.6, and Bio 53.58 hamsters. Note an increased interstitial staining in Bio 14.6 and a diffuse massive staining in Bio 53.58 hearts.

rounds and connects the cardiac myocytes (16) in hearts with dilated cardiomyopathy has not been described previously.

It was demonstrated that type III collagen expression and accumulation were markedly increased in 280-day-old hamster hearts from the Bio 53.58 strain when compared with either control F1-β or Bio 14.6 animals as a model of the hypertrophic hamster. This suggests that the rearrangement of the cardiac extracellular matrix took place in the animals with dilated cardiomyopathy. In 100-day-old hamsters, this type of collagen expression was more enhanced in the hearts of both the Bio 14.6 and Bio 53.58 hamsters than in the F1-β hamster. However, there was no significant difference between Bio 14.6 and Bio 53.58 hamsters in type III collagen expression in the heart. Thus, expression for type III collagen was at least at the same rate in these two strains until the beginning stage of hypertrophy. Our results are supported by those of Weber (4), who described idiopathic dilated cardiomyopathy in humans as accompanied by an excess proportion of thin collagen fiber, which perhaps represents type III collagen. Furthermore, the type III/type I collagen expression ratio increased in both types of cardiomyopathic hamsters from 100 days old. Thus, in the earlier phase of collagen remodeling, type III collagen accumulation is increased relative to that of type I.

The results presented here appear to be similar to what occurs in the neonatal heart (17) and in the early phase of cardiac hypertrophy (5). They also agree with findings in in vivo hypertrophy (18), in which the collagen type III/type I protein synthetic rates increase in response to stretch. In addition, the data presented here illustrate that alterations seen in the proportions of type I and type III collagen are at least partly regulated at the level of the collagen mRNA. The functional significance of changes in the relative proportions of type I and type III collagens in the interstitium has not been absolutely determined. However, several investigators have pointed out the structural differences in these collagens (4,5). Changes in the ratios of type I to type III collagen may result in altered elasticity of the heart wall.

A number of studies have illustrated the effects of various chemical factors on collagen gene expression, including transforming growth factor B (19), glucocorticoid (20), and ascorbic acids (21). Cell density (22), growth rate (23), and extracellular matrix environment (24) have also been shown to influence collagen synthesis in vitro. The data presented here show a specific increase in type III collagen in the genetically determined cardiomyopathic hamsters. However, it is not clear what kind of signal is transduced into an increase in collagen expression. Second messenger systems may be involved in these processes.

SUMMARY

The arrangement of cardiac extracellular matrix, composed predominantly of collagenous fiber, is intimately associated with cardiac function during the development of cardiomyopathy. Although some information exists regarding the morphologic organization of the extracellular matrix of the heart, little is known about the regulation and accumulation of extracellular matrix components in cardiomyopathy. We therefore examined collagen expression of messenger RNA (mRNA) in two types of cardiomyopathic hamster (Bio 14.6 and Bio 53.58) at different stages and compared it with that in normal control hamsters (F1-β). Northern blot analysis revealed the enhanced expression of mRNA for type III collagen from 100 days old in both types of cardiomyopathic hamster. This expression for type III continued up to 280 days in the Bio 53.58 hamster but not in the Bio 14.6 hamster. However, type I collagen mRNA levels were not found to change during the development in both types of experimental animals. Furthermore, we used biochemical and morphologic techniques to analyze changes in collagen accumulation in these animal models. Our studies show that type III collagen in immunofluorescence studies was diffusely observed and that collagen concentration was significantly increased in Bio strain hamsters. These results suggest that an increased deposition and mRNA expression of type III collagen may be partly responsible for altering the arrangement of myocardial architecture, structural integrity, and mechanical properties in these animals, resulting in dilation of the heart and possibly in heart failure.

ACKNOWLEDGMENTS

We thank Mrs H. Matsuki and Miss K. Haratake for their technical assistance. This study was supported by a grant-in-aid for scientific research from the Ministry of Education, Science, and Culture in Japan (03807057).

REFERENCES

1. Bajusz E, Homberger F, Baker JR, Opie LH. The heart muscle in muscle dystrophy with special reference to involvement of the cardiovascular system in the hereditary myopathy of the hamster. *Ann NY Acad Sci* 1966;138:213–31.
2. Gertz EW. Cardiomyopathic Syrian hamster: a possible model of human disease. *Prog Exp Tumor Res* 1972;16:242–60.
3. Medugorac I, Jacob R. Characterization of left ventricular collagen in the rat. *Cardiovasc Res* 1983;17:15–21.
4. Weber KT. Cardiac interstitium in health and disease: the fibrillar collagen network. *J Am Coll Cardiol* 1989;13:1636–52.
5. Weber KT, Janicki JS, Shroff SG, Pick R, Chen RM, Bashey RI. Collagen remodeling of the pressure-overloaded, hypertrophied nonhuman primate myocardium. *Circ Res* 1988;62:757–65.
6. Borg TK, Johnson LD, Lill PH. Specific attachment of collagen to cardiac myocytes: in vivo and in vitro. *Dev Biol* 1983;97:417–23.
7. Borg TK, Xuehui M, Hilenski L, Vinson N, Terracio L. The role of the extracellular matrix on myofibrillogenesis in vitro. In: Clark EB, Takao A, eds. *Developmental cardiology. Morphogenesis and function.* Mt Kisco, NY: Futura Publishing Co; 1990;175–91.
8. Bajusz E, Baker JR, Nixon CW, Hornburger F. Spontaneous hereditary myocardial degeneration and congestive heart failure in a strain of Syrian hamster. *Ann NY Acad Sci* 1969;156:105–29.
9. Bajusz E, Jasmin G. Hereditary disease model of cardiomyopathy: studies on a new line of Syrian hamsters (abstract). *Fed Proc* 1972;31:621.
10. Rona G. Catecholamine cardiotoxicity. *J Mol Cell Cardiol* 1985;17:291–306.
11. Gibbs CL, Woolley G, Kotsanas G, Gibson WR. Cardiac energetics in daunorubicin-induced cardiomyopathy. *J Mol Cell Cardiol* 1984;16:953–62.

12. Chirgwin JJ, Przbyla AE, MacDonald RJ, Rutter WJ. Isolation of biologically active ribonucleic acid from sources enriched in ribonuclease. *Biochemistry* 1979;18:5294–302.
13. Thomas PS. Hybridization of denaturated RNA transferred or dotted to nitrocellulose paper. *Methods Enzymol* 1983;100:255–66.
14. Bergman J, Loxley R. Two improved and simplified methods for the spectrophotometric determination of hydroxyproline. *Anal Chem* 1963;36:1961–5.
15. Nishimura M, Asahi M, Hayashi M, et al. Extracellular matrix in hepatic granulomatous of mice infected with *Schistosoma mansoni*. Qualitative and quantitative analysis. *Arch Pathol Lab Med* 1985;109:813–18.
16. Borg TK, Caulfield JB. Collagen on the heart. *Tex Rep Biol Med* 1979;39:321–33.
17. Zak R. Cell proliferation during cardiac growth. *Am J Cardiol* 1973;31:211–19.
18. Carver W, Nagpal ML, Nachtigal M, Borg TK, Terracio L. Collagen expression in mechanically stimulated cardiac fibroblasts. *Circ Res* 1991;69:116–22.
19. Ignotz RA, Massague J. Cell adhesion protein receptors as targets for transforming growth factor-beta action. *Cell* 1987;51:189–97.
20. Medugorac I, Jacob R. Characterization of left ventricular collagen in the rat. *Cardiovasc Res* 1983;17:15–21.
21. Walsh MJ, LeLeiko NS, Sterling KM, Jr. Regulation of type I, III, and IV procollagen mRNA synthesis in glucocorticoid-mediated intestinal development. *J Biol Chem* 1987;262:10814–18.
22. Aumailley M, Kreig T, Razaka G, Muller P, Bricaude H. Influence of cell density on collagen biosynthesis in fibroblast cultures. *Biochem J* 1982;206:505–10.
23. Hata R-I, Senoo H. L-Ascorbic acid z-phosphate stimulates collagen accumulation, cell proliferation, and formation of a three-dimensional tissue-like substrate by skin fibroblasts. *J Cell Physiol* 1989;138:1–8.
24. Mauch C, Hatamochi A, Scharffetter K, Kreig T. Regulation of collagen synthesis within a three-dimensional collagen gel. *Exp Cell Res* 1988;178:493–503.

The Cardiomyopathic Heart, edited by Makoto
Nagano, Nobuakira Takeda, and Naranjan S.
Dhalla. Raven Press, Ltd., New York © 1994.

8

Pathophysiologic Aspects of Cardiomyopathic J-2-N Hamsters

Makoto Nagano, Nobuakira Takeda, Mitsutoshi Kato,
Makoto Nagai, and Jei Yang

Department of Internal Medicine, Jikei University School of Medicine, Tokyo 125, Japan

INTRODUCTION

The cause of idiopathic cardiomyopathy is still unclear, but remarkable progress has been made in recent studies. Although Bio 14.6 strain cardiomyopathic hamsters have been used in most experiments, it is difficult to obtain newborn or embryonal and female Bio 14.6 hamsters on a commercial basis. In addition, even if they can be obtained, the reproduction rate of Bio 14.6 hamsters is low and cannibalism is prevalent when the pups are born. Therefore, studies using female fetuses or newborn hamsters are difficult to perform. In view of these problems, we have attempted over the past several years to develop hamsters without these defects in our laboratory.

METHODS AND RESULTS

We started with a male Bio 14.6 and female golden hamster, and proceeded by repeated mating with Bio 14.6 hamsters shown in Fig. 1. As a result, we obtained J-2-N cardiomyopathic white hamsters, which show a good reproduction rate and reproducible biochemical and pathophysiologic lesions such as the dilated cardiomyopathy (1). Through these matings, we also obtained a white hamster without cardiomyopathy as a control animal. Fig. 2 shows the J-2-N hamster from our laboratory; the right hamster has no cardiac lesions and thus is a normal control white hamster, whereas the left one is the J-2-N cardiomyopathic hamster. Both hamsters are 50 weeks old; the cardiomyopathic hamster has severe edema with ascites owing to cardiac failure. It was interesting to observe that at 5 weeks of age, the J-2-N hamster did not develop any cardiac damage; serum creatine phosphokinase, aldolase, and lactate dehydrogenase activities were at normal levels. This strain of hamsters included animals in which the cardiac lesion develops rather rapidly and those in which it is delayed. Nonetheless, it is possible to differentiate the hamsters that do or do not develop cardiac damage with the use of electrocardiogram (ECG) records (1).

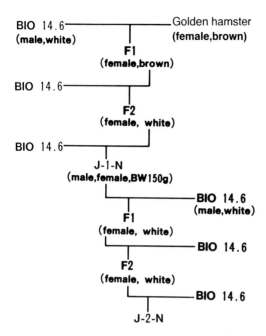

FIG. 1. Cross-breeding of a male Bio 14.6 and a female golden hamster to obtain a J-2-N hamster.

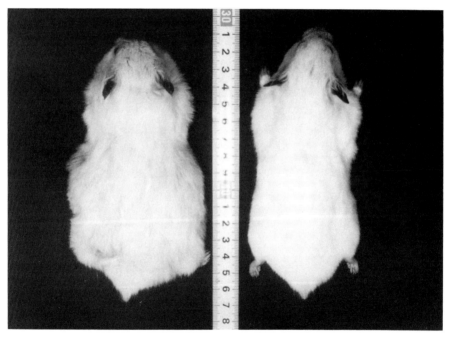

FIG. 2. J-2-N cardiomyopathic hamster and control normal hamster. **Right**, a normal white hamster without cardiac damage. **Left**, a J-2-N cardiomyopathic hamster with severe edema and ascites because of heart failure and congestive liver damage.

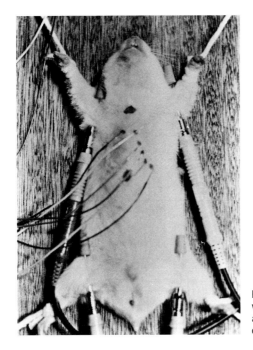

FIG. 3. Recording method of ECG, which was recorded under sodium pentobarbital anesthesia using the standard limb and chest leads.

For the ECG examination, the animal was held in place on a plate under sodium pentobarbital (Nembutal) anaesthesia and the ECG was recorded by the standard limb and chest leads, as in Fig 3. The ECG of a J-2-N hamster in Fig. 4 shows left axis deviation, abnormal Q in V_1 to V_4 heads (QS pattern), and low voltage. In comparison to this cardiomyopathic hamster, normal control white hamsters have an ECG without left axis deviation, pathologic Q, and ST-T depression. The grade of cardiac damages on the ECG was analyzed by point-of-damage score. For example, a one point score corresponds to left axis deviation, pathologic Q, ST depression, negative T, pulmonary P, low voltage, and arrhythmia. Animals with a score of 5 or more had clearly developed cardiomyopathy. This scoring system corresponds to histopathologic findings in these hearts.

Animals with scores higher than 5 showed degeneration of the myocardium and fibrosis of the interstitium, as shown in Fig. 5. The main feature of the J-2-N model is the lack of severe focal myocardial necrosis such as can be seen in Bio 14.6 and Bio 53.58 cardiomyopathic Syrian hamsters (2).

J-2-N hamsters exhibit marked dilation of both the right and left ventricles (Fig. 6). This figure shows tracings of cross-sections of hearts removed from J-2-N hamsters with advanced dilated cardiomyopathy and from control hamsters. In the J-2-N hamsters with advanced damage, marked dilation of both atria and ventricles was observed. Right ventricular failure was more severe than left ventricular failure. Pulmonary congestion was mild, but sometimes cardiac cirrhosis and nutmeg liver were seen (1).

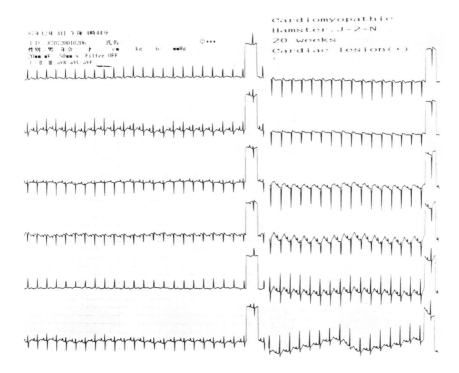

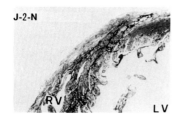

FIG. 5. Histologic findings in J-2-N cardiomyopathic hamster. Severe interstitial fibrosis is noted in the myocardium.

ECG normal J-2-N   ECG abnormal J-2-N

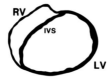

FIG. 6. Cross-sections of the heart of hamsters. **Right,** a cross-section tracing of the heart removed from a J-2-N cardiomyopathic hamster. **Left,** a tracing from a control normal hamster.

With the development of cardiac lesions in J-2-N hamsters, we observed the progressive electrocardiographic changes. When the ECG was recorded sequentially, from 4 to 5 weeks of age, left axis deviation became more severe and arrhythmias were sometimes seen. The initial r wave found in chest leads V_1 and V_2 disappeared, the height of the R wave in leads V_3 and V_4 dropped, and a QS pattern appeared. In contrast, except for left axis deviation, no such ECG changes were seen in normal control hamsters, as shown in Fig. 7.

In identifying changes in biochemical characteristics, a change of ventricular myosin isoenzyme patterns was observed (2,3). Figure 8 shows the comparison of the ventricular myosin isoenzyme pattern of cardiomyopathic J-2-N hamsters and control animals. The myosin isoenzyme pattern of the ventricles from J-2-N hamsters was remarkably shifted toward V_3 compared with the controls.

In addition, the course of the cardiac damage was evaluated by collecting blood from the vena jugularis and measuring the activities of serum creatine phosphokinase, aldolase, and lactate dehydrogenase. In conjunction with cardiac damage, these serum enzyme activities of J-2-N hamsters were increased significantly, as shown in Fig. 9 (3).

Adenosine diphosphate/adenosine triphosphate (ADP/ATP) carrier (AAC) pro-

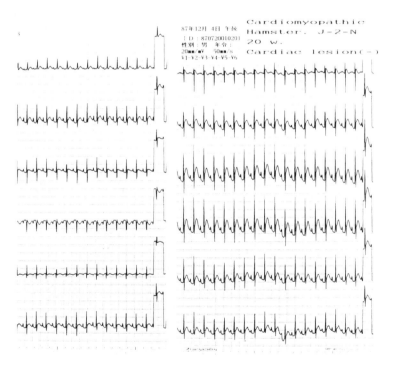

FIG. 7. ECG of control normal hamster (*left*) and J-2-N cardiomyopathic hamster (*right*).

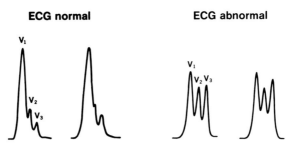

ECG normal   **ECG abnormal**

FIG. 8. The patterns of ventricular myosin isoenzyme. **Left,** a pattern of cardiac myosin iso-enzyme from a control normal hamster. **Right,** a pattern of cardiac myosin from a J-2-N cardio-myopathic hamster.

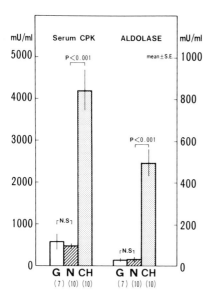

FIG. 9. Serum creatine phosphokinase (CPK) and aldolase activities of J-2-N hamsters showing significant increases. CH, J-2-N hamster; N, control normal hamster; G, golden hamster.

tein, located in the inner membrane of the mitochondria, facilitates the transport of ADP into the mitochondria to undergo phosphorylation and ATP in reverse to provide an energy supplement for the cytoplasm. Recently, in our laboratory, the AAC protein was analyzed in mitochondria of cardiomyopathic J-2-N hamster hearts. The level of AAC protein diminished in J-2-N hearts compared with normal cardiac mitochondria. The decrease in AAC protein content correlated inversely with changes in serum creatine phosphokinase levels or ECG score (4).

Finally, for investigating the functional status of the myocardium, mechanical parameters such as time to peak tension (TPT), active tension (AT) and $+dT/dt_{max}$ were examined in the isolated papillary muscles from J-2-N hamsters. The decrease in AT and increase in TPT are shown in Fig. 10. Preliminary results have been reported elsewhere (5).

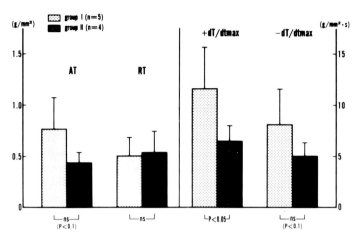

FIG. 10. Cardiac mechanics of J-2-N cardiomyopathic hamster and control normal hamster.

DISCUSSION

It is impossible to observe clinically the process of development of idiopathic cardiomyopathy from its inception. Therefore, etiologic investigations of this disease require the use of animal models. Several kinds of cardiomyopathic models exist, e.g., the cardiomyopathic Syrian hamsters and several varieties of mice, cats, and turkeys. The most widely used animal model are the Bio 14.6 hamsters. The changes noted in Bio 14.6 cardiomyopathic hamsters compared with F1-β control animals include significant weight loss from around 40 days of age. In hamsters with rapidly progressive cardiac symptoms, edema and ascites, together with early blackening of the eyeballs, appear by 60 to 90 days of age. The first early deaths caused by heart failure occur at this time. In comparison to the pathologic development in Bio 14.6, cardiac damage in J-2-N animals develops more slowly and is mild in nature. The main feature of the J-2-N model is the lack of focal myocardial necrosis such as is observed in Bio 14.6 and Bio 53.58 hamsters; the development of interstitial fibrosis is also comparatively slow. Therefore, the histopathologic changes and the elevation of serum enzyme levels are less marked than in Bio 14.6 and Bio 53.58 hamsters of the same age. J-2-N hamsters show marked dilation of both the right and left ventricles, and this animal model can be considered to most closely resemble human idiopathic dilated cardiomyopathy.

SUMMARY

Studies of idiopathic cardiomyopathy have generally used cardiomyopathic Syrian hamsters. We investigated idiopathic cardiomyopathy in the J-2-N hamster, bred in our laboratory 5 years ago. This colony has been raised to preserve the original genetic trait without cannibalism. Care has been taken to preserve the pathologic cardiac changes characteristic of this strain and its high reproduction rate. Cross-breeding between Bio 14.6 and golden hamsters was undertaken to obtain white hamsters with and without cardiomyopathy. These J-2-N hamsters were clearly differentiated from other strains by pathologic electrocardiographic findings; electrocardiographic and histopathologic changes of the heart were closely related. A marked rise in serum creatine phosphokinase, aldolase, lactate dehydrogenase, and malondialdehyde levels was established, and ventricular myosin isoenzymes were shifted toward V_3 in the cardiomyopathic heart. Isometric tension development in isolated left ventricular papillary muscles was examined; maximal developed tension showed a tendency to decrease and dT/dt_{max} was significantly depressed in the cardiomyopathic hamsters. Adenine nucleotide translocase located in the cardiac inner mitochondrial membrane diminished in J-2-N hamsters compared with hamsters without cardiomyopathy. This finding may be one of the factors involved in the pathogenesis of cardiomyopathy.

REFERENCES

1. Takeda M. Morphological and biochemical abnormalities in new cardiomyopathic Syrian hamster. *Jikeikai Med J* 1989;36:129–48.
2. Nagano M, Kato M, Nagai M, Yang J. Protective effect of ACE- and kininase inhibitor on the onset of cardiomyopathy. *Basic Res Cardiol* 1991;86[Suppl III]187–95.
3. Kato M, Takeda N, Yang J, Tanaka Y, Nagano M. The effects of ACE inhibitor and the role of the renin-angiotensin-aldosterone system in J-2-N cardiomyopathic hamster. *Jpn Circ J* 1992;56:77–85.
4. Yang J, Kato M, Takeda N, Nagano M. ADP/ATP carrier protein contents in J-2-N cardiomyopathic hamster. *J Mol Cell Cardiol* 1992;24[Suppl I]:6–16.
5. Tanamura A, Iwai T, Arino T, et al. Alterations of myocardial contractility in cardiomyopathic J-2-N hamsters. *J Mol Cell Cardiol* 1991;23[Suppl II]:100.

The Cardiomyopathic Heart, edited by Makoto
Nagano, Nobuakira Takeda, and Naranjan S.
Dhalla. Raven Press, Ltd., New York © 1994.

9

Status of β-Adrenergic Mechanisms during the Development of Congestive Heart Failure in Cardiomyopathic Hamsters (UM-X7.1)

Rajat Sethi, Vincenzo Panagia, Ken S. Dhalla, Robert E. Beamish,
*Gaetan Jasmin, and Naranjan S. Dhalla

*Division of Cardiovascular Sciences, St. Boniface General Hospital Research Centre,
Faculty of Medicine, University of Manitoba, Winnipeg R2H 2A6; and *Department of
Pathology, Faculty of Medicine, University of Montreal, Montreal H3C 3J7, Canada*

INTRODUCTION

It is now well known that the positive inotropic action of catecholamines is primarily mediated by their interaction with β-adrenergic receptors on the cardiac cell surface (1,2). The availability of selective agonists and antagonists and radioligand binding techniques have now permitted the classification of β-adrenergic receptors into two major subtypes: β_1- and β_2-adrenergic receptors (3–5). The ratio of β_1- to β_2-adrenergic receptors in the myocardium is about 4:1. The genes encoding the β_1- and β_2-adrenergic receptors have been cloned and characterized, and the probes derived from these genes have been used to examine the regulation of these receptor proteins (6–11). The sequences of β_1- and β_2-adrenergic receptors have a 71% and 54% amino acid identity in the transmembrane domain and in overall sequence, respectively (12). The β-adrenergic receptors are coupled with adenylyl cyclase through guanine nucleotide binding proteins (G proteins), and when activated by their agonists, these receptors initiate the production of cyclic adenosine monophosphate and thus regulate diverse metabolic and functional events (13). There is a family of G proteins in the membrane that serve as information transducers (14). In particular, immunodetectable levels of G_s and G_i proteins are considered responsible for stimulatory and inhibitory control of adenylyl cyclase, respectively (15). These heterotrimeric G proteins are made up of α-, β-, and γ-subunits; however, the α subunit (45 to 52 KD) of the G_s protein was found to be different from that (39 to 41 KD) of the G_i protein. Furthermore, adenosine diphosphate ribosylation of the α-subunit in the G_s protein is catalyzed by cholera toxin, whereas that in the G_i protein is catalyzed by pertussis toxin. Studies at the molecular level for both G_s and

G_i proteins have revealed that the genes for these proteins are not coregulated (16,17). Although the exact mode of coupling G protein with adenylyl cyclase is not clear, both genetic and biochemical evidence indicates that there are multiple forms of adenylyl cyclase with a molecular mass in the range of 120 to 150 KD (18–20). The catalytic subunit of the adenylyl cyclase, which is involved in the formation of cyclic AMP from adenosine triphosphate, is activated by cations such as Mn^{2+}, whereas other agents such as NaF, forskolin, cholera toxin, and pertussis toxin are considered to activate the enzyme activity through their interaction with G proteins. Thus, in view of the critical role of β-adrenergic receptors, G proteins, and the adenylyl cyclase system in influencing cardiac contractility, any change in the components of this system under pathologic conditions can be seen to impair signal transduction mechanisms in the myocardium.

β-Adrenergic Mechanisms and Cardiac Dysfunction

Several investigators have reported a wide variety of alterations in different components of the β-adrenergic receptors, G proteins, and the adenylyl cyclase system in heart dysfunction by employing various experimental animal models. For example, an increase in β-adrenergic receptor density and an increase in cyclic AMP formation due to catecholamines were reported in myocardial ischemia caused by coronary occlusion in dogs (21,22). Although other investigators also observed an increase in the β-receptor density in the ischemic myocardium of dogs and calves, the activities of adenylyl cyclase in the absence or presence of different stimulants as well as the activity of G_s protein were depressed (23–26). On the other hand, no changes in the density of β-receptors and basal adenylyl cyclase activity were observed in ischemic or hypoxic dog hearts (27,28), although a depression in isoproterenol-stimulated adenylyl cyclase activity occurred. Guinea pig ischemic hearts (29,30) showed an increase and a decrease in the β-receptor densities in cell surface and cytoplasmic membranes, respectively, whereas opposite results were obtained upon exposing neonatal rat cardiomyocytes to hypoxia (31). Although β-receptor density did not decrease, adenylyl cyclase activities due to β-receptors and G_s protein were increased in doxorubicin (Adriamycin)-induced cardiomyopathy in rabbits (32). However, no alterations in β-adrenergic receptor density, G proteins, or adenylyl cyclase activities were seen in doxorubicin-induced cardiomyopathy in rats (33). Depressions in β-adrenergic receptors and adenylyl cyclase activities in the absence or presence of various stimulants were noted in catecholamine-induced cardiomyopathy in rats (34). Rats with monocrotaline-induced right-sided heart cardiomyopathy showed depressions in $β_1$-receptor density and adenylyl cyclase activities in the presence of isoproterenol and Gpp(NH)p but no changes in the absence or presence of sodium fluoride (NaF) and forskolin or $β_2$-receptor density (35). A detailed analysis of these results reveals that changes in β-adrenergic receptors, G proteins, and adenylyl cyclase depend upon the type and stage of heart disease as well as the type of membrane preparations from failing hearts employed for investigations.

Mechanisms of the Attenuated Responses to Catecholamines

Since the positive inotropic responses to catecholamines are invariably depressed in heart failure, some efforts have been made to understand the mechanisms of attenuated responses of failing hearts to catecholamines. A decrease in the density of β-adrenergic receptors was observed in congestive heart failure in dogs with pulmonary artery constriction and tricuspid avulsion and in rats with myocardial infarction (36–38). On the other hand, congestive heart failure in guinea pigs caused by pressure overload was associated with an increase in β-adrenergic receptor density without any changes in their affinity (39). Although increased density of β-receptors was also seen in congestive heart failure in dogs, this change was associated with a loss of high affinity for these receptors as well as uncoupling of β-receptors from G proteins (40–42). Attenuated responses to isoproterenol by hearts failing owing to myocardial infarction were observed in spite of an increase in the β-receptor density in rats (43,44). In contrast to these observations, no evidence of an increase in β-receptor density or isoproterenol-stimulated adenylyl cyclase activity was seen in heart failure caused by myocardial infarction in rats (45) or dogs (46). Heart dysfunction in rats with nonocclusive coronary artery constriction without any myocardial infarction was associated with depressions in β-receptor density, G_s protein, and isoproterenol-stimulated adenylyl cyclase activity (47). Congestive heart failure due to rapid pacing in dogs was found to decrease β-receptor density, G_s protein, and adenylyl cyclase activity (48–50). Abnormalities in β-adrenergic receptors, G proteins, and adenylyl cyclase in failing human hearts seem to depend upon the cause of heart failure, including idiopathic dilated cardiomyopathy, ischemic dilated cardiomyopathy, and primary pulmonary hypertension (51–60). Experiments employing molecular biologic techniques have shown a decrease in the levels of mRNA specific for β_1-receptors (60) and an increase in the levels of mRNA for G_i protein without any changes in mRNA for G_s protein in failing human hearts (61,62). Information concerning changes in mRNA specific for adenylyl cyclase in failing hearts is still lacking.

From the foregoing information as well as in view of the existing literature on adrenergic mechanisms in heart failure reviewed elsewhere (63–67), it is evident that various components of the β-adrenergic receptors, G proteins, and adenylyl cyclase system are unchanged, up-regulated, or down-regulated in failing myocardium. Such a discrepancy in results seems to be related to the type and stage of the heart disease. However, none of the previous studies have attempted to examine the sequence of changes in these components of the adrenergic mechanisms at different stages of heart failure in any experimental model. Although most of the work in this field has been carried out on myocardial tissues from patients with heart disease, it should be recognized that all these patients were on various cardiac drugs and thus the results are difficult to interpret in terms of pathophysiologic changes in heart failure. Furthermore, information regarding the molecular mechanisms for changes in different components of the adrenergic events is just beginning to appear in the literature, and a great deal of work remains to be done before meaningful conclusions are reached. It is therefore necessary to comprehensively examine the status of events in adrenergic receptors and related molecular mechanisms at various stages of congestive heart failure in different experimental models.

Adrenergic Mechanisms in the Cardiomyopathic Hamster Heart

Extensive efforts have been made to identify abnormalities in the adrenergic system of a genetically linked hamster model of cardiomyopathy. Various investigators (68–83) have reported varying degrees of changes in adenylyl cyclase, adrenergic responses, adrenergic receptors, and G proteins in the hearts from different strains of cardiomyopathic hamsters (Table 1). Since the identification of the Bio 14.6 strain of Syrian hamsters with cardiomyopathy, several other strains of cardiomyopathic hamsters, including Bio 82.62, Bio 53.58, Bio 40.54, UM-X7.1, CHF 147, and TO have been developed (68–85). These animals have been reported to exhibit focal necrosis at the age of 30 to 40 days, which becomes maximal at 60 to 90 days. Substantial necrosis is associated with varying degrees of cardiac hypertrophy at 75 to 120 days of age, which leads to the development of different stages of congestive heart failure. Recently, another strain of cardiomyopathic (J-2-N) hamsters has been developed in which the occurrence of congestive heart failure is relatively slow (86). Thus it appears that the apparently conflicting results shown in Table 1 are attributable to differences not only in the genetic strain of cardiomyopathic hamsters but also in the extent of necrosis, hypertrophy, and congestive heart failure.

TABLE 1. *Status of adrenergic mechanisms in the cardiomyopathic hamster heart*[a]

Parameter	Increase	Decrease	No change
Adenylyl cyclase			
Basal		70	68–70,73
NaF-stimulated		68,69,71,73,74	68,69,71
Gpp(NH)p-stimulated		73	74
Forskolin-stimulated		74,78,81,83	
Catecholamine-stimulated		68,69,71,73,74,78	68,71
Adrenergic response			
β-receptor function	72	79	72,79
α-receptor function	76,77,79,80		
Adrenergic receptors			
β-receptor density	72,77,82,83	77	79
α-receptor density	72,77		76
G proteins			
G_s bioactivity		74,83	81
G_s content			74
G_s mRNA		75	74
G_i bioactivity	76,81		
G_i mRNA		75	

[a]These observations are based on the results reported in the literature by employing different strains of cardiomyopathic hamsters at various stages of cardiomyopathy. Each number in this table refers to the reference number in the text.

In order to show that changes in β-adrenergic mechanisms are dependent on the degree of congestive heart failure, we employed the UM-X7.1 strain of cardiomyopathic hamsters (70,71,73,87–91). On the basis of clinical signs, these hamsters at the age of 90 to 100 days are considered to be at the prefailure stage, whereas cardiomyopathic hamsters at 120 to 160 days, 160 to 200 days, and 200 to 280 days are grouped as at early, moderate, and severe stages of congestive heart failure, respectively. Age-matched healthy hamsters were used as controls for each group. Ventricular tissue from six to ten hamsters was pooled, and the heavy sarcolemmal fraction was isolated according to the method of Dhalla et al. (92). The adenylyl cyclase activity in the absence (basal) or presence of 2 mM NaF, 50 μM forskolin, 25 μM Gpp(NH)p, or 25 μM epinephrine was determined according to the method of Salomon (93). The determinations of K_d (dissociation constant) and B_{max} (maximal density) for both β-adrenergic receptors and α-adrenergic receptors in the sarcolemmal membrane were carried out according to the methods described elsewhere (37) by employing ^{3}H-dihydroalprenolol and ^{3}H-prazosin as radioligands, respectively. In a separate set of experiments, ventricular norepinephrine content and norepinephrine turnover rate in both control and cardiomyopathic hamsters were determined according to the procedures employed by Sole et al. (94). The data were analyzed statistically, and a p value of less than 0.05 was taken to suggest a significant difference between control and experimental preparations.

The data in Table 2 reveal no changes in the basal adenylyl cyclase activities in the sarcolemma of the cardiomyopathic hamster heart. This indicates that the catalytic site of the adenylyl cyclase is not altered in congestive heart failure in cardiomyopathic hamsters. However, when adenylyl cyclase determinations were made in the presence of 2 mM NaF, a significant depression in enzyme activity was evident at the moderate and severe stages of congestive heart failure. Likewise, the adenylyl cyclase activities in the presence of 50 μM forskolin and 25 μM Gpp(NH)p, a nonhydrolyzable analogue of guanosine triphosphate, were depressed in the cardio-

TABLE 2. *Sarcolemmal adenylyl cyclase activity in the absence or presence of NaF in cardiomyopathic hamsters (UM-X7.1) at various stages of congestive heart failure*[a]

	Adenylyl cyclase activity (pmol cyclic AMP/10 min/mg)			
	Basal		+ 2 mM NaF	
	Control	Failing	Control	Failing
Prefailure	200 ± 7.6	206 ± 5.9	421 ± 17.9	415 ± 21.4
Early failure	224 ± 15.4	221 ± 11.9	415 ± 15.4	368 ± 19.2
Moderate failure	218 ± 16.2	228 ± 15.1	429 ± 20.5	307 ± 14.3*
Severe failure	220 ± 17.1	222 ± 15.9	431 ± 18.6	271 ± 19.1*

[a]Heavy sarcolemmal preparations were employed. Each value is a mean ± standard error of six preparations. The cardiomyopathic hamsters at 90 and 100 days (prefailure), 120 to 160 days (early failure), 160 to 200 days (moderate failure), and 200 to 280 days (severe failure) of age were employed. Age-matched control hamsters were used for each group.
*$p < 0.05$.

myopathic hearts at moderate and severe stages but not at prefailure and early failure stages (Fig. 1). Since NaF, forskolin, and Gpp(NH)p are known to modify adenylyl cyclase activity through their interaction with G proteins, these results indicate some impairment or alteration of G_i or G_s protein bioactivity in cardiomyopathic hearts at moderate and severe stages of congestive heart failure.

Sarcolemmal adenylyl cyclase activity was also studied upon incubating the membrane with 25 μM epinephrine in the absence or presence of 10 μM Gpp(NH)p, and the results are shown in Fig. 2. The stimulatory effect of epinephrine was significantly decreased at moderate and severe stages but not at prefailure and early failure stages of congestive heart failure. On the other hand, β-receptor density in the membrane preparation was increased at prefailure and early failure stages, unchanged at moderate stages of failure, and depressed at severe stages of heart failure (Table 3). This pattern of changes in the density of β-adrenergic receptors was

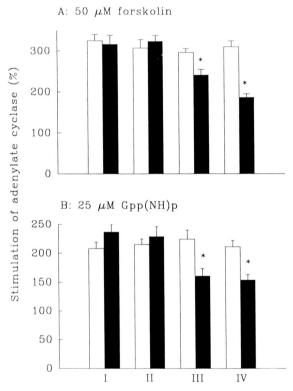

FIG. 1. Activation of sarcolemmal adenylyl cyclase by forskolin **(A)** and Gpp(NH)p **(B)** in UM-X7.1 strain of cardiomyopathic hamsters at stages of prefailure (I), early failure (II), moderate failure (III), and severe failure (IV). □, control hamsters (age-matched); ■, cardiomyopathic hamsters. Both control and cardiomyopathic hamsters at different stages of failure were within the same age range as described in Table 2. Each value is a mean ± standard error of six experiments. *$p < 0.05$.

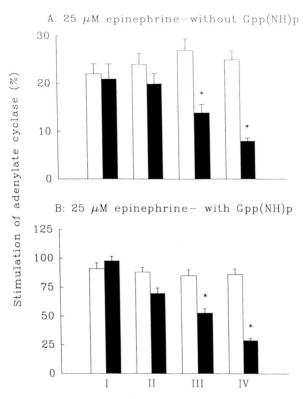

FIG. 2. Activation of sarcolemmal adenylyl cyclase by epinephrine in the absence **(A)** and presence **(B)** of 10 μM Gpp(NH)p in UM-X7.1 strain of cardiomyopathic hamsters at stages of prefailure (I), early failure (II), moderate failure (III), and severe failure (IV). □, control hamsters (agematched); ■, cardiomyopathic hamsters. Both control and cardiomyopathic hamsters at different stages of failure were within the same age range as described in Table 2. Each value is a mean ± standard error of six experiments. *$p < 0.05$.

TABLE 3. *Beta-adrenergic receptors in sarcolemma from cardiomyopathic hamsters
(UM-X7.1) at various stages of congestive heart failure*[a]

	^{3}H-Dihydroalprenolol binding			
	K_d (nM)		B_{max} (fmol/mg)	
	Control	Failing	Control	Failing
Prefailure	0.74 ± 0.05	0.73 ± 0.04	81 ± 3.2	115 ± 2.9*
Early failure	0.73 ± 0.06	0.78 ± 0.03	83 ± 4.1	104 ± 1.8*
Moderate failure	0.78 ± 0.06	0.81 ± 0.05	86 ± 3.9	82 ± 2.4
Severe failure	0.71 ± 0.07	0.76 ± 0.04	83 ± 4.0	53 ± 3.1*

[a]Heavy sarcolemmal preparations were employed. Each value is a mean ± standard error of four experiments. Both control and cardiomyopathic hamsters at different stages of failure were within the same age range as described in Table 2.
*$p < 0.05$.

specific in nature, since the density of α-adrenergic receptors was increased at pre-failure, early, moderate, and severe stages of congestive heart failure in the cardio-myopathic hamsters (Table 4). The data in Tables 3 and 4 also show no changes in the dissociation constant values of either β- or α-adrenergic receptors. Since the activation of sarcolemmal adenylyl cyclase by catecholamines is manifested through the participation of β-adrenergic receptors, the data in Fig. 2 and Table 3 indicate uncoupling of these two components. In this regard, it is noted that no change in epinephrine-stimulated adenylyl cyclase was evident at prefailure and early failure stages, although the β-adrenergic receptor density in the sarcolemmal membrane was increased. Although a decreased number of β-receptors may explain the depressed stimulation of adenylyl cyclase by epinephrine at severe stages of heart failure, no change in the density of beta-adrenergic receptors was seen when the epinephrine-stimulated adenylyl cyclase was depressed at moderate stages of congestive heart failure. Thus it appears that uncoupling of β-adrenergic receptors from adenylyl cyclase may represent a major biochemical abnormality in cardio-myopathic hearts. Alternatively, these complex changes may be attributable to varying degrees of alterations in the amounts as well as bioactivities of G_i and G_s proteins in cardiomyopathic hamster hearts.

It is generally considered that the status of β-adrenergic mechanisms in the heart is regulated by the activity of the sympathetic nervous system and the resulting levels of circulating norepinephrine. Since an increase in the activity of the sympa-thetic nervous system is considered to increase norepinephrine turnover and de-crease norepinephrine content in the heart, we determined these parameters in car-diomyopathic hamsters at different stages of congestive heart failure. The data in Table 5 indicate an increase in norepinephrine content in the myocardium at the stages of prefailure and early failure; a significant depression in this parameter was observed only at moderate and severe stages of congestive heart failure. The nor-epinephrine turnover rate in the heart was significantly increased at prefailure, early failure, and moderate failure stages but was unaltered at severe failure stages of

TABLE 4. α-Adrenergic receptors in sarcolemma from cardiomyopathic hamsters (UM-X7.1) at various stages of congestive heart failure[a]

	^{3}H-Prazosin binding			
	K_d (nM)		B_{max} (fmol/mg)	
	Control	Failing	Control	Failing
Prefailure	0.24 ± 0.03	0.25 ± 0.02	45 ± 3.8	$56 \pm 2.9^*$
Early failure	0.28 ± 0.02	0.28 ± 0.03	43 ± 2.9	$57 \pm 4.1^*$
Moderate failure	0.31 ± 0.02	0.30 ± 0.02	45 ± 2.1	$61 \pm 3.8^*$
Severe failure	0.30 ± 0.02	0.33 ± 0.03	48 ± 2.7	$64 \pm 3.6^*$

[a]Heavy sarcolemmal preparations were employed. Each value is a mean $\pm$ standard error of four experiments. Both control and cardiomyopathic hamsters at different stages of failure were within the same age range as described in Table 2.
$^*p < 0.05$.

TABLE 5. *Cardiac norepinephrine content and norepinephrine turnover rate in UM-X7.1 strain of cardiomyopathic hamsters*

	Cardiac norepinephrine (ng/g heart)		Norepinephrine turnover rate (ng/g heart/hr)	
	Control	Cardiomyopathic	Control	Cardiomyopathic
Prefailure	987 ± 31	1256 ± 47*	81 ± 4.3	152 ± 7.2*
Early failure	958 ± 45	1127 ± 36*	75 ± 3.9	137 ± 6.8*
Moderate failure	967 ± 52	702 ± 29*	80 ± 5.1	116 ± 5.4*
Severe failure	936 ± 43	413 ± 25*	87 ± 4.8	98 ± 5.9*

Each value is a mean ± SE of five experiments. Both control and cardiomyopathic hamsters at different stages of failure were within the same age range as described in Table 2.
 *$p < 0.05$.

congestive heart failure. Although these data do not show any direct relationship among changes in myocardial norepinephrine content, norepinephrine turnover rate, and adrenergic receptors, it is evident that the sympathetic activity is markedly increased at prefailure, early, and moderate stages but is decreased at severe stages of congestive heart failure in this model. It is possible that initial changes in sarcolemmal β-adrenergic receptors, G proteins, and adenylyl cyclase may be a consequence of increased sympathetic activity, whereas late changes in cardiomyopathic hearts and sympathetic activity may reflect a state of exhaustion in these animals. This view is consistent with our earlier findings that cyclic AMP content in the myocardium is increased at prefailure stages but is decreased at moderate stages of heart failure (70). Nonetheless, the data in cardiomyopathic hamsters reported in this study clearly indicate that changes in adrenergic mechanisms are complex in nature and are dependent upon the stage of congestive heart failure.

SUMMARY

The status of β-adrenergic mechanisms in the myocardium was assessed by employing cardiomyopathic hamsters (UM-X7.1 strain) 90 to 100 days old (prefailure), 120 to 160 days old (early failure), 160 to 200 days old (moderate failure), and 200 to 280 days old (severe failure). Although the basal adenylyl cyclase activity was not altered in the sarcolemma, the stimulation of enzyme activity by sodium fluoride (NaF), forskolin, Gpp(NH)p, and epinephrine was depressed in hearts from cardiomyopathic animals at moderate and severe stages of congestive heart failure. No change in basal stimulated adenylyl cyclase was observed in animals at prefailure and early failure stages. The number of β-adrenergic receptors was increased at prefailure and early failure, unchanged at moderate failure, and decreased at severe stages of congestive heart failure. On the other hand, the number of α-adrenergic receptors was increased at all stages of heart failure. The norepinephrine turnover rate was increased in all cardiomyopathic hearts except in those at severe stages of failure, whereas alterations in norepinephrine content in the heart was biphasic. These results indicate that alterations in β-adrenergic receptor mechanisms are dependent upon the stage of congestive heart failure and may be a consequence of increased sympathetic activity in cardiomyopathic hamsters. Furthermore, it is suggested that the complex alterations in β-adrenergic mechanisms in cardiomyopathic hearts are associated not only with changes in G proteins but an uncoupling of β-adrenergic receptors from adenylyl cyclase also occurs.

ACKNOWLEDGMENT

The work reported in this article was supported by a grant from the Heart and Stroke Foundation of Manitoba. Rajat Sethi was a predoctoral fellow supported by the Heart and Stroke Foundation of Canada.

REFERENCES

1. Dhalla NS, Ziegelhoffer A, Harrow JAC. Regulatory role of membrane systems in heart function. *Can J Physiol Pharmacol* 1977;55:1211–34.
2. Stiles GL, Caron MG, Lefkowitz RJ. Beta adrenergic receptors: biochemical mechanisms of physiological regulation. *Physiol Rev* 1984;64:661–743.
3. Lemonie H, Schonell H, Kaumann AJ. Contribution of β1- and β2-adrenoceptors of human atrium and ventricles to the effects of noradrenaline and adrenaline assessed with (-)-atenolol. *Br J Pharmacol* 1988;95:55–6.
4. Brodde OE, Zerkowski HR, Doetsch N, Motomura S, Khamssi M, Michel MC. Myocardial beta-adrenoceptor changes in heart failure: concomitant reduction in beta$_1$- and beta$_2$-adrenoceptor function related to the degree of heart failure in patients with mitral valve disease. *J Am Coll Cardiol* 1989;14:323–31.
5. Bunton BF, Jones CR, Molenaar P, Summers RJ. Characterization and autoradiographic localization of β-adrenoceptors subtype in human cardiac tissue. *Br J Pharmacol* 1987;92:299–310.
6. Collins S, Caron MG, Lefkowitz RJ. Regulation of adrenergic receptor responsiveness through modulation of receptor gene expression. *Ann Rev Physiol* 1991;53:497–508.
7. Kobilke BK, Dixon RA, Frielle T, et al. cDNA for the human beta2-adrenergic receptor: a protein with multiple membrane-spanning domains and encoded by a gene whose chromosomal location is shared with that of the receptor for platelet-derived growth factor. *Proc Natl Acad Sci USA* 1987;84:46–50.
8. Emorine LJ, Marullo S, Delavier Klutchko C, Kaveri SV, Durieu Trautmann O, Strosberg AD. Structure of the gene for human beta2-adrenergic receptor expression and promoter characterization. *Proc Natl Acad Sci USA* 1987;84:6995–9.
9. Saffitz, JE, Ligget SB. Subcellular distribution of β2-adrenergic receptors delineated with quantitative ultrastructural autoradiography of radioligand binding site. *Circ Res* 1992;70:1320–5.
10. Machida CA, Bunzon JR, Searles RP, et al. Molecular cloning and expression of the rat β1-adrenergic receptor gene. *J Biol Chem* 1990;265:12960–6.
11. Tate KM, Briend-Sutren MM, Emorine LJ, Delavier Klutchko C, Marullo S, Strosberg AD. Expression of three human β-adrenergic-receptor subtypes in transfected Chinese hamster ovary cells. *Eur J Biochem* 1991;196:357–61.
12. Frielle T, Collins S, Daniel KW, Caron MG, Lefkowitz RJ, Kobilke BK. Cloning of the cDNA for the human fetal-adrenergic receptor. *Proc Natl Acad Sci USA* 1987;84:7920–4.
13. Homcy CJ, Vatner SF, Vatner DE. Beta adrenergic receptor regulation in the heart in pathophysiologic states: abnormal adrenergic responsiveness in cardiac disease. *Annu Rev Physiol* 1991;53:137–59.
14. Simon MI, Strathmann MP, Gautam N. Diversity of G proteins in signal transduction. *Science* 1991;252:802–8.

15. Gilman AG. G proteins and dual control of adenylate cyclase. *Cell* 1984;36:577–9.
16. Itoh H, Toyama R, Kozasa T, Tsukamoto T, Matsuoke M, Kaziro Y. Presence of three distinct molecules species of Gi protein alpha subunit. Structure of rat cDNAs and human genomic DNAs. *J Biol Chem* 1988;263:6656–64.
17. Kozasa T, Itoh H, Tsukamoto T, Kaziro Y. Isolation and characterization of the human Gs alpha gene. *Proc Natl Acad Sci USA* 1988;2081–5.
18. Pfeuffer E, Mollner S, Pfeuffer T. Adenylate cyclase from bovine brain cortex: purification and characterization of the catalytic unit. *EMBO J* 1985;30:3675–9.
19. Livingstone MS, Sziber PP, Quinn WG. Loss of calcium/calmodulin responsiveness in adenylate cyclase of rutabaga, a drosophile learning mutant. *Cell* 1984;37:205–15.
20. Mollner S, Pfeuffer T. Two different adenylyl cyclases in brain distinguished by monoclonal antibodies. *Eur J Biochem* 1988;171:265–71.
21. Mukherjee A, Wong TM, Buja LM, Lefkowitz RJ, Willerson JT. Beta adrenergic and muscarinic cholinergic receptors in canine myocardium. Effects of ischemia. *J Clin Invest* 1979;64:1423–8.
22. Mukherjee A, Bush LR, McCoy KE, et al. Relationship between β-adrenergic receptor number and physiological responses during experimental canine myocardial ischemia. *Circ Res* 1982;50:735–41.
23. Vatner DE, Knight DR, Shen YT, Thomas JX Jr, Homcy CJ, Vatner SF. One hour of myocardial ischemia in conscious dogs increases beta-adrenergic receptor but decreases adenylate cyclase activity. *J Mol Cell Cardiol* 1988;20:75–82.
24. Susanni EE, Manders WT, Knight DR, Vatner DE, Vatner SF, Homcy CJ. One hour of myocardial ischemia decreases the activity of the stimulatory guanine-nucleotide regulatory protein Gs. *Circ Res* 1989;65:1145–50.
25. DeVos C, Robberech P, Nokin P, et al. Uncoupling between beta-adrenoceptors and adenylate cyclase in dog ischemic myocardium. *N S Arch Pharmacol* 1985;33:71–5.
26. Vatner DE, Young MA, Knight DR, Vatner SF. Beta-receptors and adenylate cyclase: comparison of nonischemic, ischemic and postmortem tissue. *Am J Physiol* 1990;258:H140–4.
27. Karliner JS, Sterens M, Norman H, Hoffman JIE. Effects of acute ischemia in the dog on myocardial blood flow, beta receptors, and adenylate cyclase activity with and without chronic beta blockade. *J Clin Invest* 1989;83:474–81.
28. Friessmuth M, Schutz W, Weindlmayer Gottel M, Zimpfer M, Spiss CK. Effects of ischemia on the canine myocardial beta adrenoceptor linked adenylate cyclase system. *J Cardiovasc Pharmacol* 1987;10:568–74.
29. Maisel AS, Motulsky HJ, Insel PA. Externalization of β-adrenergic receptors promoted by myocardial infarction. *Science* 1985;230:183–6.
30. Maisel AS, Motulsky HJ, Ziegler MG, Insel PA. Ischemia and agonist-induced changes in α and β adrenergic receptor traffic in guinea pig hearts. *Am J Physiol* 1987;253:H1159–66.
31. Rocha-singh KJ, Honbo MY, Karliner JS. Hypoxia and glucose independently regulate the β-adrenergic receptor adenylate cyclase system in cardiac myocytes. *J Clin Invest* 1991;88:204–13.
32. Calderone A, de Champlain J, Rouleau JL. Adriamycin induced changes to the myocardial beta-adrenergic system in the rabbit. *J Mol Cell Cardiol* 1991;23:333–42.
33. Fu LX, Bergh CH, Hoebeke J, et al. Effect of metoprolol on activity of beta-adrenoceptor coupled to guanine nucleotide binding regulatory proteins in Adriamycin-induced cardiotoxicity. *Basic Res Cardiol* 1991;86:117–26.
34. Corder DW, Heyliger CE, Beamish RE, Dhalla NS. Defect in the adrenergic receptor-adenylate cyclase systems during development of catecholamine-induced cardiomyopathy. *Am Heart J* 1984;107:537–42.
35. Pela G, Missali G, Raddino R, Condorelli E, Spano PF, Visioli O. β1 and β2 receptors are differentially desensitized in an experimental model of heart failure. *J Cardiovasc Pharmacol* 1990;16:839–46.
36. Fan TH, Liang CS, Kawashima S, Banerjee SP. Alterations in cardiac beta-adrenoceptor responsiveness and adenylate cyclase system by congestive heart failure in dogs. *Eur J Pharmacol* 1987;140:123–32.
37. Dixon IMC, Dhalla NS. Alterations in cardiac adrenoceptors in congestive heart failure secondary to myocardial infarction. *Coronary Artery Disease* 1991;2:805–14.
38. Dhalla NS, Dixon IMC, Suzuki S, Kaneko M, Kobayashi A, Beamish RE. Changes in adrenergic receptors during the development of heart failure. *Mol Cell Biochem* 1992;114:91–5.
39. Karliner JS, Barnes P, Brown M, Dollery C. Chronic heart failure in the guinea-pig increases cardiac α1- and β-adrenergic adrenoceptors. *Eur J Pharmacol* 1980;67:115–18.

40. Vatner DE, Homcy CJ, Sit SP, Manders WT, Vatner SF. Effects of pressure overload, left ventricular hypertrophy on adrenergic receptors and responsiveness to catecholamines. *J Clin Invest* 1984; 73:1473–82.
41. Vatner DE, Vatner SF, Fuji AM, Homcy CJ. Loss of high affinity cardiac beta adrenergic receptors in dogs with heart failure. *J Clin Invest* 1985;76:2259–64.
42. Longabaugh J, Vatner DE, Vatner SF, Homcy CJ. Decreased stimulatory guanosine triphosphate binding protein in dogs with pressure overload left ventricular failure. *J Clin Invest* 1988;81:420–4.
43. Clozel JP, Holck M, Osterrieder W, Burkard W, Da Prada MD. Effects of chronic myocardial infarction on responsiveness to isoprenaline and the state of myocardial beta adrenoceptors in rats. *Cardiovasc Res* 1987;21:688–95.
44. Mill JG, Stefanon I, Leite CM, Vassallo DV. Changes in performance of the surviving myocardium after left ventricular infarction in rats. *Cardiovasc Res* 1990;24:748–53.
45. Chasteney EA, Liang CS, Hood WB, Jr. Beta-adrenoceptor and adenylate cyclase function in the infarct model of rat heart failure. *Proc Soc Exp Biol Med* 1992;200:90–4.
46. Karliner JS, Stevens M, Grattan M, Woloszym W, Honbo N, Hoffman JIE. Beta adrenergic receptor properties of canine myocardium: effects of chronic myocardial infarction. *J Am Coll Cardiol* 1986;8:349–56.
47. Meggs LG, Haung H, Li P, Capasso JM, Anversa P. Chronic non occlusive coronary artery constriction in rats. β adrenoceptor signal transduction and ventricular failure. *J Clin Invest* 1991; 88:1940–6.
48. Calderone A, Bouvier M, Li K, Juneau C, de Champlain J, Rouleau JL. Dysfunction of the β and α adrenergic system in a model of congestive heart failure. The pacing overdrive dog. *Circ Res* 1991; 69:332–43.
49. Juneau C, Calderone A, Rouleau JL. Myocardial β-adrenergic and mechanical properties in pacing-induced heart failure in dogs. *Am J Physiol* 1992;262:H1458–67.
50. Marzo KP, Frey MJ, Wilson JR, et al. β-adrenergic receptor G-protein adenylate cyclase complex in experimental canine congestive heart failure produced by rapid ventricular pacing. *Circ Res* 1991; 69:1546–56.
51. Bristow MR, Ginsburg R, Minobe W, et al. Decreased catecholamine sensitivity and beta-adrenergic receptor density in failing human hearts. *N Engl J Med* 1982;307:205–11.
52. Bristow MR, Ginsburg R, Umans V, et al. β1 and β2 adrenergic receptor subpopulation in nonfailing human ventricular myocardium: coupling of both receptor subtypes to muscle contraction and selective β1-receptor down regulation in heart failure. *Circ Res* 1986;59:297–309.
53. Fowler MB, Laser JA, Hopkins GL, Minobe W, Bristow MR. Assessment of the β-adrenergic receptor pathway in the intact failing human heart: progressive receptor down-regulation and subsensitivity to agonist response. *Circulation* 1986;74:1280–1302.
54. Feldman AM, Cates AE, Veazey WB, et al. Increase of the 40,000 mol wt. PT substrate (G protein) in the failing human heart. *J Clin Invest* 1988;82:189–97.
55. Bristow MR, Anderson FL, Port D, et al. Differences in β-adrenergic neuro effector mechanism in ischemic versus idiopathic dilated cardiomyopathy. *Circulation* 1991;84:1024–39.
56. Anderson FL, Port JD, Reid BB, Larrabee P, Hanson G, Bristow MR. Myocardial catecholamine and neuropeptide Y depletion in failing ventricles of patients with idiopathic dilated cardiomyopathy: correlation with β-adrenergic receptor down regulation. *Circulation* 1992;85:46–53.
57. Bristow MR, Minobe W, Rasmussen R, et al. β-adrenergic neuro effector abnormalities in the failing human heart are produced by local rather than systemic mechanism. *J Clin Invest* 1992;89: 803–15.
58. Steinfath M, Daneilsen W, Von-der Leyen H, et al. Reduced alpha1- and beta2-adrenoceptor-mediated positive inotropic effects in human end stage heart failure. *Br J Pharmacol* 1992;105:463–9.
59. Bohm M, Gierschik P, Erdmann E. Quantification of Gi-proteins in the failing and nonfailing human myocardium. *Basic Res Cardiol* 1992;87 [Suppl I]:37–50.
60. Bristow MR, Feldman AM. Changes in the receptor-G protein adenylyl cyclase system in heart failure from various types of heart muscle disease. *Basic Res Cardiol* 1992;87 [Suppl I]:15–35.
61. Eschenhagen T, Mende U, Nose M, et al. Increased mRNA level of the inhibitory G protein, alpha subunit Gi 2 in human end-stage heart failure. *Circ Res* 1992;70:688–96.
62. Eschenhagen T, Mende U, Nose M, et al. Regulation and possible functional implications of G-protein mRNA expression in non failing and failing ventricular myocardium. *Basic Res Cardiol* 1992;87[Suppl I]:51–64.

63. Dhalla NS, Das PK, Sharma GP. Subcellular basis of cardiac contractile failure. *J Mol Cell Cardiol* 1978;10:363–85.
64. Dhalla NS, Pierce GN, Panagia V, Singal PK, Beamish RE. Calcium movements in relation to heart function. *Basic Res Cardiol* 1982;77:117–39.
65. Newman WH. Biochemical, structural and mechanical defects of the failing myocardium. *Pharmacol Ther* 1983;22:215–47.
66. Carafoli E, Bing RJ. Myocardial failure. *J Appl Cardiol* 1988;3:3–18.
67. Dhalla NS, Dixon IMC, Beamish RE. Biochemical basis of heart function and contractile failure. *J Appl Cardiol* 1991;6:7–30.
68. Sulakhe PV, Dhalla NS. Adenylyl cyclase activity in failing hearts of genetically myopathic hamsters. *Biochem Med* 1972;6:471–82.
69. Dhalla NS, Sulakhe PV. Adenylate cyclase activities of the sarcotubular membranes of the genetically myopathic hamsters. *Biochem Med* 1974;9:368–72.
70. Harrow JAC, Singh JN, Jasmin G, Dhalla NS. Studies on adenylate cyclase-cyclic AMP system of the myopathic hamsters' (UM-X7.1) skeletal and cardiac muscles. *Can J Biochem* 1975;53:1122–7.
71. Dhalla NS, Singh JN, Bajusz E, Jasmin G. Comparison of heart sarcolemmal enzyme activities in normal and cardiomyopathic (UM-X7.1) hamsters. *Clin Sci Mol Med* 1976;51:233–42.
72. Karliner JS, Alabaster C, Stephens H, Barnes P, Dollery C. Enhanced noradrenaline response in cardiomyopathic hamsters: possible relation to changes in adrenoceptors studied by radioligand binding. *Cardiovasc Res* 1981;15:296–304.
73. Panagia V, Singh JN, Anand-Srivastava MB, Pierce GN, Jasmin G, Dhalla NS. Sarcolemmal alterations during the development of genetically determined cardiomyopathy. *Cardiovasc Res* 1984;18:567–72.
74. Kessler PD, Cates AE, Van Dop C, Feldman AM. Decreased bioactivity of the guanine nucleotide-binding protein that stimulates adenylate cyclase in hearts from cardiomyopathic Syrian hamsters. *J Clin Invest* 1989;84:244–52.
75. Katoh Y, Konuro I, Takaku F, Yamaguchi H, Yazaki Y. Messenger RNA levels of guanine nucleotide-binding proteins are reduced in the ventricle of cardiomyopathic hamsters. *Circ Res* 1990;67:235–9.
76. Sen L, Liang BT, Colucci WS, Smith, TW. Enhanced α_1-adrenergic responsiveness in cardiomyopathic hamster cardiac myocytes. Relation to expression of pertussis toxin-sensitive G protein and α_1-adrenergic receptors. *Circ Res* 1990;67:1182–92.
77. Kagiya T, Hori M, Iwakura K, et al. Role of increased α_1-adrenergic activity in cardiomyopathic Syrian hamster. *Am J Physiol* 1991;260:H80–8.
78. Chidiac P, Nagy A, Sole MJ, Wells JW. Inefficient muscarinic transduction in cardiomyopathic Syrian hamsters. *J Mol Cell Cardiol* 1991;23:1255–69.
79. Horackova M, Beresewicz A, Rowden G, Wikinson M. Neurohumoral regulation of excitation-contraction coupling in ventricular myocytes from cardiomyopathic hamsters. *Cardiovasc Res* 1991;25:1023–34.
80. Kawaguchi H, Shoki M, Sano H, et al. Phospholipid metabolism in cardiomyopathic hamster heart cells. *Circ Res* 1991;69:1015–21.
81. Urasawa K, Sato K, Igarashi Y, Kawaguchi H, Yasuda H. A mechanism of catecholamine tolerance in congestive heart failure—alteration in the hormone sensitive adenylyl cyclase system of the heart. *Jpn Circ J* 1992;56:456–61.
82. Tawarahara K, Kurata C, Taguchi T, Kobayashi A, Yamazaki N. Augmentation of β-adrenergic receptors in cardiomyopathic hamsters (BIO 14.6) with heart failure. *Cardiovasc Res* 1992;26:526–33.
83. Ikegaya T, Kobayashi A, Houg RB, Masuda H, Kaneko M, Yamazaki N. Stimulatory guanine nucleotide-binding protein and adenylate cyclase activities in BIO 14.6 cardiomyopathic hamsters at the hypertrophic stage. *Mol Cell Biochem* 1992;110:83–90.
84. Bajusz E, Lossnitzer K. A new disease model of congestive heart failure. Studies on its pathogenesis. *Trans NY Acad Sci* 1968;30:939–48.
85. Bajusz E, Baker JR, Nixon CW, Homburger F. Spontaneous hereditary myocardial degeneration and congestive heart failure in a strain of Syrian hamsters. *Ann NY Acad Sci* 1969;156:105–29.
86. Nagano M, Kato M, Nagai M, Yang J. Protective effect of ACE- and kininase inhibitor on the onset of cardiomyopathy. *Basic Res Cardiol* 1991;86 [Suppl. III]:187–95.
87. Jasmin G, Proschek L. Hereditary polymyopathy and cardiomyopathy in the Syrian hamster. I. Progression of heart and skeletal muscle lesions in the UM-X7.1 line. *Muscle Nerve* 1982;5:20–5.

88. Proschek L, Jasmin G. Hereditary polymyopathy and cardiomyopathy in the Syrian hamster. II. Development of heart necrotic changes in relation to defective mitochondrial function. *Muscle Nerve* 1982;5:26–32.
89. Singh JN, Dhalla NS, McNamara DB, Bajusz E, Jasmin G. Membrane alterations in failing hearts of cardiomyopathic hamsters. *Recent Adv Card Struc Met* 1975;6:259–68.
90. Dhalla NS, Singh JN, Bajusz E, Jasmin G. Comparsion of heart sarcolemmal enzyme activities in normal and cardiomyopathic (UM-X7.1) hamsters. *Clin Sci Mol Med* 1976;51:233–42.
91. Panagia V, Lee SL, Singh A, Pierce GN, Jasmin G, Dhalla NS. Impairment of mitochondrial and sarcoplasmic reticular functions during the development of heart failure in cardiomyopathic (UM-X7.1) hamsters. *Can J Cardiol* 1986;2:236–47.
92. Dhalla NS, Anand-Srivastava MB, Tuana BS, Khandelwal RL. Solubilization of calcium-dependent adenosine triphosphatase from rat heart sarcolemma. *J Mol Cell Cardiol* 1981;13:413–23.
93. Salomon Y. Adenylate cyclase assay. *Adv Cyclic Nucleotide Res* 1979;10:35–55.
94. Sole MJ, Lo C-M, Laird CW, Sonnenblick EH, Wrutman RJ. Norepinephrine turnover in the heart and spleen of the cardiomyopathic Syrian hamster. *Circ Res* 1975;37:855–62.

The Cardiomyopathic Heart, edited by Makoto
Nagano, Nobuakira Takeda, and Naranjan S.
Dhalla. Raven Press, Ltd., New York © 1994.

10

β-Adrenoceptors and [12-^{3}H]-forskolin Binding Sites in the Hearts of Cardiomyopathic Bio 14.6 Syrian Hamsters

Kazuto Saito, *Atushi Kuroda, *Tetsuro Suetugu,
*Yoshiya Oku, and *Hiromitsu Tanaka

*Health Service Center, National Institute of Fitness and Sports;
and *First Department of Internal Medicine, Kagoshima University Medical School,
Kagoshima, Japan*

INTRODUCTION

Cardiomyopathic Bio 14.6 Syrian hamsters, an animal model of human idiopathic cardiomyopathy, show apparent histologic lesions, including necrosis, fibrosis, and calcification at about 30 days old, which progressively increase with
age. Death from congestive heart failure or arrhythmia generally occurs within 1
year after birth (1). Abnormalities in the β-adrenergic system of the heart may be
important in the pathogenesis of the disease and the occurrence of arrhythmias in
cardiomyopathic Syrian hamsters (2). However, alterations in the number of
β-adrenoceptors in the hearts of cardiomyopathic hamsters remain controversial (3–
5). Several reports have shown an increase in the number of β-adrenoceptors in
sarcolemma from the heart cells of cardiomyopathic Syrian hamsters with no significant differences in the affinity between control and cardiomyopathic hearts (3). On
the other hand, Kessler et al. (5) have described no significant changes in the adrenoceptors of both control and cardiomyopathic hamsters. This difference may be
attributable to variation in both the stages of cardiomyopathy and the methods used.
Since necrotic lesions, calcification, and fibrosis are not easily isolated by dissection, and it might be difficult to obtain the materials for accurate membrane ligand
studies, we used quantitative autoradiographic methods, which provide precise ana-
tomic localization, to measure the densities of β-adrenoceptors in cardiomyopathic
hamsters of various ages.

METHODS

Male cardiomyopathic (Bio 14.6 strain) and sex- and age-matched F1b control hamsters were obtained from Bio Breeder Institute (Boston, MA) and maintained in our laboratory. Experiments were carried out in accordance with the Guide for Animal Experimentation, Faculty of Medicine, Kagoshima University. We used five hamsters each of both Bio 14.6 and F1b types ages 4, 12, 26, 35, and 52 weeks. Their hearts were rapidly excised under general anesthesia with ethyl ether and immediately cut horizontally. They were frozen immediately by immersion in isopentane at $-30°C$ and were then stored at $-70°C$ for no longer than 7 days.

Frozen hearts were cut into 20-μm-thick sections transversely in a cryostat at $-20°C$. Alternate sections were thaw-mounted onto gelatin-coated slides and placed under a vacumn at 4°C for no longer than 24 hours prior to incubation. Sections were preincubated for 15 minutes at room temperature in 3 mM HEPES buffer, pH 7.4, containing 10 μM phenylmethylsulfonyl fluoride, 140 mM NaCl, 5 mM KCl, 1 mM $MgCl_2$, 1.5 mM $CaCl_2$, 11 mM glucose, and 0.001% ascorbate. To determine the number and the percentage of $β_1$- and $β_2$-adrenoceptors, we labeled tissue sections in vitro by incubation for 150 minutes at room temperature in fresh buffer containing 50 pM [^{125}I]-CYP (spec. act. 2050 Ci/mmol Amersham, Arlington Heights, IL) with or without 100 nM CGP20712A or 1 μM (-)-propranolol. The selectivity of CGP20712A was approximately 10,000 times greater for $β_1$- than for $β_2$-adrenoceptors, and the use of 100 nM CGP20712A is sufficient for estimating the percentage of $β_1$- and $β_2$-adrenoceptors in membrane preparations (6) and by autoradiography (7). Incubations were performed in parallel adjacent sections for total binding (incubated with 50 pM [^{125}I]-CYP), nonspecific binding (incubated as above with 1 μM (-)-propranolol) and nonspecific + $β_2$-adrenoceptor binding (estimated by incubation of 50 pM [^{125}I]-CYP with 100 nM CGP20712A).

Localization of adenylate cyclase was determined using [12-^{3}H]-forskolin (8). Tissue sectons were preincubated at room temperature for 10 minutes in 50 mM TRIS-HCl buffer, pH 7.7, containing 100 mM NaCl and 5 mM $MgCl_2$. Subsequently, these sections were incubated at room temperature for 10 minutes in fresh buffer containing 100 nM [12-^{3}H]-forskolin (40 Ci/mmol, New England Nuclear, Boston, MA). Nonspecific binding was determined by incubating adjacent sections under similar conditions in the presence of 100 μM unlabeled forskolin (Sigma Chemical, St. Louis, MO).

After incubation, sections were washed twice, for 2 minutes each time, at 4°C in the same buffer, rinsed for 30 seconds in ice-cold distilled water, and then immediately dried under a stream of cold air. The sections were placed in x-ray cassettes together with [^{125}I]-standards or [^{3}H]-standards and exposed to Ultrofilm (LKB Industries, Rockville, MD) for 2 days for [^{125}I]-CYP and 2 months for [12-^{3}H]-forskolin binding. After developing the film, optical densities were calculated by computerized microdensitometry. For calculations, sets of [^{125}I] and [^{3}H]-labeled standards were purchased from Amersham (Arlington Heights, IL), and the calculations were performed by interpolation on the standard curve (9,10). For histologic studies, the sections were stained using the method of van Gieson or the periodic acid–Schiff (PAS) method. All results are presented as mean ± standard error of the mean. Differences were evaluated by Student's t-test, and $p < 0.05$ was considered statistically significant.

RESULTS

The densities of $[^{125}I]$-CYP binding sites in the ventricle were inhomogeneous in the cardiomyopathic hamsters but uniform in F1b control hamsters (Fig. 1). Few $[^{125}I]$-CYP binding sites were observed in the areas that were stained strongly with PAS, but the number of these binding sites was very high in the areas immediately adjacent to the PAS-positive regions (Fig. 2). We measured the $[^{125}I]$-CYP binding sites (except PAS-positive areas) in the left ventricles of cardiomyopathic hamsters, and these binding capacities increased by about 30% to 50% in the hearts of cardiomyopathic hamsters at 12 and 26 weeks old compared with the control hamsters, without significant changes in the percentage of β_1- and β_2-subtypes (Fig. 3). In the fatal stage of the disease, these binding sites were reduced significantly in cardiomyopathic hearts, mainly owing to the decrease of β_1-subtype (Fig. 3).

$[12-^3H]$-Forskolin binding sites in the ventricle were uniform in F1b hamsters, but no binding sites were observed in the PAS-positive areas of cardiomyopathic hamsters (Fig. 4). The number of $[12-^3H]$-forskolin binding sites was not high in the area near the PAS-positive regions, which contained a large number of $[^{125}I]$-CYP binding sites (Fig. 4). The number of $[12-^3H]$-forskolin binding sites (except in PAS-positive areas) in the ventricles of the cardiomyopathic hamsters was significantly lower than in the ventricles of the F1b hamsters at 12 weeks old, and the difference between the two groups increased progressively with age (Fig. 5).

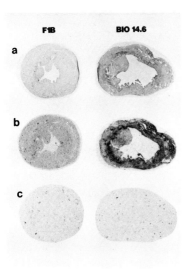

FIG. 1. Autoradiographic localization of β-adrenoceptors in the heart of a 35-week-old control (F1b) and a 35-week-old cardiomyopathic (Bio 14.6) Syrian hamster. **(A)** Sections were stained with the PAS method. **(B)** Sections were incubated with 50 pM $[^{125}I]$-CYP, as described under Methods. **(C)** Sections adjacent to B were incubated with 50 pM $[^{125}I]$-CYP in the presence of 1 μM (−)-propranolol. Original magnification is ×8.

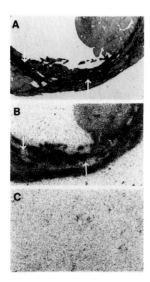

FIG. 2. Autoradiographic localization of [^{125}I]-CYP binding sites in the heart from a 52-week-old cardiomyopathic Bio 14.6 Syrian hamster. **(A)** Tissue section stained with PAS. **(B)** Section was incubated with 50 pM [^{125}I]-CYP, as described under Methods. **(C)** Section was incubated with 50 pM [^{125}I]-CYP in the presence of 1 μM (−)-propranolol. A high concentration of [^{125}I]-CYP binding sites is found in the area near the PAS-positive regions but few binding sites are seen in the PAS-positive areas (*arrows*).

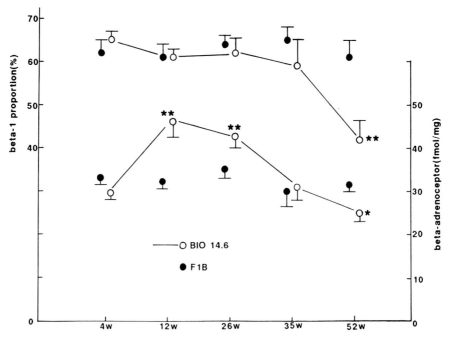

FIG. 3. Changes in the percentage of β$_1$-subtype (*upper part*) and the β-adrenoceptor density (*lower part*) of the heart from control (●) and cardiomyopathic Bio 14.6 Syrian hamsters (○) at various ages. *$p < 0.05$; **$p < 0.01$.

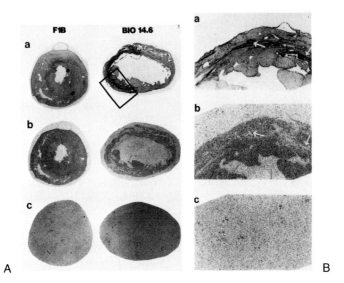

FIG. 4. Autoradiographic localization of [12-³H]-forskolin binding sites in a heart from a 35-week-old control (F1b) and a 35-week-old cardiomyopathic Bio 14.6 Syrian hamster (*left panel*) and magnified picture of black box area (*right panel*). **(a)** Tissue section stained with PAS. **(b)** Section was incubated with 100 pM [12-³H]-forskolin, as described under Methods. **(c)** Section was incubated with 100 nM [12-³H]-forskolin in the presence of 100 μM forskolin. Few binding sites are observed in the PAS-positive area (*arrows*).

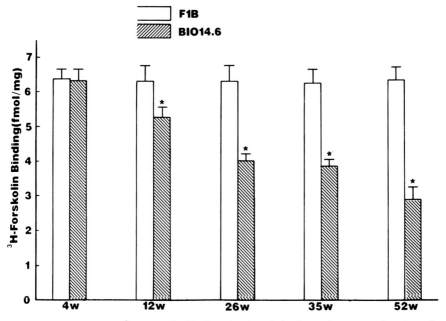

FIG. 5. Changes in [12-³H]-forskolin binding density of the heart from control and cardiomyopathic Bio 14.6 Syrian hamsters at various ages. *$p < 0.01$.

DISCUSSION

Recently, Taharahara et al. (11) have demonstrated an augmentation of β-adrenoceptors in the septal and subendocardial regions of the hearts of cardiomyopathic Syrian hamsters aged 44 weeks. However, in this study, we observed an inhomogeneous distribution of β-adrenoceptors in every part of the cardiomyopathic hearts. The number of [^{125}I]-CYP binding sites increased in the areas adjacent to the PAS-positive regions throughout the hearts of the cardiomyopathic hamsters at the ages of 12 and 26 weeks. The PAS-positive areas with few [^{125}I]-CYP binding sites contained calcification and necrosis.

The number of β-adrenoceptors in the heart is mainly regulated by circulating catecholamines. Released catecholamines activate β-adrenoceptors, and they reduce the number of receptors, a phenomenon called down-regulation (12). However, in myocardial ischemia, an increased number of β-adrenoceptors in the plasma membrane was observed, and this mechanism is mainly dependent on the loss of high-energy phosphate, resulting in a loss of β-adrenergic agonist–induced uncoupling and internalization (13–15). Previous reports have shown that the hearts of cardiomyopathic hamsters have focal myocardial ischemia caused by microvascular spasm (16). The localized high number of [^{125}I]-CYP binding sites in the ventricles of cardiomyopathic hamsters may be attributable to the depressed metabolism of high-energy phosphate, as occurs in myocardial ischemia. Severely failing hearts from 52-week-old cardiomyopathic hamsters had a reduced β-adrenoceptor density. This may be explained by the elevated circulating levels of catecholamines in heart failure (17).

Localization of adenylate cyclase was accomplished using [12-^{3}H]-forskolin, a direct stimulator of adenylate cyclase. Forskolin binding to the catalytic subunit is associated with the activation of adenylate cyclase. We observed no binding sites in the PAS-positive areas. The number of [12-^{3}H]-forskolin binding sites was not high in the area containing a high β-adrenoceptor density. After 12 weeks of age, [12-^{3}H]-forskolin binding sites, except for PAS-positive areas, were significantly lower in cardiomyopathic hearts than in control hearts. Feldman et al. (18) have demonstrated a significant decrease in adenylate cyclase activity in cardiac particulate fraction prepared from Bio 53.58 hamsters in the presence of forskolin. These data are consistent with our finding. Nonetheless, our results suggest that β-adrenoceptors bear no proportion to the adenylate cyclase system in the hearts of cardiomyopathic hamsters 12 weeks or older, especially in the areas containing high β-adrenoceptor density. Whether the decreased adenylate cyclase may result i n increasing the β-adrenoceptor density by some mechanism to normalize the action of circulating catecholamines is not clear at present.

It is well recognized that an increased calcium influx across the sarcolemma leads to cellular hypercontraction, mitochondrial calcification, and cell death (19). Activation of β-adrenoceptor is well known to increase the cyclic adenosine monophosphate (cAMP) and to phosphorylate the slow calcium channels in the sarcolemma, resulting in an increased calcium influx (20). The increased β-adrenoceptor density may induce supersensitivity to circulating catecholamines even though adenylate cyclase has been decreased, and may be followed by cell death caused by calcium overload. Furthermore, activation of the inhomogeneous β-adrenoceptors of cardiomyopathic hearts may induce a disparity of refractory periods, which play an important role in the initiation of re-entry (21), resulting in a susceptibility to arrhythmias.

In conclusion, the localized high β-adrenoceptor density in the ventricle may play an important role in the progression of the disease process and the occurrence of arrhythmias in cardiomyopathic Bio 14.6 Syrian hamsters.

SUMMARY

The localization of β-adrenoceptors and adenylate cyclase was investigated by quantitative autoradiography in the hearts of cardiomyopathic Bio 14.6 Syrian hamsters, after the incubation of tissue sections with $[^{125}I]$-iodocyanopindolol (CYP) and $[12$-$^3H]$-forskolin. Ten hamsters, (five from the Bio 14.6 and five from the F1b strain) ages 4, 12, 26, 35, and 52 weeks were used in this study. The distribution of $[^{125}I]$-CYP binding sites was uniform in the control hearts; however, it was not homogeneous in the cardiomyopathic hearts. The number of adrenergic receptors was increased at 12 and 26 weeks but was decreased at 52 weeks. $[12$-$^3H]$-forskolin binding sites decreased with age in Bio 14.6 hamsters; this binding was significantly lower than that of the controls at 12 weeks. Our results indicate that there is an inhomogeneous distribution of β-adrenoceptors that is out of proportion with adenylate cyclase in the hearts of cardiomyopathic Bio 14.6 Syrian hamsters over 12 weeks old. In conclusion, the locally high number of β-adrenoceptors may be responsible for the progression of the disease process and for the occurrence of lethal arrhythmia in cardiomyopathic Bio 14.6 Syrian hamsters.

REFERENCES

1. Bajusz E, Baker JR, Nixson CW, Homburger F. Spontaneous hereditary myocardial degeneration and congestive heart failure in a strain of Syrian hamsters. *Ann NY Acad Sci* 1969;156:105–29.
2. Sole MJ, Helke CJ, Jacobowitz DM. Increased dopamine in the failing hamster heart: transvesicular transport of dopamine limits the rate of norepinephrine synthesis. *Am J Cardiol* 1982;49:1682–90.
3. Karliner JS, Alabaster C, Stephens H, Barnes P, Dollery C. Enhanced noradrenaline response in cardiomyopathic hamsters: possible relation to changes in adrenoceptors studied by radioligand binding. *Cardiovasc Res* 1981;15:296–304.
4. Wagner JA, Reynolds IJ, Weissman HF, Dudeck P, Weisfeldt ML, Snyder SH. Calcium antagonist receptors in cardiomyopathic hamsters: selective increase in heart, muscle, brain. *Science* 1986;232: 515–18.
5. Kessler PD, Cates AV, Von Dop C, Feldman AM. Decreased bioactivity of the guanine nucleotide-binding protein that stimulates adenylate cyclase (Gs) in hearts from cardiomyopathic Syrian hamsters. *J Clin Invest* 1989;84:244–52.
6. Dooly DJ, Bittiger H, Reymann NC. CGP20712A: a useful tool for quantitating beta-1 and beta-2 adrenoceptors. *Eur J Pharmacol* 1986;130:137–9.
7. Saito K, Kuroda A, Tanaka H. Characterization of beta-1 and beta-2-adrenoceptor subtypes in the atrioventricular node of diabetic rat hearts by quantitative autoradiography. *Cardiovasc Res* 1991; 25:950–4.

8. Worley PF, Baraban JM, De Souza EB, Snyder SH. Mapping second messenger systems in the brain: differential localization of adenylate cyclase and protein kinase C. *Proc Natl Acad Sci USA* 1986;83:4053–7.
9. Nazali AJ, Gutkind JS, Saavedra JM. Calibration of ^{125}I-polymer standards with ^{125}I-brain paste standards for use in quantitative receptor autoradiography. *J Neurosci Methods* 1989;30:247–53.
10. Geary WA, Wooten GF. Quantitative film autoradiography of opiate agonist and antagonist binding in rat brain. *J Pharmacol Exp Therap* 1983;225:234–40.
11. Taharahara K, Kurata C, Taguchi T, Kobayashi A, Yamazaki N. Augmentation of beta-adrenergic receptors in cardiomyopathic hamsters (BIO 14.6) with heart failure. *Cardiovasc Res* 1992;26:526–33.
12. Limas CJ, Limas C. Rapid recovery of cardiac beta-adrenergic receptors after isoproterenol-induced "down"-regulation. *Circ Res* 1984;55:524–31.
13. Mukherjee A, Bush LR, McKoy KE, et al. Relationship between beta-adrenergic receptor numbers and physiological responses during experimental canine myocardial ischemia. *Circ Res* 1982;50:735–41.
14. Strasser RH, Krimmer J, Marquetant R. Regulation of beta-adrenergic receptors: impaired desensitization in myocardial ischemia. *J Cardiovasc Pharmacol* 1988;12[Suppl I]:s15–s24.
15. Thandroyen FT, Muntz KH, Buza LM, Willerson JT. Alterations in beta-adrenergic receptors, adenylate cyclase, and cyclic AMP concentrations during acute myocardial ischemia and reperfusion. *Circulation* 1990;82[Suppl II]:II-30–7.
16. Factor SM, Minase T, Cho S, Dominitz R, Sonnenblick EH. Microvascular spasm in the cardiomyopathic Syrian hamster: a possible cause of focal myocardial necrosis. *Circulation* 1982;66:342–54.
17. Bristow MR, Ginsburg R, Minobe W, et al. Decreased catecholamine sensitivity and beta-adrenergic receptor density in failing human hearts. *N Engl J Med* 1982;307:205–11.
18. Feldman AM, Tena RG, Kessler PD, et al. Diminished beta-adrenergic receptor responsiveness and cardiac dilatation in hearts of myopathic Syrian hamsters (BIO 53.58) are associated with a functional abnormality of the G stimulatory protein. *Circulation* 1990;81:1341–52.
19. Wrogemann K, Nylen EG. Mitochondrial calcium overloading in cardiomyopathic hamsters. *J Mol Cell Cardiol* 1978;10:185–95.
20. Sperelakis N. Cyclic AMP and phosphorylation in regulation of Ca influx into myocardial cells and blockade by calcium antagonistic drugs. *Am Heart J* 1984;107:347–57.
21. Allesie MA, Bonke FMI, Schopman FJG. Circus movement in rabbit atrial muscle as a mechanism of tachycardia II. The role of nonuniform recovery of excitability in the occurrence of unidirectional block, as studied with multiple microelectrodes. *Circ Res* 1976;39:168–77.

The Cardiomyopathic Heart, edited by Makoto
Nagano, Nobuakira Takeda, and Naranjan S.
Dhalla. Raven Press, Ltd., New York © 1994.

11

Decrease in Stimulatory Guanine Nucleotide-Binding Protein and Adenylate Cyclase Activities in Bio 14.6 Cardiomyopathic Hamsters

Masanori Kaneko, Takayoshi Ikegaya, Akira Kobayashi,
Rong Bang Hong, Hisamichi Masuda, and Noboru Yamazaki

*Third Department of Internal Medicine, Hamamatsu University School of Medicine,
Hamamatsu 431-31, Japan*

INTRODUCTION

Cardiac abnormalities in the Bio 14.6 Syrian hamster are minimal at 30 to 40 days of age but become progressively severe in 90-day-old hamsters, followed by cardiac hypertrophy and eventual congestive heart failure (1). The pathogenesis of these disorders has not yet been clearly elucidated. Some investigators have reported that both α- and β-adrenergic receptors were increased in Bio 14.6 hamsters (2,3) and that the developed tension of isolated papillary muscle was enhanced in the presence of noradrenaline but not in the presence of isoprenaline (2). Similar results indicating no changes in the response of the cardiomyopathic myocardium to β-adrenergic agonist have been reported by others (4).

The β-adrenergic receptors–adenylate cyclase system is a plasma membrane–bound protein assembly consisting of three major components (5). In the heart, the heterotrimeric guanine nucleotide–binding regulatory proteins (G proteins) couple the extracellular receptors with the enzyme and cause stimulation (G_s) or inhibition (G_i) of the AC, which regulates the intracellular concentration of the second messenger cyclic adenosine monophosphate (cAMP). Since cAMP modulates cardiac contractility (6,7), alterations in the activities of adenylate cyclase and G proteins as well as changes in β-adrenergic receptors can be seen to affect the myocardial response to both catecholamine and cardiac function. Therefore, to clarify the mechanisms for the unaltered response of cardiomyopathic hearts to β-adrenergic stimulation, we studied the norepinephrine and epinephrine contents, β-adrenergic receptor levels, AC activity, and G_s activity in the hearts of Bio 14.6 hamsters at 90 days (early hypertrophic stage) and 160 days (late hypertrophic stage) of age.

MATERIALS AND METHODS

Cardiac Membrane Preparation

Male cardiomyopathic Syrian Bio 14.6 hamsters and age-matched F1b controls were used in this study. The animals were killed by cervical dislocation at 90 and 160 days and their hearts were removed. The ventricular tissue was homogenized in 50 ml/g wet tissue of buffer (0.25 M sucrose, 5 mM TRIS-HCl, pH 7.4), using a polytron and Potter-Elvehjem homogenizer. The homogenate was centrifuged at $500 \times g$ for 10 minutes at 4°C, and the supernatant was centrifuged at $30,000 \times g$ for 10 minutes at 4°C. The resulting pellets were suspended in the buffer (50 mM TRIS-HCl, pH 7.4) and washed by centrifuging at $30,000 \times g$ for 10 minutes at 4°C. The final pellet was suspended in 20 ml/g wet tissue of 50 mM TRIS-HCl buffer, pH 7.4. The protein concentration was determined by the method of Lowry et al. (8).

Culture of S49 Lymphoma Cell cyc⁻

Lymphoma cells were cultured according to the methods of Ross et al. (9) in stationary suspension at 37°C in Dulbecco's modified Eagle's medium (4.5 g/L of D-glucose) containing 7.5% to 10% heat-inactivated horse serum.

Membrane Preparation of S49 Lymphoma Cell cyc⁻

Plasma membrane of S49 lymphoma cell cyc⁻ was prepared according to the methods of Ross et al. (9). Cells were harvested at a density of between 2.0 and 3.5×10^6/ml by low-speed centrifugation and were washed twice at room temperature in 137 mM NaCl, 5.36 mM KCl, 1.1 mM KH_2PO_4, and 1.08 mM Na_2HPO_4, pH 7.2. Subsequent steps were performed at 0°C to 4°C. Cells were suspended to 3×10^7/ml in 20 mM Na-HEPES, 2 mM $MgCl_2$, 1 mM ethylenediaminetetra-acetic acid (EDTA) (pH 8.0) (heat and moisture exchange [HME] buffer), and homogenized using the Potter-Elvehjem homogenizer. The homogenate was centrifuged at $43,000 \times g$ for 20 minutes at 4°C, and the pellet was suspended in HME buffer (the final protein concentration was approximately 2–3 mg/ml).

Assay of G_s Protein Activity

G_s activity was assessed using a reconstitution assay originally described by Sternweis et al. (10). Briefly, the technique makes use of the fact that G_s protein can be solubilized from cardiac membranes and then functionally coupled to cyc⁻ S49 mouse lymphoma cell membrane. The cyc⁻ cell line was originally described by Bourne et al. (11); it is functionally deficient in G_s but has the AC catalytic unit.

Because cardiac membranes also contain the catalytic unit of AC, we inactivated AC when measuring G_s activity by heating the membrane preparations to 37°C (12).

Heat-inactivated cardiac membranes were suspended in 20 mM TRIS-HCl (pH 8.0) containing 0.1% lubrol PX, 1 mM EDTA, 100 mM NaCl, and 1 mM dithiothreitol. Cardiac membrane suspension (10 μl) was mixed with 30 μl of cyc⁻ membrane and allowed to sit on ice for 30 minutes. Preactivation was then performed by adding 20 μl of a buffer containing 150 mM HEPES (pH 8.0), 2 mM ATP, 0.3 mg/ml bovine serum albumin, 9 mM phospho(enol)pyruvate, 15 mM $MgCl_2$, 30 μg/ml pyruvate kinase, 60 μM $AlCl_3$, 30 mM NaF, and followed by incubation at 30°C for 10 minutes. Adenylate cyclase activity was then assayed by adding 1×10^6 cpm [α-^{32}P]ATP (in a total volume of 40 μl with 125 mM HEPES (pH 8.0), 2.5 mM EDTA, 0.25 mM ATP, 0.25 mg/ml bovine serum albumin, 7.5 mM phospho(enol)pyruvate, 20 mM $MgCl_2$, 25 μg/ml pyruvate kinase, and 0.25 mM 3-isobutyl-1-methyl-xanthine, and performing incubation for an additional 30 minutes at 30°C.

The reaction was terminated by the addition of 0.9 μl of stop solution containing 2.5% sodium dodecyl sulfate, 40 mM ATP, 1.75 mM cAMP, and 10,000 cpm [^{3}H]cAMP. The amount of cAMP produced was determined as above.

Assay of Adenylate Cyclase Activity

Adenylate cyclase activity of cardiac membranes was assayed according to the method of Salomon et al. (13). The assay mixture contained the following in a final volume of 100 μl: 75 mM HEPES (pH 8.0), 1.5 mM EDTA, 500 μM ATP, 0.15 mg/ml BSA, 4.5 mM phospho(enol)pyruvate, 12 mM $MgCl_2$, 15 μg/ml pyruvate kinase, 30 μg cardiac membranes, and 1×10^6 cpm [α-^{32}P]ATP. Incubation was carried out at 30°C for 10 minutes. The reaction was stopped by the addition of 0.9 μl of a stop solution containing 2.5% sodium dodecyl sulfate, 40 mM ATP, 1.75 mM cAMP, and 10,000 cpm of [^{3}H]cAMP.

The reaction mixture was then passed through a column containing 1 ml Dowex 50AG WX8 resin. The eluate from this passage and two successive 1-ml H_2O washes was discarded. Three milliliters of H_2O was then added to the column, and the eluate was collected and passed through a column containing 1 ml of neutral almina type WN-3. The eluate from this passage and from successive washes with 1.5 ml of 0.1 M imidazole-HCl (pH 7.5) washes was discarded. Then 0.1 M imidazole-HCl (pH 7.5, 1.5 ml) was added to each column, and the eluate was collected and counted in scintillation vials containing 15 ml of toluene-based scintillation cocktail. This cocktail contained 30% (v/v) Triton-X-100, 0.4% (w/v) 2,5-diphenyl-oxazole, and 0.01% (w/v) 1,4-bis[2-(4-methyl-5-phenyl-oxazolyl)]-benzen. Recovery of added [^{3}H]cAMP was about 50%. Maximum AC activity was assessed by measuring cAMP production in the presence of 500 μM forskolin. Cardiac AC activity was saturated in the presence of 500 μM forskolin.

Assay of Cardiac Catecholamine Levels and β-Adrenergic Receptors

Tissue epinephrine and norepinephrine levels were determined according to Ueda et al. (14) using high-speed ion-exchange chromatography. [^{125} I] CYP binding was measured according to a method reported earlier (12).

Statistical Analysis

Results are presented as mean ± standard deviation. The Student t-test was used for the statistical evaluation, and $p<0.05$ was taken to reflect a significant difference.

RESULTS

Heart to Body Weight Ratio

The hearts of Bio 14.6 hamsters at 90 and 160 days of age were hypertrophied compared with those of control (F1b) hamsters 90 days old: 0.002958 ± 0.000028 versus 0.002760 ± 0.000031 g heart tissue/g body weight, $p<0.01$; 160 days old: 0.003247 ± 0.000041 versus 0.002828 ± 0.000068 g heart tissue/g body weight, $p<0.01$.

Cardiac Catecholamine Levels

The cardiac norepinephrine concentrations of Bio 14.6 hamsters were significantly elevated compared with those in control hamsters at 90 days of age (Bio 14.6 versus control: 1739 ± 120 versus 1470 ± 161 ng/g wet tissue, $p<0.05$, n=6). However, the cardiac epinephrine concentrations were similar in both groups of hamsters (Bio 14.6 versus control: 64.9 ± 9.0 versus 70.7 ± 18.3 ng/g wet tissue, n=6, not significant). Both the cardiac norepinephrine and epinephrine concentrations were similar in Bio 14.6 and control hamsters at 160 days of age (Bio 14.6 versus control: norepinephrine 1773 ± 233 versus 1793 ± 139 ng/g wet tissue, n=6: epinephrine 40.6 ± 11.5 versus 40.0 ± 5.1 ng/g wet tissue, n=6).

Cardiac β-Adrenergic Receptor Numbers

The total number of cardiac β-receptors in Bio 14.6 cardiomyopathic hamsters at 90 days of age was significantly increased compared to those in the control hamsters (Bio 14.6 versus controls: 32.0 ± 2.7 versus 23.7 ± 3.6 fmol/mg protein, $p<0.05$, n=6). However, there was no significant difference in β-receptor affinity between Bio 14.6 and control hamsters (Bio 14.6 versus control: 20.3 ± 3.6 versus 22.7 ± 7.9 pM, n=6, not significant).

TABLE 1. *Forskolin-stimulated adenylate cyclase activity in the heart of Bio 14.6 and control hamsters at 90 and 160 days of age*

	Adenylate cyclase activity (pmol cAMP/mg protein/min)	
	90 days	160 days
Control	122 ± 29^a	124 ± 28
	(n = 12)	(n = 10)
Bio 14.6	$98 \pm 24^*$	$74 \pm 13^*$
	(n = 12)	(n = 10)

[a]Each value is a mean ± standard deviation. Adenylate cyclase activity was assayed in the presence of 500 μM forskolin.
*Significantly different from control values.
($p < 0.05$).

Cardiac Adenylate Cyclase Activity

Cardiac AC activities at 90 days and 160 days of age in the presence of 500 μM forskolin were significantly lower in Bio 14.6 hamsters than in control hamsters (Table 1).

Cardiac G_s Protein Activity

To monitor changes in G_s activities in cardiac membranes, we assayed the activation of AC in a preparation containing a saturating amount of the catalytic unit of AC prepared from cyc⁻ membrane.

Figure 1 shows the ability of G_s from cardiac membranes of Bio 14.6 and control hamsters to reconstitute cyc⁻ AC over a range of concentrations of added cardiac membrane protein. The curve was linear; therefore the reconstituted activity (reflecting the G_s activity) was directly proportional to the amounts of cardiac membrane protein added. For the amounts of cardiac membrane protein within the linear range, there was a decrease of 50% in the reconstituting activity of cardiac membrane derived from Bio 14.6 hamsters when compared with that from control hamsters. Cardiac activity was calculated from the slope of the regression lines for every cardiac membrane. The cardiac G_s activities of Bio 14.6 hamsters were significantly lower than those of control hamsters at 90 days and 160 days of age (Table 2).

DISCUSSION

The Bio 14.6 Syrian hamster consistently develops cardiomyopathy and has proved to be a useful animal model for the study of human cardiomyopathy. The progression of heart disease in Bio 14.6 hamsters can be divided into four phases (1). During the first or prenecrotic phase, the animals appear healthy, and there is no pathologic evidence of disease. The second phase begins when the animals are

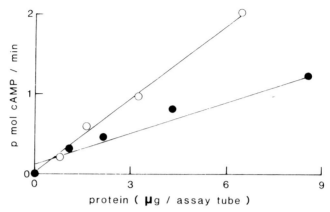

FIG. 1. Reconstitution of G_s activity from hamster cardiac membranes into cyc⁻ membranes. Various amounts of cardiac membranes from Bio 14.6 hamsters (●) and control hamsters (○) were heated at 37°C, solubilized, and reconstituted with a fixed amount of cyc⁻ membrane. Then the G_s activity stimulated by sodium fluoride was measured as described under Materials and Methods. For the various amounts of cardiac membrane added, there was a decrease of 50% in the activity reconstituted (production of cAMP from ATP) between Bio 14.6 and control hamsters, reflecting the different G_s activities of the cardiac membranes.

about 30 to 40 days of age and is characterized by the appearance of focal myocardial necrosis. By about 90 to 120 days of age, many of these necrotic lesions have healed, few new lesions appear, and cardiac hypertrophy has begun. The fourth phase is marked by cardiac dilation and eventual congestive heart failure. Cardiac failure occurs at about 180 days of age, and many animals die at about 300 days.

Sole et al. (15) reported that cardiac norepinephrine concentration was increased during the early and middle stages of cardiomyopathy (30–200 days), but not at the late stage (300 days). Our present findings on cardiac norepinephrine concentration were in agreement with the results of Sole et al. (15). Furthermore, we and other investigators have shown that cardiac cell membrane β-adrenergic receptor levels were increased in Bio 14.6 hamsters in the hypertrophic stage but not in the prenecrotic stage (2).

TABLE 2. *Cardiac G_s activity at 90 and 160 days of age in Bio 14.6 and control hamsters*

	G_s activity (pmol cAMP/mg protein/min)	
	90 days	160 days
Control	259 ± 49^a	211 ± 60
	(n = 7)	(n = 10)
Bio 14.6	$204 \pm 42^*$	$156 \pm 39^*$
	(n = 8)	(n = 11)

[a]Each value is a mean ± standard deviation.
*Significantly different from control values.
($p < 0.05$).

Stimulatory GTP-binding protein (G_s) couples β-adrenergic receptor stimulation by agonist to AC and could play an important role in positive cardiac inotropic action (16). However, Karliner et al. (2) demonstrated that isoprenaline (a β-adrenergic agonist) did not produce any augmentation of isometric tension despite the apparent increase in β-adrenergic receptor density in Bio 14.6 hamsters at 10 and 12 months of age, a time when the hamsters tested exhibited no overt signs of congestive cardiac failure. Their study showed that isoprenaline and norepinephrine stimulate the force of contraction of isolated hamster right ventricular muscle strips and that the sensitivity to norepinephrine is apparently increased in tissues derived from cardiomyopathic hamsters. The results could have been influenced at least in part by the contractile tissue preparation used, but they are expressed as a comparison between different agonists acting (-and β-agonist) on the same tissue. Therefore, it is likely that the unaltered response to β-adrenergic stimulation might be attributable to abnormalities in the postreceptor system, such as those affecting G_s protein and AC, rather than to changes in the contractile tissue.

Kessler et al. (17) have also demonstrated a functional abnormality of cardiac β-receptor-G-protein-AC complex that results from a qualitative defect in G_s protein in 29-day-old Bio 14.6 hamsters (prenecrotic stage). In contrast, cardiac levels of β-adrenoceptors and catecholamine content were not increased in 29-day-old Bio 14.6 hamsters in their study. Therefore, they suggested that the diminished G_s bioactivity was related to a genetic lesion in Bio 14.6 hamsters, because it was present before the development of the characteristic light microscopic abnormalities of cardiomyopathy. Furthermore, immunodetectable levels of Gα proteins were unchanged, suggesting a role for post-translational modification in regulating the bioactivity of G protein gene products.

Recent studies have demonstrated substantial changes in G protein function in failing human and animal hearts. In the human heart, end-stage idiopathic congestive failure was associated with a decrease in β-adrenergic receptors and an increase in G_i protein activity (18). In contrast, heart failure owing to left ventricular pressure overload was associated with increased β-adrenoceptor levels and decreased G_s protein activity (16). Furthermore, human studies have concentrated on individuals undergoing heart transplantations whose myocardial function was severely impaired as a result of idiopathic dilated cardiomyopathy; therefore the levels of β-adrenoceptors and the AC response might well be reduced in such severely damaged hearts (19). The level of β-adrenoceptors and the AC response may therefore depend on the stage of cardiomyopathy.

In this study, we investigated G_s protein and AC activity in Bio 14.6 hamsters at a later stage of cardiomyopathy than that studied by Kessler et al. (17), who used 29-day-old animals (prenecrotic stage). At 90 days of age (the early stage of cardiac hypertrophy), cardiac G_s activity and forskolin-stimulated adenylate cyclase activity were reduced despite the increased cardiac norepinephrine concentration and the raised level of β-adrenoceptors. G_s protein activity and forskolin-stimulated AC activity were also reduced at 160 days of age in Bio 14.6 hamsters (the late cardiac hypertrophic phase). These results are in agreement with those of Kessler et al.

(17), except for an increase in the number of β-adrenoceptors. The diminished G_s and AC activities might be related to the unaltered cardiac response to β-adrenergic stimulation in Bio 14.6 hamsters. In addition, the recent demonstration that G_s protein can directly activate the slow, voltage-gated calcium channel in cardiac muscle independent of protein kinase-mediated phosphorylation (20) suggests that altered G_s protein bioactivity in cardiomyopathic hamsters may contribute to the abnormal myocardial contractility.

Recent studies have shown that cAMP plays a role as a second messenger in mediating the action of growth-promoting factors (21). Muraguchi et al. (22) have demonstrated that forskolin, an agent that elevates cytoplasmic cAMP levels, selectively inhibits the progression of B cell growth factor–induced G_1 to S phase transition of B cells and also inhibits the proliferative response of B cells in a dose-dependent manner. We found a reduction of cardiac G_s and forskolin-stimulated AC activities in Bio 14.6 hamsters at the hypertrophic stage of cardiomyopathy. This phenomenon could be related to a decrease in the cytoplasmic cAMP levels despite increased levels of cardiac norepinephrine and β-adrenoceptors at this stage of cardiomyopathy. Thus, diminished G_s protein and AC activity might also affect the extent of myocardial hypertrophy in Bio 14.6 hamsters.

In conclusion, we have demonstrated functional defects in G_s protein activity and AC activity in the hearts of Bio 14.6 cardiomyopathic hamsters at 90 and 160 days of age (the hypertrophic stage of cardiomyopathy), in spite of the increased cardiac norepinephrine level and β-receptor density. These changes may be one possible mechanism leading to the unaltered response to β-adrenergic stimulation and contribute to myocardial decompensation in this animal.

SUMMARY

Although cardiac α- and β-adrenergic receptors are increased, isoprenaline does not produce an augmented response in the hearts of Bio 14.6 cardiomyopathic hamsters. Therefore, this study was undertaken to clarify the stimulatory guanosine triphosphate (GTP)–binding protein (G_s) and adenylate cyclase (AC) activities in the hearts of Bio 14.6 hamsters at 90 and 160 days of age. Cardiac norepinephrine concentration was significantly increased in Bio 14.6 hamsters compared with controls (F1b). G_s activities at 90 and 160 days of age were significantly lower in Bio 14.6 than in F1b hearts. Furthermore, forskolin-stimulated AC activities in Bio 14.6 hearts were significantly reduced at 90 and 160 days of age. These changes in G_s and AC activities may be one possible mechanism leading to the unaltered response to β-adrenergic stimulation and contribute to myocardial decompensation in Bio 14.6 cardiomyopathy.

ACKNOWLEDGMENTS

We would like to thank Professor T. Haga for his helpful advice and Dr. M. Nishimura for supplying the hamsters used in this study.

REFERENCES

1. Gertz EW. Cardiomyopathic Syrian hamster: a possible model of human disease. *Prog Exp Tumor Res* 1972;16:242–60.
2. Karliner JS, Alabaster C, Stephens H, Barnes P, Dollery C. Enhanced noradrenaline response in cardiomyopathic hamsters: possible relation to changes in adrenoceptors studied by radioligand binding. *Cardiovasc Res* 1981;15:296–304.
3. Ikegaya T, Nishiyama T, Kobayashi A, Yamazaki N. Role of α1-adrenergic receptors and the effect of bunazosin on the histopathology of cardiomyopathic Syrian hamsters of strain Bio 14.6 *Jpn Circ J* 1988;52:181–7.
4. Bohm M, Mende U, Schmitz W, Scholz H. Increased responsiveness to stimulation of α- but not β-adrenoceptors in the hereditary cardiomyopathy of the Syrian hamster. Intact adenosine- and cholinoceptor-mediated antagonistic effect. *Eur J Pharmacol* 1986;128:195–203.
5. Gilman AG. G proteins: transducers of receptor generated signals. *Annu Rev Biochem* 1987;56:615–49.
6. Epstein SE, Skelton CL, Levey GS, Entman M. Adenyl cyclase and myocardial contractility. *Ann Intern Med* 1970;72:561–78.
7. Drummond GE, Severson DL. Cyclic nucleotides and cardiac function. *Circ Res* 1979;44:145–52.
8. Lowry OH, Rosebrough HJ, Farr AL, Randall NS. Protein measurement with the Folin phenol reagent. *J Biol Chem* 1951;193:265–75.
9. Ross EM, Maquire ME, Sturgill TW, Biltonen RL, Gilman AG. Relationship between the β-adrenergic receptor and adenylate cyclase. *J Biol Chem* 1977;252:5761–75.
10. Sternweis PC, Northup JK, Smigel MD, Gilman AG. Regulatory component of adenylate cyclase; purification and properties. *J Biol Chem* 1981;256:1151–52.
11. Bourne HR, Coffino RP, Tomkins GM. Selection of a variant lymphoma cell deficient in adenylate cyclase. *Science* 1975;18:750–52.
12. Ikegaya T, Kobayashi A, Hong RB, Masuda H, Kaneko M, Yamazaki N. Stimulatory guanine nucleotide-binding protein and adenylate cyclase activities in Bio 14.6 cardiomyopathic hamsters at the hypertrophic stage. *Mol Cell Biochem* 1992;110:83–90.
13. Salomon Y, Londos C, Rodbell M. A high sensitive adenylate cyclase assay. *Anal Biochem* 1974;58:541–48.
14. Ueda E, Yoshida N, Nishimura K, et al. A semiautomated measurement of urinary catecholamines using high-speed ion-exchange column chromatography. *Clin Chim Acta* 1977;80:447–53.
15. Sole MJ, Lo CM, Laird CW, Sonnenblick EH, Wurtman RJ. Norepinephrine turnover in the heart and spleen of the cardiomyopathic Syrian hamster. *Circ Res* 1975;37:855–62.
16. Longabaugh JP, Vatner DE, Vatner SF, Homcy CJ. Decreased stimulatory guanosine triphosphate binding protein in dogs with pressure-overload left ventricular failure. *J Clin Invest* 1988;81:420–4.
17. Kessler PD, Cates AE, Dop CV, Feldman AM. Decreased bioactivity of the guanine nucleotide-binding protein that stimulates adenylate cyclase in hearts from cardiomyopathic Syrian hamsters. *J Clin Invest* 1989;84:244–52.
18. Feldman AM, Cates AE, Veazey WB, et al. Increase of the 40,000-mol wt pertussis toxin substrate (G protein) in the failing human heart. *J Clin Invest* 1988;82:189–97.
19. Bristow MR, Ginsburg R, Fowler M, et al. β1- and β2-adrenergic receptor subpopulations in normal and failing human ventricular myocardium: coupling of both receptor subtypes to muscle contraction and selective β1 receptor down-regulation in heart failure. *Circ Res* 1986;59:297–308.
20. Yatani A, Imoto Y, Codina J, Hamilton SL, Brown AM, Birnbaumer L. The stimulatory G protein of adenylyl cyclase, Gs, also stimulates dihydropiridine sensitive Ca^{2+} channels: evidence for direct regulation independent of phosphorylation by cAMP dependent protein kinase or stimulation by a dihydropiridine agonist. *J Biol Chem* 1988;263:9887–95.
21. Rozengurt E, Legg A, Strang G, Courtnay-Luck N. Cyclic AMP: a mitogenic signal for Swiss 3T3 cells. *Proc Natl Acad Sci USA* 1981;78:4392–6.
22. Muraguchi A, Miyazaki K, Kehrl JH, Fauchi AS. Inhibition of human B cell activation by diterpine forskolin: interference with B cell growth factor-induced G1 to S transition of the B cell cycle. *J Immunol* 1984;133:1283–7.

The Cardiomyopathic Heart, edited by Makoto
Nagano, Nobuakira Takeda, and Naranjan S.
Dhalla. Raven Press, Ltd., New York © 1994.

12

Inositolphosphatides Metabolism in the Cardiomyopathic Hamster

Hideaki Kawaguchi, Hitoshi Sano, Toshiyuki Kudo, Hiroshi Okada,
and Akira Kitabatake

*Department of Cardiovascular Medicine, Hokkaido University School of Medicine,
Sapporo 060 Japan*

INTRODUCTION

The Syrian cardiomyopathic hamster (Bio 14.6) displays hereditary abnormalities in cardiac and skeletal muscle that are inherited as an autosomal recessive trait (1,2). Heart involvement results in myocardial hypertrophy followed by cardiac dilation and death from congestive heart failure (3–5). Calcium overload of myocytes has been implicated in the etiology of abnormalities in cardiomyopathic hamsters because calcium uptake in the myocardium is increased, and calcium antagonist drugs are effective in improving the manifestations of the disease. Thus cardiomyopathic hamsters (Bio 14.6) are considered a useful model of human cardiac disease such as hypertrophic cardiomyopathy.

Many different hormones and neurotransmitters stimulate the breakdown of plasma membrane inositol phospholipids through receptor mediation (6–8). This so-called phosphatidylinositol (PI) turnover pathway generates two second messengers, inositol 1,4,5-trisphosphate (IP_3) and DAG. DAG stimulates membrane-bound, phospholipid-dependent, Ca^{2+}-dependent protein kinase C, whereas IP_3 releases Ca^{2+} from endoplasmic reticulum stores. Removal of IP_3 occurs by way of two different pathways: hydrolysis to inositol 1,4-bisphosphate (IP_2), and phosphorylation to IP_4. IP_4 is subsequently dephosphorylated to 1,3,4-IP_3, which is relatively inactive in releasing Ca^{2+} compared with the 1,4,5-IP_3 isomer. The physiologic significance of this extra loop of the PI turnover pathway is unknown in any mammalian cell system. Although in sea urchin eggs IP_4 has been shown to enhance Ca^{2+} entry into the cell, this phenomenon has not been proved in cardiac myocytes. We consider that this PI turnover pathway plays an important role in inducing cardiac myocyte hypertrophy. The purpose of this investigation is to study the polyphosphoinositide metabolism in the hypertrophic heart of the cardiomyopathic hamster.

MATERIALS AND METHODS

Experimental Protocol

Experiments were carried out on male cardiomyopathic hamsters (Bio 14.6) aged 8, 15, 23, 30, and 40 weeks and age-matched male control hamsters (F1b). Each age group contained ten animals. The left ventricle was excised from the heart, and blood was carefully washed out.

Subcellular Fractions

Myocardium was minced and homogenized for 60 seconds by a polytron homogenizer (PT-19, Kinematica, Switzerland) in 5 volumes (vol/wt) of 0.1 M TRIS-HCl (pH 7.4) (9). The homogenate was centrifuged at 700 g for 10 minutes, and the resultant supernatant was centrifuged at 9,000 g for 20 minutes. The pellet obtained was washed twice with the same buffer and used as the mitochondrial fraction, and the supernatant was centrifuged at 105,000 g for 60 minutes according to previously published methods (9). The pellet was washed twice with the same buffer and suspended in 0.1 M TRIS-HCl buffer (pH 8.0) and used for each assay as the microsomes. The resultant supernatant was centrifuged again at 105,000 g for 60 minutes and used as the cytosomal fraction.

Phospholipase C Activity

Each subcellular fraction was incubated with [^{14}C]arachidonic acid-labeled phospholipids (50,000 cpm/20 nmol) in 0.1 M TRIS-HCl, pH 7.0, 5 mM $CaCl_2$ for 2 minutes at 37°C (10). The released DAG and free arachidonic acid were extracted by the method of Folch et al. The chloroform phase was pooled and evaporated under a vacuum. The residues were applied to thin-layer chromatography, which was developed in diethylether-acetic acid (96:4, vol/vol) and then again in a solvent system containing petroleum ether-diethyl ether/acetic acid (v/v/v) (11). The respective spots of monoglyceride, diglyceride, triglyceride, and arachidonic acid were scraped, counted with a scintillation spectrometer, and analyzed according to previous studies (12).

PIP_2-PLC activity was determined in 50 mM TRIS-HCl (pH 6.5 and 9.0) (10), 2 mM ethylene glycol tetra-acetic acid (EGTA) and $CaCl_2$ to give 10 µM [Ca^{2+}] (30), 100 µg of cytosolic protein, and 50 µM of [^{3}H]phosphatidylinositol-4,5-bisphosphate in a final volume of 200 µl. Incubation was carried out for 2 minutes at 37°C and terminated by adding 2 ml of chloroform-methanol (2:1, v/v). The radioactivity in the aqueous phase was counted.

Inositol 1,4,5-Trisphosphate Kinase Activity

The reaction buffer contained 4 μM of [^{3}H]inositol 1,4,5-trisphosphate (a preliminary experiment revealed that V_{max} was 5.2 nmol/min/mg cytosolic protein, and K_m was 4 M), 50 mM TRIS-malate pH 7.0, 10 mM adenosine triphosphate (ATP), 20 m $MgCl_2$, 5 mM 2,3-diphosphoglycerate (2,3-DPG; this concentration of 2,3-DPG inhibited the dephosphorylation of IP_3 and IP_4 by 98%), 2 mM EGTA, and $CaCl_2$ to give 10 μM [Ca^{2+}] (13). Incubation was carried out for 2 minutes at 37°C. The reaction was terminated by the addition of 0.5 ml of ice-cold trichloroacetic acid (TCA) and 0.1 ml of 5% bovine serum albumin (BSA), after which TCA was removed by four diethylether washes and the mixture neutralized with NH_3. Inositol monophosphate, IP_2, IP_3, and IP_4 were separated by elution from AG 1-X8 columns in formate form (100 to 200 mesh; Bio-Rad) in a gradient of ammonium formate (0.2–1.2 M) plus 0.1 M formic acid. For a more detailed analysis, including separation of inositol phosphate isomers, samples were filtered and separated by high performance liquid chromatography (Whatman Partisil 10 SAX anion-exchange column with a guard column) with a gradient of ammonium formate and phosphate.

Inositol 5-Phosphatase Activity

The incubation mixture was basically the same as the IP_3 kinase incubation mixture without ATP. Incubation was carried out for 2 minutes at 37°C. The separation of IP_1, IP_2, and IP_3 was done by using the same column system as for IP_3 kinase.

Cell Preparation

Myocardial cells from hamster hearts were prepared according to a previously reported method in phosphate buffer (PB) (14) and cultured in Ham's F-10 medium with 10% fetal calf serum until use. The freshly prepared cells were maintained at 37°C in a humidified 5% CO_2-95% air atmosphere (15). Then cells were subcultured at 3×10^5 cells per dish in 1 ml of PB containing 1 mM $CaCl_2$ in 35-mm dishes for assays and used within 2 hours (16).

Cellular Response to Norepinephrine

To determine the cellular response of PLC activity to norepinephrine (NE), myocytes (3×10^5) were prelabeled with [^{3}H]myo-inositol 5 μCi for 24 hours in phosphate buffer with 0.3% fetal calf serum, then cells were washed with PB three times. Cells were incubated with the indicated concentrations of NE, 5 mM 2,3-DPG, and 10 mM lithium chloride for 2 minutes in the presence of 1 μM metoprolol (Japan CIBA-GEIGY, Osaka Japan) to exclude the effect of β-adrenergic receptor stimulation, then terminated with chloroform-methanol (2:1, v/v). The aqueous phase was applied to an AG1 × 8 column, and inositol phosphates were separated by the ammonium gradient system as described above. For determination of diacylglyceride release, cells were prelabeled with [^{3}H]-arachidonic acid (1 μCi per dish) and incubated with NE as described above. The release of DAG was determined as described earlier (11).

For IP$_3$, kinase and inositol 5-phosphatase activities after stimulation by NE were determined in permeabilized cells with saponin (10 μg/ml). This concentration of saponin did not affect either enzyme activity. Cells were preincubated with 1 μM of NE for 2 minutes, and then saponin and substrates (IP$_3$ or IP$_4$) were added and incubated for the indicated periods in cytosolic buffer (KCl 120 mM, NaCl 10 mM, KH$_2$PO$_4$ 1 mM, NaHCO$_3$ 5 mM, HEPES 10 mM, pH 7.1), EGTA 0.2 mM, and CaCl$_2$ 150 nM. Incubation was terminated with chloroform-methanol (2:1, v/v). Inositol phosphatides were separated as described above by an AG1 × 8 column and an ammonium formate gradient system.

Measurement of Ca^{2+} Flux

Cells were prepared in 35-mm Petri dishes, as described above. For determination of Ca^{2+} influx, cells were washed with Hanks' balanced salt solution with 1.26 mM calcium and incubated in 0.7 ml of Hanks' balanced salt solution (containing 1.26 mM Ca^{2+}) in the presence of NE (1 μM), and 1 μCi of ^{45}Ca^{2+} with metoprolol (1 μM) for 1 minute at 37°C. Thereafter, cells were scraped from dishes, filtered through a 0.45-μm Millipore filter, washed three times with 4 ml of Hanks' balanced salt solution, and counted in 10 ml of Ready Value (Beckman Instruments, Inc. Palo Alto, CA) (17).

Statistical Analysis

Six experiments in triplicate were analyzed in all experiments. Results are expressed as mean ± standard error of the mean (SEM). Statistical significance was estimated using the previously described method (analysis of variance) taking $p < 0.05$ as the limit of significance.

RESULTS

Left ventricular weight was increased with age. This weight in Bio 14.6 hamsters was markedly increased compared with F1b hamsters. In addition, the left ventricular wall also was markedly hypertrophic (Fig. 1).

Phosphatidylinositol-PLC activity was increased with age in both groups of animals. The increase of such activity in Bio 14.6 hamsters 23 to 40 weeks old was significant ($p < 0.001$) compared with that in Bio 14.6 hamsters 5 weeks old. In F1b hamsters at 30 to 40 weeks old, the increase was significant ($p < 0.05$) compared with F1b animals at 5 weeks, but it was smaller compared to activity in Bio 14.6 hamsters. In Bio 14.6 animals 23 to 40 weeks old, PIP$_2$-PLC activity was increased

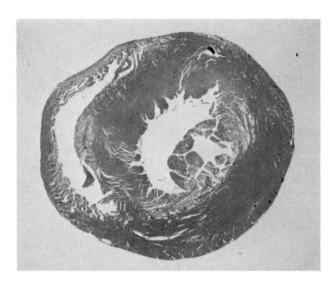

FIG. 1. Pathologic finding in Bio 14.6 hamster.

($p<0.001$) compared within Bio 14.6 hamsters 5 to 10 weeks old), and there were significant differences with F1b hamsters 23 to 40 weeks old (Fig. 2). There was also a significant increase in enzyme activity with age in F1b hamsters, but the increase was small compared with that in Bio 14.6 animals. IP_3 kinase activity was increased in 15-week-old Bio 14.6 hamsters ($p<0.001$) compared with those who were 8 weeks old. There were not significant increases in IP_3 kinase activity in Bio 14.6 hamsters 8 to 40 weeks old compared with age-matched F1b hamsters. In F1b

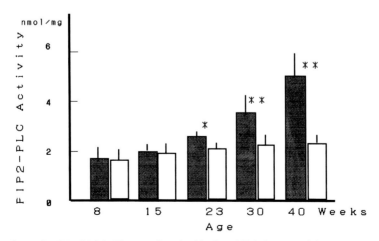

FIG. 2. Cytosolic PIP_2-PLC in Bio 14.6 (hatched bar) and F1b (open bar) hamsters was determined as described under Materials and Methods. *$p<0.05$ compared with age-matched F1b hamsters; **$p<0.001$ compared with age-matched F1b hamsters.

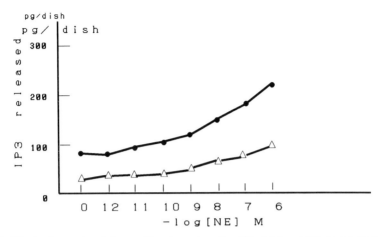

FIG. 3. Effects of norepinephrine on IP_3 release in cells of Bio 14.6 and F1b hamsters aged 10 weeks were determined as described under Materials and Methods. The effect of norepinephrine concentrations on release of IP_3 in the presence of 1 μM of metoprolol is shown. Bio 14.6 (●); F1b (△).

hamsters this activity was not increased at all ages studied. Inositol 5-phosphatase activity was increased between Bio 14.6 and F1b hamsters 8 to 40 weeks old ($p<0.05$).

Cellular Responses by Norepinephrine

When myocardial cells isolated from 10-week-old Bio 14.6 and F1b hamsters were incubated with the indicated concentrations of NE and 1×10^{-6} M of metoprolol in the presence of 10 mM lithium chloride and 5 mM of 2,3-DPG for 2 minutes, PI was markedly broken down and released IP_3 in Bio 14.6 hamsters (10^{-9}–10^{-5} M) (Fig. 3). DAG release from Bio 14.6 myocytes was markedly increased by the stimulation of NE. When cells were preincubated with the indicated concentrations of NE for 2 minutes and IP_3 was then added to permeabilized cells, IP_3 kinase activity was significantly higher in Bio 14.6 than in F1b hamsters at the NE concentrations of 10^{-9} to 10^{-5} M. The formation of IP_4 in the presence of 2,3-DPG and lithium chloride was increased for at least 10 minutes. Inositol 5-phosphatase activity was also determined after preincubation with NE for 2 minutes. Dephosphorylation of IP_3 was higher in Bio 14.6 than in F1b hamsters. The effect of NE on dephosphorylation of IP_3 was significant (at 10^{-6} M NE, $p<0.001$) compared with controls in both strains. However, there were no differences in age in stimulatory effect on IP_3 dephosphorylation by NE.

The release of IP_3 and IP_4 from [^{3}H]myoinositol prelabeled myocytes was markedly enhanced by 1 μM NE in Bio 14.6 hamsters. In NE-stimulated cells, both the PIP_2-PLC activity in isolated cells and IP_3 kinase activity in permeabilized cells were markedly enhanced in Bio 14.6 hamsters with age. IP_3 release was enhanced

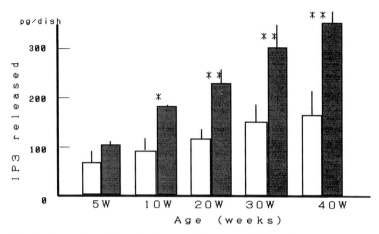

FIG. 4. Effects of norepinephrine stimulation on IP_3 release in Bio 14.6 hamsters aged 5 to 40 weeks with (hatched bar) and without (open bar) norepinephrine. Each activity was determined as described under Materials and Methods in the presence of 1 μM of metoprolol. *$p < 0.05$ compared with age-matched F1b hamsters; **$p < 0.001$ compared with age-matched F1b hamsters.

by NE from the ages of 10 to 40 weeks (Fig. 4). The basal PIP_2-PLC activity in 10-week-old Bio 14.6 hamsters was not increased compared to in 5-week-old subjects (see Fig. 2); however, at this stage the release of IP_3 caused by the response to NE was significantly activated compared to in 5-week-old Bio 14.6 hamsters. In permeabilized cells, IP_3 kinase activity was enhanced by the addition of NE at the age of 10 weeks, but there was a plateau between 10 and 40 weeks old.

We determined the effect of NE on Ca^{2+} influx into cells. The basal Ca^{2+} influx in Bio 14.6 hamsters without NE stimulation was higher than in F1b hamsters (Fig. 5A). Its influx into cells was linear within 5 minutes and then reached a plateau at 10 minutes. NE markedly stimulated Ca^{2+} influx into cells in Bio 14.6 hamsters with age (5 to 20 weeks). However, there were no differences in SR function for intracellular Ca^{2+} regulation between both strains (Fig. 5B).

DISCUSSION

We have demonstrated that cytosolic PIP_2-PLC activity was enhanced in Bio 14.6 hamster hearts compared to that in F1b hamster hearts. Furthermore, in isolated cells of Bio 14.6 subjects, PIP_2-breakdown stimulated by NE was followed by the release of IP_3, which was converted to IP; this process was markedly enhanced.

The metabolism of PIP_2 has been studied extensively in the heart, and results demonstrate that 1,4,5-IP_3 and 1,3,4,5-IP_4 are the immediate routes of metabolism. It is known that 1,4,5-IP_3 mobilizes intracellular Ca^{2+}, but whether this occurs in the heart is not known. It is also reported that 1,3,4,5-IP_4 enhances Ca^{2+} entry into

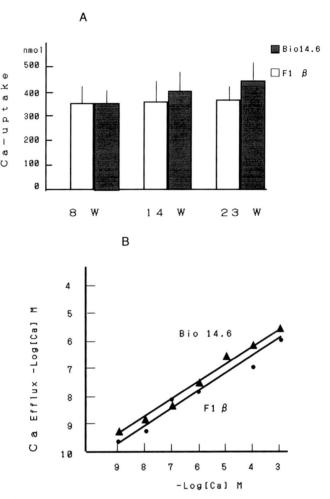

FIG. 5. **(A)** Ca^{2+} uptake into sarcoplasmic reticulum. Bio 14.6 hamsters, hatched bar, F1b hamsters, open bar. **(B)** Ca^{2+} efflux from SR of Bio 14.6 and F1b hamsters aged 14 weeks. IP_3 10 μ was added to each indicated concentration of Ca^{2+}-loaded SR. After 1 minute of incubation at 37°C, SR was filtered through a Milipore filter.

some cells and potentiates the Ca^{2+} mobilizing effect of 1,4,5-IP_3. Therefore, 1,4,5-IP_3 and 1,3,4,5-IP_4 may play an important role in controlling Ca^{2+} levels in response to hormonal stimulation, but it remains to be proved that this phenomenon exists in cardiac cells.

Irvine et al. were the first to demonstrate specific IP_3-kinase activity in a variety of animal tissues, and they reported that alterations in the kinase activity over physiologic Ca^{2+} ranges are likely to be small in rat brain. Ca^{2+} is a major mediator of the effects of the phosphoinositide system and serves as a second messenger for numerous neurotransmitters, hormones, and growth factors. IP_3 appears to bind to receptors on intracellular membranes to release Ca^{2+}. Specific binding sites for IP_3 have been demonstrated in peripheral tissues and in the brain.

In human cardiac tissue, an α_1-adrenergic receptor-mediated increase of IP_3 was reported. It has also been reported that α_1-adrenergic stimulation causes IP_4 to accumulate in adult canine myocytes. These reports suggest that the accumulations of IP_3 and IP_4 after hormonal stimulation have a physiologic role, possibly through the alteration of Ca^{2+} levels in cardiac tissue, although the accumulation of inositol polyphosphate in pathophysiologic conditions has not been studied. In our experiment, PIP_2 breakdown and IP_3 metabolism were investigated, and we clarified that basal levels of PLC and IP_3 kinase and IP_3 phosphatase activities increased in the cytosolic fraction of Bio 14.6 hamster hearts. These results led us to investigate the effect of NE on the inositolphosphatide metabolism in Bio 14.6 myocytes. We attempted to study the PI response stimulated by NE in the cardiomyopathic heart. It is reported that α_1-adrenergic stimulation plays an important role in inducing neonatal rat heart cell hypertrophy. It was shown that NE increased levels of c-*myc* encoded mRNA to tenfold over control levels. Expression of proto-oncogene c-*myc* is known to be increased in growth factor–induced cell division. This response was abolished by α_1-antagonists but was not affected by β-adrenergic antagonists. These findings show that α_1-adrenergic stimulation plays an important role in inducing neonatal cardiac myocyte hypertrophy, but it has not been clarified whether α_1-adrenergic stimulation has an effect on the development of hypertrophy in adult heart cells. As mentioned previously, PI response has an important role in the development of cell proliferation. Therefore in this study we examined the effect of NE on the metabolism of PIP_2.

The accumulations of IP_3 and IP_4 after stimulation with NE were significantly enhanced in isolated Bio 14.6 hamster myocytes. IP_3 kinase and phosphatase were also activated in permeabilized cells. The mechanisms of these enzyme activations have not been clarified. Since the activated PLC releases DAG, it may have activated protein kinase C, which could enhance these enzymes. Further experiments should be done on this point. In isolated cells of Bio 14.6 hamsters, the effect of NE on intracellular Ca^{2+} concentrations was increased. We consider that the accumulation of IP_3 and IP_4 contributed to this because the increased cytosolic free Ca^{2+} stimulated with NE was suppressed by neomycin, a PLC inhibitor (data not shown). It is not clear whether 1,3,4,5-IP_4 stimulates Ca^{2+} entry. Our data could not show whether 1,3,4,5-IP_4 affects Ca^{2+} entry.

SUMMARY

By employing the Bio 14.6 strain of cardiomyopathic hamsters, we have shown an augmentation of one of the pathways that increase the cytosolic Ca^{2+} level in the cardiomyopathic (hypertrophic) heart. These results suggest the possibility that the enhanced inositol 1,4 bisphosphate-IP_3 and IP_4-Ca^{2+} pathway and 1,2-diacylgly-cerol-DAG-PKC pathway may increase protein synthesis in the Bio 14.6 heart.

ACKNOWLEDGMENT

This study was supported in part by Grants-in-Aid for Scientific Research from the Ministry of Education, Science and Culture 01870041, 02404042 and 02454250.

REFERENCES

1. Bajusz E. Hereditary cardiomyopathy: a new disease model. 1969;77:686–96.
2. Strobeck JE, Factor SM, Bhan A, et al. Hereditary and acquired cardiomyopathies in experimental animals: mechanical, biochemical, and structural features. *Ann NY Acad Sci* 1979;317:59–88.
3. Homburger F, Baker JR, Nixon CW, Whitney R. Primary generalized polymyopathy and cardiac necrosis in an inbred line of Syrian hamsters. *Med Exp* 1962;6:339–45.
4. Bajuz E, Baker JR, Nixon CW, Homburger F. Spontaneous hereditary myocardial degeneration and congestive heart failure in a strain of Syrian hamsters. *Ann NY Acad Sci* 1969;156:105–29.
5. Gerz EW. Cardiomyopathic Syrian hamster: a possible model of human disease. *Prog Exp Tumor Res* 1972;16:242–60.
6. Fasolato C, Pandiella A, Meldolesi J, Pozzan T. Generation of inositol phosphate, cytosolic Ca^{2+}, and ionic fluxes in $PC1_2$ cells treated with bradykinin. *J Biol Chem* 1988;263:17350–9.
7. Baker KM, Singer HA. Identification and characterization of guinea pig angiotensin II ventricular and atrial receptors: coupling to inositol phosphate production. *Circ Res* 1988;62:896–904.
8. Dubyak GR, Cowen DS, Meuller LM: Activation of inositol phospholipid breakdown in HL60 cells by P2-purinergic receptors for extracellular ATP. *J Biol Chem* 1988;263:18108–17.
9. Fujii S, Kawaguchi H, Okamoto H, Saito H, Togashi H, Yasuda H. Fatty acid binding protein of cardiac muscle in spontaneously hypertensive rats: effect of hypertrophy and its regression. *J Mol Cell Cardiol* 1988;20:779–787.
10. Kawaguchi H, Yasuda H. Prostacyclin biosynthesis and phospholipase activity in hypoxic rat myocardium. *Circ Res* 1988;62:1175–81.
11. Kawaguchi H, Yasuda H. Effect of platelet-activating factor on arachidonic acid metabolism in renal epithelial cells. *Biochim Biophys Acta* 1986;875:525–34.
12. Kawaguchi H, Yasuda H. Platelet-activating factor stimulates prostaglandin synthesis in cultured cells. *Hypertension* 1986;8:192–97.
13. Shoki M, Kawaguchi H, Okamoto H, et al. Phosphatidylinositol and inositolphosphatides metabolism in hypertrophied rat heart. *Jpn Circ J* 1992;56.142–7.
14. Kawaguchi H, Iizuka K, Takahashi H, Yasada H. Inositol trisphosphate kinase activity in hypertrophied rat heart. 1990;44:42–50.
15. Kawaguchi H, Shoki M, Iizuka K, Sano H, Sakata Y, Yasuda H. Phospholipid metabolism and prostacyclin synthesis in hypoxic myocytes. 1991;1094:161–7.
16. Kawaguchi H, Yasuda H. Effect of elastase on prostacyclin synthesis in aortic smooth muscle cells. *Biochim Biophys Acta* 1986;878:42–8.
17. Kawaguchi H, Yasuda H. Effect of elastase on phospholipase activity in aortic smooth muscle cells. *Biochim Biophys Acta* 1988;958:450–9.
18. Kawaguchi H, Shoki M, Sano H, et al. Phospholipid metabolism in cardiomyopathic hamster heart cells. *Circ Res* 1991;69:1015–21.

The Cardiomyopathic Heart, edited by Makoto
Nagano, Nobuakira Takeda, and Naranjan S.
Dhalla. Raven Press, Ltd., New York © 1994.

13

Alteration of 1,2-Diacylglycerol Content in Myopathic Hamster Hearts During the Development of Cardiomyopathy and Heart Failure

Kenji Okumura, Mitsuhiko Yoshino, Yoshio Iwama, Yukio Toki,
Yutaka Miyazaki, Hidekazu Hashimoto, Takayuki Ito, and
*Junzoh Kitoh

*The Second Department of Internal Medicine and *Institute for Laboratory Animal
Research, 65 Tsuruma-cho, Showa-ku, Nagoya University School of Medicine,
Nagoya 466, Japan*

INTRODUCTION

The evolution of genetic cardiomyopathy in Bio 14.6 strain Syrian hamsters can be characterized by several distinct stages. Focal myocardial necrotic lesions appear at about 30 to 40 days of age (1). These hamsters develop cardiomyopathy with hypertrophy and dilation of the heart chambers, and most finally die from congestive heart failure at about 250 to 350 days. The primary factor initiating the cascade of events leading to congestive heart failure in this model has been attributed to a myocardial calcium overload (2,3). Furthermore, how the processes of hypertrophy and fatal heart failure are related to biochemical properties has been partially elucidated (4–7). The accumulation of 1,2-DAG, presumably generated by the action of phosphatidylinositol-specific phospholipase C, plays multiple metabolic roles through the activation of protein kinase C in the transduction of a number of agonist-stimulated events (8). However, little information is available concerning the function and role of 1,2-DAG in the myocardium. This study was carried out to determine the amount of 1,2-DAG in normal and myopathic hamsters during the development of cardiomyopathy with hypertrophy and heart failure using thin-layer chromatography and a flame ionization detector (TLC-FID) technique for the quantitation of lipids (9).

MATERIALS AND METHODS

Animals and Preparation of Samples

The experiments were performed on Bio 14.6 strain Syrian hamsters of both sexes at 30, 90, 160, and 240 days of age. Age-matched, healthy, Syrian golden hamsters were obtained from Shizuoka Animal Laboratory Center (Shizuoka, Japan). The hamsters were fed standard laboratory chow *ad libitum*, but food was withheld from the animals 8 hours prior to sacrifice. Following decapitation, the hearts were immediately excised and washed with cold normal saline. Two 40- to 60-mg tissue samples from the left ventricle near the apex were frozen in liquid N_2 in order to use one piece for neutral lipid analysis and the other for phospholipid analysis. The remaining ventricle was freeze-dried and used for the determination of RNA and DNA concentrations.

Extraction and Analysis of Lipids

The frozen tissues were homogenized for 20 seconds with a motor-driven homogenizer in a chilled chloroform/methanol mixture (2:1, v/v) containing 0.01% butylated hydroxytoluene as an antioxidant and cholesteryl acetate (0.1 mg and 0.4 mg per tube for neutral lipid analysis and phospholipid analysis, respectively) as an internal standard. The filtrate was dried under a stream of N_2 gas at 30°C. For separation of nonpolar lipids from phospholipid, crude lipids were applied to a 0.5-ml silicic acid column (minus 325 mesh), equilibrated with chloroform and eluted with 8 ml of chloroform, and evaporated under N_2 gas. The myocardial lipid contents were measured using an Iatroscan TH-10 thin-layer chromatography analyzer (Iatron Laboratories, Tokyo, Japan) and a potentiometric recorder (Chromatocorder 11, System Instrument, Tokyo, Japan) following three- or four-step development on precoated silica gel thin-layer rods, as described elsewhere (9,10). Each sample was analyzed with three or four rods, and the results were averaged. For the fatty acid compositions of 1,2-DAG and triglyceride, the remaining lipids were separated by thin-layer chromatography on silica gel plate (20 cm × 20 cm, Kieselgel 60 F_{254} from Merk, Darmstadt, Germany). The spots corresponding to standard lipids were scraped off and extracted with a chloroform-methanol mixture (9:1 for nonpolar lipids and 2:1 for phospholipids). The extract was filtered through glass fiber filters and evaporated to dryness with N_2 gas. Fatty acids in each lipid fraction were transmethylated with boron trifluoride-methanol according to the method recommended by Morrison and Smith (11). Methylated fatty acids were analyzed by gas chromatography in a GC 14-A model apparatus (Shimadzu Co., Kyoto, Japan) equipped with a flame ionization detection and an HR 20 M flexible fused silica capillary column (25 m × 0.25 mm, i.d.). Peaks were identified by comparison with standards (Nu Check Prep. Inc., Elysian, MN), and peak areas were calculated with a chromatopac C-R6A (Shimadzu Co.).

The Determination of RNA and DNA Concentrations

The ventricular tissues were homogenized in cold 10% trichloroacetic acid. The precipitate was washed with 10% trichloroacetic acid. Lipids were removed by washing with 95% ethanol and then with an ethanol-ether mixture (3:1, v/v). The precipitate was incubated in 3% KOH for 60 minutes at 37°C for base hydrolysis of the RNA. The pentose of RNA was estimated by the orcinol procedure (12). The remaining precipitate was incubated in 5% trichloroacetic acid for 15 minutes at 90°C to extract DNA (13). The amount of DNA was determined by the diphenyl-amine procedure (14).

Statistics

The results are expressed as means ± standard error of the mean, and comparisons between the two different groups were assessed with two-way analysis of variance followed by Duncan's multiple range test, except in the case of lipid fatty acid composition, for which the Mann-Whitney U-test was used. A p value of <0.05 was considered statistically significant.

RESULTS

The myopathic hamsters had significantly elevated ratios of ventricular weight to body weight by 30%, 49%, and 85% at 90, 160, and 240 days of age, respectively, compared with the ratios of the corresponding normal hamsters (Table 1). At 30 days of age, the triglyceride content in the myopathic hamster hearts was greater than in the normal hearts, but the triglyceride content in normal hearts markedly increased with the growth of the hamsters (Table 1). Therefore, the myopathic animals had only one fourth of the triglycerides of normal hamsters at 240 days of age. Major phospholipids such as phosphatidylcholine, phosphatidylethanolamine, and cardiolipin were significantly lower in the myopathic hamsters than in normal hamsters after 90 days of age. However, the difference in such phospholipids between the two groups did not increase with the development of heart failure. Phosphatidylserine and phosphatidylinositol peaks were detected, but their mass determinations by means of the TLC/FID method described here were not reliable. Age-related increases in cholesterol levels and major phospholipid contents were observed in both strains. As shown in Fig. 1, 1,2-DAG contents in 30-day-old myopathic hearts were 19% higher than in normal hearts. There was no significant difference among 90-day-old hamsters between the two groups. In contrast, the 1,2-DAG levels in the myopathic hearts were significantly lower by 21% at 160 days and 52% at 240 days than in the corresponding control animals. The oldest hamsters in both groups showed significantly lower 1,2-DAG levels than 30-, 90-, and 160-day-old hamsters despite increases in triglyceride, cholesterol, and phospholipid contents.

TABLE 1. *Body weight, ventricular weight, and myocardial lipid contents in normal and myopathic hamsters*[a]

	30-day-old		90-day-old		160-day-old		240-day-old	
	Normal	Myopathic	Normal	Myopathic	Normal	Myopathic	Normal	Myopathic
Number of hamsters	8	6	8	6	7	8	8	8
Body weight (g)	54 ± 1	50 ± 1	135 ± 2	110 ± 3**	136 ± 5	118 ± 4**	158 ± 4	106 ± 8**
Ventricular weight (mg)	172 ± 3	173 ± 3	323 ± 5	341 ± 10	308 ± 12	397 ± 18**	345 ± 10	420 ± 23*
Ventricular weight/ body weight ratio (mg/g)	3.2 ± 0.1	3.5 ± 0.1**	2.4 ± 0.1	3.1 ± 0.1**	2.3 ± 0.1	3.4 ± 0.1**	2.2 ± 0.1	4.0 ± 0.2**
Triglyceride	3.6 ± 0.3	7.7 ± 1.2**	9.1 ± 0.7	6.3 ± 0.4	28.7 ± 1.5	9.1 ± 0.9**	50.8 ± 0.9	13.2 ± 2.3**
Cholesterol	2.1 ± 0.1	1.9 ± 0.1	1.7 ± 0.1	1.9 ± 0.1	2.5 ± 0.1	2.4 ± 0.1	2.8 ± 0.2	2.9 ± 0.1
Cardiolipin	2.7 ± 0.2	2.6 ± 0.2	2.7 ± 0.2	2.4 ± 0.1	3.0 ± 0.2	2.6 ± 0.1	3.3 ± 0.1	2.8 ± 0.1**
Phosphatidylethanolamine	7.1 ± 0.4	6.3 ± 0.3	7.8 ± 0.3	6.3 ± 0.2**	10.2 ± 0.3	9.1 ± 0.2**	11.6 ± 0.5	10.0 ± 0.4**
Phosphatidylcholine	6.8 ± 0.3	7.1 ± 0.3	8.1 ± 0.4	6.7 ± 0.2*	9.5 ± 0.4	7.8 ± 0.2**	9.9 ± 0.5	8.4 ± 0.5**
Sphingomyelin	0.3 ± 0.1	0.4 ± 0.1	0.3 ± 0.1	0.3 ± 0.1	0.4 ± 0.1	0.4 ± 0.1	0.3 ± 0.1	0.3 ± 0.1

[a]Values of lipid contents are expressed as $\mu g/mg$ wet weight. Mean ± standard error of the mean.

*$p < 0.05$, compared with age-matched normal hamsters.

**$p < 0.01$, compared with age-matched normal hamsters.

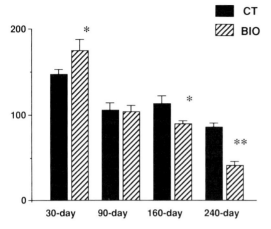

FIG. 1. 1,2-Diacylglycerol contents in normal (CT) and myopathic (BIO) hamster hearts. Each column represents the mean value ± standard error of the mean. *$p < 0.05$, **$p < 0.01$, compared with corresponding controls.

The profile of fatty acid compositions of 1,2-DAG in 240-day-old myopathic hamsters, which were found in the lowest level of 1,2-DAG, were different from those in normal hamsters (Fig. 2). The percentages of 18:0 and 20:4 (n = 6) increased and that of 18:1 (isomers) decreased by 2% to 4% in myopathic hearts. Also, differences in fatty acid composition between the two groups were found in triglycerides, and the differences were similar to those in 1,2-DAG despite different fatty acid compositions (Fig. 3).

Figure 4 shows ventricular RNA and DNA concentrations in the myocardium.

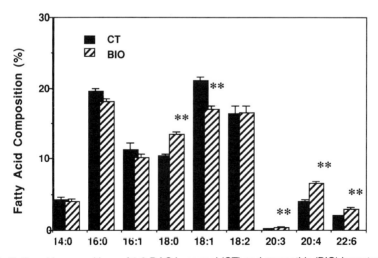

FIG. 2. Fatty acid compositions of 1,2-DAG in normal (CT) and myopathic (BIO) hamster hearts at 240 days of age. Values are presented as means ± standard error of the mean from seven to eight hamsters. The fatty acids are expressed as % area of chromatograms. ** indicates $p < 0.01$ compared with normal hamsters by the Mann-Whitney U-test.

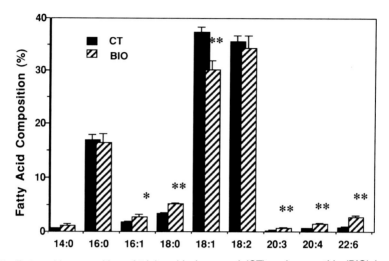

FIG. 3. Fatty acid composition of triglyceride in normal (CT) and myopathic (BIO) hamster hearts at 240 days of age. Values are presented as means ± standard error of the mean from seven to eight hamsters. The fatty acids are expressed as % area of chromatograms. *$p<0.05$ and **$p<0.01$, respectively, compared with normal hamsters by the Mann-Whitney U-test.

The RNA concentrations in the myopathic hamsters were greater at any stage of growth than in the normal animals. Higher DNA concentrations in the myopathic hamsters were also observed. Both DNA and RNA concentrations decreased with the growth of hamsters.

DISCUSSION

Studies on biologic membranes show that lipid components play an important role in providing a suitable microenvironment for the function of membrane proteins. It is conceivable that the changes in several functions, such as Ca^{2+} adenosine triphosphatase (ATPase) activity (15) and Na^{+}-Ca^{2+} exchange (16), are caused in part by the alteration of membrane phospholipids. The changes in major phospholipids observed in this study have been reported in whole homogenates of hearts (17) and in cardiac plasma membranes (15,18), but there was no significant change in prenecrotic heart tissues (17). A decrease in myocardial phospholipid content may be associated with cardiomyopathies (10). However, the abnormalities of phospholipid species were not related to the development of congestive heart failure. Moreover, these abnormalities were not noted in 30-day-old myopathic hearts, although myocardial RNA and DNA concentrations increased, indicating that the alteration of membrane phospholipids does not lead to the initiation of cardiomyopathy. Therefore, other important events may be more related to the initiation and development of cardiomyopathies and heart failure.

In this study, we observed the change in myocardial 1,2-DAG content regarding

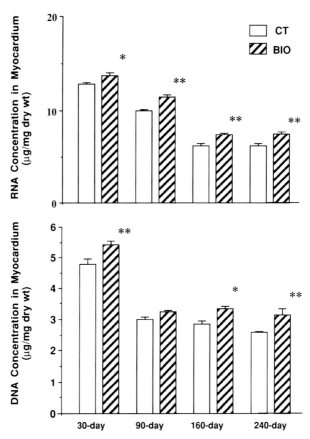

FIG. 4. RNA and DNA concentrations in normal (CT) and myopathic (BIO) hamster hearts. Each column represents the mean value ± standard error of the mean. *$p<0.05$, **$p<0.01$, compared with corresponding controls.

age in normal hearts, and such an age-related decrease in 1,2-DAG appeared to be associated with that in DNA and RNA concentrations. A significant increase in 1,2-DAG content was observed in 30-day-old myopathic hearts that did not show marked hypertrophy. There was no difference in 1,2-DAG content at 90 days of age between normal and myopathic hamsters. Then 1,2-DAG contents in myopathic hearts decreased as the stage of cardiomyopathy and heart failure progressed. At the prenecrotic stage (30 days of age), higher concentrations of DNA and RNA than in normal animals were accompanied by the increase in 1,2-DAG, which may initiate hypertrophy (19,20). At the stage of heart failure, enhanced RNA concentration appears to indicate augmented protein synthesis in heart failure (21). However, the alteration of 1,2-DAG was not directly related to changes in RNA and DNA concentrations when compared with normal hamster hearts. 1,2-DAG production is believed to result chiefly from phosphoinositide hydrolysis, which can be stimulated by several agonists via phospholipase C activation. In the myocardium, evidence that 1,2-DAG accumulation induced by norepinephrine is induced by α_1-adrenergic receptor has been shown (22), and this event is presumably accompanied by an increase in inositol trisphosphate (23). The difference in fatty acids involved in the accumulated 1,2-DAG may not be equivalent activators of protein kinase C (24). Our data show that there was a difference in fatty acid compositions not only in 1,2-DAG but also in triglyceride. Since several mechanisms of 1,2-DAG formation other than phosphoinositide hydrolysis have been proposed (25,26), it is useful to determine the source of 1,2-DAG, and fatty acid analysis of this compound may be helpful in this respect. However, it cannot be excluded that such differences in fatty acids might be attributable to differences in species of animals.

SUMMARY

We determined the level of 1,2-diacylglycerol (1,2-DAG) and its fatty acid composition in heart tissues from Bio 14.6 strain Syrian hamsters during the development of cardiomyopathy and congestive heart failure. Myopathic hearts had a 19% higher content of 1,2-DAG at a prenecrotic stage (30 days of age) than normal hamsters. No difference in 1,2-DAG content was observed at 90 days of age. However, 1,2-DAG content in myopathic hearts at 160 and 240 days of age was significantly lower by 21% and 52%, respectively, than in age-matched normal hamsters. The oldest hamsters showed reduced 1,2-DAG levels in both groups despite an age-related increase in most lipids. The 1,2-DAG fatty acid composition profile was found to be different from that of triglyceride, and there were several differences in the fatty acid composition of 1,2-DAG between the two groups at 240 days of age. Myocardial DNA and RNA concentrations in myopathic hearts were higher than those in normal hamsters, but the difference was not associated with the development of heart failure and the difference in 1,2-DAG. These results indicate that decreased levels of 1,2-DAG occur concomitantly with congestive heart failure in myopathic hamsters. Elevated 1,2-DAG levels at a prenecrotic stage might be involved in the initiation of cardiomyopathy.

ACKNOWLEDGMENTS

The authors are indebted to Dr. Takeshi Tomita (School of Agriculture, Nagoya University) for supplying Bio 14.6 strain hamsters and thank Miss Keiko Sakai for secretarial assistance in the preparation of the manuscript.

REFERENCES

1. Homburger F. Myopathy of hamster dystrophy: history and morphologic aspects. *Ann NY Acad Sci* 1979;317:2–17.
2. Borowski IFM, Harrow JAC, Pritchard ET, Dhalla NS. Changes in electrolyte and lipid contents of

the myopathic hamster (UM-X7.1) skeletal and cardiac muscle. *Res Commun Chem Pathol Pharmacol* 1974;7:443–51.

3. Lossnitzer K, Bajusz E. Water and electrolyte alterations during the life course of the BIO 14.6 Syrian golden hamster: a disease model of a hereditary cardiomyopathy. *J Mol Cell Cardiol* 1974;6:163–77.

4. Okumura K, Panagia V, Jasmin G, Dhalla NS. Sarcolemmal phospholipid N-methylation in genetically determined hamster cardiomyopathy. *Biochem Biophys Res Commun* 1987;143:31–7.

5. Weisman HF, Weisfeldt ML. Toward an understanding of the molecular basis of cardiomyopathies. *J Am Coll Cardiol* 1987;10:1135–8.

6. Kawaguchi H, Shoki M, Sano H, et al. Phospholipid metabolism in cardiomyopathic hamster heart cells. *Circ Res* 1991;69:1015–21.

7. Katoh Y, Komuro I, Takaku F, Yamaguchi H, Yazaki Y. Messenger RNA levels of guanine nucleotide-binding proteins are reduced in the ventricle of cardiomyopathic hamsters. *Circ Res* 1990;67:235–39.

8. Nishizuka Y. Studies and perspectives of protein kinase C. *Science* 1986;233:305–12.

9. Okumura K, Hashimoto H, Ito T, Ogawa K, Satake T. Quantitation of 1,2-diacylglycerol in rat heart by Iatroscan TLC/FID. *Lipids* 1988;23:253–5.

10. Okumura K, Akiyama N, Hashimoto H, Ogawa K, Satake T. Alteration of 1,2-diacylglycerol content in myocardium from diabetic rats. *Diabetes* 1988;37:1168–72.

11. Morrison WR, Smith LM. Preparation of fatty acid methyl esters and dimethylacetals from lipids with boron fluoride-methanol. *J Lipid Res* 1964;5:600–8.

12. Kerr SE, Seraidarian K. The separation of purine nucleosides from free purines and the determination of the purines and ribose in these fractions. *J Biol Chem* 1945;159:211–25.

13. Schneider WC. Determination of nucleic acids in tissues by pentose analysis. In: Colowick SP, Kaplan NO, eds. *Methods of enzymology.* New York: Academic Press, vol 3; 1957;680–4.

14. Burton K. A study of the conditions and mechanism of the diphenylamine reaction for the colorimetric estimation of deoxyribonucleic acid. *Biochem J* 1956;62:315–23.

15. Kuo TH, Tsang W, Wiener J. Defective Ca^{2+}-pumping ATPase of heart sarcolemma from cardiomyopathic hamster. *Biochim Biophys Acta* 1987;900:10–16.

16. Philipson KD, Frank JS, Nishimoto AY. Effects of phospholipase C on the Na^+-Ca^{2+} exchange and Ca^{2+} permeability of cardiac sarcolemmal vesicles. *J Biol Chem* 1983;258:5905–10.

17. Owens K, Weglicki WB, Sonnenblick EH, Gertz EW. Phospholipid and cholesterol content of ventricular tissue from the cardiomyopathic Syrian hamster. *J Mol Cell Cardiol* 1972;4:229–36.

18. Panagia V, Singh JN, Anand-Srivastava MB, Pierce GN, Jasmin G, Dhalla NS. Sarcolemmal alterations during the development of genetically determined cardiomyopathy. *Cardiovasc Res* 1984; 18:567–72.

19. Grove D, Nair KG, Zak R. Biochemical correlates of cardiac hyertrophy: III. Changes in DNA content; the relative contributions of polyploidy and mitotic activity. *Circ Res* 1969;25:463–71.

20. Gluck L, Talner NS, Stern H, Gardner TH, Kulovich MV. Experimental cardiac hypertrophy; concentrations of RNA in the ventricles. *Science* 1964;144:1244–5.

21. Paradis P, Rouleau J-L, Shenasa H, Brakier-Gingras L. Protein synthesis is increased in heart failure induced by low dose Adriamycin in rabbits. *Can J Physiol Pharmacol* 1989;67:197–201.

22. Okumura K, Kawai T, Hashimoto H, Ito T, Ogawa K, Satake T. Sustained diacylglycerol formation in norepinephrine-stimulated rat heart is associated with α_1-adrenergic receptor. *J Cardiovasc Pharmacol* 1988;11:651–6.

23. Kohl C, Schimtz W, Scholz H, et al. Evidence for α_1-adrenoceptor-mediated increase of inositol trisphosphate in the human heart. *J Cardiovasc Pharmacol* 1989;13:324–7.

24. Kerr DE, Kissinger LF, Gentry LE, Purchio AF, Shoyab M. Structural requirements of diacylglycerols for binding and activating phospholipid-dependent, Ca^{2+}-sensitive protein kinase. *Biochem Biophys Res Commun* 1987;148:776–82.

25. Kennerly DA. Diacylglycerol metabolism in mast cells: analysis of lipid metabolic pathways using molecular species analysis of intermediates. *J Biol Chem* 1987;262:16305–13.

26. Wolf BA, Williamson JR, Easom RA, Chang K, Sherman WR, Turk J. Diacylglycerol accumulation and microvascular abnormalities induced by elevated glucose levels. *J Clin Invest* 1991;87: 31–8.

The Cardiomyopathic Heart, edited by Makoto
Nagano, Nobuakira Takeda, and Naranjan S.
Dhalla. Raven Press, Ltd., New York © 1994.

14

Electrocardiographic Changes During Progression and Following Treatment of Hamster Cardiomyopathy

Gaëtan Jasmin, Libuse Proschek, *Michel Vermeulen, Fen Li, and
*René Cardinal

*Département de Pathologie, Université de Montréal, Montréal H3C 3J7, Canada; and
Centre de Recherche, Hôpital Sacré-Coeur, Montréal H4J 1C5, Canada

INTRODUCTION

The recent demonstration of dystrophin deficiency within the myocardium of the *mdx* mouse (1) has raised a good deal of interest in the etiopathology of primary cardiomyopathies. In myopathic Syrian hamsters, the genetic autosomal defect also involves the heart muscle, but the gene remains to be identified. Presumably, some essential structural protein(s) is lacking in heart cell membranes. The selective cardioprotection of certain calcium channel blockers (2,3) and the preventive action of some β-adrenoagonists and antagonists (4,5) strongly suggest defective membrane ionic regulation. Most likely, the necrotizing process in the heart in these myopathic animals relates to an abnormal energy metabolism in the mitochondria (6,7), with secondary calcium overload in myocytes and eventual loss of adrenergic tone leading to cardiac failure (8,9). Interestingly, calcium channel blockers, while preventing cardiac muscle damage, can also prolong the life span of cardiomyopathic animals (10). However, little is known, at least in these hamsters, about the preventive action of drugs on the development of heart failure. Accordingly, we undertook to evaluate the progression of myopathic changes in the heart in treated and untreated cardiomyopathic hamsters by means of ECG recordings at critical phases of the disease.

MATERIALS AND METHODS

A total of 165 male and female UM-X7.1 Syrian cardiomyopathic hamsters between 30 and 230 days old were used to study the progression of the disease by ECG recording. Fifty healthy male and female age-matched normal controls were also used. All animals were kept under optimal housing conditions (24°C with 12:12 hours light:dark cycle) and had free access to Purina Laboratory Chow and tap water. A growth curve was established by periodic weighing of normal and cardiomyopathic hamsters. At autopsy, the hearts were removed, blotted, weighed, and examined grossly for an overall estimation of necrotic changes; some hearts were fixed and processed for routine histologic examination using hemalum-phloxin-saffron as a stain (11). For therapeutic trials, we used 54 cardiomyopathic hamsters aged 200 ± 10 days with early to severe heart failure. They were treated with clentiazem, a congener of diltiazem (Nordic, Montreal, Quebec) or digitoxin (Sigma Chemicals, St. Louis, MO) for 7 to 10 days and subdivided as indicated in the table of results. The drugs were solubilized (clentiazem in physiologic saline and digitoxin in 1% carboxymethyl cellulose) and injected twice daily. Clentiazem was given intraperitoneally (AM) and subcutaneously (PM) in doses of 5 mg/kg body weight, and digitoxin subcutaneously (AM, PM) in doses of 1 mg/kg body weight. At autopsy, liver sclerosis, lung edema, and anasarca and atrial hypertrophy were scored from 0 to 3, depending upon the severity and extent of damage.

ELECTROCARDIOGRAPHIC RECORDINGS

Electrocardiographic readings, obtained by the computer averaging technique, were carried out under anesthesia (12) using sodium pentobarbital (45–50 mg/kg intraperitoneally). Ten to fifteen minutes prior to the recording, the animal was placed over a cotton pad, allowing it to rest in a natural prone position. Each of the four limbs was gently introduced into small copper tubes (9 mm id, 2-cm long) filled with conductive gel (EKG Sol, Graphic Controls Canada). These electrodes, a modification of the method of Lombard (13), were connected to bioelectric amplifiers (Nihon Kohden, Tokyo, Japan) with handwidth settings of 0.08 to 5,000 Hz to measure the three standard bipolar leads (I, II, and III). The amplifier outputs were led into a data acquisition system consisting of a digitizing board (Data Translation, Model DT-2821, Marlboro, MA) and microcomputer (Compaq Desqpro 286, Houston, TX) for A/D conversion at a sampling rate of 4,000/sec/channel. The numerical readings were transferred to the computer memory and processed on-line. After 5 minutes of an equilibration period, 60 to 90 beats were recorded, aligned, and averaged to eliminate noise (e.g., from muscular contraction, 60 Hz). The following variables were then computed: RR interval (msec), PR interval (msec), QRS width (msec), QT interval (from QRS onset to apex of T wave: QαT), and R, S, and T wave amplitudes for each lead. QαT was normalized for RR variations (QαTc = QαT/square root [RR]). To assess the reproducibility of the ECG tracings, 10 normal controls were used on different days and their ECGs recorded; no appreciable changes were noted. All animal investigations were carried out according to the guidelines for animal experimentation.

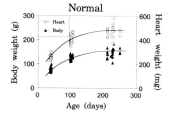

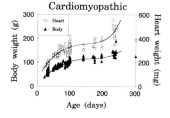

FIG. 1. Although the mean body weight values remain lower in cardiomyopathic hamsters than in normals for the total life span, the heart weight readings increase with the development and severity of terminal heart failure.

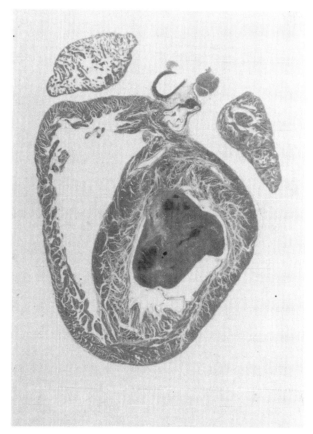

FIG. 2. Transection of a myopathic heart during the late stage of heart failure. Note the presence of a mural thrombus in the right ventricle.

RESULTS

Cardiomyopathic hamsters revealed consistently lower body weights than their age-matched normal controls. With progression of the disease, however, their hearts become dilated and heavier, indicating a cardiac hypertrophy (Fig. 1); dilation of both ventricles usually appeared after 6 months, often with formation of a wall thrombus (Fig. 2).

Representative ECG computerized tracings of younger and older adult normal and cardiomyopathic hamsters are shown in Fig. 3. The ECGs of the normal animals show taller and deeper waves and shorter intervals than those of cardiomyopathic hamsters; the earliest and most consistent changes observed in myopathic hearts were (a) progressive flattening and even inversion of the T wave; (b) a decrease in the amplitude of the R wave, mostly evident in lead III, and (c) prolongation of the intervals. A progressive decrease in heart rate with age was observed in cardiomyopathic and to a lesser extent in normal hamsters, as shown in Fig. 4A (RR interval is inversely related to heart rate). A marked early prolongation in the duration of PR and QTc intervals during the development of the disease was striking (Figs. 4B and 5A). Unexpectedly, the PR intervals were even significantly longer in cardiomyopathic females (independently of a previous pregnant state) than those in their age-matched male counterparts (Fig. 5B). Sex differences were not observed in duration of the RR interval in cardiomyopathic animals or in normal controls. Surprisingly, there were no appreciable differences in duration of the QRS

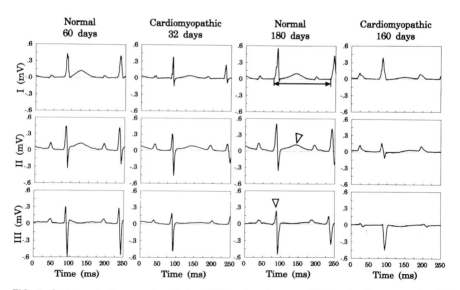

FIG. 3. Compared with normal controls, ECG tracings in myopathic hearts show a greater RR interval by 160 days of age. In addition, the amplitude of R and T waves (*arrowheads*) is significantly depressed.

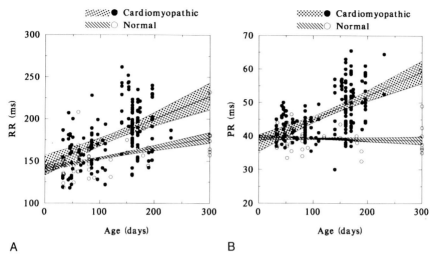

FIG. 4. Prolonged RR and PR intervals are readily seen in cardiomyopathic hamsters by 50 days of age.

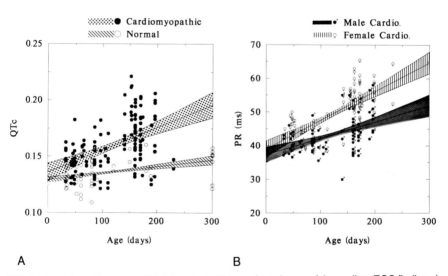

FIG. 5. The elongation of the QTc interval at 30 days of age is one of the earliest ECG findings in myopathic hamsters. On the right side, the difference in PR intervals between male and female cardiomyopathic hamsters is shown.

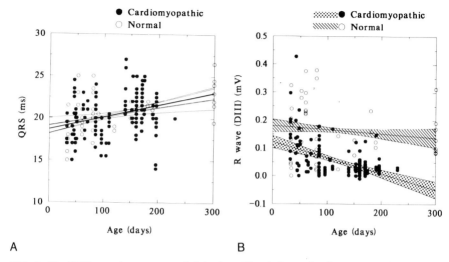

FIG. 6. The QRS complex was very slightly altered in relation to the time course of the disease, except for a relatively low amplitude of the R wave.

complex between cardiomyopathic and normal hamsters (Fig. 6A); the values were greatly scattered, sometimes overlapping and showing little relevance to age. The R wave was progressively and significantly reduced or even undetectable in lead III in cardiomyopathic hamsters with marked ascitic fluids, liver enlargement, and sclerosis. However, this phenomenon was negligible in normal controls of different ages (Fig. 6B). Similarly, the flattening or even inversion of the T wave was a prominent and regular feature in cardiomyopathic animals (Fig. 7). Most likely, this is attributable to depolarization abnormalities in cardiomyopathic hearts.

Pathologic changes during heart failure following a short treatment (7 to 10 days)

TABLE 1. *Pathologic changes during early and moderate*

Treatment (no. animals)	Dose (mg/kg/day)	Mortality (%)	Liver sclerosis	
			Severity (grade 0–3)	Incidence (%)
Untreated controls n = 12	vehicles	10	1.9 ± 1.2	58
Clentiazem n = 32	10 ip; sc	0	1.4 ± 0.8	37
Digitoxin n = 10	2 sc; sc	0	2.1 ± 0.7	70

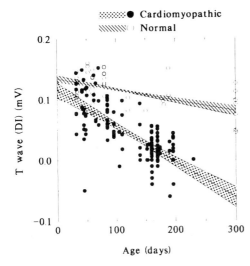

FIG. 7. The flattening of the T wave is most indicative of a defective depolarization in the myopathic heart.

with clentiazem or digitoxin are summarized in Table 1. Both clentiazem and digitoxin had a favorable effect on the life span of myopathic animals and resulted in some improvement in lung edema, anasarca, or right atrial hypertrophy. Cytoprotection was best achieved by clentiazem, as revealed by a significant reduction in liver sclerosis. In order to estimate the effect of these drugs on impaired electrical activities of cardiomyopathic hearts during heart failure, electrocardiographic readings were made before and after treatment was completed. The computed readings are shown in Fig. 8. After clentiazem treatment, the ventricular electrical activity was significantly improved, as evidenced by a greater amplitude of the R wave in lead III just like the T wave in lead II. On the other hand, the duration of intervals was almost unchanged.

stages of heart failure in cardiomyopathic treated hamsters[a]

Lung edema		Anasarca		Right atrial hypertrophy	
Severity (grade 0–3)	Incidence (%)	Severity (grade 0–3)	Incidence (%)	Severity (grade 0–3)	Incidence (%)
1.9 ± 0.8	100	1.4 ± 0.7	75	2.1 ± 0.4	72
1.2 ± 1.0	50	1.0 ± 0.8	56	1.6 ± 1.1	62
1.6 ± 0.6	100	1.1 ± 0.9	80	2.2 ± 0.7	60

[a]Means ± SE; hamsters, UM-X7.1, aged 200 ± 10 days were treated for 7 to 10 days. ip, intraperitoneally; sc, subcutaneously.

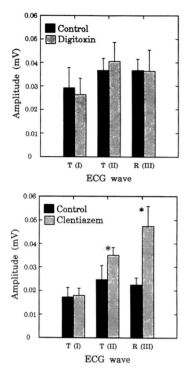

FIG. 8. A significant improvement in T(II) and R(III) wave amplitudes resulted from a 10-day treatment with clentiazem. No such effect was observed after digitoxin treatment.

DISCUSSION

In the present study, the computer averaging technique has considerably facilitated estimation of heart electrical activities in cardiomyopathic hamsters with very accurate and reliable ECG recordings. Because of the noninvasive nature of this approach, we have been able to better characterize the progression of the heart disease with or without the effect of certain cardioactive drugs. The electrical signals obtained provided a new dimension in understanding of pathologic process and possible clues to the cause and management of heart failure in these animals (14,15). The conventional ECG waves in mammals i.e., P wave (atrial depolarization), QRS complex (ventricular depolarization), and T wave (ventricular repolarization), (all but a Q wave) were identifiable in the hamster ECG, together with a well-defined isoelectrical line. To analyze the ECGs, we focused our attention primarily on the time intervals and on the amplitudes that were substantially changed (16). As a rule, all time intervals (PR, QαTc) were significantly elongated, and the amplitude tended to diminish with age, i.e., with progression of the disease in cardiomyopathic hamsters more conspicuously than in normal controls. On the other hand, only a marginal widening of the QRS complex was seen during the course of disease, without substantial differences when considering natural aging. This finding was unexpected because the QRS complex represents the elapsing time for the intraventricular conduction. It thus can be inferred that disseminated necrotic foci do not significantly impair ventricular depolarization. In fact, the cardioprotection elicited by gallopamil, a potent calcium and agonist, was unable to alter the QRS complex width (personal observation); on the contrary, the atrioventricular conduction was delayed as much as the electrical systolic changes. Hence, the hamster cardiomyopathy is characterized by a rapid and substantial lengthening of the PR interval, which is detectable at early age. This lengthening can eventually lead to atrioventricular block. In addition, we found significant differences in the PR intervals between cardiomyopathic females and males, and, surprisingly, the gap was greater in females. This finding was unexpected because no such difference exists in normal controls. The severity of heart lesions, however, is always greater in females than in males (personal observation).

The occurrence of sudden death in aging cardiomyopathic hamsters without evident clinical signs of heart failure has always been puzzling. It appears that a significant prolongation of the QTc interval indicates that the myopathic hamster heart is prone to developing lethal arrhythmia (17). A longer plateau duration of the action potential in cardiomyopathic hamsters (18) as a consequence of an altered inward Ca^{++} current (Bkaily, personal observation) most likely contributes to the prolongation of the QTc interval (19). The question of whether or not the long QT syndrome, an inherited disorder, could be implicated in hamster cardiomyopathy deserves further attention (20). No appreciable modifications in the P wave have been observed; this is not surprising, since the atria are not primarily affected in this inherited disease.

A progressive attenuation of the R wave amplitude might be attributed to a deterioration of cardiomyocytes and to an eventual change in the thoracic configuration (21). On the other hand, some old cardiomyopathic hamsters with hypertrophied hearts showed a taller R wave. Thus, the increase in muscle mass may counteract the electrophysiologic signal as a result of an overall loss of cardiocytes (22).

The flattening of the T wave as a prominent feature in the cardiomyopathic hamsters has also been reported in Duchenne's or Becker's and other forms of muscular dystrophies (23–25) and even in rats chemically treated with hydrocortisone (26). On the other hand, the lack of effect of digitoxin on ECG abnormalities supports our previous observations concerning the lack of efficacy of this treatment in the necrotization process and heart failure in cardiomyopathic hamsters. Digitoxin did not alter the heart rate as compared with the heart rate in untreated animals (310 beats/ min versus 320 beats/min, respectively). Clentiazem was better tolerated in spite of a diminution of heart rate (265 beats/min). The amplitudes of T and R waves were significantly taller than in those of untreated animals. The taller R wave is apparently not related to heart hypertrophy (22) but rather to reduction of edema in as much as to the thoracic size (21). Interestingly, treatment with clentiazem does not seem incompatible with use of a β-blocker such as propanolol.

SUMMARY

Electrocardiographic parameters were investigated in 50 normal and 165 myopathic hamsters aged between 30 and 230 days to further characterize the necrotizing and scarring process in the myocardium and the severity of heart failure. Prior to the development of necrotic changes (± 30 days), there were no appreciable changes compared with normal controls. The development of necrotic lesions at 45 days and over resulted in the depression of R- and T-wave amplitude with concomitant prolongation of QTc and PR intervals. With aging, there was a decrease in heart rate, and this was more obvious in cardiomyopathic hamsters. With the occurrence of heart failure, T and R waves were further depressed until a complete flattening occurred. On the other hand, electrocardiogram (ECG) readings were improved after treatment with clentiazem, a calcium antagonist, using a dosage of 10 mg/kg. This drug even succeeded in reducing the severity of congestive liver sclerosis. However, digitoxin given in a daily dose of 2 mg/kg, could not prevent deterioration of heart failure except in a few animals treated at an earlier stage.

Thus, ECG studies in UM-X7.1 cardiomyopathic hamsters have revealed an overall reduction of electrical activity in myopathic hearts. As a rule, the heart rate becomes slower with progression of the disease. Most striking, the PR interval was found to be elongated at the early stage of the disease, suggesting a delay in atrioventricular conduction. Myopathic hearts are prone to develop arrhythmias, as evidenced by a longer QTc interval. There was an impaired repolarization of heart ventricle as revealed by the depression of the T wave. The P wave was little altered or unaltered, indicating that atria, at least during the early stages of the disease, escape the myopathic process. Clentiazem, a calcium blocker, can prevent premature death in these animals by improving ventricular repolarization.

ACKNOWLEDGMENT

This work was supported by a grant from Nordic Laboratories Inc., Laval, Quebec, Canada. We gratefully acknowledge the secretarial and photographic work of Line Bolduc and Gaston Lambert.

REFERENCES

1. Arahata K, Ishiura S, Ishiguro T, et al. Immunostaining of skeletal and cardiac muscle surface membrane with antibody against Duchenne muscular dystrophy peptide. *Nature* 1988;333:861–3.
2. Jasmin G, Bajusz E. Polymyopathie et cardiomyopathie héréditaire chez le hamster de Syrie. Inhibition sélective des lésions du myocarde. *Ann Anat Pathol* 1973;18:49–66.
3. Jasmin G, Solymoss BC. Prevention of hereditary cardiomyopathy in the hamster by verapamil and other agents. *Proc Soc Exp Biol Med* 1975;149:193–8.
4. Jasmin G, Proschek L. The paradoxical effect of isoproterenol on hamster hereditary polymyopathy. *Muscle Nerve* 1983;6:408–15.
5. Jasmin G, Solymoss BC, Proschek L. Therapeutic trials in hamster dystrophy. *Ann NY Acad Sci* 1979;317:338–48.
6. Proschek L, Jasmin G. Hereditary polymyopathy and cardiomyopathy in the Syrian hamster. II.

Development of heart necrotic changes in relation to defective mitochondrial function. *Muscle Nerve* 1982;5:26–32.

7. Wikman-Coffelt J, Sievers R, Parmley WW, Jasmin G. Cardiomyopathic and healthy acidotic hamsters hearts: mitochondrial activity may regulate cardiac performance. *Cardiovascular Res* 1986; 20:471–81.

8. Sole MJ, Chi-Man L, Laird CW, Sonnenblick EH, Wurtman RJ. Norepinephrine turnover in the heart and spleen of the cardiomyopathic Syrian hamster. *Circ Res* 1975;37:855–62.

9. Jasmin G, Proschek L. The permissive role of catecholamines in the pathogenesis of the hamster cardiomyopathy. In: Chazov E, Sacks V, Rona G, eds. *Advances in myocardiology*. New York: Plenum Press; 1983:45–53.

10. Jasmin G, Proschek L. Comparative effects of Ca antagonists and of inotropic agents upon development of the hamster hereditary cardiomyopathy. In: Bender/Meesman, eds. *Proceedings of the International symposium on gallopamil*. Berlin: December 1986. Steinkopff Verlag Darmstadt; 1989.

11. Jasmin G, Proschek L. Hereditary polymyopathy and cardiomyopathy in the Syrian hamster. 1. Progression of heart and skeletal muscle lesions in the UM-X7.1 line. *Muscle Nerve* 1982;5:20–5.

12. Budden R, Buschmann G, Kühl UG. The rat ECG in acute pharmacology and toxicology. In: Budden R, Detweiler DK, Zbinden G, eds. *The rat electrocardiogram in pharmacology and toxicology*. Oxford: Pergamon Press; 1981:41–82.

13. Lombard Elna A. Electrocardiograms of small mammals. *Am J Physiol* 1952;171:189–93.

14. Bhattacharya SK, Crawford AJ, Pate JW. Electrocardiographic, biochemical, and morphologic abnormalities in dystrophic hamsters with cardiomyopathy. *Muscle Nerve* 1987;10:168–76.

15. Lossnitzer K, Grewe N, Konrad A, Adler J. Electrocardiographic changes in cardiomyopathic Syrian hamsters (strain BIO 8262). *Basic Res Cardiol* 1977;72:421–35.

16. Detweiler DK. The use of electrocardiography in toxicological studies with rats. In: Budden R, Detweiler DK, Zbinden G, eds. *The rat electrocardiogram in pharmacology and toxicology*. Oxford: Pergamon Press; 1981:83–115.

17. Osamu H, Mitsuoka Takao M, Yoriaki M, et al. Arrhythmogenic properties of the ventricular myocardium in cardiomyopathic Syrian hamster, BIO 14.6 strain. *Cardiovasc Res* 1991;25:49–57.

18. Rossner KL, Sachs HG. Electrophysiological study of Syrian hamster hereditary cardiomyopathy. *Cardiovasc Res* 1978;12:436–43.

19. Spear JF. Relationship between the scalar ECG and cellular electrophysiology of the rat heart. In: Budden R, Detweiler DK, Zbinden G, eds. *The rat electrocardiogram in pharmacology and toxicology*. Oxford: Pergamon Press; 1981:29–40.

20. Vincent GM, Timothy KW, Leppert M, Keating M. The spectrum of symptoms and QT intervals in carriers of the gene for the long-QT syndrome. *N Engl J Med* 1992;327:846–52.

21. Jensen RA, Acton EM, Peters JH. Doxorubicin cardiotoxicity in the rat: comparison of electrocardiogram, transmembrane potential, and structural effects. *J Cardiovasc Pharmacol* 1984;6:186–200.

22. Hodgkins BC, Nelson CV, Angelakos ET. Cardiac electrical resultant dipole moment of spontaneously hypertensive rats. *Am J Physiol* 1981;241:H541–6.

23. Perloff JH. Cardiac rhythm and conduction in Duchenne's muscular dystrophy: a prospective study of 20 patients. *J Am Coll Cardiol* 1984;3:1263–78.

24. Sanyal SK, Johnson WW. Cardiac conduction abnormalities in children with Duchenne's muscular dystrophy: ECG features and morphologic correlates. *Circulation* 1982;66:853–63.

25. Fitzpatrick AP, Shapiro LM, Rickards AF, Poole-Wilson PA. Familial restrictive cardiomyopathy with atrioventricular block and skeletal myopathy. *Br Heart J* 1990;63:114–18.

26. Badarau G, Wasserman L, Dolinesco S. Recherche sur les relations entre les modifications électrocardiographiques et les processus morphopathologiques au cours de l'évolution des myocardodystrophies expérimentales chez le rat. *Rev Roum Méd Int* 1969;6,2:121–30.

The Cardiomyopathic Heart, edited by Makoto Nagano, Nobuakira Takeda, and Naranjan S. Dhalla. Raven Press, Ltd., New York © 1994.

15

Effect of Angiotensin-Converting Enzyme Inhibitor on Myocardial Collagen Metabolism in Cardiomyopathic Hamsters

Tsutomu Araki, Masami Shimizu, Norihiko Sugihara, Hiroyuki Yoshio, Hidekazu Ino, and Ryoyu Takeda

The Second Department of Internal Medicine, School of Medicine, Kanazawa University, Takara-machi 13-1, Kanazawa 920, Japan

INTRODUCTION

Collagen is the major component of the cardiac interstitium, and its quantitative and qualitative changes are thought to exert some influence on cardiac structure and function. Recently, Weber et al. (1) emphasized the significance of the cardiac interstitium, especially collagen, and proposed the new terms of "*interstitial heart disease*" and "*cardiopathy*" in lieu of cardiomyopathy. Myocardial collagen metabolism has been extensively studied in hypertrophied hearts. Recently, much attention has been paid to qualitative changes in collagen, especially collagen types, and the association between the collagen types and cardiac function, which Weber et al. (2) described using the new term of "*collagen remodeling.*"

On the other hand, the cardiomyopathic hamster is frequently used as an animal model of human cardiomyopathy. In this model, the increase in the interstitial fibrosis of the myocardium, mostly composed of collagen, is commonly observed with aging (3). However, the details of myocardial collagen metabolism in the cardiomyopathic hamster are still unclear.

In the present study, to clarify myocardial collagen metabolism in the cardiomyopathic hamster, the collagen content, as quantitative changes in collagen, was measured by determining the collagen-specific amino acid, hydroxyproline. The ratio of type I to type III collagen (type I/III ratio), as qualitative changes in collagen, was determined by SDS-PAGE. In addition, the effects of the ACE inhibitor captopril on the collagen content and type I/III ratio were studied.

MATERIALS AND METHODS

Experimental Animals

Five-week-old male Bio 14.6 cardiomyopathic hamsters were treated with the ACE inhibitor captopril (20 mg/kg/day) in drinking water for 20 weeks, and the heart weight to body weight ratio, collagen content, and type I/III ratio at 25 weeks were measured and compared with those in 5- and 25-week-old untreated Bio 14.6 and normal F1b hamsters. Each group contained 6 hamsters. All hamsters were weighed, and then the hearts were removed immediately after anesthesia with diethylether and washed in ice-cold 0.05 M TRIS-HCl buffer (pH 7.4) containing 5 mM ethylenediaminetetra-acetic acid (EDTA) and 1 M NaCl. The atria and great vessels were separated from the heart, and the remaining ventricular wet weights were measured as the heart weight. A small part of the left ventricle was selected for determination of the hydroxyproline content and histologic examination.

Extraction of Collagen

The tissue was cut into small pieces and homogenized in ice-cold 0.05 M TRIS-HCl buffer (pH 7.4) containing 5 mM EDTA and 1 M NaCl with a homogenizer. The homogenates were washed in the same buffer for 24 hours and centrifuged at 3,000 g for 15 minutes at 4°C. The precipitates were suspended and washed in 0.5 M acetic acid for 24 hours and centrifuged at 3,000 g for 15 minutes at 4°C. The precipitates were digested with pepsin (10 mg pepsin/g wet weight of tissue) in 0.05 M acetic acid (10 ml acetic acid/g wet weight of tissue) for 24 hours and centrifuged at 10,000 g for 60 minutes at 4°C, and the first supernatants were obtained. The remaining precipitates were again digested with pepsin as described above, and the second supernatants were added to the first ones. The pepsin in the supernatants was inactivated with NaOH for 24 hours at room temperature, and the gelatinous precipitates, predominantly consisting of types I and III collagens, were observed and separated by centrifugation at 10,000 g for 60 minutes at 4°C. The separated collagens were resolubilized in 5 mM acetic acid and analyzed by SDS-PAGE.

Sodium Dodecylsulfate–Polyacrylamide Gel Electrophoresis

The types of pepsin-extracted collagen were analyzed by SDS-PAGE in the presence of 3 M urea according to the method described by Hayashi and Nagai (4) with some modifications. Briefly, SDS-PAGE consisted of 3% stacking gel and 5% separating gel in TRIS-glycine buffers. Electrophoresis was carried out with a constant current of 20 mA per gel until Bromphenol Blue reached the bottom. Standard purified types I and III collagen extracted from porcine skin were used as a control and 0.1 M dithiothreitol was used for reduction. After electrophoresis, the gels were stained with Coomassie Brilliant Blue R 250 and subsequently destained in a solu-

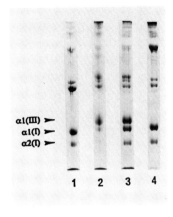

FIG. 1. SDS-PAGE of pepsin-extracted collagen from the myocardium of the hamster. Lanes 1 and 2 show the electrophoretic pattern of the standard type I and type III collagen (reduced) from porcine skin as a control. Lanes 3 and 4 are those of pepsin-extracted collagen from the myocardium of the hamster that was reduced (lane 3) and not reduced (lane 4).

tion of acetic acid and methanol. Under the conditions of electrophoresis in the presence of urea, clear separation of α_1 and α_2 chains of type I collagen and α_1 chains of type III collagen was achieved (Fig. 1), although α_1 chains of type I and III collagen move at the same rate in the absence of urea. The stained gels were scanned using a densitometer, and the recordings of the areas under each peak were determined using a planimeter. The areas representing α_1 chains were used to calculate the relative percentages of types I and III collagen.

Collagen Content

Myocardial tissues for determination of the hydroxyproline content were heated with 6 N HCl at 110°C for 24 hours to hydrolyze collagen into its component amino acids. The hydroxyproline content was measured spectrophotometrically by its reaction with Ehrlich's reagent according to the method described by Inayama et al. (5). The collagen content was calculated by multiplying the hydroxyproline content by the constant 7.46 and expressed as milligrams of collagen per gram ventricular wet weight.

Histologic Examination

Myocardial tissues for light microscopy were immediately submerged in 20% neutral buffered formalin (pH 7.4), embedded in paraffin, cut into sections 4-μm thick, and stained with Mallory-Azan stain to assess the degree of fibrosis.

Statistical Analysis

All results were expressed as mean ± standard deviation, and intergroup differences were evaluated by analysis variance followed by Scheffe's multiple comparison. Statistical significance was defined as $p < 0.05$.

TABLE 1. *Effects of captopril on myocardial collagen metabolism in cardiomyopathic hamsters*

	Normal F1b		Untreated Bio 14.6		Captopril-treated Bio 14.6
	5 weeks	25 weeks	5 weeks	25 weeks	25 weeks
BW (g)	127 ± 14	139 ± 12	91 ± 12	120 ± 16	106 ± 10
HW (mg)	384 ± 46	439 ± 19	331 ± 57	529 ± 66	412 ± 37*
HW/BW (mg/g)	3.04 ± 0.30	3.17 ± 0.17	3.64 ± 0.23	4.42 ± 0.11	3.91 ± 0.27*
Collagen content (mg/g)	3.11 ± 0.31	3.46 ± 0.31	3.80 ± 0.52	6.14 ± 0.48	4.53 ± 0.48**
Type I/III ratio	1.62 ± 0.32	2.07 ± 1.08	0.93 ± 0.11	0.81 ± 0.21	1.32 ± 0.22

*$p < 0.05$ and **$p < 0.01$ compared with 25-week-old untreated Bio 14.6 hamster.
BW, body weight; HW, heart weight; HW/BW, heart weight to body weight ratio.

RESULTS

Heart Weight to Body Weight Ratio

All results are shown in Table 1. There was a marked increase in the heart weight to body weight ratio with aging in the untreated Bio 14.6 as compared with the F1b hamster. Captopril treatment for 20 weeks significantly decreased this ratio in Bio 14.6 animals ($p < 0.05$).

Collagen Content

There was a marked increase in the collagen content with aging in the untreated Bio 14.6 as compared with F1b hamsters. Captopril treatment for 20 weeks significantly reduced the collagen content in Bio 14.6 animals ($p < 0.01$).

Type I/III Ratio

The type I/III ratio tended to increase (that is, type I collagen dominant) in F1b and decrease (that is, type III collagen dominant) in the untreated Bio 14.6 hamsters with aging. Captopril treatment for 20 weeks tended to retard the increase in the proportion of type III collagen and normalize the type I/III ratio in Bio 14.6 hamsters.

Histologic Findings

Histologic findings of the left ventricle in 25-week-old hamsters in each group are shown in Fig. 2. There was a marked increase in interstitial fibrosis and calcification in the untreated Bio 14.6 as compared with the F1b hamster. Captopril treatment decreased the interstitial fibrosis and calcification.

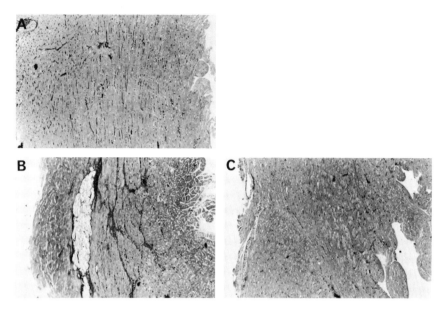

FIG. 2. Histologic findings of the myocardium in 25-week-old hamsters. **(A)** Normal F1b hamsters; **(B)** untreated Bio 14.6 hamsters; **(C)** captopril-treated Bio 14.6 hamsters. (Mallory-Azan stain, original magnification ×25.)

DISCUSSION

Human dilated cardiomyopathy is characterized by chamber dilatation and decreased myocardial contractility. Histologically, a marked increase in interstitial fibrosis is observed with the hypertrophy and degeneration of myocytes. Recently, Weber et al. (1,6) reported an increase in the proportion of type III collagen, which is thinner and has less tensile strength than type I collagen, by using the polarized light and picrosirius red technique, and they suggested an association between the increase in the proportion of type III collagen and chamber dilatation and decreased myocardial contractility in human dilated cardiomyopathic hearts. Cardiomyopathic hamster Bio 14.6 is an animal model of human cardiomyopathy. In this model, although a marked increase in interstitial fibrosis of the myocardium is commonly observed with aging, there have been no reports on myocardial collagen metabolism, especially changes in collagen types. In this paper, we clarified the myocardial collagen metabolism in the cardiomyopathic hamster by measuring the collagen content as quantitative changes in collagen and determining the type I/III ratio as qualitative changes in collagen. In summary, increases in the collagen content and proportion of type III collagen were observed with aging in cardiomyopathic hamsters as compared with normal hamsters. These results suggest the presence of quantitative and qualitative disorders of myocardial collagen metabolism in the cardiomyopathic hamster, and further, an association between the increase in the proportion of type III collagen and the deterioration of cardiac function in the cardio-myopathic hamster as well as in human dilated cardiomyopathy.

On the other hand, Weber et al. (7) have paid much attention to the association between fibrosis and the cardiac renin-angiotensin-aldosterone system in hyper-trophied hearts. They reported that angiotensin II or aldosterone was responsible for cardiac fibroblast proliferation and enhanced collagen synthesis, and that the ACE inhibitor captopril or the aldosterone antagonist spironolactone prevented fibrosis. Mukherjee et al. (8) examined the effects of captopril on the collagen content and type I/III ratio in spontaneously hypertensive rats and reported that captopril treat-ment did not significantly reduce the collagen content but did normalize the type I/III ratio. Kato et al. (9) examined the effects of captopril on the onset of cardio-myopathy in the cardiomyopathic J-2-N hamster and reported a decrease in the percentage of fibrosis by histologic examination. However, there have been no reports of the effects of captopril on myocardial collagen metabolism, especially changes in collagen types, in the cardiomyopathic hamster. In this paper, we also studied the effects of captopril on myocardial collagen metabolism in the cardio-myopathic hamster. In summary, the increases in the collagen content and propor-tion of type III collagen observed in the untreated cardiomyopathic hamster were suppressed by captopril treatment. These results suggest that captopril improves myocardial collagen metabolism in the cardiomyopathic hamster not only quan-titatively but also qualitatively, and that the mechanism of this improvement may be related to the cardiac renin-angiotensin-aldosterone system in cardiomyopathic hearts as well as in hypertrophied hearts.

In summary, we clarified the quantitative and qualitative derangements of myo-cardial collagen metabolism in the cardiomyopathic hamster and the improvement of these disorders by captopril treatment. We speculate that the interstitial fibrosis of the myocardium is related to the cardiac renin-angiotensin-aldosterone system in cardiomyopathic hearts.

SUMMARY

To clarify myocardial collagen metabolism in the cardiomyopathic hamster, which is an animal model of human cardiomyopathy, the collagen content, as quan-titative changes in collagen, was measured by determining the hydroxyproline con-tent. The ratio of type I to type III collagen (type I/III ratio), as qualitative changes in collagen, was determined by sodium dodecyl sulfate–polyacrylamide gel electro-phoresis (SDS-PAGE). In addition, the effects of an angiotensin-converting enzyme (ACE) inhibitor on the collagen content and type I/III ratio were studied. Five-week-old Bio 14.6 cardiomyopathic hamsters were treated with captopril (20 mg/kg/day) in their drinking water for 20 weeks, and the collagen content and type I/III ratio at 25 weeks are compared with those in 25-week-old untreated Bio 14.6 and normal F1b hamsters. Quantitatively, the collagen content markedly increased with aging in the untreated Bio 14.6 as compared with the F1b hamster. Qualitatively, the type I/III ratio tended to increase (that is, type I collagen became dominant) in F1b hamsters and decrease (that is, type III collagen became dominant) in the untreated Bio 14.6 hamsters significantly with age. Captopril treatment for 20 weeks reduced the collagen content significantly and tended to retard the increase in the proportion of type III collagen and normalize the type I/III ratio in the cardiomyopathic hamster. These results suggest that captopril improves myocardial collagen metabolism in the cardiomyopathic hamster not only quantitatively but also qualitatively, and that the mechanism of this improvement may be related to the cardiac renin-angiotensin-aldosterone system.

REFERENCES

1. Weber KT. Cardiac interstitium in health and disease: the fibrillar collagen network. *J Am Coll Cardiol* 1989;13:1637–52.
2. Weber KT, Janicki JS, Shroff SG, Pick R, Chen RM, Bashey RI, Collagen remodeling of the pressure-overloaded, hypertrophied nonhuman primate myocardium. *Circ Res* 1988;62:757–65.
3. Cohen-Gould L, Robinson TF, Factor ST. Intrinsic connective tissue abnormalities in the heart muscle of cardiomyopathic Syrian hamsters. *Am J Pathol* 1987;127:327–34.
4. Hayashi T, Nagai Y. Separation of the α chains of type I and III collagens by SDS-polyacrylamide gel electrophoresis. *J Biochem* 1979;86:453–9.
5. Inayama S, Shibata T, Ohtsuki J, Saito S. A new microanalytical method for determination of hydroxyproline in connective tissues. *Keio J Med* 1978;27:43–6.
6. Weber KT, Pick R, Janicki JS, Gadodia G, Lakier JB. Inadequate collagen tethers in dilated cardiopathy. *Am Heart J* 1988;116:1641–6.
7. Weber KT, Brilla CG. Pathological hypertrophy and cardiac interstitium. Fibrosis and renin-angiotensin-aldosterone system. *Circulation* 1991;83:1849–65.
8. Mukherjee D, Sen S. Collagen phenotypes during development and regression of myocardial hypertrophy in spontaneously hypertensive rats. *Circ Res* 1990;67:1474–80.
9. Kato M, Takeda N, Takeda A, Ohkubo T, Nagai M, Nagano M. Inhibitory effects of captopril on the onset of cardiomyopathy in cardiomyopathic hamsters. In: Korecky B, Dhalla NS, eds. *Subcellular basis of contractile failure*. Boston: Kluwer Academic Publishers; 1990:193–208.

The Cardiomyopathic Heart, edited by Makoto
Nagano, Nobuakira Takeda, and Naranjan S.
Dhalla. Raven Press, Ltd., New York © 1994.

16

Effects of an Angiotensin-Converting Enzyme Inhibitor, Cilazapril, on Congestive Heart Failure in Cardiomyopathic Hamsters

Fumiaki Nakamura, Masahiro Nagano, Ryuichi Kobayashi,
Jitsuo Higaki, Hiroshi Mikami, *Naomasa Kawaguchi,
*Shunzo Onishi, and Toshio Ogihara

*Department of Geriatric Medicine, Osaka University Medical School, Suita 565; and
*Department of Pathology, College of Biomedical Technology, Osaka University,
Toyonaka 560, Japan*

INTRODUCTION

In patients with congestive heart failure, the sympathetic nervous system and the renin-angiotensin system are activated to compensate for the cardiac dysfunction (1). However, the activation of these systems induces fluid retention and systemic vasoconstriction, resulting in further deterioration of ventricular function (2). Theoretically, pharmacologic inhibition of these systems would be beneficial in the treatment of congestive heart failure. Actually, ACE inhibitors are used for the treatment of congestive heart failure as first-line drugs (3), and their effectiveness in reducing mortality and morbidity has been widely recognized (4,5). However, the renin-angiotensin system essentially increases cardiac contractility through the angiotensin II (Ang II) receptor in the cardiac myocyte (6). Therefore, it appears paradoxical that its inhibition leads to an improvement of cardiac function. Since ACE inhibitors possess diuretic and inhibitory action of the sympathetic nervous system, these agents can also exert beneficial effects in the treatment of heart failure through these mechanisms.

This study was designed to elucidate the cardioprotective mechanisms of ACE inhibitor in heart failure, with special focus on the role of the cardiac renin-angiotensin system. We hypothesized that long-term inhibition of ACE may affect the cardiovascular response to Ang II, resulting in an improvement of cardiac performance in heart failure. The Bio cardiomyopathic hamster was used as a model of congestive heart failure because Ang II receptor has been shown to be present in cardiac tissue (7). Cilazapril was administered for 80 days in order to examine the chronic effects of ACE inhibition on cardiac performance.

MATERIALS AND METHODS

Animals and Drug Treatment

One-hundred-and-twenty-day-old male cardiomyopathic hamsters (Bio 14.6) and age-matched normal golden Syrian hamsters from Bio-Breeders (Pittsburgh, PA) were used. They were allowed free access to regular rat chow (Oriental Kobo Ltd., Osaka, Japan) and tap water and were housed under identical conditions before the experiments. Cardiomyopathic and golden Syrian hamsters were each randomly divided into two groups. Group 1 was given tap water (vehicle group) and Group 2 (cilazapril-treated group) was given cilazapril (donated by Eizai Co. Ltd., Tokyo, Japan) once a day (10 mg/kg body weight per day) by gastric gavage, beginning at 160 through 240 days of age.

Contraction Experiments

After the treatment period, hamsters were heparinized (1,000 U intraperitoneally) and anesthetized with sodium pentobarbital (50 mg/kg intraperitoneally). Then the heart and the thoracic aorta were removed ($n = 6$, for each of four groups). The heart was rapidly dissected out and placed in cold Krebs-Henseleit bicarbonate buffer (pH 7.4) solution saturated with 95% oxygen/5% carbon dioxide. The heart was perfused by the Langendorff method at 37°C with oxygenated modified Krebs-Henseleit buffer at a pressure of 60 mmHg, which was monitored with a blood pressure amplifier (AP-641G, Nihon Kohden Co., Tokyo, Japan) located at the level of the aortic valve. The hearts were electrically paced (electronic stimulator, SEN-3301, Nihon Kohden Co., Tokyo, Japan) at 270 beats/min via platinum electrodes spaced 3 mm apart and placed in contact with the base of the right ventricle. The duration of the stimulus was 5 msec at 2 to 3 volts. The left ventricle was catheterized with a 5F Mikro-tip catheter transducer (model MPC-500, Millar Instruments, Houston, TX) via the mitral valve for the measurement of left ventricular pressure. Thirty minutes was allowed for equilibration. Data obtained included left ventricular pressure and its first derivative, $LV + dP/dt_{max}$, monitored continuously and recorded on a pressure processor (model EQ-601G, Nihon Kohden Co., Tokyo, Japan). Left ventricular performance was assessed by determining the ability of the isolated heart to respond to infusion of Ang II. Ang II was infused continuously via a syringe pump (model STC-525, Terumo Ltd., Tokyo, Japan) into a cannula positioned just above the aortic stump at eight graded infusion rates (10^{-7}, 3×10^{-7}, 5.2×10^{-7}, 10^{-6}, 1.7×10^{-6}, 3×10^{-6}, 5.2×10^{-6}, and 10^{-5} M), for 5 minutes each.

Vascular contraction experiments were performed on thoracic aortic ring segments. Each aortic ring segment (2 mm) was mounted on stirrups in a 25-ml tissue bath. The resting tension of the aorta was set at 1 g, and the tension was recorded isometrically (FD pick up, model TB-612T, Nihon Kohden Co., Japan). The mounted vascular segment was bathed at 37°C in Krebs' solution bubbled with 95% O_2 and 5% CO_2. Aortic contractile responses to exogenous Ang II and norepinephrine were assessed. After 60 minutes of equilibration, KCl solution was injected into the tissue bath at a final concentration of 20 mM. At 30 minutes after KCl injection, the tissues were washed three times over 30 minutes in Krebs' solution to allow the tension to return to the basal level. Ang II or norepinephrine was then injected as a bolus (Ang II, 250 μl; norepinephrine, 450 μl) in five graded concentrations (Ang II, 10^{-10}, 10^{-9}, 10^{-8}, 10^{-7}, and 10^{-6}; NE, 10^{-8}, 10^{-7}, 10^{-6}, 10^{-5}, and 10^{-4} M), for 10 minutes each. Contractile responses to Ang II and to norepinephrine were expressed as a ratio to maximum contraction produced by 20 mM KCl.

Measurement of Angiotensin II

In another series of experiments, hamsters were used for assessment of the renin-angiotensin system (n = 6 for each of four groups). Hamsters were weighed and decapitated, and blood was collected in chilled polyethylene tubes with ethylenediaminetetra-acetic acid disodium (EDTA.2Na). Blood was centrifuged at 3,000 g for 15 minutes and 2 ml of plasma was immediately applied to a minicolumn to extract Ang II. Cardiac and aortic Ang II were measured as described previously by us (8). Briefly, hamsters were perfused with heparinized saline (20 U/ml) from the apex of the heart to remove any contamination of blood. The heart and thoracic aorta were removed. The left ventricle was isolated (including the interventricular septum), frozen on dry ice, and stored at −70°C until assay. For extraction of Ang II, the heart was thawed, weighed, and homogenized by Polytron (Brinkman Instruments, Westbury, NY) in 0.1 N hydrochloric acid. The tissue supernatant, obtained by centrifugation of the homogenate at 20,000 g for 30 minutes, and plasma were applied to a minicolumn (500 mg; Amprep C8, Amersham, Buckinghamshire, UK) to extract Ang II. Ang II measurement was performed by high-performance liquid chromatography coupled with radioimmunoassay (9).

Histologic Study

Samples of myocardium from cardiomyopathic hamsters after the treatment were fixed in buffered 10% formalin, embedded in paraffin, and stained with hematoxylin and eosin, Masson trichrome, or Sirius red for microscopic observations (n = 4 for vehicle and cilazapril-treated groups).

Statistical Analysis

All data were expressed as mean ± standard error of the mean. Differences between golden Syrian and cardiomyopathic hamsters and between vehicle and cilazapril treatment were assessed by two-factor analysis of variance (ANOVA) (10). When the interaction was significant, one-way ANOVA followed by Bonferroni's test was applied to assess the difference among groups.

RESULTS

Activities of the circulating and the tissue renin-angiotensin system, assessed by measurement of its active peptide Ang II in normal (golden Syrian) and cardio-myopathic hamsters are shown in Table 1. In vehicle-treated hamsters, plasma Ang II was higher in cardiomyopathic than in golden Syrian hamsters. Treatment with cilazapril reduced plasma Ang II in cardiomyopathic but not in golden Syrian hamsters. Using two-factor ANOVA, no independent effect of strain or treatment on plasma Ang II was detected (Table 1). In contrast, left ventricular Ang II was higher in cardiomyopathic than in golden Syrian hamsters and was decreased by cilazapril in both cardiomyopathic and golden Syrian hamsters. Neither strain nor treatment difference affected aortic Ang II.

Cardiomyopathic hamsters were lighter than golden Syrian hamsters in body weight (Table 2). Treatment with cilazapril did not affect body weight in either animal. Left ventricular weight in cardiomyopathic hamsters treated with vehicle was higher than that in golden Syrian hamsters. Liver and lung weights did not differ among the four groups.

Figure 1 shows the changes in left ventricular contractile response to Ang II infusion in golden Syrian and cardiomyopathic hearts. Responses of left ventricular pressure and left ventricular positive max dP/dt ($LV + dP/dt_{max}$) were significantly lower ($p < 0.05$) in cardiomyopathic than in golden Syrian hamsters. Treatment with cilazapril significantly improved the responses of left ventricular pressure and $LV + dP/dt_{max}$ to Ang II in both groups.

TABLE 1. *Plasma and tissue angiotensin II[a]*

	Plasma Ang II (pg/ml)	LV Ang II (pg/g tissue)	Ao Ang II (pg/g tissue)
GS-Veh	12.2 ± 2.2	96.5 ± 13.3	164.9 ± 32.6
GS-CLZ	8.8 ± 0.9	79.9 ± 2.0	107.2 ± 24.5
CM-Veh	23.5 ± 1.6[*]	145.9 ± 5.2	204.2 ± 36.8
CM-CLZ	15.7 ± 0.8[†]	115.4 ± 6.4	176.9 ± 13.4
Interaction	[#]	NS	NS
GS vs. CM	—	[#]	NS
Veh vs. CLZ	—	[#]	NS

[a]Values are mean ± standard error of the mean.
[#]$p < 0.05$ by two-factor ANOVA.
[*]$p < 0.05$ versus GS-Veh.
[†]$p < 0.05$ versus CM-Veh by Bonferroni.
LV, left ventricle; Ao, aorta; GS, normal golden Syrian hamster; CM, Bio 14.6 cardiomyopathic hamster; Ang II, angiotensin II; Veh, vehicle; CLZ, cilazapril at 10 mg/kg/day; NS, not significant.

TABLE 2. Body and tissue weights[a]

	Body weight (g)	Heart weight (mg/g BW)	Liver weight (mg/g BW)	Lung weight (mg/g BW)
GS-Veh	162.3 ± 3.8	3.1 ± 0.1	42.3 ± 1.8	5.1 ± 0.8
GS-CLZ	158.1 ± 3.1	3.3 ± 0.1	34.4 ± 1.5	5.2 ± 0.2
CM-Veh	104.7 ± 3.6	5.8 ± 0.5[*]	34.8 ± 1.6	5.6 ± 0.3
CM-CLZ	103.4 ± 2.2	4.7 ± 0.2[†]	35.2 ± 0.4	4.8 ± 0.4
Interaction	NS	[#]	NS	NS
GS vs. CM	[#]	—	NS	NS
Veh vs. CLZ	NS	—	NS	NS

[a]Values are mean ± standard error of the mean.
[#]$p < 0.05$ by two-factor ANOVA.
[*]$p < 0.05$ versus GS-Veh.
[†]$p < 0.05$ versus CM-Veh by Bonferroni.
GS, normal golden Syrian hamster; CM, Bio 14.6 cardiomyopathic hamster; Veh, vehicle; CLZ, cilazapril at 10 mg/kg/day; NS, not significant.

Aortic contractile responses to Ang II and to norepinephrine are shown in Fig. 2. There was no strain difference or treatment effect in the developing pressure response to either Ang II or norepinephrine.

Histologically, cardiomyopathic hearts showed cell disarray, eosinophilic degeneration, and myocardial hypertrophy (Fig. 3A). Treatment with cilazapril tended to improve these abnormalities in cardiomyopathic hamster hearts (Fig. 3B).

DISCUSSION

In this study, we evaluated the effects of chronic ACE inhibition on cardiac performance in cardiomyopathic hamsters. From microscopic findings of Bio 14.6 hamster hearts, the progress of cardiomyopathy can be divided into six chronologic stages: (a) stages of immaturity (until 1 month after birth), (b) cardiomyolysis (1–2 months), (c) granulation (2–3 months), (d) fibrosis (3–4 months), (e) hypertrophy (4–6 months), and (f) insufficiency (over 6 months) (11). Since the purpose of this study was to investigate the preventive effect on the progression of left ventricular failure, cilazapril was administered to Bio 14.6 hamsters from 160 to 240 days of age when they were in the transition stage from hypertrophy to insufficiency.

The renin-angiotensin system is activated in human heart failure (12,13) by intravascular dehydration and by stimulation of the sympathetic nervous system (1). In the present study, cardiomyopathic hamsters showed higher plasma Ang II concentrations than normal hamsters, suggesting that the cardiomyopathic hamsters used in this study had a renin angiotensin profile similar to that in humans and that they are suitable models for the evaluation of the role of the renin-angiotensin system in heart failure.

Chronic treatment with cilazapril improved the response to Ang II with the reduction of Ang II concentration in the plasma and the cardiac tissue. In cardio-

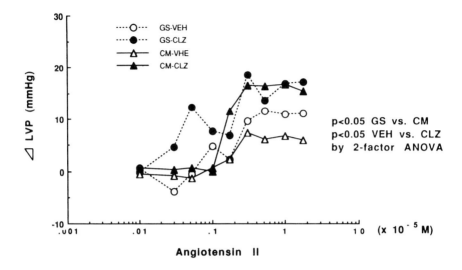

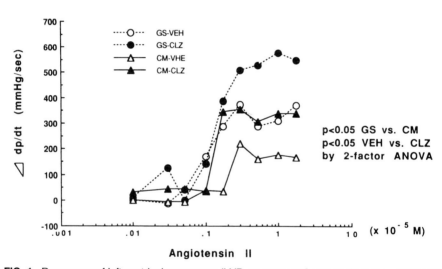

FIG. 1. Responses of left ventricular pressure (LVP, *upper panel*) and positive max dP/dt (dP/dt, *lower panel*) to angiotensin II. GS, normal golden Syrian hamster; CM, cardiomyopathic hamster; VEH, vehicle; CLZ, cilazapril; ANOVA, analysis of variance.

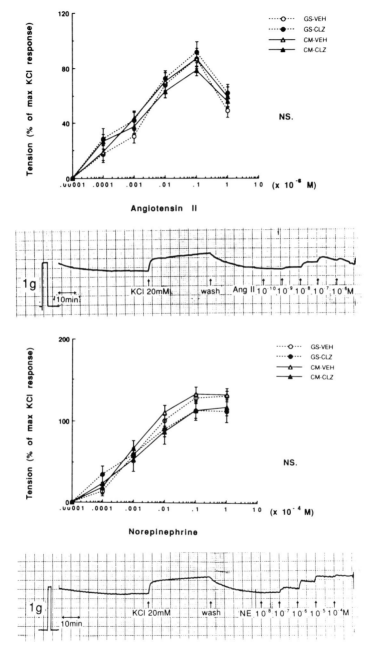

FIG. 2. Aortic contractile responses to angiotensin II (Ang II, *upper panel*) and to norepi-nephrine (NE, *lower panel*). GS, normal golden Syrian hamster; CM, cardiomyopathic hamster; VEH, vehicle; CLZ, cilazapril; NS, not significant.

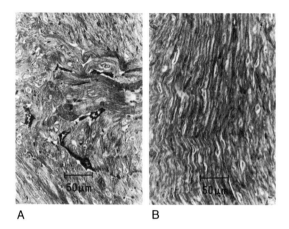

A   B

FIG. 3. Micrographs (×400) of left ventricles from (**A**) vehicle-treated cardiomyopathic hamster and (**B**) cilazapril-treated cardiomyopathic hamster.

myopathic hamsters, cilazapril significantly decreased plasma Ang II, indicating that the dose used in this study was enough to suppress the increased plasma level of Ang II. Elevation of the renin-angiotensin system was reported to correlate with the severity of heart failure in humans (14). Therefore, if the activation of the renin-angiotensin system is related to the deterioration of cardiac function, the decrease in plasma Ang II may account for the improvement of cardiac contractile response in the cardiomyopathic hamster. However, cilazapril also increased the cardiac response to Ang II in the golden Syrian hamster, in which plasma Ang II was not decreased. No decrease in plasma Ang II by ACE inhibitor was also reported by Mento et al. (15), in a study in which long-term administration of enalapril did not reduce plasma Ang II. These results suggest that inhibition of the circulating renin-angiotensin system does not solely explain the improvement of cardiac function by cilazapril.

The extrarenal tissue renin-angiotensin system in the heart has been recently demonstrated (16,17) and is postulated to play an important role in physiologic and pathologic states (16). We therefore evaluated the tissue renin-angiotensin system in the cardiomyopathic heart in this study. Similarly to the one in the plasma, left ventricular Ang II was higher in cardiomyopathic than in golden Syrian hamsters. These data confirm the previous results of Haleen et al. (18), who showed higher ventricular ACE activity in cardiomyopathic hamsters. The mechanism of elevated Ang II in the heart is not clear. One possible explanation is that elevated Ang II may compensate the cardiac dysfunction. Treatment with cilazapril resulted in a decrease of cardiac tissue Ang II levels in both golden Syrian and cardiomyopathic animals. Haleen et al. (18) also demonstrated that the higher activity of ventricular ACE in cardiomyopathic hamsters was inhibited by quinapril. These data suggested a good correlation between inhibition of ventricular ACE activity and cardioprotection. By combining these and our data, we may conclude that inhibition of the cardiac renin-angiotensin system may account for the beneficial effect of ACE inhibitors in hamsters.

The level of aortic Ang II was not different between golden Syrian and cardiomyopathic hamsters or between vehicle- and cilazapril-treated hamsters. This might relate to the similar contractile responses of aorta to Ang II and norepinephrine among the four groups. These results indicate that the vascular renin-angiotensin system may not be important in the dysfunction of cardiac contraction and in cardiovascular action of cilazapril in heart failure. The mechanism of cardioprotection by ACE inhibitors is multifactorial. It has been demonstrated that ACE inhibitors cause (a) systemic and coronary vasodilation, (b) diuresis and natriuresis, and (c) paradoxical dipsogenic action (19). All of these could affect the cardiac performance in heart failure in vivo. Therefore, these may also be possible factors contributing to the improvement of cardiac contractility by cilazapril.

Body weight was significantly lower in cardiomyopathic animals, which is consistent with the findings of Rossner (20) and Hirakata et al. (7). The lower body weight in cardiomyopathic hamsters may be explained by the fact that the progressive loss of skeletal muscle and adipose tissue exceeded the generalized fluid retention caused by heart failure (20). Cilazapril administration at 10 mg/kg/day did not change the body weight, suggesting that this dose did not have a toxic effect. There was no difference in the ratio of liver weight to body weight between cardiomyopathic and golden Syrian hamsters. In the study of Rossner (20), the liver of cardiomyopathic hamsters weighed significantly less than that of normal hamsters. Histologically, the liver of cardiomyopathic hamsters showed chronic passive congestion and fatty infiltration (20). The use of hamsters older (400 to 458 days old) than those in the present study (240 days old at the time of the experiment) may have resulted in the difference in liver weight. No significant difference in lung weight was found between the two strains, which is consistent with previous data (20). We showed that the ratio of heart weight to body weight was significantly greater in cardiomyopathic hamsters than in golden Syrian hamsters and was decreased by cilazapril in cardiomyopathic hamsters. Previous studies (7,20) also showed that the heart weight of cardiomyopathic hamsters was significantly greater than that of normal hamsters. It was reported that the heart from the cardiomyopathic hamster was dilated and had thin walls, and white streaks were seen in the myocardium (20). Haleen et al. (18) showed that ventricular volume was significantly greater in cardiomyopathic than in golden Syrian hamsters. Chronic quinapril treatment in the cardiomyopathic hamster prevented the increase in ventricular wall and chamber volume. These results suggest that the reduction in heart weight could be related to the prevention of cardiac dysfunction by cilazapril.

Hirakata et al. (7) reported that the affinity of cardiac Ang II receptor was 35% higher in cardiomyopathic hamsters than in golden Syrian hamsters. Higher plasma Ang II in the cardiomyopathic hamster was demonstrated in this study. Thus, deteriorated response to Ang II may be explained by a postreceptor mechanism. Chronic inhibition of ACE may produce up-regulation of Ang II receptor, resulting in an improvement of contractile response to Ang II.

Histologically, treatment with cilazapril tended to be less effective in the presence of cell disarray, eosinophilic degeneration, and myocardial hypertrophy, which are usually observed in cardiomyopathic hamsters. Treatment with a calcium channel blocker, verapamil, started from 20 days old for 70 days, prevented the fibrosis and calcification in cardiomyopathic hamsters (21). In this study, we used 160-day-old hamsters in which fibrosis and calcification were already seen (11). The later start of the drug treatment may have prevented the cardioreparative effect of the ACE inhibitor.

Ang II acts on a membrane-bound receptor and activates the inositol 1,4,5-triphosphate (IP_3) and 1,2-diacylglycerol pathways, leading to an increase in intracellular calcium (22–24). ACE inhibitors possess a calcium channel blocking property (25), which may result in histologic improvement. ACE inhibitors have been shown to reduce coronary arterial resistance (26). Haleen et al. (18) reported that administration of quinapril prevented the decline of coronary flow in cardiomyopathic hamsters. Increase in myocardial blood flow may also account for the cardioprotective effect of cilazapril.

In summary, isolated heart from cardiomyopathic hamsters showed deterioration of the cardiac response to Ang II with increase in plasma and cardiac Ang II. Chronic treatment with cilazapril decreased cardiac Ang II and improved left ventricular performance. From these results, it is concluded that decreases in cardiac Ang II may explain the improvement in left ventricular contractile response to Ang II, thus accounting for the cardioprotective effect of the ACE inhibitor, cilazapril, in congestive heart failure. Further studies using Ang II receptor antagonist are required to clarify the direct effect of inhibition of the renin-angiotensin system in congestive heart failure.

SUMMARY

In order to examine the cardioprotective mechanism of angiotensin-converting enzyme (ACE) inhibitors in heart failure, the cardiac and vascular responses to angiotensin II (Ang II) were assessed in the Bio 14.6 cardiomyopathic hamster. The study included cardiomyopathic male hamsters (160 days old, n = 32) and golden Syrian hamsters (n = 32) as controls. Vehicle or cilazapril (10 mg/kg/day) was given orally for 12 weeks. Isolated heart was perfused retrogradely using the Langendorff method. Contractile responses of the heart and thoracic aorta to exogenous Ang II (10^{-7} to 10^{-5} M) were examined. Ang II levels in the plasma, heart, and aorta were measured by radioimmunoassay. Cardiac wet weight was higher in cardiomyopathic than in golden Syrian hamsters; cilazapril decreased cardiac weight. In vehicle-treated hamsters, plasma Ang II was higher in cardiomyopathic than that in golden Syrian hamsters. Treatment with cilazapril reduced plasma Ang II in cardiomyopathic but not in golden Syrian hamsters. Left ventricular Ang II in cardio-myopathic hamsters was higher than in golden Syrian hamsters but was decreased by cilazapril in both groups. No strain or treatment differences were found with use of aortic Ang II. Responses of left ventricular pressure and $LV + dP/dt_{max}$ were significantly lower ($p < 0.05$) in cardiomyopathic compared with golden Syrian hamsters. The increase in both left ventricular pressure and $LV + dP/dt_{max}$ from baseline values was significantly greater in cilazapril-treated hearts in cardio-myopathic hamsters compared with that in vehicle-treated cardiomyopathic ham-sters. In contrast, no significant difference was found in the aortic contractile re-sponse to Ang II and to norepinephrine between strains and between treatments. These findings suggest that decrease in cardiac Ang II may explain the improvement in left ventricular contractile response to Ang II, thus accounting for the cardio-protective effect of ACE inhibitor on heart failure.

ACKNOWLEDGMENT

The authors gratefully acknowledge Ms. Misako Masumoto for her excellent technical assistance.

REFERENCES

1. Bristow MR, Gilbert EM. Anti-adrenergic actions of angiotensin converting enzyme inhibitors. *Curr Opin Cardiol* 1989;4[Suppl 2]:45–50.
2. Curis C, Cohen JN, Vrobel T, Franciosa JA. Role of the renin angiotensin system in the systemic vasoconstriction of chronic congestive heart failure. *Circulation* 1978;58:763–70.
3. Packer M. Therapeutic options in the management of chronic heart failure. Is there a drug of first choice? *Circulation* 1989;79:198–204.
4. CONSENSUS Trial Study Group. Effects of enalapril on mortality in severe congestive heart fail-ure. *N Engl J Med* 1987;316:1429–35.
5. Pfeffer MA, Pfeffer JM, Steinberg C, Finn P. Survival after an experimental myocardial infarction: beneficial effects of long-term therapy with captopril. *Circulation* 1985;72:406–12.
6. Arnal J-F, Cudek P, Plouin P-F, Guyenne T, Michel J-B, Corvol P. Low angiotensinogen levels are related to the severity and liver dysfunction of congestive heart failure: implications for renin mea-surements. *Am J Med* 1991;90:17–22.
7. Hirakata H, Fouad-Tarazi FM, Bumpus FM, et al. Angiotensins and the failing heart. Enhanced positive inotropic response to angiotensin I in cardiomyopathic hamster heart in the presence of captopril. *Circ Res* 1990;66:891–9.
8. Nagano M, Higaki J, Nakamura F, et al. Role of cardiac angiotensin II in isoproterenol-induced left ventricular hypertrophy. *Hypertension* 1992;19:708–12.
9. Shimamoto K, Ishida H, Nakahashi Y, et al. A very sensitive direct radioimmunoassay system for plasma angiotensin II and its clinical application in various hypertensive diseases. *Jpn Circ J* 1984;48:1228–35.
10. Wallenstein S, Zucker CI. Some statistical methods useful in circulation research. *Circ Res* 1980; 47:1–7.
11. Onishi S, Wada A. Heredofamilial factor as a cause of myocardial damage. In: Sekiguchi M, Olsen EGJ, Goodwin JF. *Heart and Vessels* 1985[Suppl 1]:34–8.
12. Francis GS, Benedict C, Johnstone DE, et al. Comparison of neuroendocrine activation in patients with left ventricular dysfunction with and without congestive heart failure. A substudy of the Studies of Left Ventricular Dysfunction (SOVLD). *Circulation* 1990;82:1724–9.

13. MacAlpine HM, Morton JJ, Leckie B, Rumley A, Gillen G, Dargie HJ. Neurogendocrine activation after myocardial infarction. *Br Heart J* 1988;60:117–24.
14. Arnal J-F, Cudek P, Plouin P-F, Guyenne T, Michel J-B, Corvol P. Low angiotensinogen levels are related to the severity and liver dysfunction of congestive heart failure: implications for renin measurements. *Am J Med* 1991;90:17–22.
15. Mento PF, Wilkes BM. Plasma angiotensins and blood pressure during converting enzyme inhibition. *Hypertension* 1987;7[Suppl III]:III-42–III-48.
16. Dzau VJ. Cardiac renin-angiotensin system: molecular and function aspects. *Am J Med* 1988; 84[Suppl 3A]:22–7.
17. Wikes BM, Mento PM, Pearl AR, et al. Plasma angiotensins in anephric humans: evidence for an extrarenal angiotensin system. *J Cardiovasc Pharmacol* 1991;17:419–23.
18. Haleen SJ, Weishaar RE, Overhiser RW, et al. Effects of quinapril, a new angiotensin converting enzyme inhibitor on left ventricular failure and survival in the cardiomyopathic hamster. Hemodynamic, morphological, and biochemical correlates. *Circ Res* 1991;68:1302–12.
19. Schiffrin EL, Genest J. Mechanism of captopril-induced drinking. *Am J Physiol* 1982;242:R136–40.
20. Rossner KL. Calcium current in congestive heart failure of hamster cardiomyopathy. *Am J Physiol* 1991;260:H1179–86.
21. Kobayashi A, Yamshita T, Kaneko M, Nishiyama T, Hayashi H, Yamazaki N. Effects of verapamil on experimental cardiomyopathy in the Bio 14.6 Syrian hamster. *J Am Coll Cardiol* 1987;10:1128–34.
22. Smith JB, Smith L, Brown ER, et al. Angiotensin II rapidly increases phosphatidate-phosphoinositide synthesis and phosphoinositide hydrolysis and mobilizes intracellular calcium in cultured arterial muscle cells. *Proc Natl Acad Sci USA* 1984;81:7812–16.
23. Nabika T, Velletri PA, Lovenberg W, Beaven MA. Increase in cytosolic calcium and phosphoinositide metabolism induced by angiotensin II and [Arg] vasopressin in vascular smooth muscle cells. *J Biol Chem* 1985;260:4661–70.
24. Alexander RW, Brock TA, Gimbrone MA, Jr, Rittenhouse SE. Angiotensin II increases inositol triphosphate and calcium in vascular smooth muscle. *Hypertension* 1985;7:447–51.
25. Gill J, Jeremy JY, Dandona P. Captopril inhibits the influx of calcium into platelets. *Eur J Pharmacol* 1989;162:193–4.
26. Ferrone RA, Herran CL, Antonaccio MJ. Comparison of the acute and chronic hemodynamic effects of captopril and guanethidine in spontaneously hypertensive rats. *Clin Exp Hypertens* 1980;2:247–72.

The Cardiomyopathic Heart, edited by Makoto
Nagano, Nobuakira Takeda, and Naranjan S.
Dhalla. Raven Press, Ltd., New York © 1994.

17

Effects of Angiotensin-Converting Enzyme Inhibitors and Prostaglandin E_1 Derivatives on the Cardiomyopathic Hamster

Mitsutoshi Kato, Jie Yang, Takaaki Iwai, Akira Tanamura,
Nobuakira Takeda, and Makoto Nagano

*Department of Internal Medicine, Aoto Hospital, Jikei University School of Medicine,
6-41-2, Aoto, Katsushika-ku, Tokyo 125, Japan*

INTRODUCTION

A wide range of results has been obtained from clinical as well as fundamental research using experimental animals; however, the cause of idiopathic cardiomyopathy is still unclear. In order to obtain further information on this point, we administered three kinds of cardioprotective agents, e.g., captopril and enalapril, angiotensin-converting enzyme (ACE) inhibitors, and OP-1206-αCD for prostaglandin E_1 derivative to J-2-N cardiomyopathic hamsters. Male J-2-N hamsters were divided randomly into two groups. One group was left untreated, whereas the treated group received captopril, enalapril, and OP-1206-αCD. It should be pointed out that attention has been focused on the use of ACE inhibitors in the treatment of heart failure, and there have been several reports published on the efficacy of captopril for congestive heart failure. The present study examined the roles of the RAA and kallikrein-kinin systems in idiopathic cardiomyopathy on the basis of the effects of these ACE inhibitors. The indices used were the electrocardiogram (ECG), histopathologic findings, serum MDA, creatine kinase and aldolase levels, and the ventricular myosin isoenzyme patterns.

MATERIALS AND METHODS

J-2-N Cardiomyopathic Hamster (1)

In our laboratory, we bred a male cardiomyopathic Bio 14.6 hamster (2) with a female golden hamster, and the F_1 female obtained was bred with the same Bio 14.6 hamster. The F_2 female thus obtained was bred with the same Bio 14.6 male parent, and the resultant F_3 hamster was a cardiomyopathic hamster with a higher reproduction rate than the Bio 14.6 hamster. This hamster was designated as the J-1-N cardiomyopathic hamster, and healthy J-2-N hamsters were obtained after some generations of interbreeding with a new Bio 14.6 cardiomyopathic hamster.

Healthy J-2-N hamsters or golden hamsters showed a normal electrocardiogram (ECG) except for left axis deviation, whereas the cardiomyopathic animals exhibited QS patterns in the limb or chest leads. In the normal ECG group, the serum creatine kinase level was the same as that in the golden hamsters, but the hamsters with abnormal ECGs showed a marked rise in these levels.

Administration of ACE Inhibitors

At 5 weeks of age, 28 male J-2-N cardiomyopathic hamsters were divided randomly into two groups. The captopril group received 15 mg/kg of captopril orally for 10 weeks, dissolved in their drinking water. The other group was left untreated. Body weights were periodically determined from the beginning to the end of the experimental period. ECGs were recorded using both limb and chest leads from around the beginning of the experimental period.

For the second experiment, following the captopril experiment, 24 5-week-old male cardiomyopathic J-2-N hamsters were divided into two groups, and one group received 1.5 mg/kg of enalapril for 10 weeks and the other group was left untreated. Since the enalapril group did not show improvement in ECG findings at 10 weeks, the administration period was extended to 15 weeks.

OP-1206-αCD Administration (4)

For OP-1206-αCD administration, male J-2-N cardiomyopathic hamsters were divided randomly into two groups. The OP-1206-αCD group received 200 mg/kg of OP-1206-αCD orally for 10 weeks, dissolved in their drinking water. The other group was left untreated.

At the end of the experimental period, blood of each group was obtained under sodium pentobarbital anesthesia and the serum creatine kinase, aldolase, lactate dehydrogenase, and MDA (5,6) levels were determined. Hearts were studied biochemically. In the biochemical analysis, the myocardial ventricular myosin isoenzyme patterns were compared. In addition, we prepared sarcolemmal membranes using a modification of the method of Reeves et al. (7), and the Na^+-K^+-adenosine triphosphatase activity of this membrane was measured (8).

For cardiac myosin isoenzyme determination, native myosin was extracted from 40 mg of tissue of both ventricles in accordance with the method of Martin et al. (9). Myosin isoenzymes were separated by pyrophosphate gel electrophoresis using the method of Hoh et al. (10). Samples of myosin solution were placed on the gels, and electrophoresis was performed for 27 hours at 2°C; then the gels were stained and examined by a densitometer.

RESULTS

None of the hamsters receiving captopril died during the drug administration period. Three animals in the untreated group died, possibly of heart failure.

Figure 1 shows the serum creatine kinase and aldolase levels. In the untreated group, serum creatine kinase rose markedly, whereas in the captopril group, the elevation was inhibited significantly. Serum aldolase levels showed similar changes. However, administration of enalapril tended to inhibit the rise in creatine kinase levels (25% inhibition in enalapril-treated group), but the difference was not significant.

Figure 2 shows percentages of the left and right ventricular myosin isoenzymes V3 in the untreated, captopril, and enalapril groups. In the untreated group, an increase in V3 myosin was observed. In contrast, the captopril group displayed ventricular myosin isoenzyme patterns similar to those in control hamsters.

Figure 3 shows serum MDA levels in the captopril and enalapril groups. The MDA levels were markedly elevated in untreated cardiomyopathic animals. MDA

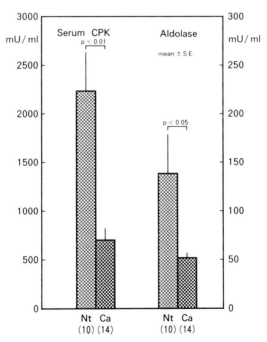

FIG. 1. Serum creatine kinase and serum aldolase levels in the captopril administration experiments. In the untreated J-2-N cardiomyopathic hamster group, serum creatine kinase and aldolase levels rose significantly, but this rise was markedly inhibited by captopril administration. Nt, untreated group of J-2-N cardiomyopathic hamsters; Ca, captopril administration group. Values represent means ± standard error of the mean.

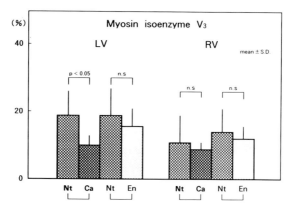

FIG. 2. Percentages of the left and right ventricular myosin isoenzymes V3 in the untreated and enalapril groups. In the untreated group, an increase in V3 myosin was observed. In contrast, the treated group displayed similar ventricular myosin isoenzyme patterns of control hamsters. Nt, untreated group of J-2-N cardiomyopathic hamsters; Ca, captopril-treated group; En, enalapril-treated group. Values show the mean ± standard deviation.

levels were reduced by the administration of captopril but not by treatment with enalapril.

The sarcolemmal Na^+-K^+-ATPase activity was depressed in cardiomyopathic hearts. Only a slight improvement was seen in the Na^+-K^+-ATPase activity of sarcolemmal membrane in the enalapril group. However, the measurement of the enzyme activity upon treating the membrane with detergent, enalapril group showed no improvement of the Na^+-K^+-ATPase activity (Fig. 4). Figure 5 shows

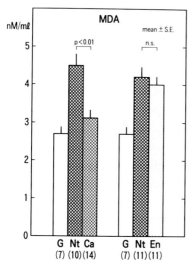

FIG. 3. Serum MDA levels in the captopril- and enalapril-treated groups. MDA concentrations were reduced by the administration of captopril but not by treatment with enalapril. G, golden hamster (control); nt, untreated group; En, enalapril group. Values represent means ± standard error of the mean.

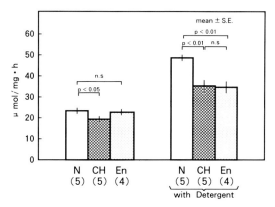

FIG. 4. Na$^+$-K$^+$-ATPase activities of sarcolemmal membrane of enalapril-treated and control hamsters. Only a slight improvement was seen in the Na$^+$-K$^+$-ATPase activity of sarcolemmal membrane without detergent. However, in the measurement with detergent, the enalapril group showed no improvement of Na$^+$-K$^+$-ATPase activity. N, normal hamster; CH, cardiomyopathic hamster; En, enalapril-treated group. Values represent means ± standard error of the mean.

the serum creatine kinase, aldolase, and MDA levels in the OP-1206-αCD treatment experiment at 15 weeks. In the untreated group, serum creatine kinase, aldolase, and MDA levels were higher in cardiomyopathic animals, whereas the OP-1206-αCD group showed tendency toward some beneficial effect ($p<0.1$). Some improvement was seen in other parameters of the OP-1206-αCD group, but these effects were not significant.

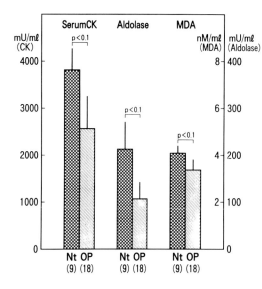

FIG. 5. Serum creatine kinase, aldolase, and MDA levels in OP-1206-αCD treatment experiment at 15 weeks. In the untreated group, serum creatine kinase, aldolase, and MDA levels rose as this figure, whereas in the OP-1206-αCD group, a beneficial effect could be seen. Nt, untreated group; OP, OP-1206-αCD treated group. Values represent means ± standard error of the mean.

DISCUSSION

J-2-N cardiomyopathic hamsters have different characteristics from the Bio 53.58 and Bio 14.6 strains (11). J-2-N hamsters are characterized by the relatively slow progression of interstitial fibrosis, without any of the focal necrosis seen in Bio 53.58 and Bio 14.6 hamsters. The histopathologic changes and serum creatine kinase increases are milder than those seen in Bio 53.58 and Bio 14.6 hamsters. However, J-2-N hamsters show marked dilation of both ventricles, and they are a model of dilated cardiomyopathy.

Recently, several studies have been carried out on the protective effects of ACE inhibitors on the cardiovascular system resulting from their effects on the myocardium in addition to their antihypertensive effect. Captopril stimulates an increase in the synthesis of prostaglandin E_2 (PGE_2) in cultured rabbit renomedullary interstitial cells. However, enalapril and enalaprilic acid did not increase prostaglandin E_2 levels, even at 1,000-fold high concentrations (12). These results suggested the importance of the sulfhydryl group of captopril in the production of prostaglandin E_2 and also suggested that this action is not an ordinary effect of ACE inhibitors.

Some other drugs for treatment of cardiomyopathy were also used in Bio 14.6, Bio 53.58, and UM-X7.1 cardiomyopathic models. For example Factor et al. (13,14) reported that verapamil alleviated myocardial damage. They stated that its effect was attributable to the prevention of small blood vessel contraction, which leads to the advancement of myocyte necrosis during the initial stages of cardiomyopathy. Waagstein et al. (15) reported that metoprolol therapy of dilated cardiomyopathy showed an improvement in both subjective and objective symptoms as well as a reduction in mortality. However, the evaluation of metoprolol is still not definitive, and a careful administration of this drug for selected cases of cardiomyopathy is being carried out at present. Data on the experimental use of β-blockers are relatively few, but Tominaga et al. (16) reported the beneficial effects of carteolol on a murine model of viral myocarditis and dilated cardiomyopathy caused by the encephalomyocarditis virus.

As the cardiomyopathy progresses in cardiomyopathic hamsters, the renin-angiotensin-aldosterone system is activated, angiotensin II causes an increase in peripheral vascular resistance, and aldosterone produces sodium retention, which leads to hypervolemia. These changes lead to aggravation of heart failure and poor circulation. Captopril improves the poor circulation, and its inhibition of angiotensin II also reduces the progression of cardiomegaly. However, the increase in tissue kinins and vasodilatory prostaglandins is assumed to play a major role in cardiomyopathy based on the finding that enalapril had less effect than captopril in J-2-N hamsters. OP-1206-αCD (prostaglandin E_1) was administered to J-2-N hamsters, but the differences between the OP-1206-αCD group and the untreated group were not significant; however, some beneficial effects were seen. Thus the results from the prostaglandin E_1 administration experiment show the importance of kallikrein-kinin systems in the cardiomyopathic hamster.

SUMMARY

We administered captopril or enalapril to 5-week-old J-2-N cardiomyopathic hamsters and investigated the roles of the renin-angiotensin-aldosterone (RAA) and kallikrein-kinin systems in the onset and progress of cardiomyopathy. Also we administered OP-1206-αCD, a prostaglandin E_1 derivative. In the untreated group, serum creatine kinase levels increased in accordance with the progression of cardiomyopathy, but this increase was markedly inhibited by the administration of captopril. The rise in serum aldolase levels was similarly inhibited. Serum malondialdehyde (MDA) levels were significantly reduced by the administration of captopril. Electrocardiographic findings and the ventricular myosin isoenzyme patterns were also markedly improved by captopril. The improvement in all these parameters was less with administration of enalapril. These differences between captopril and enalapril suggest that increases in tissue bradykinin and vasodilatory prostaglandins may play an important role in the beneficial effects of captopril. When OP-1206-αCD was administered to J-2-N hamsters, some tendency to beneficial effects was observed. These results suggest the importance of the kallikrein-kinin system in the development of cardiomyopathy in J-2-N cardiomyopathic hamsters.

REFERENCES

1. Kato M, Nagano M. Experimental animal models of cardiomyopathy. In: Opie LH, Sugimoto T, eds. *Cardiomyopathy update-4. Metabolic and molecular aspects of cardiomyopathy.* Tokyo: University of Tokyo Press; 1991:69–84.
2. Strobeck JE, Factor SM, Bhan A. Hereditary and acquired cardiomyopathies in experimental animals: mechanical, biochemical and structural features. *Ann NY Acad Sci* 1979;59:59–85.
3. Kato M, Takeda N, Yang J, Nagano M. The effects of angiotensin converting enzyme inhibitors and the renin-angiotensin-aldosterone system in J-2-N cardiomyopathic hamsters. *Jpn Circ J* 1992; 56:77–85.
4. Fujitani B, Watanabe M, Kuwashima J, Tsuboi T, Kadokawa T, Kitagawa T. Effect of a prostaglandin E_1 derivative (OP-1206) and acetylsalicylic acid on electrically induced thrombosis in guinea-pig mesenteric artery and its modification by an inhibitor of prostaglandin I_2 synthetase, tranylcypromine. *Jpn J Pharmacol* 1986;40:31–5.
5. Ohkawa H, Ohishi N, Yagi K. Assay for lipid peroxides in animal tissues by thiobarbituric acid reaction. *Anal Biochem* 1979;95:351–8.
6. Kato M, Kako KJ. Effects of N-(2-mercaptopropionyl)glycine on ischemic-reperfused dog kidney in vivo and membrane preparation in vitro. *Mol Cell Biochem* 1987;78:151–9.
7. Reeves JP, Bailey CA, Hale CC. Redox modification of sodium-calcium exchange activity in cardiac sarcolemmal vesicles. *J Biol Chem* 1986;261:4948–55.
8. Kato M, Kako KJ. Orientation of vesicles isolated from baso-lateral membranes of renal cortex. *Mol Cell Biochem* 1987;78:9–16.
9. Martin AF, Pagani ED, Solaro RJ. Thyroxine-induced redistribution of isoenzymes of rabbit ventricular myosin. *Circ Rec* 1982;50:117–24.
10. Hoh JFY, Mcgrath PA, Hale PT. Electrophoretic analysis of multiple forms of rat cardiac myosin: effects of hypophysectomy and thyroxine replacement. *J Moll Cell Cardiol* 1978;10:1053–76.
11. Bajusz E. Hereditary cardiomyopathy: a new disease model. *Am Heart J* 1969;77:686–96.

12. Zusman RM. Effects of converting-enzyme inhibitors on the renin-angiotensin-aldosterone, brady-kinin, and arachidonic acid-prostaglandin systems: correlation of chemical structure and biologic activity. *Am J Kidney Dis* 1987;5:13–23.
13. Factor SM, Cho S, Scheuer J, Sonnenblick E, Malhotra A. Prevention of hereditary cardiomyopathy in the Syrian hamster with chronic verapamil therapy. *J Am Coll Cardiol* 1988;12:1599–1604.
14. Factor SM, Sonnenblick EH. Microvascular spasm in the cardiomyopathic Syrian hamster as a cause of focal necrosis and myocardial failure. In: Kawai C, Abelmann WH, eds. *Cardiomyopathy update-1. Pathogenesis of myocarditis and cardiomyopathy*. Tokyo: University of Tokyo Press; 1978: 63–78.
15. Waagstein F, Hjilamarson A, Varnauskas E, Wallentis I. Effects of chronic beta-adrenergic receptor blockade in congestive cardiomyopathy. *Br Heart J* 1975;37:1022–36.
16. Tominaga M, Matsumori A, Okada I, Yamada T, Kawai C. β-blocker treatment of dilated cardiomyopathy. *Circulation* 1991;83:2021–28.

The Cardiomyopathic Heart, edited by Makoto Nagano, Nobuakira Takeda, and Naranjan S. Dhalla. Raven Press, Ltd., New York © 1994.

18

Role of Lipid Peroxidation in the Early Stage of Cardiomyopathy in the Bio 14.6 Syrian Hamster

Akira Kobayashi, Masanori Kaneko, Terumoto Fukuchi, and Noboru Yamazaki

The Third Department of Internal Medicine, Hamamatsu University School of Medicine, 3600, Handa-cho, Hamamatsu, 431-31, Japan

INTRODUCTION

Highly reactive oxygen species can cause lipid peroxidation and have been shown to play a role in producing myocardial damage in a variety of conditions, such as catecholamine-induced cardiomyopathy (1), alcoholic cardiomyopathy (2), and doxorubicin-induced cardiomyopathy (3).

The Bio 14.6 cardiomyopathic Syrian hamster (Bio 14.6 hamster) is a well-known animal model of congestive cardiomyopathy. Histologic studies have shown that myocardial degeneration in Bio 14.6 hamsters resembles reperfusion necrosis, and functional spasm of the small intramyocardial coronary arteries has been demonstrated (4) to occur in this animal model. Furthermore, it has been reported that the myocardial levels of free radicals and lipid peroxides are significantly increased in Bio 14.6 hamsters (5,6). Thus, there are several lines of evidence to suggest the involvement of free radicals and lipid peroxidation in the pathogenesis of cardiomyopathy in this hamster model.

It has been shown that tissues and cells can be damaged if the formation of free radicals and/or the extent of lipid peroxidation exceeds the capacity of the natural protective mechanisms (7). The toxic effects of free radicals are prevented by radical scavenging systems, and the antioxidant status of a tissue constantly varies with the pathophysiologic conditions imposed. Therefore, to evaluate the contribution of a deficit in the antioxidant reserve to the pathogenesis of cardiomyopathy in Bio 14.6 hamsters, we examined the myocardial activity of GSHPx and superoxide dismutase (SOD) as well as the myocardial selenium concentration. In addition, we evaluated the effect of α-tocopherol treatment on myocardial damage in the early stage of cardiomyopathy (up to 90 days) in this hamster model.

165

MATERIALS AND METHODS

Animals

The cardiomyopathic Bio 14.6 Syrian hamster is an inbred strain carrying the autosomal recessive cardiomyopathic gene, *cm*. Animals were obtained from Bio Breeders Inc. (MA) and were maintained at the Institute for Experimental Animals at Hamamatsu University School of Medicine. A newly established strain (designated Bio 14.6 HAM) was used as normal control hamsters (8). All experiments conformed to the Hamamatsu University School of Medicine regulations governing the care and use of laboratory animals.

Tissue Preparation for Assay of GSHPx and SOD Activity

Bio 14.6 Syrian hamsters and Bio 14.6 HAM hamsters 30 and 90 days old were lightly anesthetized with diethylether according to the method of Guarnieri et al. (9), and then their hearts were removed. The hearts were immediately perfused retrogradely via the aorta, rinsed in ice-cold saline, trimmed to remove connective tissue, and then weighed. All subsequent procedures were carried out at a temperature below 4°C. The hearts were cut into small pieces with scissors, and the pieces were washed once with ice-cold isolation medium (0.25 mM sucrose and 50 mM potassium phosphate, pH 7.2). The minced tissue was then homogenized in 10 volumes of ice-cold isolation medium using a Polytron homogenizer. Preliminary experiments showed that this homogenization procedure was satisfactory for the measurement of GSHPx and SOD activity. A portion of the homogenate was diluted with a twofold volume of isolation medium and then frozen in liquid nitrogen and stored at $-80°C$ until use.

GSHPx Activity

Glutathione peroxidase was assayed by a modification of the method of Guarnieri et al. (9). In brief, the assay mixture (2 ml) constituted 50 mM TRIS/HCl (pH 7.3), 0.2% Triton X-100, 1 mM NaN_3, 1 mM glomerular-stimulating hormone (GSH), 0.16 mM nicotinamide-adenine dinucleotide phosphate (NADPH), 1 U/ml of GSH reductase, and 30 µl of tissue homogenate. Addition of 0.2% Triton X-100 enabled monitoring of changes in the absorbance of the tissue homogenate without affecting the enzyme activity. After 5 minutes of preincubation at 37°C, the reaction was started by the addition of 0.2 mM cumene hydroperoxide, and the rate of disappearance of NADPH was monitored at 340 nm. A blank that contained isolation medium instead of tissue homogenate was incubated simultaneously to correct for the nonenzymatic oxidation of GSH or NADPH by cumene hydroperoxide. The GSH and cumene hydroperoxide concentrations used approximately corresponded to the Km values of hamster heart GSHPx for the respective substrates, but since the rate of nonenzymatic oxidation of GSH increased linearly with the substrate concentration, the assay conditions were chosen in a preliminary experiment to allow a reproducible procedure. One unit of enzyme was defined as the amount that catalyzed the oxidation of 1 μM of NADPH per minute. Protein concentrations were measured by the biuret procedure (10).

Superoxide Dismutase Activity

Superoxide dismutase activity was assayed by the nitrite method of Oyanagi (11), which is based on the ability of SOD to inhibit nitrite formation from hydroxylamine in the presence of superoxide. In brief, the reaction mixture (1 ml) consisted of 4 mM Na tetraborate, 6 mM potassium phosphate, 0.1 mM ethylenediaminetetra-acetic acid, 1 mM hydroxylamine, and 0.4 mM hypoxanthine (pH 8.2). After addition of the cardiac tissue homogenate, the reaction was initiated by adding xanthine oxidase. The reaction was allowed to proceed for 30 minutes at 37°C and then was stopped by the addition of 2 ml of 25% acetic acid containing 30 μM *N*-I naphthylethylenediamine and 450 μg/ml of sulfanilic acid (coloring reagent). The mixture was allowed to stand for 30 minutes at room temperature, and the absorbance was measured at 550 nm within 3 hours. In every experiment, the xanthine oxidase activity was checked and the amount added was chosen so as to generate sufficient superoxide to give an absorbance of 0.25 to 0.30 at 550 nm in the absence of SOD. One unit of enzyme was defined as the amount necessary to achieve 50% inhibition of nitrite formation.

Effects of α-Tocopherol on Myocardial Damage in Bio 14.6 Hamsters

Twelve 21-day-old Bio 14.6 hamsters were divided into two groups and treated as follows: the α-tocopherol group (n = 9) received intraperitoneal α-tocopherol (70 mg/kg per day) for 70 days, whereas the control group (n = 9) received the same volume of the vehicle alone. Animals were killed at 90 days of age (n = 6 in each group), and the morphologic changes in their hearts were assessed as described previously (12). In brief, transverse 5-mm slices were cut at the midpoint of both ventricles, fixed in 10% buffered formalin for 2 days, and then embedded in paraffin. Sections 3 μm in thickness were stained with hematoxylin-eosin, Mallory-Heidenhain triple stain, and von Kossa's stain. Photographs of the three differently stained sections were taken at 60 times magnification, and the damaged areas of myocardium were traced and measured with an image analyzer (Konton, Germany). The proportion of myocardial damage in both groups was then compared to assess the protective effect of α-tocopherol in the early stage of Bio 14.6 cardiomyopathy.

Statistical Analysis

All data were expressed as the mean ± standard deviation and were statistically evaluated by Student's t-test, with $p<0.05$ indicating statistical significance.

RESULTS

Glutathione Peroxidase Activity

The cardiac GSHPx activity in Bio 14.6 hamsters at ages 30 and 90 days was compared with that in age-matched normal controls. The specific activity of GSHPx in 30-day-old Bio 14.6 hamsters was significantly higher than that in the control hamsters (0.066 ± 0.016 versus 0.032 ± 0.004 U/mg protein, $p<0.01$) (Fig. 1). However, there was no significant difference between the two groups of hamsters at 90 days of age (0.031 ± 0.002 versus 0.033 ± 0.002 U/mg protein, not significant). There was also no significant difference in the apparent Km values of GSHPx for GSH and cumene hydroperoxide determined at a fixed concentration of GSHPx at 90 days of age (Km for GSF with 0.2 mM cumene hydroperoxide: 1.62 [Bio 14.6] versus 1.06 [control] mM; Km for cumene hydroperoxide with 1 mM GSH: 0.103 versus 0.144).

Myocardial Selenium Concentration

Since glutathione peroxidase requires selenium for its activity to be expressed, myocardial selenium concentrations were also measured. The selenium concentration in Bio 14.6 hamsters was 227 ± 26 ng/g wet tissue and that in controls was 236 ± 37 ng/g, indicating no significant difference between the two groups.

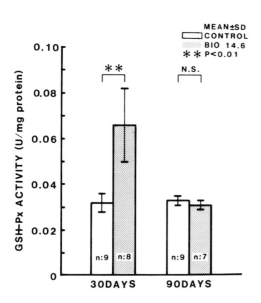

FIG. 1. GSHPx activity at different stages of development in control hamsters and Bio 14.6 cardiomyopathic hamsters. The specific GSHPx activity at 30 days of age was significantly higher in Bio 14.6 than in control hamsters. N.S., not significant.

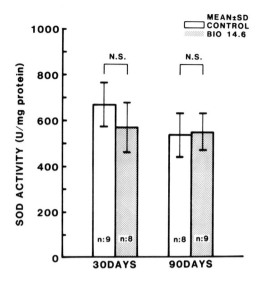

FIG. 2. SOD activity at different stages of development in control and Bio 14.6 cardiomyopathic hamsters. There were no significant changes. N.S., not significant.

Superoxide Dismutase Activity

The specific SOD activity in the hearts of Bio 14.6 and control hamsters at 30 and 90 days of age showed no significant differences (30 days: 571 ± 109 versus 669 ± 109 U/mg protein, p = not significant; 90 days: 549 ± 90 versus 537 ± 102 U/mg protein, p = not significant) (Fig. 2).

Effect of α-Tocopherol on Myocardial Damage

Morphometric analysis was used to assess the degree of protection against myocardial damage. The total and damaged areas of the myocardium were measured, and the proportion of damage was compared in the two groups. The total damaged area (%) in the α-tocopherol-treated group was significantly smaller than that in the control group ($1.82 \pm 0.77\%$ versus $2.96 \pm 0.99\%$, $p<0.05$) (Fig. 3). The calcified area (%) in the α-tocopherol-treated group was also significantly smaller than that in the control group ($0.37 \pm 0.25\%$ versus $1.38 \pm 0.65\%$, $p<0.01$) (Fig. 4). Furthermore, the areas of fibrosis were smaller in the α-tocopherol-treated group, although there was no significant difference between the two groups. These results indicated that α-tocopherol treatment in the early stage of cardiomyopathy development (21 to 90 days of age) could reduce the severity of myocardial damage in Bio 14.6 hamsters.

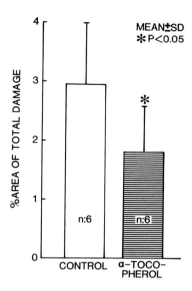

FIG. 3. Effect of α-tocopherol on the percentage of area of total myocardial damage. Treatment with α-tocopherol significantly reduced myocardial damage in Bio 14.6 cardiomyopathic hamsters.

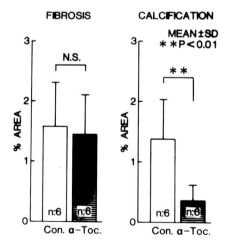

Con. : CONTROL
a-Toc. : a-TOCOPHEROL

FIG. 4. Effect of α-tocopherol on the area of fibrosis and calcification in Bio 14.6 cardiomyopathic hamsters. N.S., not significant.

TABLE 1. *Myocardial histologic lesions and free radical and antioxidant activities in Bio 14.6 hamsters at different ages*[a]

Age (days)	Histologic lesions (20)	Free radicals	Antioxidant
<25	Normal	?	?
30~40	Necrotic lesions occur	Free radicals ↑	GSHP × ↑, SOD→
60	Incidence of lesions is 100%	Lipid peroxide ↑	α-Tocopherol ↓
90	Healing of myolytic lesions (fresh lesions continue to occur)	Free radicals ↑ Lipid peroxide ↑	GSHP ×→, SOD→

[a]These data are based on the results reported in refs. (5) and (6).

DISCUSSION

We have previously shown that the myocardial concentrations of lipid peroxide and free radicals (Table 1) are increased in Bio 14.6 hamsters (5). Since the major endogenous enzymatic antioxidant defense mechanism in myocytes involves SOD and GSHPx, we investigated the activities of these two enzymes in this study. At 30 days of age, myocardial GSHPx activity in Bio 14.6 hamsters was approximately twice that in the normal controls, and treatment with α-tocopherol significantly reduced myocardial damage.

The antioxidant status of a living tissue is a dynamic property that is constantly adjusting to various physiologic and/or pathophysiologic conditions. It is well known that failure of this compensatory antioxidant mechanism, due to the increased production of free radicals and/or reduced activity of the antioxidant enzymes, can lead to cellular damage. In this regard, a number of authors have reported changes in antioxidant enzymes under a wide range of physiologic conditions, such as aging and exercise (13). GSHPx activity increases following the administration of lipid peroxides (14). In addition, Gupta et al. (15) have suggested that myocardial adaptation to an increased pressure load is accompanied by increased activity of radical scavenging enzymes, and they proposed that this greater antioxidant capacity may reduce lipid peroxidation and help maintain cardiac function during a period of higher oxidative stress. Therefore, the increased GSHPx activity in Bio 14.6 hamsters at 30 days of age may have been a compensatory response to oxidative stress. On the other hand, myocardial SOD activity did not change. It is possible that an increase in oxyradicals (H_2O_2) led to the inhibition of SOD activity (16) so that no increase was noted. In fact, the concentration of mitochondrial free radicals is significantly increased in Bio 14.6 hamsters (5). It has also been reported that glutathione reductase and catalase activity was increased, whereas SOD activity was unchanged in dystrophic skeletal muscle from Bio 14.6 hamsters (17). However, the increase in cardiac GSHPx activity does not seem to be sufficient to inhibit lipid peroxidation in the Bio 14.6 hamster. If there is a relative antioxidant deficit in the Bio 14.6 heart, and if free radicals are involved in the pathogenesis of cardiomyopathy at an early stage, we would expect an improvement of myocardial damage to follow the administration of antioxidants at this stage.

Myers et al. (18) and Singal et al. (1) have demonstrated that pretreatment of animals with α-tocopherol significantly reduced myocardial damage caused by doxorubicin or isoproterenol. Walton (19), however, reported that neither vitamin E nor antioxidants could retard the pathologic muscular changes in human muscular dystrophy. Myers et al. (18) and Singal et al. (1) obtained good results by the prior treatment of animals with α-tocopherol; Walton (19) studied patients with chronic muscular dystrophy in whom treatment was started in the late stages. In this study, we started treatment with α-tocopherol at 21 days of age because the Bio 14.6 heart is almost normal at this stage (20). We found a protective effect of α-tocopherol therapy in Bio 14.6 hamsters treated during the early stage of cardiomyopathy (up to 90 days). Sakanashi et al. (6) have reported vitamin E deficiency in the myocardium of Bio 14.6 hamsters at 60 days of age and have suggested that it might be related to the increase in lipid peroxide. These results indicate that free radicals and/or lipid peroxidation may play a significant role in the early pathogenesis of cardiomyopathy in Bio 14.6 hamsters. Furthermore, the relative antioxidant deficit reflects an increase in the levels of free radicals and lipid peroxides rather than a true deficiency of antioxidants.

SUMMARY

An increase in myocardial glutathione peroxidase (GSHPx) activity was observed at the early stage of cardiomyopathy (30 days of age) in Bio 14.6 hamsters. However, despite this compensatory response of GSHPx, there is a relative deficit in the antioxidant reserve, i.e., the antioxidant reserve is insufficient to protect the heart from the toxic effects of increased free radicals and lipid peroxidation. On the other hand, the administration of α-tocopherol can prevent the progression of myocardial damage at the early stage of cardiomyopathy in Bio 14.6 hamsters. These findings suggest a role for free radicals in the early pathogenesis of cardiomyopathy in Bio 14.6 hamsters.

REFERENCES

1. Singal PK, Kapur N, Dhillon KS, Beamish RE, Dhalla NS. Role of free radicals in catecholamine-induced cardiomyopathy. *Can J Physiol Pharmacol* 1982;60:1390–7.
2. Edes I, Piros G, Forster T, Csanady M. Alcohol-induced congestive cardiomyopathy in adult turkeys: effects on myocardial antioxidant defense systems. *Basic Res Cardiol* 1987;82:551–6.
3. Tomlinson CW, Godin DV, Rabkin SW. Adriamycin cardiomyopathy: implications of cellular changes in a canine model with mild impairment of left ventricular function. *Biochem Pharmacol* 1985;34:4033–41.
4. Factor S, Sonnenblick EH. Microvascular spasm as a cause of cardiomyopathies. *Cardiovasc Rev Rep* 1983;4:1177–82.
5. Kobayashi A. Yamashita T, Kaneko M, Nishiyama T, Hayashi H, Yamazaki N. Effects of verapamil on experimental cardiomyopathy in the Bio 14.6 Syrian hamster. *J Am Coll Cardiol* 1987; 10:1128–34.
6. Sakanashi T, Sako S, Nozuhara A, et al. Vitamin E deficiency has a pathological role in myocytolysis in cardiomyopathic Syrian hamster (BIO 14.6). *Biochem Biophys Res Commun* 1991; 181:145–50.

7. Freeman BA, Crapo JD: Biology of disease; free radicals and tissue injury. *Lab Invest* 1982;47:412–26.
8. Fukuchi T, Kobayashi A, Kaneko M, Ichiyama A, Yamazaki N. Possible involvement of free radicals and antioxidants in the early stages of the development of cardiomyopathy in BIO 14.6 Syrian hamster. *Jpn Heart J* 1991;32:655–66.
9. Guarnieri C, Flamigni F, Caldarera CM: Role of oxygen in the cellular damage induced by re-oxygenation of hydroxic heart. *J Mol Cell Cardiol* 1980;12:797–808.
10. Gornall AG, Bardawill CJ, David MM: Determination of serum proteins by means of the biuret reaction. *J Biol Chem* 1949;177:751–62.
11. Oyanagi Y: Reevaluation of assay methods and establishment of kit for superoxide dismutase activity. *Anal Bioche* 1984;142:290–6.
12. Yamashita T, Kobayashi A, Yamazaki N, Miura T, Shirasawa H: Effects of L-carnitine and verapamil on myocardial carnitine concentration and histopathology of Syrian hamster Bio 14.6. *Cardiovasc Res* 1986;20:614–20.
13. Kanter MM, Hamlin RL, Unverferth DV, Davis HW, Merola AJ: Effect of exercise training on antioxidant enzymes and cardiotoxicity of doxorubicin. *J Appl Physiol* 1985;59:1298–1303.
14. Reddy K, Tappel AL: Effect of dietary selenium and autooxidized lipids on the glutathione peroxidase system of gastro-intestinal tract and other tissues in the rat. *J Nutr* 1974;104:1069–78.
15. Gupta M, Singal PK: Higher antioxidative capacity during a chronic stable heart hypertrophy. *Circ Res* 1989;64:398–406.
16. Hodgson EK, Fridovich I: The interaction of bovine erythrocyte superoxide dismutase with hydrogen peroxide: inactivation of the enzyme. *Biochemistry* 1975;14:5294–99.
17. Salminen A, Kihlstrom M: Increased susceptibility to lipid peroxidation in skeletal muscles of dystrophic hamsters. *Experientia* 1989;45:747–9.
18. Myers CE, McGuire WP, Liss RH, Ifrim I, Grotzinger K, Young RC. Adriamycin; the role of lipid peroxidation in cardiac toxicity and tumor response. *Science* 1977;197:165–7.
19. Walton JN, Nattrass FJ: On the classification, natural history and treatment of the myopathies. *Brain* 1954;77:169–75.
20. Gertz EW: Cardiomyopathic Syrian hamster: a possible model of human disease. *Prog Exp Tumor Res* 1972;16:242–60.

The Cardiomyopathic Heart, edited by Makoto
Nagano, Nobuakira Takeda, and Naranjan S.
Dhalla. Raven Press, Ltd., New York © 1994.

19

Molsidomine, Isosorbide Dinitrate, and Antithrombotic Agents Do Not Prevent Cardiomyopathy in the Syrian Hamster

Hans-Georg Olbrich, Hans-Joachim Woltersdorf, Nikolai Aldag,
Kazimierz Krupinski, *Markward Schneider, Martin Kaltenbach,
†Ernst Mutschler

*Zentrum der Inneren Medizin, *Zentrum der Pathologie, and †Pharmakologisches Institut
für Naturwissenschaftler der Johann Wolfgang Goethe-Universität, Theodor-Stern-Kai 7,
60596 Frankfurt am Main, Germany*

INTRODUCTION

Since its first description 30 years ago (1), the cardiomyopathic Syrian hamster has become widely used as a model for cardiomyopathy leading to congestive heart failure. During the last 10 years a great deal of progress has been made toward the understanding of the pathogenesis of cardiomyopathy. Early pathognomonic features are myocardial calcium overload and necrotic lesions (2,3).

Among the biochemical abnormalities found in cardiomyopathic hamsters, (a) an increase in cardiac sympathetic activity (4–6) as well as a hypersensitivity of both vascular smooth muscle cells and cardiac myocytes to catecholamine stimulation (7–9) and (b) an increase in numbers of receptor binding sites for calcium channel blockers in heart and smooth muscle indicating augmented numbers of calcium channels in these tissues (10) are considered to play crucial roles in the pathogenesis of the disease. Both abnormalities may be the reason for vascular spasms in the cardiomyopathic hamster heart (11,12), which may damage the myocardium by intermittent ischemia-reperfusion injuries (13) and may affect myocardial cells directly, leading to calcium overload.

Catecholamines are well known to induce myocardial necrosis (14), and intravascular platelet aggregation is considered to be involved in this process (15,16). However, in the cardiomyopathy of the Syrian hamster, it is unknown whether platelet function has any pathogenetic relevance. With respect to circulatory disturbances in hamster cardiomyopathy, we investigated whether vasodilators of coronary conductance vessels, such as isosorbide dinitrate and molsidomine, can influ-

175

ence the course of the disease. Furthermore, to test the contribution of thrombocytes to hamster cardiomyopathy, we examined the effect of platelet aggregation inhibition using acetylsalicylic acid. In addition, the influence of heparin on hamster cardiomyopathy was studied.

MATERIALS AND METHODS

Animals

A total of 148 30-day-old cardiomyopathic Syrian hamsters (strain Bio 82.62) weighing 41 to 54 g were used.

Drugs Tested

Molsidomine, isosorbide dinitrate, and verapamil were kindly provided by Cassella Riedel Pharma GmbH (Frankfurt am Main, Germany). Acetylsalicylic acid was purchased from Bayer AG (Leverkusen, Germany), and unfractionated mucosa sodium salt heparin was purchased from Hoffmann-La Roche (Grenzach-Wyhlen, Germany). Treatment was given for 30 days from day 30 to day 60.

Effect of Molsidomine, Isosorbide Dinitrate, and Verapamil

In a first series, cardiomyopathic hamsters were divided into six groups. Group I (n = 20) received placebo treatment with isotonic saline. Groups II to IV (n = 20 each) received molsidomine, 0.1, 1.0, and 10 mg/kg, respectively. Group V (n = 20) received treatment with verapamil, 10 mg/kg. Group VI (n = 20) received treatment with isosorbide dinitrate, 10 mg/kg. Molsidomine, isosorbide dinitrate, and verapamil were dissolved in isotonic saline. Since molsidomine is sensitive to light, this drug was handled in the dark.

Effect of Acetylsalicylic Acid and Heparin

In a second series, cardiomyopathic hamsters were divided into three groups. Group I (n = 8) received placebo treatment with isotonic saline. Group II (n = 10) received acetylsalicylic acid, 10 mg/kg. Group III (n = 10) received heparin, 100 IU/kg.

The substances were administered by subcutaneous injection every 12 hours. The animals were sacrificed at 60 days of age, and their hearts were excised rapidly. After removal of the atria, a cross-section of each heart was fixed in 4% buffered formaldehyde for histopathologic processing. The remaining heart tissue was frozen at $-20°C$ for subsequent calcium measurement.

Morphologic Analysis

Morphometric evaluation of myocardial necrosis was performed on hematoxylin-eosin stained sections according to the point-counting method described by Weibel et al. (17).

Calcium Measurement

The calcium content of the myocardium was determined by flameless atomic absorption spectrophotometry (Perkin-Elmer Atomabsorption Spectrophotometer 5000).

Platelet Function Tests

Platelet count and function tests were performed on platelet-rich plasma (18). Platelet count was measured by electronic particle counting using a Blood Cell Counter Ultra-Flow 100 (Clay-Adams). The collagen (Equine-Kollagen-Reagenz Horm, Munich, F.R.G.)-induced platelet aggregation test (19) was performed on an Automated Aggregation Clotting Timer (Laborgeräte and Analysensyteme Vertriebsgesellschaft mbH, Ahrensburg, Germany). The final collagen concentration used in the test amounted to 1 μg/ml. Platelet adhesion to extracellular matrix was studied using bovine subendothelial extracellular matrix (20) purchased from IBT Int. Bio-Technologies LTD (Kiryat Hadassah, Jerusalem, Israel).

Statistical Analysis

The data are expressed as mean ± standard deviation. The data of each series were analyzed by analysis of variance. Subsequently, differences between placebo and real treatments were tested by the Wilcoxon U-test adjusted to multiple comparisons according to Bonferroni-Holm (21). A p value <0.05 was accepted as significant. The study was approved by the regional German authorities for animal experiments.

RESULTS

Morphology

In general, the area of necrotic lesions was quite discrete in all cardiomyopathic hamsters. In the placebo-treated animals, it ranged from 0 to 4.2% (mean 1.3 ± 1.3%) in the first series (Fig. 1A) and from 0.3 to 4.4% (mean 2.5 ± 1.4%) in the second series (Fig. 2A).

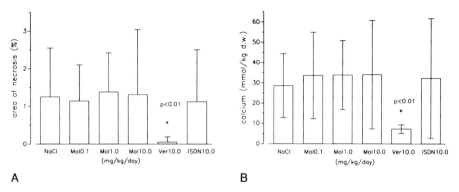

FIG. 1. Area of myocardial necrosis (**A**) and total myocardial calcium content (**B**) measured by atomic absorption spectrophotometry in 60-day-old cardiomyopathic hamsters under treatment with molsidomine (Mol), 0.1, 1.0, and 10.0 mg/kg, verapamil (Ver), 10.0 mg/kg, isosorbide dinitrate (ISDN), 10.0 mg/kg, and placebo (NaCl). *$p<0.01$ versus all other groups.

Molsidomine, Isosorbide Dinitrate, and Verapamil

The myocardium of the molsidomine-treated animals showed $1.14 \pm 0.96\%$ area of necrosis with 0.1 mg/kg/day, $1.38 \pm 1.04\%$ with 1.0 mg/kg/day, and $1.31 \pm 1.73\%$ with 10.0 mg/kg/day molsidomine (Fig. 1A). A similar amount of necrosis was found in the animals treated with isosorbide dinitrate with a mean of $1.12 \pm 1.38\%$. These data did not differ from those produced in placebo-treated animals. As expected, only a few myocardial necrotic areas were present in the verapamil-treated hamsters (mean $0.05 \pm 0.14\%$, $p<0.01$ versus statistics in placebo animals).

Acetylsalicylic Acid and Heparin

In the myocardium of the acetylsalicylic acid–treated and heparin–treated animals, $3.0 \pm 1.8\%$ and $2.4 \pm 1.7\%$ areas of necrotic lesions were observed, respectively (Fig. 2A). There were no differences compared with placebo treatment.

Calcium in the Myocardium

The myocardium of the placebo-treated hamsters contained 28.6 ± 15.8 mmol Ca/kg dry weight in the first series (Fig. 1B) and 33.1 ± 26.3 mmol Ca/kg dry weight in the second series of experiments (Fig. 2B).

Molsidomine, Isosorbide Dinitrate, and Verapamil

The myocardium of the molsidomine-treated animals contained 33.6 ± 21.4 mmol Ca/kg dry weight with 0.1, 33.8 ± 17.0 mmol Ca/kg dry weight with 1.0, and

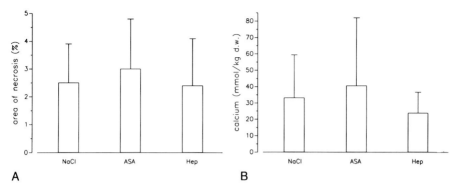

FIG. 2. Area of myocardial necrosis (**A**) and total myocardial calcium content (**B**) measured by atomic absorption spectrophotometry in 60-day-old cardiomyopathic hamsters under treatment with acetylsalicylic acid (ASA), 10 mg/kg, heparin (Hep), 100 IU/kg, and placebo (NaCl).

34.0 ± 26.2 mmol Ca/kg dry weight with 10.0 mg/kg/day molsidomine (Fig. 1B). Hamsters treated with isosorbide dinitrate showed a myocardial calcium content of 32.3 ± 29.4 mmol Ca/kg dry weight. This treatment did not change the myocardial calcium content compared with in placebo treatment. A significantly reduced myocardial calcium content was observed only after treatment with verapamil (7.3 ± 2.1 mmol Ca/kg dry weight, $p < 0.01$ versus placebo treatment).

Acetylsalicylic Acid and Heparin

No significant differences were observed after treatment with acetylsalicylic acid or heparin compared with placebo treatment. The myocardial calcium content amounted to 40.5 ± 41.5 mmol Ca/kg dry weight with acetylsalicylic acid and 23.7 ± 12.9 mmol Ca/kg dry weight with heparin (Fig. 2B).

Platelet Function Tests

The platelet count in the placebo-treated cardiomyopathic hamsters ranged from 115.0 to 900.0/nl, mean 591.5 ± 255.8/nl (Fig. 3A). Treatment with acetylsalicylic acid or heparin did not significantly influence the number of platelets, resulting in platelet counts of 385.2 ± 276.8/nl and 432.4 ± 198.7/nl, respectively.

Acetylsalicylic acid and, to a lesser extent, heparin, significantly inhibited the platelet adhesion to extracellular matrix by 23.2 ± 9.8% and 10.5 ± 2.1%, respectively, as compared with 1.6 ± 1.2% in placebo treatment ($p < 0.01$) (Fig. 3B).

Collagen-induced platelet aggregation was reduced by acetylsalicylic acid, showing an α slope of 33.2 ± 2.2° and a maximum amplitude of 36.7 ± 4.4 mm versus 41.3 ± 2.5° and 44.5 ± 4.6 mm, respectively, compared with placebo treatment ($p < 0.01$) (Fig. 3C). There was no effect on platelet aggregation with heparin.

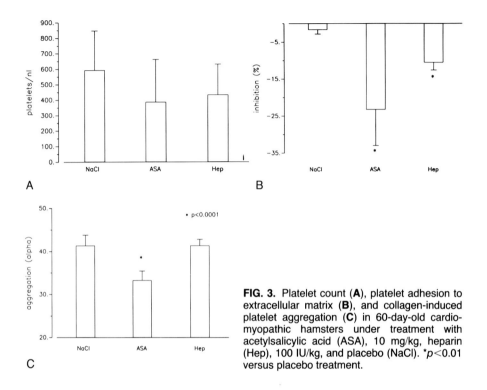

FIG. 3. Platelet count (**A**), platelet adhesion to extracellular matrix (**B**), and collagen-induced platelet aggregation (**C**) in 60-day-old cardiomyopathic hamsters under treatment with acetylsalicylic acid (ASA), 10 mg/kg, heparin (Hep), 100 IU/kg, and placebo (NaCl). *$p<0.01$ versus placebo treatment.

DISCUSSION

Considerable evidence has been presented for a pathogenetic role of microcirculatory disorders in the course of the hereditary cardiomyopathy of the Syrian hamster (5,11,12,22). The aim of this investigation was to obtain more knowledge on the nature of the circulatory disturbances by examining the efficacy of the nitratelike compound molsidomine as well as isosorbide dinitrate, the platelet aggregation inhibitor acetylsalicylic acid, and the anticoagulant heparin in preventing cardiomyopathy.

According to our data, none of these compounds was able to prevent the progression of the disease. Only the calcium antagonist verapamil inhibited the manifestation of the pathognomonic features of the disease, calcium overload, and myocardial necrosis. The beneficial effect of verapamil in preventing hamster cardiomyopathy is well known from the studies of Jasmin and Bajusz (22) as well as that of Lossnitzer et al. (23).

Isosorbide dinitrate and molsidomine are dilators of arterial and venous smooth muscle, both exerting their action by stimulating guanylate cyclase via the release of nitric oxide (24,25). Both are potent dilators of coronary conductance vessels (26, 27), including reversal of vasospasm in variant (Prinzmetal's) angina (28); however, they have little effect on coronary resistance vessels (29,30). Verapamil, on the other hand, has little effect on large epicardial conductance vessels (31); however, it has a high potency in decreasing coronary vascular resistance (32).

An increasing number of data suggest that enhanced sympathetic activity (4), in particular α_1 adrenergic activity (6), and a hereditary hypersensitivity of both vascular smooth muscle and cardiac myocytes to α-adrenergic stimulation (5,6,9) are responsible for the microcirculatory disturbances, i.e., microvascular spasms, in hamster cardiomyopathy. This hypothesis is supported by the finding that α-adrenoceptor blocking agents are effective in reducing the pathologic features of the disease (5,6). We would also like to emphasize that nitrates have been shown to prevent coronary artery constriction induced by α-adrenoceptor stimulation (31). Thus, the lack of influence of isosorbide dinitrate and molsidomine on hamster cardiomyopathy suggests that coronary conductance vessels are not involved in the pathogenesis of the disease.

In another experimental model, the inhibition of platelet function has been shown to protect against catecholamine-induced myocardial necrosis (15,16). This finding has led to the assumption that platelet-dependent microvascular alterations play a crucial role in the development of catecholamine-induced cardiac necroses. In the cardiomyopathy of the Syrian hamster, the question arose as to whether these mechanisms are of pathogenetic relevance in this disease as well.

Acetylsalicylic acid significantly inhibited collagen-induced aggregation and platelet adhesion to extracellular matrix. Platelet adhesion to subendothelial structures or to damaged endothelial cells probably is one of the first reactions in intravasal thrombogenesis. The antithrombotic effect of acetylsalicylic acid is thought to derive from inhibition of thromboxane A_2 production (33). Thromboxane A_2 is formed from arachidonic acid in platelets and is a potent vasoconstrictor and platelet agonist (34). Heparin was used in a low-dose administration. In a previous study, comparable amounts of unfractionated heparin also reduced platelet adhesion to extracellular matrix to a certain extent (35), which is confirmed by the present investigation. Platelet count was not changed by either acetylsalicylic acid or heparin. The anticoagulant activity of heparin was not documented.

The failure of inhibition of platelet function to influence the course of the hamster cardiomyopathy demonstrates that platelet function is not involved in the pathogenesis of this disease.

SUMMARY

Microvascular spasms are considered to contribute substantially to the pathogenesis of the cardiomyopathy of the Syrian hamster. These may be caused by an increase in calcium channels in vascular smooth muscle cell membrane and/or by increased sympathetic activity in the heart. This study was designed to examine (a) the effects of coronary conductance vessel dilators such as molsidomine (0.1, 1, and 10 mg/kg) and isosorbide dinitrate (10 mg/kg), and (b) the influence of platelet aggregation inhibition by acetylsalicylic acid (10 mg/kg) on hamster cardiomyopathy (strain Bio 82.62). In addition, the effect of heparin (100 IU/kg) was examined. The drugs were applied subcutaneously twice a day. Verapamil (10 mg/kg) and equivalent amounts of saline served as controls. Myocardial necrosis and tissue calcium content were the parameters for the progression of the cardiomyopathy. Whereas verapamil completely prevented myocardial necrosis and calcium overload (7.3 ± 2.1 [standard deviation] versus 28.6 ± 15.8 mmol Ca^{2+}/kg dry weight with saline), molsidomine, isosorbide dinitrate, acetylsalicylic acid, and heparin did not influence the course of the disease. In conclusion, the lack of beneficial effects of nitrate-like vasodilators or inhibition of platelet aggregation suggests that (a) coronary conductance vessels and (b) platelet function are not involved in the pathogenesis of hamster cardiomyopathy.

ACKNOWLEDGMENT

The authors gratefully appreciate the helpful discussions with Professor Gisbert Kober, M.D., Bad Nauheim, Germany.

REFERENCES

1. Homburger F, Baker JR, Nixon W, Wilgram G. A new hereditary disease of Syrian hamsters: primary generalized polymyopathy and cardiac necrosis. *Arch Intern Med* 1962;110:660–2.
2. Bajusz E, Lossnitzer K. A new disease model of chronic congestive heart failure: studies on its pathogenesis. *Trans NY Acad Sci* 1968;30:939–48.
3. Lossnitzer K, Steinhardt B, Grewe N, Stauch M. Characteristic electrolyte changes in the hereditary myopathy and cardiomyopathy of the Syrian golden hamster. *Basic Res Cardiol* 1975;70:508–20.
4. Lund DD, Schmid PG, Bhatnagar RK, Roskoski R, Jr. Changes in parasympathetic and sympathetic neurochemical indices in hearts of myopathic hamsters. *J Auton Nerv Syst* 1982;5:237–46.
5. Sole MJ, Factor SM. Hamster cardiomyopathy. A genetically transmitted sympathetic dystrophy? In: Beamish RE, Panagia V, Dhalla NS, eds. *Pathogenesis of stress-induced heart disease.* Boston: Martinus Nijhoff; 1984:34–43.
6. Kagiya T, Hori M, Iwakura K, et al. Role of increased alpha 1-adrenergic activity in cardiomyopathic Syrian hamsters. *Am J Physiol* 1991;260:H80–88.
7. Lossnitzer K, Janke J, Hein B, Stauch M, Fleckenstein A. Disturbed myocardial calcium metabolism—a possible pathogenetic factor in the hereditary cardiomyopathy of the Syrian hamster. *Recent Adv Stud Cardiac Struct Metab* 1975;6:283–90.
8. Karliner JS, Alabaster C, Stephens H, Barnes P, Dollery C. Enhanced noradrenaline response in cardiomyopathic hamsters: possible relation to changes in adrenoreceptors studied by radioligand binding. *Cardiovasc Res* 1981;15:296–304.
9. Böhm M, Mende U, Schmitz W, Scholz H. Increased responsiveness to stimulation of α- but not β-adrenoceptors in the hereditary cardiomyopathy of the Syrian hamster. Intact adenosine- and cholinoceptor-mediated isoprenaline antagonist effect. *Eur J Pharmacol* 1986;128:195–203.
10. Wagner JA, Reynolds IJ, Weisman HF, Dudeck P, Weisfeldt ML, Snyder SH. Calcium antagonist receptors in cardiomyopathic hamsters: selective increases in heart muscle brain. *Science* 1986; 232:515–18.
11. Factor SM, Minase T, Cho S, Dominitz R, Sonnenblick EH. Microvascular spasm in the cardiomyopathic Syrian hamster: a preventable cause of focal myocardial necrosis. *Circulation* 1982; 66:342–54.
12. Figulla HR, Vetterlein F, Glaubitz M, Kreuzer H. Inhomogenous capillary flow and its prevention by verapamil and hydralazine in the cardiomyopathic Syrian hamster. *Circulation* 1987;76:208–16.

13. Geft IL, Fishbein MC, Ninomiya K, et al. Intermittent brief periods of ischemia have a cumulative effect and may cause myocardial necrosis. *Circulation* 1982;66:1150–3.
14. Rona G, Chappel Cl, Balazs T, Gaudry R. An infarct-like myocardial lesion and other toxic manifestations produced by isoproterenol in the rat. *AMA Arch Pathol* 1959;67:443–52.
15. Haft JI, Gershengorn K, Kranz PD, Oestreicher R. Protection against epinephrine-induced myocardial necrosis by drugs that inhibit platelet aggregation. *Am J Cardiol* 1972;30:838–43.
16. Kammermeier H, Ober M. Essential contribution of thrombocytes to the occurrence of catecholamine-induced cardiac necroses. *J Mol Cell Cardiol* 1985;17:371–6.
17. Weibel ER, Kistler GS, Scherle WF. Practical stereological methods for morphometric cytology. *J Cell Biol* 1966;30:23–38.
18. Kitek A, Breddin K. Optical density variations and microscopic observations in the evaluation of platelet shape change and microaggregate formation. *Thromb Haemost* 1980;44:154–8.
19. Born GVR. Quantitative investigation into the aggregation of blood platelets. *J Physiol* 1962; 162:67–8.
20. Vlodavsky I, Eldor A, HyAm E, Atzom R, Fuks Z. Platelet interaction with the extracellular matrix produced by cultured endothelial cells: a model to study the thrombogenicity of isolated subendothelial basal lamina. *Thromb Res* 1982;28:179–91.
21. Holm S. A simple sequentially rejective multiple test procedure. *Scand J Statist* 1979;6:65–75.
22. Jasmin G, Bajusz E. Prevention of myocardial degeneration in hamsters with hereditary cardiomyopathy. In: Fleckenstein A, Rona G, eds. *Recent advances in studies on cardiac structure and metabolism, vol VI.* Baltimore: University Park Press; 1975:219–28.
23. Lossnitzer K, Mohr WS, Konrad A, Guggenmoos R. The hereditary cardiomyopathy in the Syrian golden hamster—influence of verapamil as calcium antagonist. In: Kaltenbach M, Loogen F, Olsen EGJ, eds. *Cardiomyopathy and myocardial biopsy.* Berlin, Heidelberg, New York: Springer Verlag; 1978:2–37.
24. Rapaport RM, Murad F. Endothelium-dependent and nitrovasodilator-induced relaxation of vascular smooth muscle: role for cyclic GMP. *J Cyclic Nucleotide Protein Phosphorylation Res* 1983;9:281–96.
25. Noak E, Martin F. Molecular aspects underlying the vasodilator action of molsidomine. *J Cardiovasc Pharmacol* 1989;14[Suppl 11]:S1–5.
26. Feldman RL, Pepine CJ, Conti CR. Magnitude of dilatation of large and small coronary arteries by nitroglycerin. *Circulation* 1981;64:324–32.
27. Schulz W, Kober G, Bernauer R, Kaltenbach M. Active and passive changes in coronary diameter after vasodilation with SIN-1, the active metabolite of molsidomine. *Am Heart J* 1985;10:694–99.
28. Murao S, Mashima S. Shimomura K, Uchida Y, Yoshimoto N. Pathophysiology of variant angina pectoris and effects of anti-anginal drugs—clinical and experimental study. *Jpn J Med* 1978; 17:284–5.
29. Winbury MM, Howe BB, Hefner MA. Effect of nitrates and other coronary dilators on large and small coronary vessels: hypothesis for the mechanism of action of nitrates. *J Pharmacol Exp Ther* 1969;168:70–95.
30. Fiedler VB, Nitz RE. Effects of molsidomine, nitroglycerin, and isosorbide dinitrate on the coronary circulation, myocardial oxygen consumption, and hemodynamics in anaesthetized dogs. *Naunyn Schmiedebergs Arch Pharmacol* 1981;317:71–7.
31. Brown G. Response of normal and diseased epicardial coronary arteries to vasoactive drugs: quantitative arteriographic studies: *Am J Cardiol* 1985;56:23E–29E.
32. Schlepper M, Witzleb E. Tierexperimentelle Untersuchungen über die Veränderungen von Coronardurchblutung und Sauerstoffverbrauch des Herzens nach α-Isopropyl-α-[(N-methyl-N-homoveratryl)- -amino-propyl]-3,4-dimethoxyphenylacetonitril. *Arzneimittelforschung* 1962;12:559–61.
33. Reilly IAG, FitzGerald GA. Aspirin in cardiovascular disease. *Drugs* 1988;35:154–76.
34. Hamberg M. Samuelsson B. Prostaglandin endoperoxides, novel transformations of arachidonic acid in human platelets. *Proc Natl Acad Sci USA* 1974;71:3400–04.
35. Krupinski K, Basic-Micic, M, Lindhoff E, Breddin HK. Inhibition of coagulation and platelet adhesion to extracellular matrix by unfractionated heparin and a low molecular weight heparin. *Blut* 1990;61:289–94.

The Cardiomyopathic Heart, edited by Makoto
Nagano, Nobuakira Takeda, and Naranjan S.
Dhalla. Raven Press, Ltd., New York © 1994.

20

Subcellular Basis for Increased Diastolic Stiffness in Experimental Cardiomyopathies

Valery I. Kapelko, *Mikhail I. Popovich, Vladimir I. Veksler,
†Renee Ventura-Clapier, Zaza A. Khuchua, and Valdur A. Saks

*Cardiology Research Center, 15A Cherepkovskaya Street, 121552 Moscow, Russia;
*Institute of Prophylactic and Clinical Medicine, 20 Kubinskoi Revolutsii St.,
Kishinev, Moldova; and †University Paris-Sud, 91405 Orsay, France*

INTRODUCTION

The pathogenesis of cardiomyopathies has been extensively studied in the last decades; however, the precise sequence of events leading to cardiac contractile failure still remains uncertain. Among several experimental models, the hamster hereditary cardiomyopathy as well as doxorubicin-induced cardiomyopathy have been given more attention (1–3), possibly because of their close relevance to human cardiomyopathy. Other models, such as that induced by alcohol ingestion, diabetes, and catecholamine administration, have been studied less frequently (1,2,4).

Despite different mechanisms underlying the various types of cardiomyopathies, they share a common feature of structural alterations in which irreversibly damaged cardiomyocytes are replaced by connective tissue. The cardiac performance of these hearts, however, is determined by partially damaged but still surviving cells, and characterization of their state contributes to an understanding of the pathogenesis of this disease. We performed functional, metabolic, and ultrastructural studies in several cardiomyopathic models (5–14), the results of which are briefly reviewed in this chapter.

MATERIALS AND METHODS

Experimental Models

Most of these studies were done in rats treated with doxorubicin (10 weeks) or noradrenaline (4 weeks), whereas other models included autoimmunization of rats with heart antigen, prolonged pesticide administration (12 weeks), and spontaneously occurred smallpox virus infection. The scheme of treatment is presented in detail elsewhere (8,10). Also hamster derivatives of the Bio 14.6 hamster hereditary cardiomyopathic line—namely, the UM-X7.1 (6) and CMF 146 (11–14) strains (ages 160–200 days)—were studied.

Heart Perfusion

Hearts were perfused according to Neely's working heart model at 37°C with Krebs' solution saturated with 95% O_2 and 5% CO_2, pH 7.3 to 7.4. The aortic output was measured by electromagnetic flowmeter 501D, Caroline Medical Electronics. A steel needle was introduced into the left ventricular chamber through its wall, and left ventricular pressure and aortic pressure were monitored by a Gould 2600S recorder. The left ventricular diastolic stiffness was estimated by determining the ratio between increments of diastolic pressure and volume for a given diastole (7–10).

Isolated Atria

The right atria were superfused with the same solution in thermostated cell at 29°C. Their ends were clipped, and one of them was connected to an isotonic lever and opposed by a light load. The lever's movements during atrial contractions were paced by the Grass stimulator and detected with an MTI fotonic sensor and monitored by the Gould 2200 recorder (5).

Energy Metabolites

At the end of each experiment, the heart was clamped by Wollenberger's clamps cooled in liquid nitrogen, and the contents of myocardial adenine nucleotides, phosphocreatine, and free creatine were determined enzymatically (7–10).

Mitochondrial Studies

Endocardial fibers were skinned with saponin (40 mcM/mL), and the rate of oxygen consumption was determined with the Yellow Springs Instruments Oxygraph, as described elsewhere (11–14). The activity of creatine kinase was assessed by the reverse reaction.

RESULTS AND DISCUSSION

Cardiac Contractile Function

The cardiac pump function was significantly depressed in all models studied (8–10). Reductions in heart rate, cardiac and aortic outputs, and left ventricular systolic pressure were common findings, indicating cardiac pump insufficiency. Also, the ability of the heart to raise its function to withstand increased volume or pressure loads was markedly depressed. Remarkably, at the lowest left atrial filling pressure, some cardiomyopathic hearts could pump an even higher cardiac output than control hearts (10). This finding probably reflects a dilation of the left ventricular chamber, as the same models have shown most prominent dystrophic alterations (8). However, at maximal filling pressure, the maximal cardiac output in all experimental groups was reduced by 26% to 55%.

A moderate rise in left ventricular systolic pressure caused by increased hydrostatic resistance was accompanied by a substantial decrease in cardiac output only in myopathic hearts. The cardiac work reached its maximum in control experiments at complete clamping of the aortic outline. Cardiomyopathic hearts showed a 42% to 56% reduction in this value (10). Thus, both maximal left ventricular pressure development and the ability to maintain high levels of cardiac output were substantially depressed in cardiomyopathic hearts.

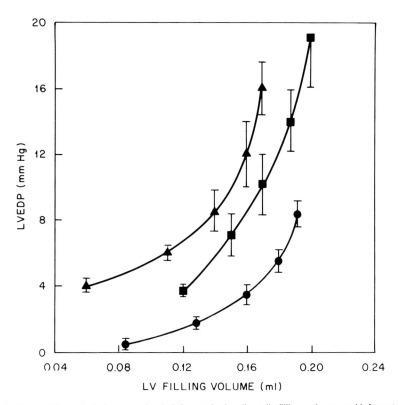

FIG. 1. The relationship between a rise in left ventricular diastolic filling volume and left ventricular end diastolic pressure during a stepwise increase in left atrial filling pressure from 5 to 25 cm of water. Controls (●); doxorubicin-treated hearts (■); noradrenaline-treated hearts (▲); each value is mean ± standard error of six to nine experiments. *LVEDP*, left ventricular end diastolic pressure.

Markedly increased values of left ventricular pressure throughout the diastole as well as left ventricular diastolic stiffness were the most consistent findings in all experimental groups (7–10). Both values were twofold to fourfold higher than in control groups. The relationship between the rise in diastolic volume and pressure during increased volume loading showed a clear shift of the curve up and to the left (Fig. 1). The left ventricular diastolic stiffness was also found to increase stepwise during an elevation of aortic resistance. These data provide evidence for substantially decreased left ventricular distensibility, which contributes to cardiac pump failure in experimental groups. An increased diastolic stiffness was also observed in isovolumetric cardiomyopathic hamster hearts (6).

The most plausible explanation for decreased diastolic distensibility is the fibrosis that is always observed in cardiomyopathic hearts. However, fibrotic tissue creates much more resistance to stretch than do cardiomyocytes; therefore fibrotic tissue can be considered a very strong series elastic component contributing to the pressure-volume diastolic curve only at increased volumes, whereas within normal range, the cardiac distensibility should be determined by the surviving cardiomyocytes.

The ultrastructural study revealed that most myofibrils were relaxed, but in some cells, the contraction band formation of sarcomeres was observed, whereas adjacent sarcomeres in the same cell were overdistended (7). This finding was frequently observed in various experimental models as well as in human cardiomyopathy (1) and is usually considered to be the result of calcium retention in myofibrils. It obviously should create an increased resistance of sarcomeres to distention.

Calcium-Related Inotropic Events

It is well known that the contracture of sarcomeres can be caused by both failure of sarcoplasmic reticulum (SR) to accumulate calcium and insufficient adenosine triphosphate (ATP) supply to myofibrils. An increased functional load on SR can be induced at high frequency rates. An example of such a test (Fig. 2) clearly shows that the rise in left ventricular minimal diastolic pressure is accompanied by a dramatic reduction in left ventricular filling pressure–time area. This incomplete relaxation contributes to decreased cardiac output at increased heart rates. A deteriorating effect of higher frequencies was also reported in isovolumetric hamster hereditary cardiomyopathy (15).

The force-frequency relationship in a broader range was studied in isolated atria taken from doxorubicin-treated rats (5). Atria had sizes and weights similar to those of controls, but the maximal extent of shortening in slightly loaded contractions was roughly half that of control atria. Doxorubicin-treated atria also responded to increased simulation frequency by a substantial rise in the degree of incomplete relaxation; this value at the highest rate—5 Hz—was approximately five times higher than that of control atria. This finding is also in accordance with the suggestion of inappropriate function of SR in this model (16). However, the results of the other functional test—paired pulse stimulation—do not support this suggestion. The po-

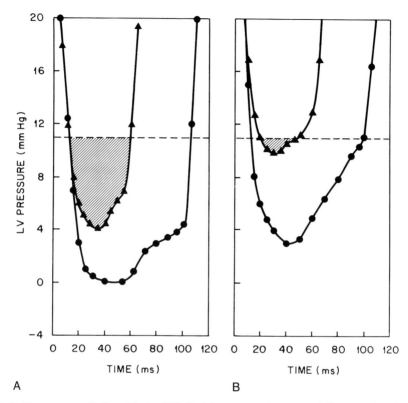

FIG. 2. Time course of left ventricular (*LV*) diastolic pressure in representative experiments at a normal (240/min) heart rate (●) and an increased (360/min) heart rate (▲). **A**: Control. **B**: Doxorubicin treatment. The horizontal lines indicate the level of stable left atrial filling pressure, whereas the shaded areas show the left ventricular filling pressure time integral.

tentiation of the extent of shortening in doxorubicin-treated atria was much more apparent, and at maximal potentiation, the difference in contractile amplitude between groups completely disappeared (Fig. 3).

Because paired pulse potentiation is widely believed to be determined by an ability of the SR to accumulate and release an additional quantity of calcium ions, the observed finding may be considered indicative of unchanged function of SR. There are some other indications of almost undisturbed SR function. In fact, SR and T-tubules were found to be more prominent in hamster cardiomyopathy, the relaxation velocity of isolated myocytes was normal, and these cells could maintain roughly normal myoplasmic calcium concentrations (17). Furthermore, the relaxation constant of left ventricular pressure was unchanged in doxorubicin-treated rat hearts (9). Also, the calcium-binding function of the SR was reported to be unchanged in human cardiomyopathy, as evidenced by studies both in isolated vesicles (18) and in skinned myocardial fibers (19).

If the function of SR is really almost unchanged, the contractile failure that was

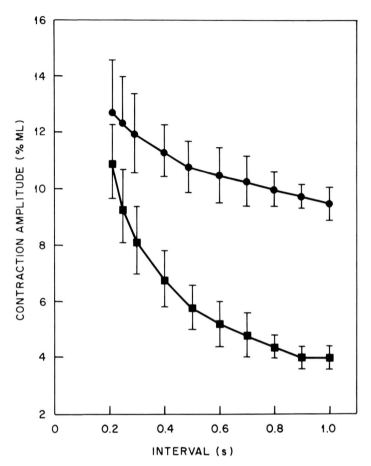

FIG. 3. Potentiation of contractile amplitude of isolated right atria induced by paired pulse stimulation at varied delays. Control (●); doxorubicin treatment (■). Each value is mean ± standard error of five to seven experiments.

consistently observed in isolated hearts and atria as well as in isolated myocytes at normal external calcium concentrations (17) may be determined by either impaired response of the contractile apparatus to calcium or decreased calcium myoplasmic concentration.

Maximal force developed by myofibrils in skinned myocardial fibers at saturating calcium concentrations and optimal energy supply was reported to be unchanged in most experimental models (5,10,14) and in the human cardiomyopathic heart (19). Myofibrillar calcium sensitivity varied from being mildly increased (5,10,14) to remaining almost unchanged (19) but was not found to be decreased in any of the studies. These data indicate that some changes in myofilament protein structure can occur that result in tighter calcium retention in troponin complexes. Such changes may include a shift from "fast" V1 isoenzyme of myosine to a "slow" V3 form that possesses lower adenosine triphosphatase (ATPase) activity (20). This shift may be particularly important for rat and hamster hearts with a predominantly V1 form.

The other main determinant of myocardial contractility—myoplasmic calcium concentration—was reported to be normal in isolated beating myocytes from hamster cardiomyopathic hearts at normal or increased external calcium concentrations, and was found to be increased at lower external calcium levels (17). Nevertheless, the contractile amplitude of these cells was reduced at normal or elevated external calcium levels. Thus, other factors apart from myoplasmic calcium or myofibrillar calcium sensitivity seem to determine the depressed contractility in cardiomyopathic cells.

Myofibrillar Energy Supply

An insufficient supply of ATP to myofibrils can decrease both myofibrillar contractility by inhibitory action of increased inorganic phosphate (P_i) on Ca^{2+}-troponin binding and distensibility by incomplete rephosphorylation of adenosine diphosphate (ADP) which, in turn, results in an increased quantity of attached actomyosin bonds. The latter factor may be facilitated in vivo by some retention of calcium ions in myofibrils resulting from their increased calcium sensitivity. Markedly lower levels of ATP and phosphocreatine (PCr) were observed in almost all models studied (6–10,12,13,21,22). PCr seems to be more sensitive than ATP (6,8). A definite inverse correlation between depletion of ATP or PCr content and increased left ventricular diastolic stiffness, observed for various models (6,8,10), supports the suggestion of insufficient ATP supply to myofibrils in situ.

In normal cardiomyocytes, the mitochondria and creatine kinase system determine energy production and utilization in the cell. Mitochondrial function in saponin-skinned myocardial fibers from hamster hearts was evaluated by measuring oxygen consumption in the presence of natural controlling substances.

Four principal findings were found (11–14). First, although maximal oxygen consumption was similar in control and myopathic fibers—43.5 and 42.7 ng atoms O_2/min/mg of mitochondrial protein, respectively—the content of cytochrome aa$_3$ per milligram of myocardial mass was reduced by 38% at the normal ratio of cytochrome to mitochondrial protein. This suggests that the cardiomyopathic heart has a lower content of mitochondria without any changes in their maximal capacity of oxygen consumption. Because the fractional volume occupied by mitochondria in cardiomyocytes was found to be unchanged in the same model (23), these data indicate a partial loss of cardiomyocytes. In fact, a 13% cellular loss, as determined by cell counting, was reported for this stage of disease (24).

Second, mitochondrial respiration stimulated by creatine addition at low physiologic levels of ADP was found to be 40% to 70% lower in various experimental series as compared with the control groups (12–14). This finding, evidencing decreased activity of mitochondrial creatine kinase, has been supported by electrophoretic data revealing a twofold decrease in mitochondrial creatine kinase isoenzyme, whereas that of the BB form increased fourfold (12).

Third, total creatine kinase activity in cardiomyopathic hearts was only 62% of that in control hearts, and this was accompanied by a twofold decline of the flux through creatine kinase, as measured by the ^{31}P-NMR saturation technique (12).

Fourth, myofibrillar creatine kinase activity was also found to be decreased (14). It was assessed in skinned fibers that developed contracture at lower MgATP concentrations; in the presence of PCr, the value of pMgATP at which half-maximal contracture occurred was 0.2 units less for cardiomyopathic myocardium. Also, when fibers were supplied with PCr + ADP regenerating system in the absence of ATP, their tension recovery after quick stretch was markedly slowed, the time constant being 37% more than in normal fibers. When both PCr and ATP were present, no difference was observed (14). These data form evidence for reduced potency of myofibrillar creatine kinase isoenzyme to transform PCr into ATP.

Taken together, these findings indicate a depressed functional activity of the creatine kinase system in cardiomyocytes of hamsters with hereditary cardiomyopathy. However, it remains to be established whether these changes are primary or secondary. In fact, they may occur as a result of depressed myocardial contractility followed by decreased myofibrillar energy demand.

Clinical Implications

Many of the features observed in experimental models of cardiomyopathy have also been observed in human studies (25–28). Cardiac contractile failure in vivo is combined with elevated left ventricular diastolic pressure and decreased chamber distensibility. Isolated trabeculae can develop normal maximal force at low rates of contraction, and skinned myocardial fibers have calcium sensitivity similar to fibers from other patients who do not have cardiomyopathy (26,28). Moreover, myoplasmic diastolic and systolic calcium concentration in failing myocardium seems not to be different from that in controls (28).

However, as in animals, the contractile function of human cardiomyopathic myocardium is disturbed as a result of abnormal intracellular calcium handling. The force developed by isolated trabeculae becomes less than that in corresponding controls at higher frequencies when fusion of calcium transients and isometric twitches occurs (27). A remarkable finding in these studies was the observation of a delayed reduction in myoplasmic calcium concentration (26,27). The time course of such calcium transients is similar to the prolonged action potential of these fibers, and the authors hypothesized that the second slow component of the transient might be caused by prolonged calcium entry.

Relatively less is known about energy metabolism in human cardiomyopathy. The ratio of PCr/ATP, as studied by ^{31}P-NMR, was found to be 19% less in these patients than in healthy subjects (29). Some functional and metabolic data were obtained in our study of 39 patients with dilated cardiomyopathy of three functional

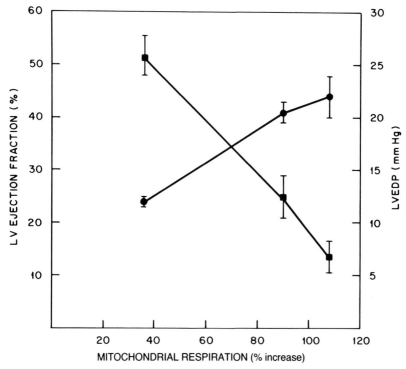

FIG. 4. The relationships between creatine-stimulated respiration of in situ mitochondria of endomyocardial samples, ejection fraction (●), and left ventricular end diastolic pressure (*LVEDP*) (■) in patients with dilated cardiomyopathy of different functional classes. Each value is mean-± standard error of 3 to 24 observations. Reproduced with permission from Saks et al., ref. 13.

classes (13). Endomyocardial biopsies, as well as echocardiographic and angiographic studies, were performed. The maximal respiration rate of saponin-treated fibers was similar in classes I and II and was 22% less in class III. Creatine-stimulated respiration was depleted in class III by 17% and in class II by 67% compared with class I. The most interesting finding of this study was the relationship between creatine-stimulated respiration of mitochondria and hemodynamic parameters. Almost linear inverse correlation was observed between a depletion of creatine-stimulated respiration and increased left ventricular end diastolic pressure (Fig. 4) in these patients. A slightly worse correlation was observed for the ejection fraction.

SUMMARY

Despite obvious limitations in correspondence between experimental models and human disease, the main findings obtained in experimental and clinical studies are similar. They both show diastolic and systolic myocardial dysfunction that may be attributed to both abnormal intracellular calcium handling and disturbances in energy production and utilization.

REFERENCES

1. Factor SM, Sonnenblick EH. The pathogenesis of clinical and experimental congestive cardiomyopathies: recent concepts. *Progr Cardiovasc Dis* 1985;27:395–420.
2. Goodwin JF. Mechanisms in cardiomyopathies. *J Mol Cell Cardiol* 1985;17[Suppl 2]:5–9.
3. Singal PK, Deally CMR, Weinberg LE. Subcellular effects of Adriamycin in the heart: a concise review. *J Mol Cell Cardiol* 1987;19:817–28.
4. Dhalla NS, Pierce GN, Innes IR, Beamish RE. Pathogenesis of cardiac dysfunction in diabetes mellitus. *Can J Cardiol* 1985;1:263–81.
5. Kapelko VI, Veksler VI, Gorina MS, Golikov MA. Calcium-dependent changes of the myocardial contractile function at chronic Adriamycin treatment. *Acta Physiol Pol* 1988;39:166–74.
6. Kapelko VI, Parmley WW, Wu S, Stone RD, Jasmin G, Wikman-Coffelt J. Increased left ventricular diastolic stiffness in the early phase of hereditary cardiomyopathy. *Am Heart J* 1988;116:765–70.
7. Kapelko VI, Popovich MI, Sharov, VG, et al. The ultrastructural, metabolic and functional alterations of the heart at prolonged Adriamycin treatment. *J Appl Cardiol* 1989;4:79–89.
8. Kapelko VI, Veksler VI, Popovich MI. Cellular mechanisms of alterations in myocardial contractile function in experimental cardiomyopathies. *Biomed Sci* 1990;1:77–83.
9. Kapelko VI, Golikov MA, Novikova NA, Popovich MI. Cardiac contractile changes induced by acute and chronic Adriamycin administration. *CV World Rep* 1990;3:60–4.
10. Kapelko VI, Veksler VI, Popovich MI, Ventura-Clapier R. Energy-linked functional alterations in experimental cardiomyopathies. *Am J Physiol* 1991;261[Suppl]:39–44.
11. Khuchua ZA, Ventura-Clapier R, Kuznetsov AV, Grishin MN, Saks VA. Alterations in the creatine-kinase system in the myocardium of cardiomyopathic hamsters. *Biochem Biophys Res Commun* 1989;165:748–57.
12. Khuchua ZA, Kuznetsov AV, Vasilyeva EV, et al. The creatine kinase system and cardiomyopathy. *Am J Cardiovasc Pathol* 1992;4:223–34.
13. Saks VA, Belikova YO, Kuznetsov AV, et al. Phosphocreatine pathway for energy transport: ATP diffusion and cardiomyopathy. *Am J Physiol* 1991;261[Suppl]:30–8.
14. Veksler VI, Ventura-Clapier R, Lechene P, Vassort G. Functional state of myofibrils, mitochondria and bound creatine kinase in skinned ventricular fibers of cardiomyopathic hamsters. *J Mol Cell Cardiol* 1988;20:329–42.
15. Markiewitz W, Wu S, Sievers R, et al. Influence of heart rate on metabolic and hemodynamic parameters in Syrian hamster cardiomyopathy. *Am Heart J* 1987;114:362–8.
16. Panagia V, Lee SL, Singh A, Pierce GN, Jasmin G, Dhalla NS. Impairment of mitochondrial and sarcoplasmic reticulum functions during the development of heart failure in cardiomyopathic (UM-X 7.1) hamsters. *Can J Cardiol* 1986;2:236–47.
17. Sen L, O'Neill M, Marsh JD, Smith TW. Myocyte structure, function, and calcium kinetics in the cardiomyopathic hamster heart. *Am J Physiol* 1990;259:H1533–43.
18. Movsesian MA, Bristow MR, Krall J. Calcium uptake by cardiac sarcoplasmic reticulum from patients with idiopathic dilated cardiomyopathy. *Circ Res* 1987;65:1141–4.
19. D'Agnolo A, Luciani GB, Mazzucco A, Gallucci V, Salviati G. Contractile properties and calcium release activity of the sarcoplasmic reticulum in dilated cardiomyopathy. *Circulation* 1992;85:518–25.
20. Takeda N, Nakamura I, Hatanaka T, Ohkubo T, Nagano M. Myocardial mechanical and myosin isoenzyme alterations in streptozotocin-diabetic rats. *Jpn Heart J* 1988;29:455–63.
21. Sievers R, Parmley WW, James T, Wikman-Coffelt J. Energy levels at systole vs. diastole in normal hamsters vs. myopathic hamster heart. *Circ Res* 1983;53:759–66.
22. Whitmer JT. Energy metabolism and mechanical function in perfused hearts of Syrian hamsters with dilated and hypertrophic cardiomyopathy. *J Mol Cell Cardiol* 1986;18:307–17.
23. Perennee J, Willemin M, Pocholle P, Hatt PY, Crozatier B. Cardiac ultrastructural abnormalities in Syrian hamsters with spontaneous cardiomyopathy or subjected to cardiac overloads. *Basic Res Cardiol* 1992;87:54–64.

24. Sorenson AL, Tepper D, Sonnenblick EH, Robinson TF, Capasso JM. Size and shape of enzymatically isolated ventricular myocytes from rats and cardiomyopathic hamsters. *Cardiovasc Res* 1985;19:793–9.
25. Grossman W, Lorell B, eds. *Diastolic relaxation of the heart.* Boston: Martinus Nijhoff Publishing;1988.
26. Gwathmey JK, Copelas L, MacKinnon R, et al. Abnormal intracellular calcium handling in myocardium from patients with end-stage heart failure. *Circ Res* 1987;61:70–6.
27. Morgan JP, Erny RE, Allen PD, Grossman W, Gwathmey JK. Abnormal intracellular calcium handling, a major cause of systolic and diastolic dysfunction in ventricular myocardium from patients with heart failure. *Circulation* 1990;81[Suppl III]:21–32.
28. Perreault CL, Meuse AJ, Bentivegna LA, Morgan JP. Abnormal intracellular calcium handling in acute and chronic heart failure: role in systolic and diastolic dysfunction. *Eur Heart J* 1990;11[Suppl C]:8–21.
29. Hardy CJ, Weiss RG, Bottomley PA, Gerstenblith G. Altered high-energy phosphate metabolites in patients with dilated cardiomyopathy. *Am Heart J* 1991;122:795–801.

The Cardiomyopathic Heart, edited by Makoto
Nagano, Nobuakira Takeda, and Naranjan S.
Dhalla. Raven Press, Ltd., New York © 1994.

21

Force-Frequency Relationship in the Nonfailing and End-Stage Failing Human Myocardium: Influence of Positive Inotropic Interventions

B. Pieske, G. Hasenfuss, Ch. Holubarsch, M. Büchler,
*H. Posival, and H. Just

*Medizinische Klinik III, University of Freiburg, 7800 Freiburg, Germany; and
Herzzentrum Bad Oeynhausen, Germany

Since the first investigations of Bowditch in 1871, it had been known that in many animal species force of contraction increases with increasing heart rates. This phenomenon has been shown in isolated mammalian myocardium (1,2) and in whole-heart experiments (3,4), and has been termed the "treppe" phenomenon or positive force-frequency relationship. It is related to a frequency-dependent increase in the transmembranous Ca^{2+} fluxes (5,6).

Experiments of Sonnenblick and colleagues (7) in the intact human heart suggested a positive velocity-frequency relationship. The situation in the isolated human myocardium has been evaluated recently under physiologic conditions. The former results of Sonnenblick's group could be extended, because in nonfailing human myocardium not only shortening velocity but also isometric twitch tension increases with increasing stimulation frequencies (8,10). However, it became obvious that the force-frequency relationship is inverse in heart failure owing to DCM (8–10). Similar results have been obtained in in vivo investigations, in which hemodynamic parameters, such as cardiac index, increase in patients without heart failure but decrease in patients with dilated cardiomyopathy at high heart rates (11,12).

There is no conclusive information on the subcellular defects that lead to the inverse force-frequency relationship in DCM. However, some alterations at the level of the myocyte in DCM that have been investigated during the last years may contribute to the inversion of the force-frequency relationship. Excitation-contraction coupling is impaired by a decrease in β-adrenoceptor density (13–15) and changes on the level of the G proteins (16,17), thus leading to a decrease in adenylate cyclase activity and intracellular cyclic adenosine monophosphate (cAMP)

197

content (11,18). A reduced cAMP content may decrease the amount of Ca^{2+} entering the cell as well as the rate of Ca^{2+} reuptake by the sarcoplasmic reticulum (SR). Furthermore, a decrease in SR Ca^{2+}-adenosine triphosphatase (ATPase) messenger RNA (mRNA) expression (19) has been shown to occur in the failing human myocardium. These changes may lead to the reported reduced uptake capacity of the SR for Ca^{2+} (20). As a consequence, the amount of Ca^{2+} stored in the SR, and thus the amount of Ca^{2+} released during systole for activation of the contractile proteins, may also be reduced (21,22).

In the failing myocardium, force of contraction can be increased by distinct positive inotropic interventions that act by stimulating the myocytes on different intracellular levels. In order to investigate whether positive inotropic interventions normalize the inverse force-frequency relationship in the failing human heart, muscle strips were exposed to either a cAMP-independent (Ca^{2+}) or cAMP-dependent (isoproterenol) positive inotropic intervention prior to the investigation of the force-frequency relationship. Both interventions increased the amount of activator Ca^{2+} available to the contractile proteins. In addition, isoproterenol, by phospholamban phosphorylation, was found to increase the activity of the SR Ca^{2+} pumps (23,24).

MATERIALS AND METHODS

Myocardial Muscle Strips

Human left ventricular papillary muscle strips were obtained from three nonfailing hearts that could not be transplanted for technical reasons and from six end-stage failing hearts secondary to dilated cardiomyopathy at the time of heart transplantation. Coronary heart disease and valvular disease had been excluded in all failing hearts prior to transplantation. In the DCM group, all patients were clinically classified as having New York Heart Association IV failure, the mean age was 58 ± 3 years, and the mean ejection fraction was $22 \pm 1\%$. No cardiac catheterizations had been performed in the organ donor group, but all donors had normal left ventricular function. Their mean age was 47 ± 5 years.

Preparation Procedure

Left ventricular papillary muscle strips were prepared and mounted to an isometric force transducer as described elsewhere (10). Briefly small pieces of papillary muscles were excised immediately after explantation and stored in a special cardioplegic solution containing 30 mM of 2,3-butanedione monoxime, bubbled with carbogen (95% O_2, 5% CO_2, pH of 7.4) at room temperature. Upon arrival in the laboratory, small (cross-sectional area <0.6 mm^2) muscle strips were dissected exactly along fiber orientation with the help of a stereomicroscope and specially designed preparation chambers. All preparation steps were carried out in the presence of the cardioprotective solution, which minimizes cutting injury (25). The muscle strips were then mounted horizontally in an organ bath (Hugo Sachs Electronics, March-Hugstetten, Germany) and connected to an isometric force transducer. Signals were recorded using a chart strip recorder (Graphtec Lineacorder, Yokohoma, Japan). Muscles were superfused with a carbogen-bubbled (pH of 7.4) modified Krebs-Henseleit solution of the following composition (in mM): Na^+, 152; K^+, 3.6; Cl^-, 135; Ca^{2+}, 2.5; Mg, 0.6; HCO^{3-}, 25; H^2PO^{4-}, 1.3; SO^{4--}, 0.6; glucose, 11.2; and insulin, 10 IU/L at 37°C. After initially prestretching the muscle strips with 1 mN, they were stimulated by field stimulation using a voltage 20% above threshold, at a frequency of 1 Hz. After 1 hour of equilibration, the cardioprotective solution was completely washed out, and the muscles were stretched along their length-tension curve in 0.05-mm steps until force of contraction was maximal. Then, the force-frequency relationship was obtained in each muscle by changing stimulation rates, in increments of 0.25 Hz, from 0.5 to 3 Hz (30 to 180 beats per minute). Force-frequency relationships were obtained either at basal conditions (Ca^{2+} of 2.5 mM) or after prestimulating force of contraction with either Ca^{2+}, 7.2 mM or isoproterenol, 0.03 μM. At the end of each experiment, a test for adequate oxygenation (26) was performed by changing the carbogen to 80% O_2, 5% CO_2, and 15% N_2 at the stimulation rate at which force of contraction was maximal. This procedure lowered oxygen tension significantly in the bathing solution, and muscle strips in which force of contraction declined by more than 10% during 30 minutes under these conditions were considered hypoxic and were discarded from the evaluation. By the end of the experiment, muscle length and wet weight were measured and cross-sectional area was determined by dividing wet weight by muscle length.

Statistical Analysis

Average values are given as mean ± standard error of the mean. Mean values of peak twitch tension of the different groups at each stimulation frequency were compared using Student's t-test and the Bonferroni-Holms procedure. Differences were considered significant if p was <0.05.

RESULTS

The force-frequency relationship was investigated in nonfailing and end-stage failing human myocardium caused by DCM under basal (Ca^{2+}, 2.5 mM) conditions and after positive inotropic interventions. Figure 1 shows typical recordings of experiments performed in a left ventricular papillary muscle strip from a nonfailing heart (*upper trace*) and from a heart with DCM (*lower trace*) at a basal Ca^{2+} concentration of 2.5 mM. Stimulation frequency was increased stepwise from 0.5 to 3.0 Hz (30 to 180 beats per minute). In nonfailing myocardium, force of contraction increased continuously with increasing stimulation frequencies and was maximal at 2.0 Hz. In DCM, force of contraction was maximal at 0.75 Hz and then declined

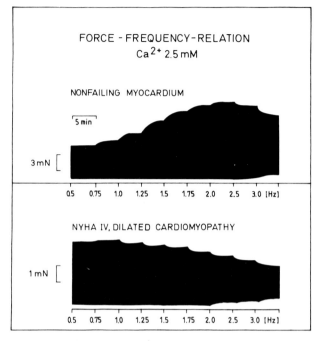

FIG. 1. Original recordings of typical experiments showing the influence of stimulation frequency on isometric force of contraction of human papillary muscle strips from a nonfailing (*upper panel*) and an end-stage failing heart secondary to dilated cardiomyopathy (New York Heart Association IV classification) (*lower panel*). Stimulation frequency has been increased stepwise from 0.5 to 3.0 Hz.

continuously. There was a small rise in diastolic tension in both preparations at the highest frequencies.

The averaged values for the experiments are summarized in Fig. 2. Force of contraction is given in percent change from baseline at 30 beats per minute. In nonfailing myocardium, force of contraction increased continuously up to $250 \pm 24\%$ at a stimulation rate of 120 beats per minute ($p < 0.05$ at 0.75 Hz versus 0.5 Hz) and then declined slightly. In DCM, force of contraction was maximal at 45 beats per minute ($104 \pm 2\%$) and then declined continuously with higher stimulation rates ($p < 0.05$ at 90 versus 30 beats per minute).

For the experiments after positive inotropic interventions, the effects of a half-maximal concentration of Ca^{2+} (7.2 mM) or isoproterenol (0.03 μM) on nonfailing and end-stage failing human myocardium at a stimulation frequency of 1 Hz were tested. A Ca^{2+} concentration of 7.2 mM exerted a significant positive inotropic effect in both groups, which was about 30% less in the DCM group compared with the controls (Fig. 3, *left panel*). In nonfailing human myocardium, isoproterenol exerted a similar positive inotropic effect at a Ca^{2+} concentration of 7.2 mM. However, in end-stage failing myocardium, the positive inotropic effect of isoproterenol

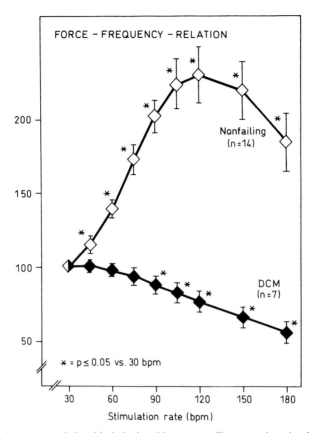

FIG. 2. Force-frequency relationship in isolated human papillary muscle strips from nonfailing hearts (◇) and from end-stage failing hearts secondary to dilated cardiomyopathy (DCM) (◆) under control conditions (Ca^{2+}, 2.5 mM). Force of contraction (ordinate) is given in percent of the baseline value at 30 beats per minute (bpm) for each group. Stimulation frequency (abscissa) was increased stepwise from 0.5 to 3.0 Hz.

was reduced by 60% as compared with in nonfailing myocardium (Fig. 3, *right panel*).

Figure 4 summarizes the effect of increasing stimulation frequencies in nonfailing myocardium after prestimulation with Ca^{2+}, 7.2 mM (☐). The results at control conditions (Ca^{2+}, 2.5 mM), as shown in Fig. 2, are given for comparison (◇). The data indicate that, after prestimulation with Ca^{2+}, 7.2 mM, the percent increase in force of contraction is slightly reduced at high stimulation frequencies, but the shape of the force-frequency relationship remains the same. Because the values are given in percent from baseline at 30 beats per minute, the plot does not show the positive inotropic effect of the increased Ca^{2+} concentration.

The same type of experiment after prestimulating nonfailing human myocardium with isoproterenol (○) is shown in Fig. 5. Again, the control curve at a Ca^{2+} con-

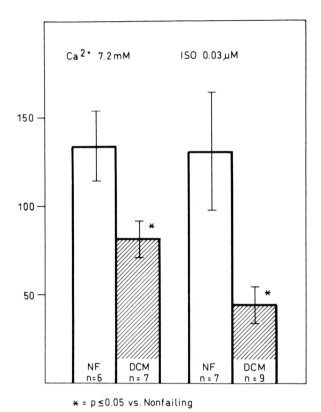

FIG. 3. Positive inotropic effect of a half-maximal concentration of Ca^{2+} (7.2 mM; *left side*) and isoproterenol (0.3 µM; *right side*) in isolated papillary muscle strips from nonfailing (NF) and end-stage failing secondary to dilated cardiomyopathy [DCM] myocardium at a stimulation frequency of 30 beats per minute. Increase in force of contraction is given in percent of the baseline value before the drug was applied.

centration of 2.5 mM is given for comparison, and the change in contractile force is given in percent from the baseline value at 30 beats per minute. As with a Ca^{2+} concentration of 7.2 mM, the increase in force of contraction with higher stimulation rates is slightly reduced with isoproterenol, but the shape of the positive force-frequency relationship remains unchanged.

Figures 6 and 7 show the same experiments in papillary muscle strips from end-stage failing myocardium from hearts with DCM. Again, the change in force of contraction is given in percent of the baseline values, set 100% at 30 beats per minute. In Figure 6, force of contraction has been prestimulated with Ca^{2+}, 7.2 mM (■), and the control curve at a Ca^{2+} concentration of 2.5 mM is given for comparison (◆). The results show that, at a Ca^{2+} concentration of 7.2, the decline of the isometric twitch tension is even more pronounced with increasing stimulation frequencies as compared with control conditions (Ca^{2+}, 2.5 mM). However, after

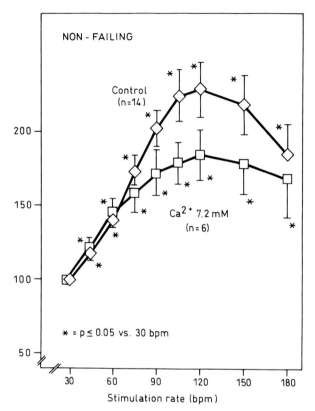

FIG. 4. Force-frequency relationship in isolated papillary muscle strips from nonfailing human myocardium before (◇) and after prestimulating force of contraction with Ca^{2+}, 7.2 mM (□). Force of contraction (ordinate) is given in percent change of the baseline value at 30 beats per minute (bpm) for each group. Stimulation frequency (abscissa) was increased stepwise from 30 beats per minute to 180 beats per minute.

prestimulating force of contraction with isoproterenol (Fig. 7, ●), in contrast to the control experiments, force of contraction increases with increasing stimulation frequencies in the lower frequency range. In the higher frequency range, the decrease in force of contraction is less pronounced compared with the control experiments at a Ca^{2+} concentration of 2.5 mM.

DISCUSSION

The frequency dependence of myocardial contractility has been studied extensively in myocardium from different animal species during the last decades (1,2). Because human myocardium has become available as a result of the increasing number of heart transplantations in the last years and since advances in myocardial

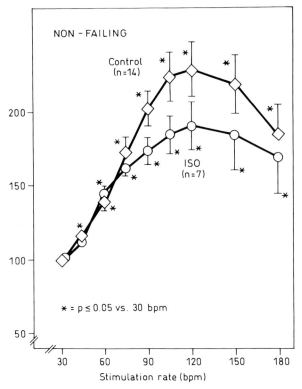

FIG. 5. Force-frequency relationship in isolated papillary muscle strips from nonfailing human myocardium before (◊) and after prestimulation with isoproterenol, 0.03 μM (o). Force of contraction (ordinate) is given in percent change of the baseline value at 30 beats per minute (bpm). Stimulation frequency (abscissa) was increased stepwise from 30 beats per minute to 180 beats per minute.

conservation and preparation techniques have allowed sufficiently thin and stable muscle preparations to be obtained, the effects of stimulation frequency on force of contraction has been investigated in isolated human myocardium (8–10). From these studies, it is known that isometric force of contraction continuously increases with increasing stimulation frequency in nonfailing human papillary muscle strips, but it decreases in end-stage failing myocardium owing to DCM. However, the effects of positive inotropic interventions on the force-frequency relationship in human myocardium are not well characterized.

The present study was designed to investigate the influence of an increased extracellular Ca^{2+} concentration and isoproterenol on the force-frequency relationship in the nonfailing and end-stage failing human heart. An increase in the extracellular Ca^{2+} concentration raises force of contraction independently of cAMP by an increased trans-sarcolemmal Ca^{2+} influx during depolarization and thus by an increased Ca^{2+} availability to the contractile proteins (27). In contrast to previous

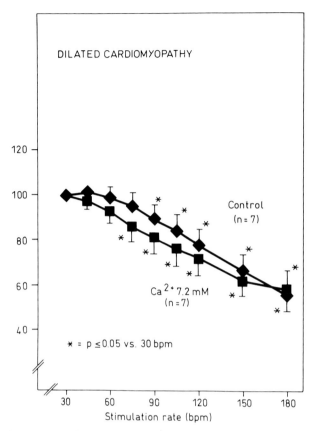

FIG. 6. Force-frequency relationship in isolated papillary muscle strips from end-stage failing human myocardium secondary to dilated cardiomyopathy before (♦) and after (■) prestimulation with Ca^{2+}, 7.2 mM. The change in force of contraction (ordinate) is given in percent from the baseline value at 30 beats per minute (bpm). Stimulation frequency (abscissa) was increased stepwise from 30 beats per minute to 180 beats per minute.

reports (11), the positive inotropic effect of Ca^{2+} was reduced by about 30% in papillary muscle strips from failing hearts compared with controls at a stimulation frequency of 1 Hz. This finding in DCM may be attributable to a reduction in myofibrillar protein content (21,28) and defects in intracellular Ca^{2+} handling (21,22), although the sensitivity of the contractile proteins remains unchanged (29). However, the positive inotropic effect of Ca^{2+} was pronounced in the failing myocardium, but this cAMP-independent intervention was not able to normalize the inverse force-frequency relationship. There was even a tendency for further deterioration of the muscle strip function at higher stimulation frequencies.

With the cAMP-dependent inotrope isoproterenol, the positive inotropic effect was reduced by about 60% in papillary muscle strips from end-stage failing hearts

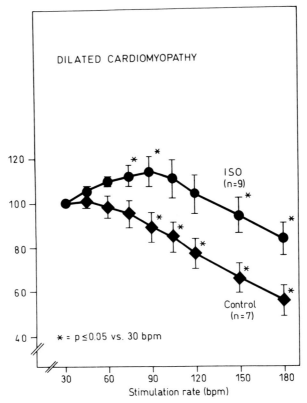

FIG. 7. Force-frequency relationship in isolated papillary muscle strips from end-stage failing human myocardium secondary to dilated cardiomyopathy before (♦) and after (●) prestimulating force of contraction with isoproterenol (0.03 μM). The change in force of contraction (ordinate) is given in percent change from baseline value at 30 beats per minute (bpm). Stimulation frequency (abscissa) was increased stepwise from 30 beats per minute to 180 beats per minute.

as compared to nonfailing myocardium. This finding confirms previous reports of diminished in vitro effects of catecholamines in end-stage failing myocardium (13,14), which may be attributable to β-adrenoceptor down-regulation (13) and changes in β-adrenoceptor coupling to adenylate cyclase by G proteins (16,17). However, the results of our study show that isoproterenol did not change the shape of the force-frequency relationship in nonfailing myocardium but partially normalized the force-frequency relationship in the failing myocardium in the lower frequency range.

It has been hypothesized that one major defect in DCM is a disturbed SR Ca^{2+} handling with a diminished capacity of SR Ca^{2+} uptake and, thus, a diminished release of Ca^{2+} from the SR in early systole (12,22,30). The results of our study may be interpreted in terms of defective SR Ca^{2+} handling. In nonfailing myocardium, force of contraction rises with increasing stimulation frequencies because the net Ca^{2+} inward current increases owing to the increasing number of depolarizations per unit of time. Because SR Ca^{2+} uptake capacity is normal, this leads to an increased loading of the SR with Ca^{2+} and thus to an increased calcium release during the next twitch. After prestimulating force of contraction with either Ca^{2+} or isoproterenol, the shape of the force-frequency relationship is preserved on a higher level of twitch tension, reflecting the high capability of the SR for Ca^{2+} cycling, even at high stimulation frequencies.

In DCM, a decrease in the expression of SR Ca^{2+} ATPase mRNA (19) and a decrease in the SR Ca^{2+} uptake capability (20) have been reported. These defects may lead to a reduced loading of the SR with Ca^{2+}. This may become even more relevant at high stimulation frequencies, when diastole shortens and thus the time for SR Ca^{2+} uptake decreases. As a consequence, at the following beat, less Ca^{2+} may be released from the SR for activation of the contractile proteins, leading to the negative force staircase.

Phospholamban plays an important role in the regulation of the activity of the SR Ca^{2+} pumps and thus in the reuptake capacity of the SR for Ca^{2+} (31). Phospholamban phosphorylation by a cAMP-dependent protein kinase leads to an increase in the Ca^{2+} transport capacity of the SR (23,24). The present results may reflect the functional importance of phospholamban phosphorylation in dilated cardiomyopathy. Despite the positive inotropic effect after Ca^{2+}, the force-frequency relationship was found to deteriorate further, possibly because of the increased intracellular Ca^{2+} concentration and the further stress on the partially defective Ca^{2+} transport systems. By contrast, after administration of isoproterenol, an increase in the intracellular cAMP concentration with protein kinase activation led to an additional phospholamban phosphorylation (24) with a stimulation of the remaining SR Ca^{2+} pumps. This might explain the partial normalization of the negative staircase in the lower frequency range after isoproterenol administration. Therefore, for future investigations, it would be challenging to speculate that a pure phospholamban phosphorylation, without increasing the trans-sarcolemmal Ca^{2+} influx, might be able to normalize the negative force-frequency relationship in DCM even more efficiently.

SUMMARY

The force-frequency relationship (30 to 180 beats per minute) was investigated in isometric contracting left ventricular papillary muscle strips from nonfailing and end-stage failing human hearts secondary to dilated cardiomyopathy (DCM) under basal (Ca^{2+}, 2.5 mM) conditions and after prestimulating force of contraction with either isoproterenol (0.03 μM) or Ca^{2+}, 7.2 mM. Under basal conditions, force of contraction increased continuously with increasing stimulation frequencies in nonfailing myocardium but decreased in end-stage failing myocardium (inverse force-frequency relationship). Increasing the extracellular Ca^{2+} concentration to 7.2 mM exerted a positive inotropic effect in both groups. Under this condition, the shape of the force-frequency relationship was unchanged in nonfailing myocardium but its decline was even more pronounced in DCM. With administration of isoproterenol, there was a significant positive inotropic effect in both groups, which was, however, much smaller in the DCM group compared to the control group. Isoproterenol did not change the shape of the positive force-frequency relationship in nonfailing myocardium. However, in DCM, the inverse force-frequency relationship became positive in the low-frequency range and was inverse only at frequencies higher than 1.5 Hz. These data indicate that (a) in contrast to nonfailing myocardium, the force-frequency relationship is negative in end-stage failing human myocardium caused by DCM; (b) the inversion of the force-frequency relationship gets accentuated with an increased extracellular Ca^{2+} concentration in DCM; and (c) isoproterenol improves the force-frequency relationship in DCM in the lower frequency range.

REFERENCES

1. Blinks JR, Koch-Weser J. Analysis of the effects of changes in rate and rhythm upon myocardial contractility. *J Pharmacol Exp Ther* 1961;134:373–89.
2. Parmley WW, Sonnenblick EH. Relation between mechanics of contraction and relaxation in mammalian cardiac muscle. *Am J Physiol* 1969;216:1084–91.
3. Freeman GL, Little WC, O'Rourke RA. Influence of heart rate on left ventricular performance in conscious dogs. *Circ Res* 1987;61:455–64.
4. Mitchell JH, Wallac AG, Skinner NS, Jr. Intrinsic effects of heart rate on left ventricular performance. *Am J Physiol* 1963;205:41–8.
5. Allen DG, Blinks JR. Calcium transients in aequorin-injected frog cardiac muscle. *Nature* 1978; 273:509–13.
6. Winegard S, Shanes AM. Calcium flux and contractility in guinea pig atria. *J Gen Physiol* 1962;45: 371–94.
7. Sonnenblick H, Morrow A, Williams J. Effects of heart rate on the dynamics of force development in the intact human ventricle. *Circulation* 1966;33:945–51.
8. Mulieri LA, Leavitt BJ, Hasenfuss G, Allen PD, Alpert NR. Contraction frequency dependence of twitch and diastolic tension in human dilated cardiomyopathy. *Bas Res Cardiol* 1992[Suppl 1]:199–211.
9. Mulieri LA, Hasenfuss G, Leavitt B, Allen PD, Alpert NR. Altered myocardial force-frequency relation in human heart failure. *Circulation* 1992;85:1743–50.
10. Pieske B, Hasenfuss G, Holubarsch Ch, Schwinger R, Böhm M, Just H. Alterations of the force-frequency-relationship in the failing human heart depend on the underlying cardiac disease. *Bas Res Cardiol* 1992[Suppl 1]:213–221.
11. Feldman MD, Copelas L, Gwathmey JK, et al. Deficient production of cyclic AMP: pharmacologic evidence of an important cause of contractile dysfunction in patients with endstage heart failure. *Circulation* 1987;75:331–9.
12. Hasenfuss G, Holubarsch Ch, Hermann HP, Astheimer K, Pieske B, Just H. Veränderte Beziehung zwischen Herzfrequenz und Hämodynamik bei Patienten mit dilatativer Kardiomyopathie. *Klin Wochenschr* 1992;96[Suppl 28]:166.
13. Bristow M, Ginsburg R, Minobe W, et al. Decreased catecholamine sensitivity and β-adrenergic-receptor density in failing human hearts. *N Engl J Med* 1982;307:205–11.
14. Böhm M, Diet F, Feiler G, et al. Subsensitivity of the failing human heart to isoprenaline and milrinone is related to β-adrenoceptor downregulation. *J Cardiovasc Pharmacol* 1988;12:726–32.
15. Brodde OE, Zerkowski HR, Borst HG, Maier W, Michel MC. Drug- and disease-induced changes of human cardiac β1- and β2-adrenoceptors. *Eur Heart J* 1989;10[Suppl B]:38–44.
16. Feldman AM, Cates AE, Veazey WB, et al. Increase of the 40.000-mol wt pertussis toxin substrate (G-protein) in the failing human heart. *J Clin Invest* 1988;82:189–97.
17. Böhm M, Gierschik P, Jakobs KH, et al. Increase of Gi in human hearts with dilated but not ischemic cardiomyopathy. *Circulation* 1990;82:1249–65.

18. Bristow M, Hershberger R, Port D, Minobe W, Rasmussen R. β1- and β2-Adrenergic receptor-mediated adenylate cyclase stimulation in nonfailing and failing human ventricular myocardium. *Mol Pharmacol* 1989;35:295–303.
19. Mercadier JJ, Lompre AM, Duc P, et al. Altered sarcoplasmic reticulum Ca2 + -ATPase gene expression in the human ventricle during end-stage heart failure. *J Clin Invest* 1990;85:305–9.
20. Limas CJ, Olivari M, Goldenberg IF, Levine TB, Benditt DG, Simon A. Calcium uptake by cardiac sarcoplasmic reticulum in human dilated cardiomyopathy. *Cardiovasc Res* 1987;21:601–5.
21. Hasenfuss G, Mulieri LA, Leavitt BJ, Allen PD, Haeberle JR, Alpert NR. Alteration of contractile function and excitation-contraction coupling in dilated cardiomyopathy. *Circ Res* 1992;70:1225–32.
22. Beuckelmann DJ, Näbauer M, Erdmann E. Intracellular calcium handling in isolated ventricular myocytes from patients with terminal heart failure. *Circulation* 1992;85:1046–55.
23. Kranias EG, Solaro RJ. Phosphorylation of troponin I and phospholamban during catecholamine stimulation of rabbit heart. *Nature* 1982;298:182.
24. Lindemann JP, Jones LR, Hathaway DR. β-adrenergic stimulation of phospholamban phosphorylation and Ca2 + -ATPase activity in guinea pig ventricles. *J Biol Chem* 1983;258:464.
25. Mulieri LA, Hasenfuss G, Ittleman F, Blanchard EM, Alpert NR. Protection of human left ventricular myocardium from cutting injury with 2,3-butanedion monoxime. *Circ Res* 1989;65:1441–4.
26. Paradise NF, Schmittler JL, Surmitis JM. Criteria for adequate oxygenation of isometric kitten papillary muscle. *Am J Physiol* 1981;241:H348–53.
27. Carafoli E. Intracellular calcium homeostasis. *Ann Rev Biochem* 1987;56:395–433.
28. Pagani ED, Alousi AA, Grant AM, Older TM, Dziuban SW Jr, Allen PD. Changes in myofibrillar content and Mg-ATPase activity in ventricular tissues from patients with heart failure caused by coronary artery disease, cardiomyopathy, or mitral valve insufficiency. *Circ Res* 1988;63:380–5.
29. Wankerl M, Böhm M, Morano I, Rüegg JC, Eichhorn M, Erdmann E. Calcium sensitivity and myosin light chain pattern of skinned cardiac fibers from patients with various kinds of cardiac disease. *J Mol Cell Cardiol* 1990;22:1425–38.
30. Morgan JP, Erny RE, Allen PD, Grossman W, Gwathmey JK. Abnormal intracellular calcium handling, a major cause of systolic and diastolic dysfunction in ventricular myocardium from patients with heart failure. *Circulation* 1990;81[Suppl III]:III21–32.
31. Tada M, Kirchberger MA, Katz AM. Phosphorylation of a 22,000 dalton component of the cardiac sarcoplasmic reticulum by adenosine 3′,5′-monophosphate dependent protein kinase. *J Biol Chem* 1975;250:2640.

The Cardiomyopathic Heart, edited by Makoto
Nagano, Nobuakira Takeda, and Naranjan S.
Dhalla. Raven Press, Ltd., New York © 1994.

22

Myocardial Metabolic Derangement of Keshan Disease: A Noncoronary Myocardial Injury

Tongshu Yang, Yibing Ouyang, Jie Yang, Gonghe Dai, Xiuqi Bai,
Lizhong Hou, Shaowei Li, Jingxin Wang, and Ping Zhu

*Institute of Preclinical Sciences, N. Bethune University of Medical Sciences, National Key
Laboratory of Enzyme Engineering, Jilin University, Chang Chun, China*

In recent years, the development of cellular and molecular cardiology has greatly promoted the understanding of the nature of heart diseases. In the studies of ischemic and anoxic heart injuries, new concepts such as "oxygen paradox," "calcium paradox," "oxygen free radical injuries," "reperfusion disorders," and "myocardial stunning" have emerged and gradually deepened our knowledge of myocardial injury mechanisms. In light of these achievements, we have explored some new fields in cardiology at cellular and molecular levels (1). The studies on noncoronary primary myocardial injuries described in this chapter are examples of this exploration.

It is clear that ischemic heart disease is the most common cardiac disorder. This necrotic and denatured myocardial disease had been considered to be the result of circulatory disorders of coronary arteries. Recently, however, experimental pathologists have successfully set up many kinds of animal models with myocardial injuries without coronary damage (2,3). This research has indicated that noncoronary primary myocardial injuries may exist. In fact, the hereditary cardiomyopathy that occurs in hamsters, human cardiomyopathy, and KD (the last is well known in China) (4) are considered pathomorphologically with or without mild coronary damage. Currently, studies of noncoronary primary myocardial injuries have created new interest in the field of cardiology.

In this field, KD is a kind of endemic cardiomyopathy characterized by myocardial necrosis (5). Pathologically, it is not accompanied by obstruction and injuries of the coronary vessel, and it is also essentially different from obstructive vascular or reperfusion injuries (6). Biochemically, KD has many metabolic characteristics (7–9). For many years, we have performed biochemical studies of populations from areas with high concentrations of KD, as well as metabolic studies on the hearts of people with KD (85 patients with KD and controls) as well as on more than 2,000 KD animal models. The major results follow.

METABOLIC DEVIATION OF THE POPULATION IN AREAS MARKED BY A HIGH INCIDENCE OF KD

Results of the biochemical analysis of the myocardial marker enzymes of the healthy populations from KD areas are evidently different from findings in the control population (Table 1). The aberrant metabolism suggests that the potential for injury already exists in the myocardium of the "healthy population" from KD areas. It showed, at the population level, the primary characteristics of the myocardial injuries in KD.

EVIDENT DYSFUNCTION IN THE MYOCARDIAL MITOCHONDRIA IN KD

In 1980, we first discovered a decrease in activities of myocardial respiratory enzymes succinic dehydrogenase (SDH) and cytochrome oxidase (CCO) in patients with KD (10–12). The activities of CCO and SDH in the myocardium in patients with subacute KD (ten cases) were remarkably decreased, and the average activity of SDH was only 21.2% compared with that of the control group (28 cases), and CCO was 40.8% compared with that of the control group (Table 2). The respiratory enzyme activities in the patients with chronic KD (two cases) also decreased but to a somewhat lesser extent than in patients with subacute KD. These results, which

TABLE 1. *The serum enzymatic spectrum of patients with subacute Keshan disease (KD) and of coupling healthy controls (mean value)*

	Glutamic oxaloacetic transaminase (IU/L)	Glutamate pyruvate transaminase (IU/L)	Creatine kinase (IU/L)	Lactate dehydrogenase (IU/L)
Healthy controls from nonendemic areas (n = 36)	35.81	30.69	133.2	270.5
Healthy controls from endemic areas (n = 54)	30.76	15.31	147.2	243.4
Coupling healthy controls (n = 19)[a]	40.57[b]	34.81	156.1[b]	327.1[b]
Patients with subacute KD (n = 19)	73.70	21.11	509.0[b]	487.1[b]

[a]The coupling analysis on the serum enzymatic spectrum of hospitalized patients with subacute KD and healthy children inhabiting the same areas.
[b]Compared with that of healthy controls of the nonendemic or endemic areas, the statistical difference is significant ($p < 0.05$).

TABLE 2. Activities of respiratory enzymes in the myocardium in Keshan disease (KD)

Group	n	Succinic dehydrogenase (Δ O$_2$ mm Hg)[a]	Cytochrome oxidase (Δ O$_2$ mm Hg)[b]
Subacute KD	10	18.4 ± 11.8	12.6 ± 10.1
Chronic KD	3	56.5 ± 44.4	27.3 ± 21.7
Control (1)	2	78.4 ± 13.9	30.9 ± 2.6
Control (2)	3	71.5 ± 7.3	45.3 ± 10.6

[a]O$_2$ mm Hg/6 min/15 mg wet weight.
[b]O$_2$ mm Hg/3 min/7.5 mg wet weight.
Note: 1 mm Hg = 133.32 Pa.

support the facts cited earlier (12), not only indicate the imbalance of oxygen supply and requirements in patients with KD, but also suggest a disorder in the requirement for oxygen, indicating that KS patients have oxygen consumption disturbances in their bodies (Table 3).

In the comprehensive research survey of Chuxiong, Yunnan province, in 1984 to 1986, we also found that the mitochondrial oxidative phosphorylation of the myocardium of patients with KD was apparently injured (13). The state 3 respiration rate of the mitochondrial oxidative phosphorylation in the myocardium of nine patients with subacute KD and three patients with chronic KD was remarkably decreased. Meanwhile, their state 4 respiration rate increased compared with that of controls (six patients): the state 4 respiration rate in the chronic group increased more than fourfold, and it increased 3.44-fold in the subacute group. The decrease in state 3 respiration rate and the increase in state 4 respiration rate reflect a functional disorder in the regulation of myocardial mitochondria to the intracellular respiration. The respiration control indexes (RCIs) of both the subacute group and the chronic KD group were 2.40 ± 0.875 and 2.86 ± 0.648, respectively; these values were lower than those reported in the control group (8.65 ± 1.32), indicating severe impairment of the regulation function of myocardial mitochondrial respiration in the patients with KD. These results suggest that, without adenosine diphosphate (ADP) stimulation, the myocardial mitochondria of patients with KD still consumed a very high quantity of oxygen, resulting in the oxygen leak phenomenon (Fig. 1).

The oxygen leak from the respiration chain could not effectively reduce the four

TABLE 3. Activities of mitochondrial respiratory enzyme in the myocardium of patients with Keshan disease (KD)

Group	n	Succinic dehydrogenase	Cytochrome oxidase
		(Δ O$_2$ mm Hg/mg protein)	
Subacute KD	7	8.8 ± 4.4	13.6 ± 8.7
Control (healthy)	6	23.6 ± 8.1	32.3 ± 15.9
t-Test		$p < 0.02$	$p < 0.05$

Note: 1 mm Hg = 133.32 Pa.

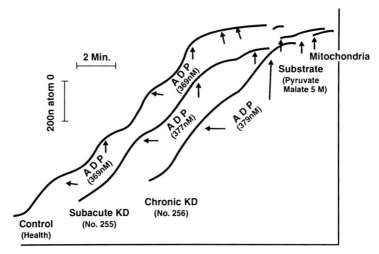

FIG. 1. Oxidative phosphorylation of mitochondria in the myocardium of patients with Keshan disease (KD). *ADP*, adenosine diphosphate.

electrons to water; therefore, it partially accomplished its reduction through single, double, or triple electrons, producing a series of reactive oxygen species, such as superoxide anion radicals, hydrogen peroxide, and hydroxyl radicals (14):

a. The four-electron reduction of the oxygen molecule reduced the oxygen directly to water (with participation of the CCO complex):

$$O_2 + 4H^+ + 4e \rightarrow 2H_2O$$

b. The single, double, and triple electrons reduced the oxygen molecule (non-enzymatic reduction) into reactive oxygen species:

$$O_2 \xrightarrow{e} O_2 - \cdot \xrightarrow{e, 2H^+} H_2O_2 \xrightarrow{e, H^+} \cdot OH + H_2O$$

The excessive reactive oxygen species produced by myocardial respiration dysfunction became the important triggering factor in the myocardial necrosis of KD.

DAMAGE TO THE MYOCARDIAL MEMBRANE

In the biomembrane system of the KD hearts, in addition to the previously described mitochondrial disorder, evident dysfunction occurred in the myocardial plasma membrane. This was manifested as follows:

a. The permeability of enzymes in the myocardial plasma membrane prominently increased (15,16). In our experiments, we found that, in the hearts of both patients with KD and animal models with KD, the activities of myocardium-

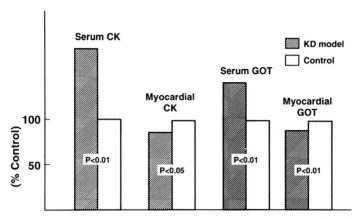

FIG. 2. Enzyme permeability of myocardial membrane in animal model with Keshan disease (KD). *CK*, creatine kinase; *GOT*, glutamic-oxaloacetic transaminase.

enriched enzymes, such as creatine kinase (CK) and glutamic-oxaloacetic transaminase (GOT) were apparently decreased, although their activities in serum were increased remarkably (Fig. 2). In addition, when a large-molecular-weight enzyme, such as horseradish peroxidase (HRP), was injected into the blood of the animal models with KD, the entry of HRP from the blood into the myocardial cells was much greater than that in the control group (Table 4) (17).

b. There were abnormalities of membrane-bound enzyme activity, membrane receptor activity, and membrane fluidity. If the plasma membrane was directly isolated from the myocardial cells of animal models with KD, the activities of Na^+, K^+-adenosine triphosphatase (ATPase) and ouabain receptors were found to be greatly decreased. Detecting the myocardial membrane with a DPH probe, we observed that the lipid fluorescent polarized amplitude reflecting the fluidity of the lipid bilayer was increased (Fig. 3) in these experimental models (18).

These experimental results strongly suggest that KD hearts are extremely susceptible to free radicals, which produce evident changes in the function and constituents of the biomembrane system.

TABLE 4. *Horseradish peroxidase perfused from blood into the myocardial cells of Keshan disease (KD) animal models*

	2 Months		3 Months	
Group	n	Number of positive cells	n	Number of positive cells
Nonendemic grains	7	5	16	63.5
Endemic grains	7	52	16	180.5
t-Test		$p<0.05$		$p<0.01$

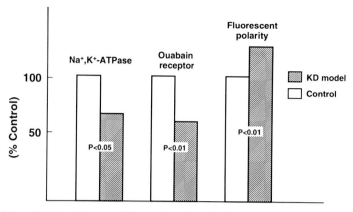

FIG. 3. Characteristics of myocardial membrane in animal models with Keshan disease (KD).

DISORDER OF MYOCARDIAL CONTRACTILE PROTEINS

In addition to the changes in energy supply, free radical metabolism, and Ca^{2+} concentration described earlier (19,20), alterations in contractile protein may be directly associated with the heart failure in KD.

From the results in Table 5, it can be seen that the myosin isoenzymes shifted from V1 to V3; the ratio of light chain-2 to light chain-1 increased in subacute KD. In addition, decreased activity of myosin light chain kinase and decreased super-precipitation activity of the actomyosin molecular model were found (21,22).

As there are two kinds of heavy chains—α and β—myosin molecules may exist in three kinds of dimers of $\alpha\alpha$, $\alpha\beta$, and $\beta\beta$, which are called V1, V2, and V3, respectively, in the rat and hamster. Therefore, the shift of myosin isozyme distribution in patients and animals with KD may be accompanied by changes in their α and β myosin heavy chain gene expression and thus may lead to changes in myosin ATPase activities. Table 6 provides the results of myosin ATPase activity and myosin heavy chain gene expression in animals with KD with increasing periods of feeding with KD-area grains. The results indicate that the α-CMHC mRNA contents were decreased and β-CMHC mRNA contents were increased with increases in the period of feeding with KD-area grains. These results were significant after KD grains were fed for 2 months.

TABLE 5. *The alterations in contractile protein of Keshan disease (KD)*

Group	Myosin isoenzyme (V2 + V3)V1	Myosin light chain (LC) LC2/LC1
Subacute KD	1.25 (n = 6)[a]	0.73 ± 0.18 (n = 6)[a]
Control	0.5 (n = 7)	0.57 ± 0.15 (n = 6)

[a]$p < 0.01$.

TABLE 6. *Changes of myosin ATPase activities and myosin heavy chain gene expression in the rats fed KD-area grains*

Group (month)	Myosin ATPase (% control)	α-CMHC mRNA (% control)	β-CMHC mRNA (% control)
1 (n = 6)	98.98	96.67	100.20
2 (n = 6)	85.71[a]	95.15[a]	103.94[a]
3 (n = 6)	74.51[b]	44.26[b]	136.36[b]

[a]$p<0.05$.
[b]$p<0.01$.

The changes in α- and β-CMHC mRNA were parallel, not only with the shift of myosin isoenzymes distribution, but also with the myosin ATPase activity. As shown in Table 6, the decreased myosin ATPase activity was positively correlated with the content of α-CMHC mRNA and negatively correlated with the β-CMHC mRNA. These alterations may contribute to the decrease in myocardial contractility in KD (23).

Ca^{2+}-activating ATPase is related to the contractile velocity of the myocardium, and the numbers of myosin molecules bridged with actin determine the myocardial contractility. Therefore, the series of alterations in the function-metabolism coupling, such as "cardiac hemodynamics-myocardial contractility-myosin Ca^{2+}-ATPase-myosin isoenzymes regulation of myosin light chain kinase" formed the molecular biologic basis of myocardial contractile disturbances in KD.

FREE RADICAL METABOLISM OF MYOCARDIUM

Because of the observed decreases in GSHPx activity and vitamin E and selenium levels in the blood of patients with KD and of the inhabitants of endemic KD areas (24–30), we proposed that KD was closely related to low selenium intake and free radical metabolism. In Chuxiong, Yunnan province, we directly studied the free radical metabolism in the hearts of patients with KD. The results indicated that these patients had disorders in free radical metabolism (Table 7).

TABLE 7. *Disturbances of free radical metabolism in the myocardium with Keshan disease (KD)*

Group	Electron spin resonance value (peak/peak)	Lipid peroxide (nmol MDA/ç wet weight)	XOD (U/g wet weight)	Superoxide dismutase (U/g wet weight)
Subacute KD	1.61 ± 0.23[a]	98.1 ± 29.0[a]	315.0 ± 131.9[a]	420.4 ± 122.2[a]
(n)	(6)	(7)	(7)	(7)
Chronic KD		59.1	603.8	606.1
(n)		(1)	(1)	(1)
Control (healthy)	1.08 ± 0.09	60.9 ± 4.7	530.0 ± 151.6	769.3 ± 146.5
(n)	(4)	(6)	(6)	(6)

[a]$p<0.05$ compared with control group.

Using ESR techniques, we made a direct estimation of the free radical levels in the myocardium of six patients with subacute KD. The ESR value was found to be much higher (about 1.5 times) in this group than in controls. The activities of the enzymes that remove free radicals, including SOD, were decreased in the myocardium of the patients with subacute KD (seven cases), whereas the lipid peroxide (LPO) content in these patients was greatly increased.

Studies of animal models with KD (rats fed on grain from endemic areas for 75 days) further indicated that the following changes occur in the free radical metabolism of KD hearts (Fig. 4):

a. Increased free radical content. The ESR value of the control group (seven cases) was 1.40 ± 0.14, whereas that of the experimental group (eight cases) was 1.75 ± 0.39 (peak/peak value).

b. Increased LPO content. In the control group (eight cases), the LPO level (nmol MDA/g net weight) was 146.6 ± 11.5, whereas in the experimental group (10 cases), it was 168.4 ± 14.8.

c. Decreased GSHPx activity. In the control group (eight cases), GSHPx activity (IU/g wet weight) was 6.44 ± 1.84, whereas in the experimental group, it was 2.45 ± 0.49 (ten cases).

d. Decreased SOD activity. In the control group (eight cases), SOD activity (IU/g wet weight) was 537.5 ± 142.2, whereas in the experimental group, it was 487.0 ± 111.8. There was no significant difference between these two groups.

e. No obvious changes in xanthine oxidase activity. In the analysis of the animal blood, the GSHPx activity in the experimental group (7.88 ± 3.36 IU/mL) was found to be much lower than that in the control group (10.64 ± 3.56 IU/mL), whereas the SOD activity in the former group (327.6 ± 140.5 IU/mL) was apparently lower than that in the latter (685.5 ± 77.6 IU/mL).

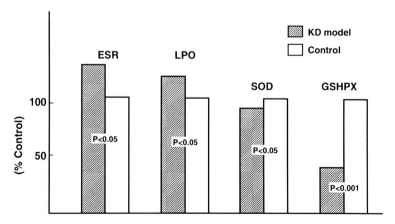

FIG. 4. Free radical metabolism of myocardium in animal models with Keshan disease (KD). *ESR*, electron spin resonance; *LPO*, lipid peroxide; *SOD*, superoxide dismutase; *GSHPX*, glutathione peroxidase.

These changes in the free radical metabolism in the animal models of KD were essentially compatible with the regularity of the myocardial changes in the patients with KD. Therefore, this indicated that in the grain consumed in endemic areas or in the areas of KD patients, certain factors might be present that could cause free radical metabolic disorders. These factors could trigger metabolic reaction of oxidative stress in the organism in nature. Although the same obvious biochemical abnormalities occurred in the animal models with KD, the results of pathologic examinations were basically normal. Thus the oxygen free radical disorders can be considered to be early metabolic changes in the myocardial injuries in KD. Since the free radical does not result from myocardial necrosis, it must play an initiating role in the etiology of the disease.

CONCLUSION

We have concluded that, whether at the population and individual level, or at the level of the molecules that directly carry out the function of the damaged target organ, the heart in both patients with KD and animal models of KD is subject to primary disorders in myocardial metabolism; this indicates that KD is a kind of primary metabolic cardiomyopathy with mitochondrial injury as its main characteristic. KD is a kind of human cardiomyopathy; it is also the predominant human cardiomyopathy in the world. Therefore, studies of the myocardial metabolism associated with KD not only provide evidence for what is the primary mechanism of the Keshan disease, but also are of great referent value in studies of noncoronary myocardial injury disease and other heart diseases. It is our hope, then, that an increasing number of cardiologists will direct their attention to this disease and take part in studies in the field.

SUMMARY

In China, Keshan disease (KD) is a kind of endemic cardiomyopathy characterized by myocardial necrosis and particular metabolic properties in biochemistry. For many years, we have devoted ourselves to studying the myocardial damage in patients as well as animals with KD. Mitochondrial respiration disturbances have been observed in KD myocardium, indicating a decrease in the respiratory enzyme activities and the obstruction of oxidative phosphorylation characterized by the oxygen leakage phenomenon. The sarcolemmal alterations in the activities and distribution of enzymes, the membrane permeability, and the lipid components and membrane fluidity have been studied. Examination of the free radical system revealed that the glutathione peroxidase superoxide dismutase (GSHPx-SOD) activities decreased and the catalase activity increased in KD myocardium; the net contents of free radicals apparently increased as well, as demonstrated by electron spin resonance (ESR) analysis; selenium contents decreased, but lipid peroxide increased.

The alterations of contractile proteins were also shown in KD myocardium. Similar results were obtained in both patients and animal models with KD.

REFERENCES

1. Yang T, Li S, Yang J. Advances in the studies of cellular and molecular cardiology. In: *Progress in Medical Sciences*. Ministry of Health of China; 1991;63.
2. Bajusz E, Hereditary cardiomyopathy. A new disease model. *Am Heart J* 1969;77:686.
3. Nagano M, Takdea N, Kato M, Nagai M, Yang J. Pathophysiological aspect of cardiomyopathy hamster J-2N in this proceedings. 1992.
4. Hou L, Yang T, Zhou Z. Biochemical analysis on the population of Keshan disease endemic areas. In: Ministry of Public Health of China, ed. *Collected work of comprehensive scientific survey on Keshan Disease in Chu-Xiong prefecture.* Peking: People's Health Publication; 1988:236.
5. Yu W, Zeng S, Zeng X. Researches of Keshan disease at the present and the past and its future. In: Ministry of Public Health of China, ed. *Scientific research on prevention and treatment of Keshan disease in China.* Peking: Environmental Science Publishers of China, 1987;161.
6. Wang F, Li G, Kang D, Yang T, Zhang H. Pathologic characteristics and etiological significance of Keshan disease. In: Ministry of Public Health of China, ed. *Scientific research on prevention and treatment of Keshan disease in China.* Peking: Environmental Science Publishers of China, 1987; 283.
7. Li F. Biochemical metabolic characteristics and significance of Keshan disease. In: Ministry of Public Health of China, ed. *Scientific research on prevention and treatment of Keshan disease in China.* Peking: Environmental Science Publishers of China, 1987.
8. Yang T. Metabolic disorders of myocardial cells in Keshan disease. In: Ministry of Public Health of China, ed. *Scientific research on prevention and treatment of Keshan disease in China.* Peking: Environmental Science Publishers of China; 1987;227.
9. Ouyang Y, Yang T. Free-radical metabolism of myocardium of the patients with Keshan disease. *Chin J Endemiol* 1987;6:193.
10. Bai S, Yang T. Disorders of the respiratory enzymes of the myocardium from the patients with Keshan disease. *Commun Endemiol* 1982;3:1.
11. Yang T. Keshan disease and anoxia. *J Jilin Med Univ* 1973;1:37.
12. Bai S, Dai G, Zou Z. Analysis of the myocardial respiratory enzymes of the patients with Keshan disease in the endemic areas of Chu-xiong, Yunan. *J N Bethune Univ Med Sci.* 1984;10[Suppl: Myocardial Metabolism]:115.
13. Yang T, Zhu P, Dai G, Bai X, Zhao Y. Characteristics of metabolism in Keshan disease. *J Mol Cell Cardiol* 1987;1[Suppl]:41.
14. Marklund SL. Role of toxic effects of oxygen in reperfusion damage. *J Mol Cell Cardiol* 1988; 20[Suppl]:2.23.
15. Zhao Y, Yang T. Changes in isoenzyme distribution and CK activity of the rats fed on grains from Keshan disease endemic areas. *J N Bethune Univ Med Sci* 1984;10 [Suppl: Myocardial Metabolism]:135.
16. Hou L, Zhao Y, Yang T. Properties of serum enzymatic spectrum of the rats fed on grains from Keshan disease endemic areas. *J N Bethune Univ Med Sci* 1984;10 [Suppl: Myocardial Metabolism]:54.
17. Li C, Wang L, Li Z, Zhang L, Li Z, Zhao Z. Effect of grains from Keshan disease endemic areas on the membranous permeability of myocardial cells in rats. *J N Bethune Univ Med Sci* 1985;11:250.
18. Yang J. Biochemical studies on the plasma membrane of cardiac cells. *J N Bethune Univ Med Sci* 1986;12[Suppl]:6.
19. Yang F, Lin Z. Keshan disease is a kind of cardiac mitochondrial disease. In: Ministry of Public Health of China, ed. *Collected work of comprehensive scientific study on Keshan disease in Chu-Xiong prefecture.* Peking: People's Health Publication; 1988:184.
20. Zhao J, Yang T, Zhang X. Studies on the activity of cytochrome C oxidase in the cardiac cells of the patients with Keshan disease. *Chin J Endemiol* 1992;11:68.
21. Zhu P, Yang T. The changes in myocardial structural proteins of rats fed on grains from Keshan disease areas and its significance. *J Mol Cell Cardiol* 1987;19[Suppl 1]: 42.

22. Zhu P, Yang T. Studies on the cardiac contractile proteins. Changes of cardiac myosin ATPase in rats fed on grains from Keshan disease endemic areas. *Chin J Endemiol* 1985;4[Suppl]:93.

23. Guan J, Huang S, Li F. Analysis of selenium and glutathione peroxidase in the myocardium and red blood cells in the patients suffering from Keshan disease. Ministry of Public Health of China, ed. *Collected work of comprehensive scientific survey of Keshan disease in Chu-Xiong prefecture*. Peking: People's Health Publication; 1988:222.

24. Xia Y, Bai J, Yang G. Selenium and Keshan disease. In: Ministry of Public Health of China, ed. *Scientific research on prevention and treatment of Keshan disease in China*. Peking: Environmental Science Publishers of China 1987;167.

25. Xu G, Xie J. Water and soil in the etiology of Keshan disease—prevention of Keshan disease by sodium selenite and the relationship between selenium deficiency and the occurrence of Keshan disease. In: Ministry of Public Health of China, ed. *Scientific research on prevention and treatment of Keshan disease in China*. Peking: Environmental Science Publishers of China 1987;173.

26. Li S, Zhao Y. Analysis on the light chains of the myocardial myosin in the patients with subacute Keshan disease. In: Ministry of Public Health of China, ed. *Collected work of comprehensive scientific survey on Keshan disease in Chu-Xiong prefecture*. Peking: People's Health Publication; 1988;205.

27. Zhao J, Yang T. Analysis on the activity of superoxide dismutase in the red blood cells of the children from Chu-Xiong endemic areas. Ministry of Public Health of China, ed. *Collected work of the comprehensive scientific survey on Keshan disease in Chu-Xiong prefecture*. Peking: People's Health Publication; 1988:210.

28. Ouyang Y, Yang T. Free-radical metabolism of the animal model with Keshan disease. Ministry of Public Health of China, ed. *Collected work of comprehensive scientific survey on Keshan disease in Chu-Xiong prefecture*. Peking: People's Health Publication; 1988:213.

29. An R, Li G, Zhang G, Zhang L. Effect of grains from Keshan disease endemic areas on the metabolism of certain elements in myocardium. *J N Bethune Univ Med Sci* 1984;10 [Suppl: Myocardial Metabolism]:183.

30. Li G, Yang J. Lipid metabolic disorders in the children of Keshan disease endemic areas. Ministry of Public Health of China, ed. *Collected work of comprehensive scientific survey on Keshan disease in Chu-Xiong Prefecture*. Peking: People's Health Publication, 1988;247.

The Cardiomyopathic Heart, edited by Makoto
Nagano, Nobuakira Takeda, and Naranjan S.
Dhalla. Raven Press, Ltd., New York © 1994.

23

Alterations of the Cardiac Sarcolemma in Keshan Disease Models and Their Pathogenic Significance as Compared with Those in Cardiomyopathic J-2-N Hamsters

Jie Yang, *Yibing Ouyang, †Nobuakira Takeda, †Mitsutoshi Kato,
*Guang-qu Li, Makoto Nagano, and *Tongshu Yang

*Biochemistry Department, China-Japan Friendship Hospital, Beijing, China;
*N. Bethune University of Medical Sciences, Changchun, China; and †Department of
Internal Medicine, Jikei University School of Medicine, Tokyo, Japan*

Keshan disease (KD) is a type of endemic cardiomyopathy occurring primarily in China. It is also the most common human cardiomyopathy worldwide. Accordingly, considerable effort has been made to study and prevent the disease (1). Clinically, KD is characterized by myocardial injury and heart failure thought to result from a series of alterations in myocardial and general metabolism; however, this study focuses only on abnormality of the cardiac membrane, especially the heart sarcolemma, in animals with KD.

Numerous biochemical studies conducted over the last 30 years have demonstrated several abnormalities of myocardial metabolism in KD (2). Some studies showing increases in serum creatine kinase (CK), lactate dehydrogenase (LDH), and glutamic oxaloacetic transaminase (GOT) activities (3) have suggested that the abnormality of the cardiac sarcolemma in the acute state of KD is similar to that in myocardial infarction. Increased intracellular Ca^{2+} that may be associated with sarcolemmal function has also been found in animals with KD (4), as under physiologic conditions, the sarcolemma, sarcoplasmic reticulum (SR), and mitochondria are responsible for the control of intracellular Ca^{2+} concentration. However, elimination of Ca^{2+} from the cell relies primarily on the Ca^{2+} pump and Na^+-Ca^{2+} exchange, and the latter is further involved in the operation of sarcolemmal Na^+, K^+-ATPase. The Ca^{2+} pump, which is generally considered to consist of Ca^{2+}-stimulated ATPase, is also located in the cardiac sarcolemma.

In addition, the heart sarcolemma is fundamentally involved not only in cell organization but also in the electrical and chemical processes of myocardial cells, as it acts as a barrier against a variety of substances such as ions and large molecules.

Therefore, alterations of this membrane may contribute to intracellular abnormality. Because of the endemic character of KD, its pathogenesis may involve the absence of certain elements or the presence of abnormal material in food and water consumed by individuals in affected areas; in fact, this has been partly confirmed by epidemiologic studies (5). Therefore, some external pathogen may initially affect the sarcolemma of the cell.

Much less is known about the role of membrane damage in other forms of cardiomyopathy. However, in doxorubicin- and alcohol-related cardiomyopathies, a direct membrane effect of the exogenous materials is probably of pathogenic significance in myocardial damage. In the ischemic heart, the release of intracellular enzymes may be the result of membrane damage caused by the action of lipase, which hydrolyzes membrane phospholipids, and also the result of the effect of free radicals (6).

For these reasons, the present study was undertaken to determine (a) whether there are changes in the heart sarcolemma in animals with KD, especially before necrosis occurs; (b) the nature of the membrane changes, if present, and their pathogenic significance in myocardial abnormalities; and (c) the possible pathogenetic mechanism of the membrane damage, with emphasis on comparison with the J-2-N cardiomyopathic hamster.

MATERIALS AND METHODS

Animal Model

Keshan disease model rats were established by providing them with feed produced by Bethune Medical University using plants and other materials taken from the disease area. Normal rats of the same age were used as controls. The J-2-N hereditary cardiomyopathic hamster was developed and bred at Aoto Hospital, Jikei Medical University, and age-matched golden hamsters were used as controls (7).

Distribution of Enzymes and Creatine Kinase Isoenzymes

After separating mitochondria and other cell organelles, the cytosol and serum were used for intracellular and extracellular enzyme analysis, respectively. The CK isozyme distribution was determined by electrophoresis using 1% agarose gel and 50 mM TRIS-barbital buffer (pH of 8.9). After staining, the gel was scanned with a densitometer.

Isolation and Characterization of the Cardiac Sarcolemma

The cardiac sarcolemma was isolated from heart tissue of animals with KD by the method of Dhalla and associates (8). Purification of the sarcolemmal membrane was confirmed by measurement of marker enzymes. The activity of Na^+, K^+-ATPase in the membrane was 8.9-fold enriched compared with that of the homogenate. Contamination with other cellular organelles was also examined. The presence of mitochondria was determined on the basis of SDH and CCO activities in the sarcolemma preparation, and that of the SR was determined using glucose-6-phosphatase (G-6-P) activity (9,10). No SDH or CCO activity was evident; but 12.6% G-6-P activity was found in the membrane preparation.

Characterization of the Sarcolemmal Membrane in Keshan Disease

Na^+, K^+-ATPase was determined by the method of Kai et al. (11), and protein concentration was determined using the technique of Lowry and colleagues (12). 5′-Nucleotidase activity was tested as previously described (13).

Membrane fluidity was assayed by measuring the polarization of membrane labeled with a DPH fluorescent probe, using excitation and emission wavelengths of 365 nm and 425 nm, respectively. P is the value of polarizing fluorescence and is defined as follows:

$$P = (I_H - I_1)/(I_H + I_1)$$

The intensity of fluorescence is represented by I, and P is a parameter of membrane order, which is negatively correlated with the fluidity of the membrane (14).

Free Radical Metabolism

ESR was used to determine the free radical content. The ESR spectra were recorded using a JES-FEI spectrometer. The measurement parameters were temperature: room temperature; frequency (9.4 GHz); modulation amplitude (5.0 gauss); field (3800 + 100 gauss). Under these conditions, the signals observed in animals with KD and controls were similar, differing only in signal intensity. Because the intensity of the ESR signal is directly proportional to the free radical content of the sample, the relative height of the peak was used to represent the content of free radical. SOD was examined according to the method of Iwamoto et al. (15). GSHPx activity measurement was done by the method described elsewhere (16). Lipid peroxide content was determined according to Ohkawa (17).

Mitochondrial Functions

H^+-ATPase activity was measured by the method of Pande and Blanchaer (18). Inorganic phosphate and protein determinations were done in the same way as determinations of Na^+, K^+-ATPase. The ADP/ATP carrier protein content was measured using a method we had developed (19). SOD and CCO were determined by methods described earlier (9).

RESULTS AND DISCUSSION

The results of our studies confirmed the presence of changes in membrane permeability and their association with alterations in the biochemical characteristics of membrane-bound enzymes and membrane lipids. The possible pathogenesis of these membrane alterations is also discussed.

Confirmation of Sarcolemmal Injury

Examination of serum and intracellular enzymes indicated their redistribution between intracellular and extracellular fluids in animals with KD (Fig. 1). The higher activities in serum and lower activities in intracellular fluid suggested leakage of myocardial enzymes from myocytes. Our morphologic study indicated the intact nature of the myocardial cells in these animals, as shown in Fig. 2, and the ultrastructural appearance of the myocardium also confirmed their macrophage contact (20). Therefore, the "enzyme leakage" may result from increased permeability of the sarcolemma but may not be the outcome of membrane damage in the myocardial cells, such as the obvious necrosis seen in myocardial infarction.

Leakage of intracellular enzymes may affect the metabolism of myocardial cells. For example, loss of CK may cause derangement of energy metabolism, especially the transport of intracellular energy. In animals with KD, the distribution of the CK isozymes, CK-MM and CK-MB, appeared to be altered (Table 1); this may be involved in the special energy demand of the myocardium secondary to enzyme

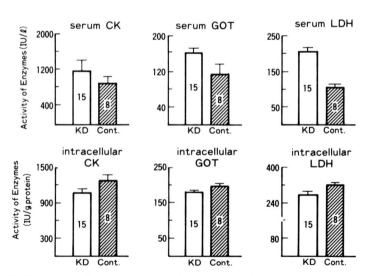

FIG. 1. Distribution of cellular content—notably enzymes—between serum and intracellular fluid in Keshan disease models. *CK*, creatine kinase; *GOT*, glutamic oxaloacetic transaminase; *LDH*, lactic dehydrogenase; *Cont.*, control.

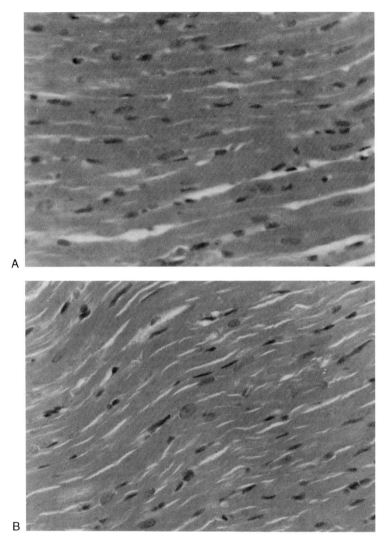

FIG. 2. Top: Section of myocardium from Keshan disease models that were used in this study. **Bottom**: Myocardium from a control animal.

leakage and may also contribute to the derangement of cell metabolism and even cardiocyte death.

To establish animal models that correspond to the different kinds and extents of KD, pathologists have developed a series of useful methods. The animal model used in this study was characterized by increased susceptibility to KD, but without any obvious changes in morphology (20). This characteristic is very useful for studies of membranes because macrography contact was a prerequisite for examin-

TABLE 1. *Comparison of myocardial energy supply between animals with Keshan disease (KD) and J-2-N cardiomyopathic hamsters*

	KD animal (% control)	J-2-N (% control)
Ouabain-sensitive Na,K-ATPase	71.75**	55*
Intracellular enzyme redistribution	Serum CK, GOT, LDH ↑ Intracellular CK, GOT, LDH ↓	Serum CK, GOT ↑ Intracellular CK, GOT ↓
CK isoenzymes	CK-MM ↑, CK-MB ↓	CK-MM ↑
OSCP H$^+$-ATPase	58.7**	121*
SDH, CCO activities	23.5 SDH** 40.1 CCO**	
AAC content		86.8*

$^a p<0.05$, $**p<0.01$.
OSCP, oligomycin-sensitivity-conferring-protein; CCO, cytochrome oxidase; SDH, succinic dehydrogenase; CK, creatine kinase; AAC, ADT/ATP carrier; GOT, glutamic oxaloacetic transaminase; LDH, lactate dehydrogenase.

ing the ion gradient and permeability of intracellular enzymes or cations. Our previous study also indicated some difference between acute myocardial damage and chronic KD-associated myocardial injury with regard to the extent and characteristics of the membrane enzyme changes (21). Some studies have noted this kind of change—that is, increased membrane permeability—but without any obvious change in morphology (22).

Despite the lack of obvious alteration in the morphology of the cardiac sarcolemma, the redistribution of the enzymes indicates increased permeability of the membrane in KD. This suggests that a study to identify possible biochemical abnormalities of the membrane proteins and membrane lipids would be warranted.

Characterization of the Sarcolemmal Alteration

As shown in Table 2, the activities of Na$^+$, K$^+$-ATPase, 5'-nucleotidase, ouabain receptor and membrane fluidity decreased in the heart sarcolemma of animals with KD. Among these, Na$^+$, K$^+$-ATPase plays a vital role in the physiology of

TABLE 2. *Alterations in the cardiac sarcolemma of animals with Keshan disease (KD)*

	KD animal	Control
Na,K-ATPase (Pi/mg pro./hr)	48.82 ± 1.81 (n = 12)*	54.84 ± 2.32 (n = 12)
Ouabain receptor (% control)	71.75% (n = 12)*	100% (n = 12)
5'-AMPase (Pi/mg pro./hr)	4.16 ± 0.34 (n = 12)*	6.09 ± 0.18 (n = 12)
Fluidity (fluorescent polarity)	0.232 ± 0.017 (n = 12)*	0.188 ± 0.055 (n = 12)

$*p<0.01$.

cardiac cells, such as the control of ion balance, membrane potential, and intracellular pH. In KD, an increase in the intracellular Ca^{2+} ion concentration (4), mitochondrial calcification, and a decrease in mitochondrial Ca^{2+} absorption ability have been confirmed (23). The increase in Ca^{2+} concentration may be a result of increased intracellular Na^+ secondary to inactivity of Na^+, K^+-ATPase (24). In cardiac cells, this function plays a more important role than in other tissues. Normally, inhibition of Na^+, K^+-ATPase induces an increase in intracellular Na^+ to a level of about 100 mM. However, in heart cells, such inhibition causes intracellular Na^+ to increase to only about 30 mM. In this case, intracellular Na^+ is controlled by net Na^+ extrusion produced by Na^+-Ca^{2+} exchange. Certainly, under pathologic conditions, the increase in intracellular Na^+ also results in an increase in intracellular Ca^{2+} owing to Na^+-Ca^{2+} exchange. The increased intracellular Ca^{2+} concentration may induce severe functional and structural alterations, such as calcium precipitation in mitochondria, myolysis, and necrosis of cells, as demonstrated in cardiomyopathic hamsters (25,26) and KD (4). Such loss of myocytes increases the burden on remaining cells, thus increasing sympathetic stimulation and leading to myocytic hypertrophy and further cell loss, which may develop in myocardial failure. Certainly, before the changes in Na^+-Ca^{2+} exchange and the Na^+-K^+ pump, there may be alterations in other Ca^{2+} channels, such as Ca^{2+}-pumping ATPase (27). This indicates that the increase in $[Ca^{2+}]$ is a result of many intracellular system actions. Besides the increased Ca^{2+} concentration in the cell, Na^+-Ca^{2+} exchange is also involved in determining the membrane potential and pH of the cell.

Normally, Na^+, K^+-ATPase hydrolyzes one molecule of ATP for the transport of three Na^+ ions out of the cell, and it pumps in two K^+ ions. Therefore, the Na^+-K^+ pump is electrogenic. This transport process produces part of the membrane potential and the depolarization of the membrane. In KD, it has been shown that the membrane potential is decreased in the myocardium, and this may involve inactivity of Na^+, K^+-ATPase. The correlation of the change in Na^+, K^+-ATPase with electrophysiologic alterations has also been demonstrated in animals fed a magnesium-deficient diet (28). The decreased enzyme activity leads to an increase in intracellular Na^+, resulting in a change in membrane potential as well as arrhythmias.

In addition, 5′-nucleotidase, as a membrane-bound protein, is a marker of sarcolemmal membrane, and also participates in the degradation of intracellular and extracellular ATP, together with sarcolemmal ATPase. Therefore, the decreased activity of the enzyme may contribute to the variety of physiological effects observed in KD.

Possible Mechanism of Sarcolemmal Alteration in KD

Heart sarcolemmal alterations of membrane enzymes and membrane lipids have been confirmed in animals with KD. What, then, are the pathogenetic mechanisms underlying these membrane alterations, which could be of significance for the prevention and treatment of KD? Study results indicate two possible mechanisms: (a) abnormal free radical metabolism and associated sarcolemmal alteration in KD, and (b) disordered intracellular energy supply.

Free Radical Metabolism Abnormality and Its Mediated Sarcolemmal Alteration in KD

This mechanism is, in part, similar to the mechanism underlying some other cardiomyopathies and heart diseases, such as ischemia-reperfusion injury (29,30). Therefore, the mechanism may be relatively widespread in cases of membrane damage. Moreover, different diseases have their own unique pathogenetic features. In the present work, we investigated whether the membrane changes were associated with alterations of free-radical scavengers, contents of free radicals, and/or lipid peroxide content. As shown in Table 3, the activities of SOD and GSH-Px were decreased in animals with KD because they form a line of membrane defense through their antioxidative action. The content of free radicals was increased compared with normal controls, as revealed by ESR spectroscopy, and the lipid peroxide content was increased.

These results suggest a disorder of free-radical metabolism in KD, thus affecting the membrane-bound protein and membrane lipids. For example, in membrane lipids, the increased lipid peroxidation in KD may be a result of these disorders, and thus may induce membrane phospholipid destruction (31) and decreased membrane fluidity. These changes lead to increased permeability to cations (32) and enzymes, as well as changes in membrane potential. An arrhythmogenic effect of lipid peroxidation has also been demonstrated directly in isolated auricles. This effect is thought to result from derangement of Na^+, K^+-ATPase because the enzyme plays

TABLE 3. *Disorders of free radical metabolism in animals with Keshan disease (KD)*

	KD animal	Control
Free radical content (ESR value, peak/peak)	1.75 ± 0.39 (n = 8)*	1.40 ± 0.14 (n = 7)
SOD activities (IU/g.w.w.)	487 ± 111.8 (n = 10)*	537.6 ± 142.2 (n = 8)
GSH-Px activities (IU/g.w.w.)	2.45 ± 0.49 (n = 10)***	6.44 ± 1.84 (n = 8)
GSH-Px after adding selenium (% control)	103.4 ± 1.98 (n = 10)**	100 (n = 10)
Peroxide lipid (TBA) (nM MDA/g.w.w.)	168.4 ± 14.8 (n = 10)**	146.6 ± 11.5 (n = 8)

$*p < 0.05$; $**p < 0.01$; $***p < 0.001$.
ESR, electron spin resonance spectroscopy; SOD, superoxide dismutase; GSH-Px, glutathione peroxidase.

a key role in maintaining the transmembrane potential and electrochemical stability of the myocardium (33).

Free radicals may also affect membrane-bound proteins, leading to the decreased enzyme activity observed in KD animals. Although the exact mechanism is not clear, it may be associated with alterations in the phospholipid microenvironment of the enzyme, such as a decrease in lipid peroxidase-mediated fluidity. This may affect the conformation of the membrane-bound enzyme, thus inducing the decrease in activity. For example, it has been shown that removal of membrane lipid interrupts the conformation of the enzyme (34). Certainly, free radicals also affect membrane enzyme activity directly, as they can induce the oxidation of sulfhydryl groups of enzyme proteins.

Table 3 shows the changes in the antioxidative enzymes in animals with KD. In comparison with GSH-Px, the change in SOD does not seem very great, although in the blood of the animals, SOD was elevated markedly (35). It is interesting that similar results have also been obtained in cardiomyopathic hamsters (36). The addition of selenium to the diet produced recovery of the decreased GSH-Px activity in KD animals, and this was accompanied by a decrease in lipid peroxidase and free radical content (36).

According to the results described earlier, it appears that an increase of free radicals and a decrease of scavengers may contribute to the abnormalities observed in membrane proteins and membrane phospholipids, and thus may influence membrane permeability, membrane fluidity, and enzyme activities.

Disordered Intracellular Energy Supply

The second possible mechanism underlying the membrane alterations that occur in KD involves a disordered intracellular energy supply, which may play a special role in KD, perhaps differentiating it from other heart diseases. Decreased Na^+, K^+-ATPase activity has been shown in many heart diseases, such as bacterial endocarditis (37), ventricular failure in hypertrophy (38), myocardial ischemia (39), and the cardiomyopathic hamster (40). However, it is quite evident that there are different mechanisms in the pathogenesis of these diseases.

To clarify the mechanism, we compared a KD model with the cardiomyopathic hamster J-2-N, which was developed and bred by Nagano (7). From Table 1, it can be seen that similar changes occur in the heart sarcolemma of animals with KD and that of J-2-N cardiomyopathic hamsters. These changes include decreased Na^+, K^+-ATPase activity and redistribution of intracellular enzymes.

However, in mitochondria, the activities of H^+-ATPase showed different alterations—that is, the activities were decreased in KD and increased in J-2-N hamsters as compared with their respective controls. In addition, animals with KD demonstrated an obvious disorder of oxidative phosphorylation; SDH and CCO activities, and the stage 3 respiration rate of mitochondrial oxidative phosphorylation, were remarkably decreased (41). For this reason, the intracellular ATP concentration was also decreased (42). However, in the cardiomyopathic hamster, no obvious decrease in ATP concentration could be found, or only the creatine phosphate:creatine ratio was decreased (43). In the J-2-N hamster, the mitochondrial ADP/ATP carrier (AAC) protein content was decreased compared with controls. The AAC protein plays a central role in linking the thermodynamically divergent metabolisms of the intramitochondrial and extramitochondrial compartments. A recent report has also indicated the possibility of an autoantibody against the ADP-ATP carrier that not only binds to the mitochondrial membrane but also cross-reacts with antigenic determinants on the heart plasma membrane (44).

These results suggest that, in the J-2-N hamster, the disorder of energy supply occurs primarily during energy transport, not during the production of energy. However, in KD, the disorder of energy metabolism starts at the point of mitochondrial oxidative phosphorylation and leads to a deficiency in intracellular ATP supply.

It is worth considering that energy status may affect membrane function. For example, the energy cost for Na^+, K^+-ATPase may account for 20% of the total cellular energy. The intracellular free energy, ΔG, depends on the hydrolysis of ATP; therefore, a decrease in ATP will decrease the energy available to the enzymes and affect their functions. For example, in the Na^+-K^+ pump, if the ΔG is less than the energy required by the pump, the $[Na]_i$ and $[K]_o$ will lead to change. In the ischemic heart, intracellular Na^+ increased, although in initial ischemia, the $[Na^+]$ level remained at 4.7 to 7.6 mM after 10 to 15 minutes of ischemia; this corresponds to a relatively slow decrease in the ATP level owing to conversion of ADP to AMP and ATP, as well as glycolysis (45). Thus, it has been shown that KD is an ischemic cardiomyopathy by pathologic analysis, and that this may contribute to the observed membrane alterations.

SUMMARY

An attempt was made to determine the nature of the abnormality of the cardiac sarcolemma in Keshan disease (KD), a kind of endemic cardiomyopathy occurring primarily in China. Redistribution of the cellular contents, notably enzymes, between the serum and intracellular fluid, and the morphologic observation of intact macrophages in the cells, indicated increased membrane permeability and suggested the possibility of membrane injury. Examination of the isolated sarcolemma indicated a decrease in Na, K-adenosine triphosphatase (ATPase), ouabain receptor, 5'-nucleotidase activity, and membrane fluidity in KD animal models. Therefore, some abnormalities in the myocardial metabolism of KD are suggested; these include increased $[Ca^{2+}]$ and Ca precipitation in mitochondria and cell necrosis. Two pathogenic mechanisms of membrane damage involving free radical metabolism and intracellular energy supply are possible. The increased free radical content revealed by electron spin resonance spectroscopy (ESR) and a decrease of free radical scavengers, superoxide dismutase (SOD) and glutathione peroxidase (GSHPx), indicated a disorder of free radical metabolism in KD. These may contribute to the increased lipid peroxide level and may further induce the dysfunction of membrane permeability, membrane fluidity, and membrane-bound enzyme activities. Measurement of H^+-ATPase, succinate dehydrogenase (SDH), cytochrome oxidase (CCO), and adenosine triphosphate (ATP) content demonstrated a disorder of energy supply in KD animal models. Unlike the situation in J-2-N cardiomyopathic hamsters, the disorder in KD starts at ATP synthesis, which reduces the intracellular ATP concentration. However, J-2-N hamsters are characterized by hereditary cardiomyopathy, and the disorder of energy supply is located primary at the intracellular energy transport step, such as a decrease in the content of mitochondrial adenosine diphosphate (ADP)/ATP carrier and myocardial creatine kinase (CK) level.

REFERENCES

1. Sun J. Review of the basic research and clinic works in Keshan disease. In: Ministry of Public Health of China, eds. *Scientific research on prevention and treatment of Keshan disease*. Peking: Environmental Science Publishers of China; 1987:1–24 (in Chinese).
2. Yang T. Metabolic disorder of myocardium in Keshan disease. In: Ministry of Public Health of China, eds. *Scientific research on prevention and treatment of Keshan disease*. Peking: Environmental Science Publishers of China; 1987:227–232.
3. Hou LZ, Yang TS, Zhou ZJ. Serum biochemical assay in population of Keshan disease. *J Mol Cell Cardiol* 1992;24 (Suppl I):221.
4. An RG, Li GS, Zhang GT, Zhang LC. Effect of grains from Keshan disease endemic areas on the metabolism of some elements in myocardium. *J N Bethune Univ Med Sci* [Supplement: Myocardial Metabolism]:1984; 183–185 (in Chinese).
5. Zhao TL. Report on the examination of Keshan disease in Chu Xong. In: Ministry of Public Health of China, eds. *Scientific research on prevention and treatment of Keshan disease*. Peking: Environmental Science Publishers of China; 1987;186–192.
6. Katz AM, Freston JW, Messineo FC, Herbette LG. Membrane damage and the pathogenesis of cardiomyopathies. *J Mol Cell Cardiol* 1985;17[Suppl]:11–20.
7. Nagano M, Takeda N, Kato W, Nagai M, Yang J. Pathophysiological aspect of cardiomyopathic hamster J-2-N. *J Mol Cell Cardiol* 1992;24[Suppl II]:418.
8. Dhalla NS, Lee SL, Anand MB, Chanhan MS. Effect of acebutolol, practolol, and propanolol on rat heart sarcolemma. *Biochem Pharmacol* 1977;26:2050–2060.
9. Dai GH, Yang TS. Changes of cellular respiration in myocardium from animals fed with cereals from KD areas. Yang TS, ed. *J N Bethune Univ Med Sci* 1984; [Supplement: *Myocardial Metabolism*]:125–128.
10. Aronson NN Jr, Touster O. Isolation of rat liver plasma membrane fragments in isotonic sucrose. *Methods Enzymol* 1974;31:93–102.
11. Kai M, White G, Hawthorne J. The phosphatidylinositol kinase of rat brain. *Biochem J* 1966; 101:328–337.
12. Lowry OH, Rosebrough NJ, Farr AL, Randall RJ. Protein measurement with the Folin phenol regent. *J Biol Chem* 1951;193:265–275.
13. Post RL, Sen AX. Sodium and potassium-stimulated ATPase. *Methods Enzymol* 1967;10:762–768.
14. Yang Y, Guo PC, Wang DH. Study on the liposome inlaid with isolated membrane protein. *Chin Sci(B)* 1983;6:519.
15. Iwamoto Y, Mifuchi I. Superoxide dismutase activity of lactobacilli. *Chem Pharm Bull* 1982; 30:237–241.
16. KD Research Group of Chinese Medical Academy. A method for measuring GSHPX activity. *Health Res* 1977;6:61–66.
17. Ohkawa H, Ohishi N, Yagi K. Assay for lipid peroxidation in animal tissues by thiobarbituric acid reaction. *Anal Biochem* 1979;95:351–358.

18. Pande SU, Blanchaer MC. Reversible inhibition of mitochondria adenosine diphosphate phosphorylation by long chain acyl coenzyme A esters. *J Biol Chem* 1971;246:401–411.

19. Yang J, Kato M, Takeda N, Nagano M. Alterations of mitochondria ADP/ATP carrier protein in heredity cardiomyopathic hamster J-2-N. In: Tanaka N, Nagano M, eds. *Cardiac structure and metabolism*, Vol 14. Lopoo Press; 1991:251–257 (in Japanese).

20. Wang F, Li GS, Kang DR, Yang TS, Zhang HY. Pathologic characteristics and etiological significance of Keshan disease. In: Ministry of Public Health of China, eds. *Scientific research on prevention and treatment of Keshan disease*. Peking: Environmental Science Publishers of China; 1987; 238–248.

21. Yang J, Mai YC, Yang TS. Alterations of cardiac sarcolemma in different myocardial injuries. *Prog Biochem Biophys* 1991;18:132 (in Chinese).

22. Rossi MA, Silva JS. Permeability alteration of the sarcolemmal membrane, particularly at the site of macrophage contact in experimental chronic *Trypanosoma crizi* myocarditis in mice. *Int J Exp Pathol* 1990;71:545–555.

23. Win W Qiu, Yang TS. Activity of ^{45}Ca uptake by myocardial mitochondria from rats fed with grains from KD areas. *J Mol Cell Cardiol* 1992;24[Suppl I]:209.

24. Norgaard A, Baandrup U, Larsen JS, Kjeldsen K. Heart Na^+,K^+-ATPase activity in cardiomyopathic hamster as estimated from K^+-dependent 3-O-MFPase activity in the crude homogenates. *J Mol Cell Cardiol* 1987;19:589–594.

25. Olbrich HG, Borgers M, Thone F, et al. Ultrastructural localization of calcium in the myocardium of cardiomyopathic Syrian hamster. *J Mol Cell Cardiol* 1988;20:753–762.

26. Sole MJ, Liew CC. Catecholamines, calcium and cardiomyopathy. *Am J Cardiol* 1988;62:20G–24G.

27. Kuo TH, Tsang W, Wiener J. Defective Ca^{2+}-pumping ATPase of heart sarcolemma from cardiomyopathic hamster. *Biochim Biophys Acta* 1987;900:10–16.

28. Fischer PW, Giroux A. Effects of dietary magnesium on sodium potassium pump in the heart of rats. *J Nutr* 1987;117:2091–2095.

29. Weisfeldt ML. Reperfusion and reperfusion injury. *Clin Res* 1987;35:13–20.

30. Mailer K, Macleod I, Morris W. Age-related change in anti-oxidative enzymes in cardiomyopathic hamster hearts. *Mech Ageing Dev* 1991;59:37–45.

31. Freeman BA, Crapo JD. Biology of disease: free radicals and tissue injury. *Lab Invest* 1982;47:412–426.

32. Nagata XX, et al. Effect of lipid peroxidation on mitochondria membrane function. *Biochemistry* 1978;50:861 (in Japanese).

33. Meerson FZ, Belkina LM, Sazontova TG, Saltykova VA, Arkhipenko YuV. The role of lipid peroxidation in pathogenesis of arrhythmias and prevention of cardiac fibrillation with antioxidants. *Basic Res Cardiol* 1987;82:123–137.

34. Akera T, Brody TM. Myocardial membranes. Regulation and function of sodium pump. *Annu Rev Physiol* 1982;44:375.

35. Ouyang YB, Yang TS. Free radical metabolism of myocardium from the patients with Keshan disease. *Chin J Endemiol* 1987;6:193–196.

36. Li GQ, Yang TS. Effect of organic selenium on the metabolism of myocardial free radical in rats fed with grain from KD areas [abstract]. *Proceedings of IUBMB conference, Biochemistry of Disease*. Nagoya: IUBMB, 1992;284.

37. Tomlinson CW, Lee SL, Dhalla NS. Abnormality in heart membrane and myofibril during bacterial infective cardiomyopathy in rabbit. *Circ Res* 1976;39:82–92.

38. Yazaki Y, Fujii J. Depressed Na,K-ATPase activity in the failing rabbit heart. *Jpn Heart J* 1972; 13:73–83.

39. Beller GA, Conroy J, Smith T. Ischemia-induced alteration in myocardial (Na,K) ATPase and cardiac glycoside binding. *J Clin Invest* 1976;57:341–350.

40. Dhalla NS, Singh JN, Bajusz E, Jasmin G. Comparison of heart sarcolemmal enzyme activities in normal and cardiomyopathic (UM-X7.1) hamsters. *Clin Sci Mol Med* 1976;51:233–242.

41. Yang TS, Dai GH. Changes in mitochondria respiratory enzymes of myocardium from rats fed with grain of KD area. *Chin J Endemiol* 1982;1:108–111.

42. Zhao Y, Tang TS. Influence of KD endemic area cereals on myocardial ATP contents in animals. *Chin J Endemiol* 1985;4:101–104.

43. Wrogemann K, Blanchare MC, Jacobson BE. Oxidative phosphorylation at various stages of the

genetically determined cardiomyopathy in the Syrian hamster. *Recent Adv Study Cardiac Struct Metab* 1973;467–478.

44. Kuhl U, Melzner B, Schafer B, Schultheiss HP, Strauer BE. The channel as cardiac autoantigen. *Eur Heart J* 1991;12[Suppl D]:99–104.

45. Kleber G. Resting membrane potential. Extracellular potassium activity and intracellular sodium activity during acute global ischemia in isolated perfused Guinea pig hearts. *Circ Res* 1983;52:442–450.

The Cardiomyopathic Heart, edited by Makoto
Nagano, Nobuakira Takeda, and Naranjan S.
Dhalla. Raven Press, Ltd., New York © 1994.

24

Possible Stages of Adaptive Remodeling of Myocardial Cells

László Szekeres

*Institute of Pharmacology, Albert Szent-Györgyi Medical University,
H-6720, Szeged, Hungary*

INTRODUCTION

Cardiac hypertrophy resulting from chronic mechanical overload represents a cardiophysiologic adaptation to a disease, such as congestive heart failure (1). This adaptation may induce remodeling of the heart, including both metabolic and morphologic changes, which may ultimately lead to cardiomyopathy. Changes include abnormal gene expression, such as isoform changes of structural and nonstructural myocardial proteins (2).

The stimulus for altered gene expression seems to depend on the factor eliciting the cardiac hypertrophy (3). There is, however, increasing evidence for the importance of the adrenergic system in this process. Thus, chronic infusion of subhypertensive doses of norepinephrine in the dog induced left ventricular hypertrophy (4). Long-term treatment with low doses of isoproterenol stimulated in vivo cardiac hypertrophy without evidence of necrosis (5). There is also evidence that catecholamines increase the rate of protein synthesis in the heart (6) and stimulate nucleic acid metabolism in cardiac cells (7). Dubus and colleagues (8) have shown that low doses of β-adrenergic agonists stimulate the synthesis of noncontractile proteins, but not of contractile proteins, in cultured myocytes isolated from adult rat heart, whereas high doses had a toxic effect. This type of adaptation, characterized by a gradual increase in myocardial mass, develops slowly, and requires a period of weeks or even months.

The aim of the present study is to investigate other, more rapidly developing types of adaptation and to analyze possible similarities and dissimilarities with the adaptation process leading to cardiac hypertrophy. The most rapidly developing adaptation to moderate stress (brief coronary occlusion or a brief period of rapid cardiac pacing)—so-called "preconditioning"—protects against the consequences of a subsequent, more severe (ischemic) stress within 30 minutes after preconditioning (9–12).

As shown by the author's group in 1983 (13), a more slowly developing type of adaptation is the late-appearing cardioprotection that occurs in response to moderate stress and lasts for a few days. This protection can be evoked by a single dose of prostacyclin or its stable analog 7-oxo-prostacyclin (14), or by a series of rapid cardiac pacings (15). Accordingly, the following questions were studied:

a. What kind of changes occur in these more rapidly developing adaptation processes resulting in cardioprotection?
b. What is their possible mechanism?
c. What are the possible common factors concerning the nature of moderate stresses that elicit the adaptation process?
d. Are there common signal transduction pathways for altered gene expression?

RESULTS AND CONCLUSIONS

Changes Appearing in the More Rapidly Developing Adaptation Processes

Brief preconditioning stimuli (brief coronary occlusion or rapid pacing) may initiate a short-lasting (30–60 min) adaptation process, protecting against the consequences of a more severe myocardial ischemia (e.g., a longer period of coronary artery occlusion). Thus these stimuli may delay lethal cell injury and reduce infarct size (9,10), and may prevent or moderate postocclusion or reperfusion arrhythmias (11,12).

The late-appearing, more prolonged cardioprotection induced by variform, moderate, ischemic stresses (e.g., prostacyclin, 7-oxo-prostacyclin, or a series of rapid cardiac pacings) represents a dose- and time-dependent process, with maximal protection occurring 24 to 48 hours after the inducing stress (14). It prevents or moderates the following:

a. Global and local myocardial ischemia (13,16,17)
b. Early postocclusion and reperfusion arrhythmias (13,17)
c. Late postinfarction arrhythmias (18)
d. Ischemic loss of K^+ and accumulation of Na^+ (and after reperfusion accumulation of Ca^{2+}) in the myocardium (19)
e. Early morphologic changes secondary to ischemia and reperfusion (19)
f. Toxic effects of cardiac glycosides (20)

Possible Mechanisms of Adaptation Resulting in Cardioprotection

The short-term cardioprotection initiated by brief preconditioning stimuli is probably attributable to the preconditioning-induced release of endogenous cardioprotective substances, such as adenosine (21), prostacyclin (22), nitric oxide (23). Formation of stress proteins has also been suggested (24,25). In terms of the mechanism(s) involved in the late-appearing, more prolonged cardioprotection, there is evidence that the following factors have a role:

(a) Reduced sensitivity to β-adrenergic stimuli (26)
(b) Increased activity and amount of sarcolemmal Na^+,K^+-ATPase (27), moderate ischemia- and reperfusion-induced loss of K^+, and increased Na^+ and Ca^{2+} levels in the myocardium, leading to a reduction in the toxicity of ouabain (19,20).
(c) Increased activity of myocardial cyclic guanosine monophosphate (cGMP)-hydrolyzing PDE I, which moderates the inhibitory effect of cGMP on cAMP-hydrolyzing PDE III (28), the latter of which is capable of splitting excess cAMP.
(d) Antiarrhythmic electrophysiologic changes, such as prolongation of the effective refractory period (ERP) and the action potential duration (APD) (29,30), which represents an endogenous Class III antiarrhythmic action.
(e) Hemodynamic changes that reduce myocardial oxygen demand, such as a moderate bradycardia, a slight decline in blood pressure and contractility, moderation of the ischemic rise of left ventricular end diastolic pressure (LVEDP), and moderation of the ischemic diminution of coronary flow (17,31).

Possible Common Factors of Stresses Eliciting the Process of Adaptation

Careful investigation of the changes evoked by the rapidly developing, short-lasting cardiac adaptation; by the later-appearing, more prolonged cardioprotection; and by adaptation to chronic mechanical overload, as well as their possible mechanisms, reveals the key role of the adenylate-cyclase/cAMP pathway. This pathway is activated to a different extent and for different periods of time by stresses inducing adaptation in all the three forms just mentioned.

Thus, single or multiple brief coronary occlusions, or brief rapid pacings, cause transient myocardial ischemia and the release of catecholamines and other endogenous substances, such as prostacylin, which may activate the adenylate-cyclase/cAMP system. Administration of prostacyclin or of its stable analogs at the optimal dose, or a series of rapid cardiac pacings, may stimulate the adenylate-cyclase/cAMP system even more vigorously, whereas long-lasting mechanical overload leading to cardiac hypertrophy is nearly always linked with elevated blood catecholamine levels. Several studies have reported a correlation between plasma catecholamine levels and left ventricular mass (32).

Signal Transduction and Possible Role of Increased Synthesis of Proteins

Common to all three types of adaptation processes discussed thus far is the fact that signal transduction involves the adenylate-cyclase/cAMP pathway. As stated earlier, catecholamines increase the rate of protein synthesis in the heart (6), and low doses of β-adrenergic agonists stimulate the synthesis of noncontractile myo-cardial proteins (8). To this latter category belong the stress proteins induced in mammalian heart by heat shock (33) and ischemia (34), which appear a few hours after the cardiac insult. Moreover, the enzymes Na^+,K^+-ATPase and cGMP-de-pendent PDE I have been shown to play a major role in the mechanism of prolonged cardioprotection (27,28).

In the rapid and short-lasting adaptation induced by brief preconditioning stimuli, the role of preconditioning-induced stress proteins is still questionable. In isolated rabbit hearts, functional and biochemical protection from heat stress has been dem-onstrated (35). However, in in vivo studies of rabbits, no reduction in infarct size has been demonstrated (36). Protein synthesis inhibitors, such as dactinomycin and cycloheximide, were reported not to attenuate preconditioning in rabbits (37). There is convincing evidence to support the premise that protection is related to the release of endogenous cardioprotective substances (21–23).

In the more slowly developing adaptation process that results in cardioprotection lasting for a few days, there is evidence for activation and induction of essential enzymes, such as Na^+,K^+-ATPase (27) or cGMP-hydrolyzing PDE I (28). This occurs via the adenylate-cyclase/cAMP pathway.

Cardiac hypertrophy represents a very gradual, slowly developing adaptation pro-cess as compared to the types of adaptation discussed earlier. The development of hypertrophy involves both qualitative and quantitative changes in gene expression. The genes are normal, but the way in which they are regulated is modified (38). The role of adrenergic stimulation in cardiac hypertrophy has been discussed earlier in this chapter.

On the basis of the presented data, the conclusion can be drawn that the adenyl-ate-cyclase/cAMP pathway plays a key role in the adaptation process. It is likely that a certain threshold level of cAMP is needed for signal transduction, leading to induction of enzymes and contractile proteins. The author's research indicates that, up to now, no attempt has been made to define these threshold values for the differ-ent types of adaptation discussed.

Another issue that has not been investigated is the importance of the repeated application of stresses of low intensity. This fractionated application should be used to avoid unwanted side effects caused by a stimulus sufficiently intensive to activate and induce enzymes. Whether summation of stress fractions will reach the threshold required to initiate transcription remains to be elucidated.

SUMMARY

Cardiac hypertrophy represents a physiological adaptation to chronic mechanical overload leading to congestive heart failure. This adaptation could induce remodel-ing of the heart, involving both metabolic and morphologic changes resulting in cardiomyopathy. These changes include altered gene expression, such as isoform changes of structural and nonstructural myocardial proteins. The stimulus for altered gene expression seems to be a moderate but lasting disturbance of oxidative processes, together with an activation of the adrenergic system. Thus, long-term treatment with catecholamines induces cardiac hypertrophy; indeed, a correlation has been found between plasma catecholamine level and the extent of cardiac hypertrophy. The present study investigates this and other, more rapidly developing types of adaptation in an attempt to identify the common mechanisms. The short-term adaptation initiated by brief preconditioning stimuli protects against myocardial ischemia, delays lethal cell injury, reduces infarct size, and prevents or moderates postocclusion and reperfusion arrhythmias. This cardioprotection is mediated by the ischemic release of endogenous substances (e.g., catecholamines, prostacyclin), activating the cyclooxygenase/cyclic adenosine monophosphate (cAMP) system. The later-appearing, more prolonged cardioprotection induced by various forms of more severe (but not injurious) stimuli, such as an optimal dose of prostaglandin I_2 (PgI_2) or its stable analogs, or a series of rapid cardiac pacings, considerably moderates myocardial ischemia, early and late postocclusion and reperfusion arrhythmias, early ischemia- and reperfusion-induced morphologic changes 24 to 48 hours after the inducing stimulus. The stimulus activates the adenylate-cyclase/cAMP system, and a certain threshold level of cAMP triggers induction of enzymes shown to be essential in this type of cardioprotection. The presented data allow the conclusion that the adenylate-cyclase/cAMP pathway plays a key role in the process of adaptation.

REFERENCES

1. Swynghedauw B. Remodeling the heart in chronic pressure overload. In: Smits JFM, De Mey JGR, Daemen MJAP, Struyker XX, Boudier HAJ, eds. *Pharmacology of cardiac and vascular remodeling*. Darmstadt, Germany: Steinkopff Verlag; 1991:99–106.
2. Katz AM. Pathogenesis of impaired pump function in congestive heart failure. In: Brachmann J, Dietz R, Kübler W, eds. *Heart failure and arrhythmias*. Berlin: Springer-Verlag; 1990:8–16.
3. Zimmer HG, Peffer H. Metabolic aspects of the development of experimental cardiac hypertrophy. In: Jacob R, ed. *Controversial issues in cardiac pathophysiology*. Darmstadt, Germany: Steinkopff Verlag; 1986:127–138.
4. Laks MM, Morady F, Swan HJ. Myocardial hypertrophy produced by chronic infusion of subhypertensive doses of NE in the dog. *Chest* 1973;64:75–78.
5. Taylor P, Tang Q. Development of isoproterenol-induced cardiac hypertrophy. *Can J Physiol Pharmacol* 1984;62:384–389.
6. Mallow S. Effect of sympathomimetic drug on protein synthesis in rat heart. *J Pharmacol Exp Ther* 1973;187:482–487.
7. Wood NY, Lindenmayer GC, Schwartz A. Myocardial synthesis of ribonucleic acids. Stimulation with isoproterenol. *J Mol Cell Cardiol* 1971;3:127–133.
8. Dubus I, Samuel JL, Marotte F, Delcayre C, Rappaport L. β-adrenergic agonists stimulate the synthesis of noncontractile but not contractile proteins in cultured myocytes isolated from adult rat heart. *Circ Res* 1990;66:867–874.
9. Murry CE, Jennings RB, Reimer KA. Preconditioning with ischemia: a delay of lethal cell injury in ischemic myocardium. *Circulation* 1986;74:1124–1136.
10. Schott RJ, Rohmann S, Braun ER, Schaper W. Ischemic preconditioning reduces infarct size in swine myocardium. *Circ Res* 1988;66:1133–1142.
11. Végh Á, Komori S, Szekeres L, Parratt JR. Antiarrhythmic effects of preconditioning in anaesthetised dogs and rats. *Cardiovasc Res* 1992;26:487–495.

12. Végh Á, Szekeres L, Parratt JR. Transient ischaemia induced by rapid cardiac pacing results in myocardial preconditioning. *Cardiovasc Res* 1991;25:1051–1053.
13. Szekeres L, Krassói I, Udvary É. Delayed antiischaemic effect of PgI2 and of a new stable PgI2 analogue 7-oxo-PgI2-Na in experimental model angina in dogs. *J Mol Cell Cardiol* 1983;15[Suppl 1]:394.
14. Szekeres L, Pataricza J, Szilvássy Z, Udvary É, Végh Á. Cardioprotection: endogenous protective mechanisms promoted by prostacyclin. In: Gülch RG, Kissling G, eds. *Current topics in heart failure*. Darmstadt, Germany: Steinkopff Verlag; 1991:215–221.
15. Szekeres L, Szilvássy Z, Udvary É, Végh Á. Rapid pacing evoking myocardial ischaemia induces both short-term and delayed cardioprotection. *J Mol Cell Cardiol* 1991;23[Suppl 5]:S72.
16. Szekeres L, Koltay M, Pataricza J, Takáts I, Udvary É. On the late antiischaemic action of the stable PgI2 analogue: 7-oxo-PgI2-Na and its possible mode of action. *Biomed Biochim Acta* 1984;43:135–142.
17. Udvary É, Szekeres L. Prostacyclin: antiischaemic or cardioprotective? In: Kecskeméti V, Gyires K, Kovács G, eds. *Prostanoids: Proceedings of the 4th Congress of the Hungarian Pharmacological Society*, Vol 3. Budapest: Akadémiai Kiadó; 1985:333–338.
18. Végh Á. 7-oxo-PgI2 induced delayed protective action from late postocclusion arrhythmias in conscious dogs. In: Slezak J, ed. *Ischemia and reperfusion injury of the heart. Proceedings of the ISHR East European Subsection Meeting*. Smolenice, Czechoslovakia; May, 1990: 93.
19. Szekeres L, Bálint Z, Karcsu S, Tósaki Á. Delayed protection by 7-oxo-PgI2 against cardiac transmembrane ion shifts and early morphological changes due to ischaemia and reperfusion. *Cardioscience* 1990;1:280–286.
20. Szilvássy Z, Szekeres L, Udvary É, Végh Á. On the 7-oxo-PgI2 induced lasting protection against ouabain arrhythmias in anaesthetized guinea pigs. *Biomed Biochim Acta* 1988;47:35–38.
21. Liu GS, Thornton J, Van Winkle DM, Stanley AWH, Olsson RA, Downey JM. Protection against infarction afforded by preconditioning is mediated by A1 adenosine receptors in rabbit heart. *Circulation* 1991;84:350–356.
22. Végh Á, Szekeres L, Parratt JR. Protective effects of preconditioning of the ischemic myocardium involve cyclo-oxygenase products. *Cardiovasc Res* 1990;24:1020–1023.
23. Végh Á, Szekeres L, Parratt JR. Does nitric oxide play a role in ischaemic preconditioning? *J Mol Cell Cardiol* 1991;23[Suppl 5]:S72.
24. Yellon DM. The role of stress proteins in myocardial protection. *J Mol Cell Cardiol* 1992;24[Suppl 2]:S7.
25. Schaper W, Brand T, Frass O, Sharma HS, Zimmermann R, Verdouw P, Andres J. Gene expression is markedly changed in stunned and preconditioned myocardium. *J Mol Cell Cardiol* 1992;24[Suppl 2]:S10.
26. Szekeres L, Németh M, Szilvássy Z, Tósaki Á, Udvary É, Végh Á. On the nature and molecular basis of prostacyclin induced late changes. *Biomed Biochim Acta* 1988;47:6–11.
27. Dzurba A, Ziegelhöffer A, Breier A, Vrbjar N, Szekeres L. Increased activity of sarcolemmal (Na,K)-ATPase is involved in the late cardioprotective action of 7-oxo-prostacyclin. *Cardioscience* 1991;2:105–108.
28. Krause EG, Bartel S, Luthardt G, Szilvássy Z, Szekeres L. The cytoprotective effect of 7-oxo-prostacyclin (7-oxo) is related to a rise in particulate cGMP-hydrolysing PDE activity in the myocardium. *J Mol Cell Cardiol* 1990;22[Suppl 3]:S33.
29. Szekeres L, Németh M, Papp JGY, Udvary É. Short incubation with 7-oxo-prostacyclin induces long-lasting prolongation of repolarization time and effective refractory period in rabbit papillary muscle preparation. *Cardiovasc Res* 1990;24:34–41.
30. Szekeres L, Szilvássy Z, Udvary É, Végh Á. 7-oxo-PgI2 induced late appearing and long-lasting electrophysiological changes in the heart in situ of the rabbit, guinea-pig, dog and cat. *J Mol Cell Cardiol* 1989;21:545–554.
31. Udvary É, Végh Á, Szekeres L. 7-oxo-PgI2-induced late appearing and long lasting antiischemic action in dogs. *Pharmacol Res Commun* 1989;20[Suppl 1]:171–172.
32. Corea L, Bentivoglio M, Verdecchia P, Matalese M. Plasma norepinephrine and left ventricular hypertrophy in hypertension. *Am J Cardiol* 1984;53:1299–1303.
33. Currie WR, Karmazyn M, Kloc M, Mailer K. Heat-shock response is associated with enhanced postischemic ventricular recovery. *Circ Res* 1988;63:543–549.
34. Mestril R, Dillmann WH. Heat shock and adaptive response to ischemia. *Trends Cardiovasc Res* 1991;1:240–244.

35. Yellon DM, Pasini E, Ferrari R, Downey JM, Latchman DS. Whole body heat stress protects the isolated perfused rabbit heart. *Circulation* 1990;82[Suppl 3]:463.
36. Schott RJ, Nao B, Strieter R, Groh M, Kunkel S, McClanahan T, Schaper W, Gallagher K. Heat shock does not precondition canine myocardium. *Circulation* 1990;82[Suppl 3]:464.
37. Thornton J, Striplin S, Liu GS, Swafford A, Stanley AWH, Van Winkle DM, Downey JM. Inhibition of protein synthesis does not block myocardial protection afforded by preconditioning. *Am J Physiol* 1990;259 [Supplement: Heart Circulation and Physiology, Vol 28]H1822–H1825.
38. Boheler KR, Schwartz K. Gene expression in cardiac hypertrophy. *Trends Cardiovasc Med* 1992; 2:176–182.

The Cardiomyopathic Heart, edited by Makoto
Nagano, Nobuakira Takeda, and Naranjan S.
Dhalla. Raven Press, Ltd., New York © 1994.

25

Vinculin-Containing Costameres: Parts of Contraction Forces Transmitting Sites of Cardiomyocytes

Kyoko Imanaka-Yoshida, *Barbara A. Danowski, *Jean M. Sanger
and *Joseph W. Sanger

*The First Department of Internal Medicine, Mie University School of Medicine,
Tsu, Mie 514 Japan; and *Department of Anatomy, Pennsylvania Muscle Institute,
School of Medicine, University of Pennsylvania, Philadelphia, Pennsylvania 19104, USA.*

INTRODUCTION

The heart is a biologic pump primarily composed of cardiomyocytes and connective tissue. Collagen fibers are the major component of the connective tissue. They form a continuous hierarchical network, extending from pericardium to endomysium, surrounding individual cardiomyocytes, so that they coordinate the delivery of the contraction forces of myocytes to the whole ventricular chamber (1). How, then, are the contraction forces of myofibrils inside the cells transmitted to connective tissue? Are there any special sites of communication of myocytes with extracellular matrix? The earlier electron microscopic data, as well as more recent antibody studies, have identified vinculin-rich submembranous ribs called costameres, which have been proposed to play a role in anchoring the Z lines to the cell membrane (2–4) and transmitting contraction forces from myofibrils to the extracellular substrates (5,6); however, direct functional evidence for this linkage has been lacking.

In this study, we examined the relationship between costameres and the transmission of contraction force of cultured cardiomyoctyes using the flexible silicone rubber substratum technique, developed by Harris and colleagues (7,8). This silicone rubber substratum is thin, optically clear, and easily deformable. Thus, contraction forces of individual cells, transmitted to the substratum through cell-substratum adhesions, result in the formation of wrinkles in the silicone rubber sheet (8). Adult rat cardiomyocytes grown on the flexible silicone rubber substratum were microinjected with either fluorescently labeled α-actinin or vinculin. We then compared the pattern of substratum wrinkles generated by these cells during contraction with the

245

locations of both the Z lines of the myofibrils and the costameres. Our observations revealed that contraction forces are exerted on the substratum through the costameres.

MATERIALS AND METHOD

Cell Culture

Cells were obtained from the hearts of male rats weighing 200 to 225 g (Wistar, VAF/ + ; Charles River, Wilmington, MA) using the process of retrograde perfusion with collagenase, as previously published (9). The cardiomyocytes were cultured onto either glass-bottomed dishes (MatTek Corporation, Ashland, MA) covered with 20 μg of laminin (Gibco-BRL, Gaithersburg, MD), or silicone rubber substrata that had previously been exposed to a drop of laminin (20 μg).

Silicone Rubber Substrata

Flexible rubber substrata were prepared as follows (10): a thin layer of silicone fluid, (poly [dimethyl siloxane], 30,000 cP, Dow Corning, Midland, MI) was spread onto the bottom of glass-bottomed dishes. The dish was then placed upside down over the flame of a Bunsen burner for approximately 1 second. This process polymerizes the uppermost layer of the silicone fluid covering the bottom of the culture dish. The flexible rubber substrata remains stable for many days.

Preparation of Fluorescent Probes and Microinjection

Alpha-actinin and vinculin were prepared from frozen chicken gizzards (11) and labeled with iodacetamidotetramethyl rhodamine (IATR) (Molecular Probes, Eugene, OR), or rhodamine, succinimidyl ester (SR) (Molecular Probes, Eugene, OR), respectively (12). Microinjection of the labeled proteins into living cells was accomplished using high-pressure techniques, as previously described (13).

Microscopy and Image Processing

Interference Reflection Microscopy (IRM). Contacts between a cell and the substratum were detected in living cells and fixed cells, using a Nikon Diaphot inverted microscope with a filter cube containing a half-silvered mirror (Omego Optics, Brattleboro, VT). The image produced indicated the distances between the cells' ventral surfaces and the substratum: very dark or black areas indicated distances of approximately 10 to 15 nm, gray areas indicated distances of approximately 30 nm, and light or white areas indicated distances of 100 nm or more (14,15).

Image Acquisition and Processing. Sequences of cells containing fluorescently labeled, injected proteins were recorded onto ¾-inch videotape using a Dage SIT camera. Subsequently, images were summed and processed using the Image 1 image processing program (Universal Imaging, West Chester, PA).

Immunofluorescence

Monoclonal antibody to vinculin was purchased from Sigma (St. Louis, MO). Cells were washed with phosphate-buffered saline (PBS) and fixed for 3 minutes in 4% paraformaldehyde plus 0.1% Triton X-100 in PIPES-buffered saline (10 mM of PIPES, 150 nM of NaCl, pH of 7.2). All subsequent washing steps were done with PIPES-buffered saline plus 0.1% Triton. The cells were permeabilized in 0.5% Triton X-100 for 5 minutes, rinsed several times with the saline solution, and then incubated with antivinculin antibody for 2 hours at room temperature. After extensive washing to remove any unbound primary antibodies, the cells were incubated for 1 hour in DTAF-goat-anti-mouse IgG (Jackson Immunologicals, West Grove, PA), and rinsed with the saline solution. The coverslips were then dipped in distilled water before mounting in a drop of MOWIOL (Calbiochem, La Jolla, CA).

RESULTS

Heart cells isolated from adult rats were plated onto the prepared silicone rubber substrata and were examined daily to determine the extent of spreading of the cells and the initiation of the deformation of the substratum. Most of the cardiomyocytes were well spread and beating after 7 to 10 days. We observed some cells forming pleatlike wrinkles of silicone rubber substratum during contraction (Fig. 1b). These deformations appeared as evenly and closely spaced pleats underneath the cell during contraction and disappeared under relaxation. The spacings between the pleatlike wrinkles were between 1.8 and 2.0 μm, identical to the measured spacing between Z lines of sarcomeres. Thus, these observations suggested that wrinkles were formed between adjacent Z lines of contracting myofibrils. In order to test this, we microinjected fluorescently labeled α-actinin (IATR-α-actinin) into cells growing on silicone rubber substrata. Fluorescently labeled α-actinin is incorporated rapidly into existing Z lines of cardiac and skeletal muscle cells (12,16). Images of the same injected cell were recorded using phase contrast and fluorescence microscopy. By alternating between phase and fluorescence optics, we directly compared the positions of the Z lines and the substratum wrinkles (Fig. 1a,b). An enlarged area of the cell depicted in Figure 1 is illustrated in Figure 2. The paired lines or calipers observed in the figures are a feature of the Image 1 Image Processing software that allows a marked distance on one digitally stored image to be superimposed at the same coordinates on a second digitally stored image. The calipers were adjusted by aligning them with α-actinin-positive Z lines on the fluo-

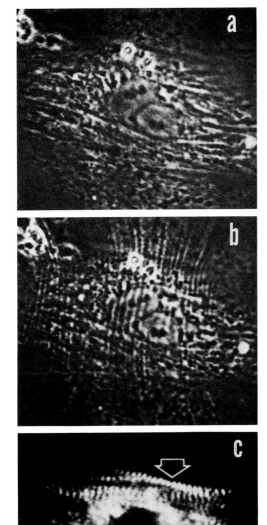

FIG. 1. A live cardiomyocyte cultured for 8 days on silicone rubber substratum. Closely spaced, pleatlike wrinkles appear during contraction **(b)** and disappear during relaxation **(a)**. Fluorescently labeled α-actinin was microinjected into live cells and imaged with a low-light-level (SIT) camera **(c)**. Scale bar = 10 μ. (Reproduced with copyright permission of Rockefeller University Press, ref. 34.)

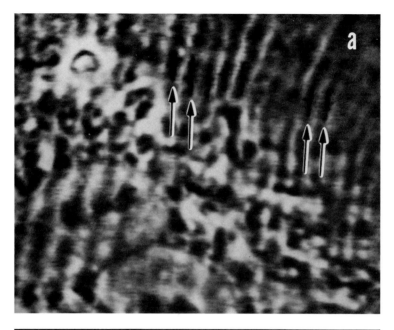

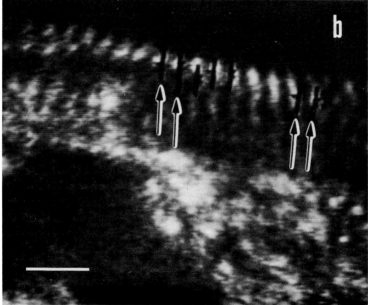

FIG. 2. Enlarged images of the area indicated by the arrow in Figure 1c. Calipers (indicated by arrows) were adjusted by measuring distances between α-actinin positive Z lines (**b**) and then overlaid onto the phase contrast image of the cell and wrinkles (**a**). Scale bar = 10 μ. (Reproduced with copyright permission of Rockefeller University Press, ref. 34.)

rescent image (Fig. 2b). The resulting overlay of the calipers on the phase contrast image is shown in Figure 2a, indicating that the wrinkles form between adjacent Z lines.

In order to examine the relationship between substratum wrinkles and vinculin localization, we microinjected SR-labeled vinculin into contracting cardiomyocytes cultured on the flexible substrata. The distribution of injected vinculin varied considerably from cell to cell. We found that some cells formed pleatlike wrinkles in which vinculin had a costameric distribution, as defined by Pardo and colleagues (2,3); that is, they were aligned in bands at Z lines (Fig. 3a,b). In some cells, vinculin did not appear to have a costameric distribution, but it localized instead to small streaks, similar in appearance to the adhesion plaques of nonmuscle cells. In addition, there were some instances in which cells showed a costameric distribution of vinculin but did not produce pleatlike wrinkles. However, no cells that were found that produced pleatlike wrinkles that did not have costameric vinculin distribution. Therefore, it appears that the ability to generate pleatlike wrinkles upon contraction is correlated with the presence of costameres.

To ascertain whether costameres are sites of cell-substratum adhesion, we used IRM. Cells that had been grown on laminin-coated glass coverslips were fixed and stained with an antivinculin antibody, and were examined using both fluorescence and IRM optics. Although the staining pattern varied according to the distribution of injected vinculin, we found some instances in which the costameres colocalized with dark bands in the IRM image (Fig. 4). Cells that possessed vinculin-positive costameres but lacked a corresponding pattern of close contacts were also observed. However, it should be noted that the number of cells containing both a costameric distribution of vinculin and a corresponding IRM image of close contacts increased with time in culture.

DISCUSSION

Costameres are vinculin-containing, electron-dense plaques that exist between the cell membrane and Z lines of skeletal and cardiac muscles (2–4). These are thought to link myofibrils to the cell membrane (2–4). Vinculin is a major component of adhesion plaques in many cultured cells (17,18). Adhesion plaques, also known as focal adhesions or focal contacts (19), are usually located at the termini of actin-containing stress fibers, and are also the sites where the cells' contractile forces are transmitted to their substratum (19). In recent years, it has become apparent that costameres have many characteristics common to adhesion plaques. Both of them are membrane-associated plaques and are enriched not only in vinculin, but in talin (19–21) and integrins (19,22). These similarities have suggested that costameres are also sites where forces are transmitted to the substratum, like adhesion plaques. Using electron microscopy, Street demonstrated that some contraction forces of frog sartorius muscle are transmitted laterally across the muscle fiber (6). On the other hand, it has been shown that intercellular collagen struts terminate on

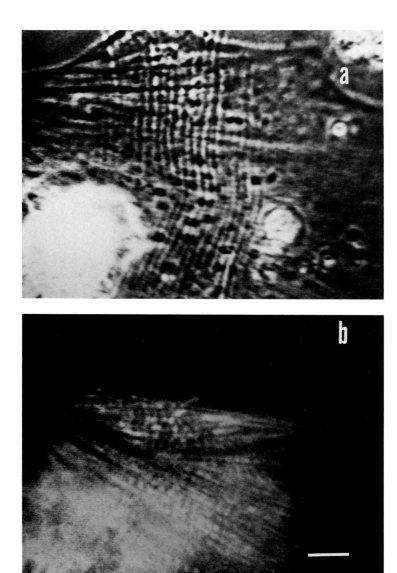

FIG. 3. A contracting cardiomyocyte cultured for 10 days and microinjected with rhodamine-labeled vinculin. Phase contrast (**a**) and fluorescent (**b**) images of the same area. Pleatlike wrinkles of silicone rubber substratum (a) are associated with costamere, a periodic distribution (b). Scale bar = 10 μ. (Reproduced with copyright permission of Rockefeller University Press, ref. 34.)

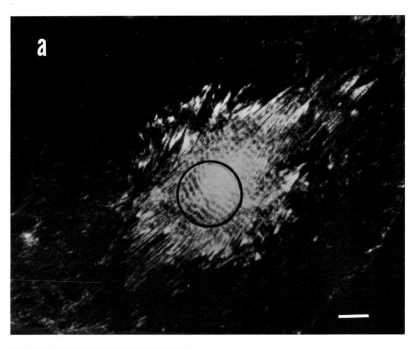

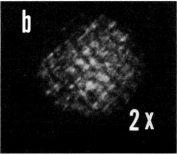

FIG. 4. **a**: Cardiomyocytes were fixed and stained with antivinculin antibody. **b**: The enlarged IRM image of the encircled area of Figure 4a. Banded dark close contacts, colocalizing with costameres, are clearly shown. Scale bar = 10 μ. (Reproduced with copyright permission of Rockefeller University Press, ref. 34.)

the surface of myocytes just lateral to Z lines of myofibrils (23). This unique association and the configurational changes of the struts observed in various contracted states (23) have also supported the idea that costameres are sites of force transmission. Using the flexible silicone rubber technique (7,8) and microinjection of fluorescently labeled cytoskeletal proteins, we have found that: (a) pleatlike wrinkles form in the flexible substratum between adjacent Z lines as the cells beat; (b) the presence of pleatlike wrinkles is always associated with a periodic distribution of vinculin, costameres; and (c) the cells develop a banded pattern of dark focal con-

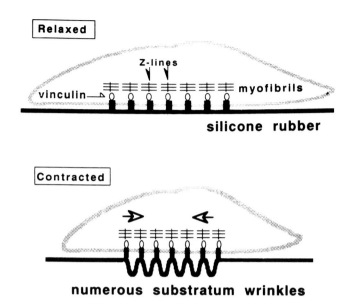

FIG. 5. Diagram showing the authors' hypothesis of the force-transmitting mechanism of cardiomyocytes. Individual Z lines are anchored to silicone rubber by the attachment complexes, which include vinculin (*top*). When the myofibrils contract (*bottom*), the forces are transmitted through the attachment complexes and cause pleatlike wrinkles.

tacts (as determined by IRM) that correspond to costameres. These results show that Z lines are linked not only to sarcolemma, but also to extracellular matrix, by costameres, and that contraction forces are transmitted through these sites (Fig. 5). Furthermore, the findings that all cells with costamere-distributed vinculin do not cause pleatlike wrinkles suggest vinculin localization alone is not sufficient for effective force transmission to the extracellular matrix. This invites the speculation that costameres function as "attachment complexes," composed not only of vinculin, but also of α-actinin, talin, integrin, and probably other as yet unidentified proteins. In addition, other proteins, which are usually not present at adhesion plaques, such as spectrin (24,25), clathrin (26), intermediate filament proteins (24,27), and dystrophin (28), have also been found at costameres. It is known that they are involved with membrane-cytoskeletel interactions (29,30), although the precise roles of each protein at costameres, or their interaction, are unclear. However, they might be also involved in forming the attachment complex, or costamere.

The results presented here suggest that costamere complex could prevent cardiomyocytes from slippage during contraction, allowing the heart to work effectively as one pump. Thus these linkages could be important determinants of the efficiency of cardiac contractions or myocardial stiffness. It is known that the defects in dystrophin or alterations in dystrophin isoforms may contribute to specific cardiomyopathy (30–32). Similarly, deficiency or mutation of other proteins composing the costamere complex might produce some sorts of cardiomyopathies. Future studies of these attachment complexes will provide a new approach to analyzing various heart diseases.

SUMMARY

A technique using an easily deformable flexible silicone rubber is useful for observing contraction forces of cultured cells. When adult rat cardiomyocytes are cultured on the silicone rubber substratum, they form a series of fine pleatlike wrinkles of the substratum in response to beating. How do the wrinkles relate to myofibrils and the distribution of the adhesion plaque protein vinculin? In order to answer this question, we microinjected fluorescently labeled α-actinin and vinculin to visualize Z lines and costameres, respectively. The periodicity of the wrinkles were coincident with the spacing of the Z lines, as determined by the localization of fluorescent α-actinin. A costamere, a banded pattern of vinculin that colocalizes with Z lines, was detected in the area where pleatlike wrinkles formed. Interference reflection microscopic images of the cells showed banded dark close contacts corresponding to costameres. These results indicate that myofibrils are linked to substratum at Z lines by costameres containing vinculin, and that contraction forces can also be transmitted to extracellular matrix through costameres.

ACKNOWLEDGMENTS

This work was supported by the National Institutes of Health (HL-15835 to the Pennsylvania Muscle Institute) and the National Science Foundation (DCB 90-08704 to Dr. J. M. Sanger). Dr. B. A. Danowski was supported on an NIH postdoctoral training grant (HL-07499 to Dr. J. W. Sanger), and was the recipient of an NIH Individual Postdoctoral Fellowship (GM-14142).

REFERENCES

1. Katz AM. Cardiac interstitium in health and disease: the fibrillar collagen network. *J Am Coll Cardiol* 1989;13:1657–1662.
2. Pardo JV, Siciliano JD, Craig SW. A vinculin-containing cortical lattice in skeletal muscle: transverse lattice elements ("costameres") mark sites of attachment between myofibrils and sarcolemma. *Proc Natl Acad Sci USA* 1983;80:1008–1012.
3. Pardo JV, Siciliano JD, Craig SW. Vinculin is a component of an extensive network of myofibril-sarcolemma attachment regions in cardiac muscle fibers. *J Cell Biol* 1983;97:1081–1088.
4. Koteliansky VE, Gneushev GN. Vinculin localization in cardiac muscle. *FEBS Lett* 1983;159:158–160.
5. Shear CR, Bloch RJ. Vinculin in subsarcolemmal densities in chicken skeletal muscle: localization and relationship to intracellular and extracellular structures. *J Cell Biol* 1985;101:240–256.
6. Street SF. Lateral transmission of tension in frog myofibers: a myofibrillar network and transverse cytoskeletal connections are possible transmitters. *J Cell Physiol* 1983;114:346–364.
7. Harris AK, Wild P, Stopak D. Silicone rubber substrata: a new wrinkle in the study of cell locomotion. *Science* 1980;208:177–179.

8. Harris AK. Stopak D, Wild P. Fibroblast traction as a mechanism for collagen morphogenesis. *Nature* 1981;290:249–251.

9. LoRusso SM, Imanaka-Yoshida K, Shuman H, Sanger JM, Sanger JW. Incorporation of fluorescently-labeled contractile proteins into freshly isolated living adult cardiac myocytes. *Cell Mot Cytoskel* 1992;21:111–122.

10. Harris AK. Fibroblasts and myofibroblasts. *Methods Enzymol* 1988;163:623–642.

11. Feramisco JR, Burridge K. A rapid purification of α-actinin, filamin, and a 130,000-dalton protein from smooth muscle. *J Biol Chem* 1980;255:1194–1199.

12. Sanger JM, Mittal B, Pochapin M, Sanger JW. Myofibrillogenesis in living cells microinjected with fluorescently labeled alpha-actinin. *J Cell Biol* 1986;102:2053–2066.

13. Sanger JM, Pochapin M, Sanger JW. Midbody sealing after cytokinesis in embryos of the sea urchin *Arabacia punctulata*. *Cell Tiss Res* 1985;240:287–292.

14. Izzard CS, Lochner LR. Formation of cell-to-substrate contacts during fibroblast motility: an interference reflexion study. *J Cell Sci* 1980;42:81–116.

15. Gingell D, Todd I. Interference reflection microscopy: A quantitative theory for image interpretation and its application to cell-substratum separation measurement. *Biophys J* 1979;26:507–526.

16. Sanger JW, Mittal B, Sanger JM. Formation of myofibrils in spreading chick cardiac myocytes. *Cell Mot Cytoskel* 1984;4:405–416.

17. Geiger B. A 130K protein from chicken gizzard: its localization at the termini of microfilament bundles in cultured chicken cells. *Cell* 1979;18:193–205.

18. Geiger B, Tokuyasu KT, Dutton AH, Singer SJ. Vinculin, an intracellular protein localized at specialized sites where microfilament bundles terminate at cell membranes. *Proc Natl Acad Sci USA* 1980;77:4127–4131.

19. Burridge K, Fath K, Kelly T, Nuckolls G, Turner C. Focal adhesions: transmembrane junctions between the extracellular matrix and the cytoskeleton. *Ann Rev Cell Biol* 1988;4:487–525.

20. Belkin AM, Koteliansky VE, Zhidkova NI. Localization of talin in skeletal and cardiac muscles. *FEBS Lett* 1986;200:32–36.

21. Terracio L, Gullberg D. Rubin K, Craig S, Borg TK. Expression of collagen adhesion proteins and their association with the cytoskeleton in cardiac myocytes. *Anat Rec* 1989;223:62–71.

22. Terracio L, Rubin K, Gullberg D, Balog E, Carver W, Jyring R, Borg TK. Expression of collagen-binding integrins during cardiac development and hypertrophy. *Circul Res* 1991;68:734–744.

23. Robinson TF, Factor SM, Capasso JM, Wittenberg BA, Blumenfeld OO, Seifter S. Morphology, composition and function of struts between cardiac myocytes of rat and hamster. *Cell Tissue Res* 1987;249:247–255.

24. Craig SW, Pardo JV. Gamma actin, spectrin, and intermediate filament proteins colocalize with vinculin at costameres, myofibril-to-sarcolemma attachment sites. *Cell Motil* 1983;3:449–462.

25. Messina DA, Lamanski LF. Immunocytochemical studies of spectrin in hamster cardiac tissue. *Cell Mot Cytoskel* 1989;12:139–141.

26. Kaufman SF, Bielser D, Foster RF. Localization of anti-clathrin antibody in the sarcomere and sensitivity of myofibril structure to chloroquine suggest a role for clathrin in myofibril assembly. *Exp Cell Res* 1990;191:227–238.

27. Granger BL, Lazarides E. The existence of an insoluble Z-disc scaffold in chicken skeletal muscle. *Cell* 1978;15:1253–1268.

28. Porter GA, Dmytrenko M, Winkelmann JC, Bloch RJ. Dystrophin colocalizes with β-spectrin in distinct subsarcolemmal domains in mammalian skeletal muscle. *J Cell Biol* 1992;117:997–1005.

29. Bennett V. Spectrin-based membrane skeleton: a multipotential adaptor between the plasma membrane and the cytoplasm. *Physiol Rev* 1990;70(4):1029–1065.

30. Brodsky FM. Living with clathrin: its role in intracellular membrane traffic. *Science* 1988; 242:1396–1402.

31. Koenig M, Monaco AP, Kunkel LM. The complete sequence of dystrophin predicts a rod-shaped cytoskeletal protein. *Cell* 1988;53:219–228.

32. Bies RD, Chamberlain JS, Cartez MD, Roberts R, Caskey CT. Dystrophin expression in diaphragm and cardiac purkinje fibers: evidence that alternative spliced isoforms are involved in disease. *J Cell Biochem* 1991[Suppl 15C]:187.

33. Towbin JA, Brink P, Gelb B, Zhu XM, Chamberlain JS, McCabe ERB, Swift M. X-linked cardiomyopathy: muscular genetic evidence of linkage to the Duchenne muscular dystrophy locus. *J Cell Biochem* 1991[Suppl 15C]:165.

34. Danowski BA, Imanaka-Yoshida K, Sanger JM, Sanger JW. Costameres are sites of force transmission to the substratum in adult rat cardiomyocytes. *J Cell Biol* 1992;118:1411–1420.

The Cardiomyopathic Heart, edited by Makoto
Nagano, Nobuakira Takeda, and Naranjan S.
Dhalla. Raven Press, Ltd., New York © 1994.

26

Metabolically Deranged Cardiomyopathy of the Trauma-Sepsis Syndrome

Heinz Rupp, *Ursula Müller, and *Karl Werdan

Institute of Physiology II, University of Tübingen, D-7400 Tübingen, Germany;
*Department of Medicine I, Klinikum Grosshadern, University of München,
D-8000 München, Germany

INTRODUCTION

Despite the development of new classes of antibiotics, the mortality from sepsis and septic shock remains as high as 20% to 60% and has not been reduced within the last several decades. During the trauma-sepsis syndrome, the integrity of the organism deteriorates, leading to multiple organ failure. Until recently, it was thought that the heart was affected little during multiple organ failure. However, it appears that even if the cardiac output is increased during initial stages of the trauma-sepsis syndrome, the myocardial performance is depressed (1,2). Because the myocardial dysfunction occurs as a result of systemic disease, it is referred to as secondary cardiomyopathy. Although most patients exhibiting multiple organ failure have bacterial infections, other disease states can also induce the typical sepsis response of macrophages, monocytes, and granulocytes. Because sepsis mediators and cardiodepressive factors act in conjunction with a markedly perturbed neuroendocrine status of the body, the specific role of the individual factors is difficult to assess in animal experiments. In this overview, we attempt to examine the role of various sepsis mediators using cell culture experiments. Emphasis is placed on data with relevance to the pathogenesis of septic cardiomyopathy.

CARDIOVASCULAR FUNCTION DURING THE TRAUMA-SEPSIS SYNDROME

It remains an intriguing clinical finding that the function of the cardiovascular system becomes rapidly impaired during the trauma-sepsis syndrome. Of major pathogenetic importance is the peripheral vasodilation that results in a reduction of peripheral resistance of up to 30% (3). The vasodilation cannot be attributed to fever (Fig. 1), but arises from vascular degeneration and interstitial edema (4). Vascular

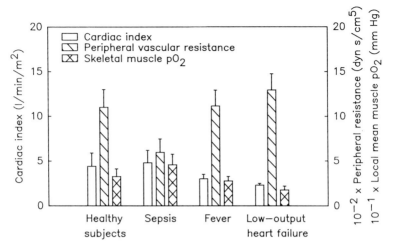

FIG. 1. Cardiovascular parameters and skeletal muscle partial oxygen pressure (pO_2) in intensive care patients with sepsis (meeting at least five of the nine criteria for sepsis), with fever without sepsis (meeting less than five criteria for sepsis), or with low-output heart failure. The healthy subjects were nonsmoking volunteers. (Data adapted from Boekstegers and Werdan, ref. 3.)

responsiveness to α-adrenergic agonists, angiotensin, and calcium entry blockers is depressed, rendering pharmacologic vasoconstrictive interventions inefficient (4). In an adaptive response, the cardiac output of the intact heart should increase by a factor of 2 to 3; however, this is not the case in septic cardiomyopathy owing to myocardial depression (see Fig. 1). Accompanying impaired myocardial function are reduced ejection fraction and an increased end diastolic pressure. Although the peripheral oxygen supply is increased, as can be deduced from the tissue oxygen partial pressure of skeletal muscle (see Fig. 1), an energy deficit exists in various organs owing to disturbances in oxygen diffusion and utilization. Thus, the impaired cardiac performance associated with inadequate rise of cardiac output might have detrimental consequences for the oxidative metabolism of peripheral organs. Although the causes of the depressed myocardial performance are multifactorial, coronary hypoperfusion does not play a role (5). It appears, however, that alterations in cardiac metabolism are of great relevance.

GENERAL METABOLIC STATUS OF THE BODY DURING THE TRAUMA-SEPSIS SYNDROME

The primary cause of the detrimental effects of the trauma-sepsis syndrome arising from various toxins (Table 1) is seen in the liberation of sepsis mediators from the macrophage-monocyte cell lines and granulocytes (Table 2). Although these cytokines have various actions (see Table 2), the present discussion will be limited

TABLE 1. *Effect of bacterial and fungal toxins on cardiac contractility*

Toxin	Origin	Intact heart	Myocyte pulsation amplitude	Myocyte beating rate
Endotoxin (6–8)	Escherichia coli, Pseudomonas aeruginosa	(−)	100 μg/mL: (±)	100 μg/mL: (±)
Exotoxin A (7,9–11)	P. aeruginosa	(−)	0.1 μg/mL: (−)	0.1 μg/mL: (−)
Streptolysin O (12,13)	Streptococcus pyogenes	(−)	1 μg/mL: (−)	0.01 μg/mL: (−)
Staphylococcal α toxin (14,15)	Staphylococcus aureus	(−)	100 μg/mL: (−)	100 μg/mL: (−)
T-2 toxin (16)	Fusarium fungi	(−)	500 μg/mL: (−)	500 μg/mL: (−)

The concentrations represent the lowest values required for observing significant effects. (−), depressive action; (±), no significant effect. (For a detailed discussion, see Werdan et al., ref. 2.)

to their metabolic effects. In addition to the sepsis mediators, blood catecholamine, glucagon, and cortisol concentrations are increased (28). This neuroendocrine imbalance results in various metabolic disturbances. Thus, interleukin-1 (IL-1) stimulates proteolysis (29), which is further potentiated by the effect of the increased glucagon and cortisol levels (28). The ensuing protein catabolism affects not only skeletal muscle, particularly endangering the respiratory system, but would be expected to influence heart muscle as well. The increased amino acids are used for protein synthesis of so-called acute phase and shock proteins (Table 2) and for gluconeogenesis (28). The increased blood glucose level provides the fuel for glu-

TABLE 2. *Effect of sepsis mediators on cardiac contractility*

	Main action	Intact heart	Myocyte pulsation amplitude	Myocyte beating rate
TNF$_\alpha$ (2,17–19)	Stress proteins (+), adenylyl cyclase (−)/(+)	(−)	5 ng/mL: (−)	5 ng/mL: (−)
IL-1,2 (18,20)	Adenylyl cyclase (−), 30-kD stress protein (+)	(±)	1,000 U/mL: (±)	1,000 U/mL: (−)
Interferon τ (21,22)	Histocompatibility complex	(−)	(?)	(?)
Complement (23,24)	Altered permeability Lysis	(?)	40 μg/mL: (+) 350 μg/mL: (−)	40 μg/mL: (+) 350 μg/mL: (−)
PAF (25–27)	Phosphoinositol pathway (+) I_{K1} current (−)	(−)	1 nM PAF: (−)	1 nM PAF: (+)

IL, interleukin; complement, membrane attack complex C5b-9; PAF, platelet activating factor. The concentrations represent the lowest values required for observing significant effects. (−), depressive action; (+), stimulatory action; (±), no significant effect. (For a detailed discussion, see Werdan et al., ref. 2.)

cose-dependent cells. Glucose uptake by the major glucose-utilizing organ of the body, the skeletal muscle, becomes gradually depressed during sepsis, however. The main cause is the reduced activity of the pyruvate dehydrogenase (PDH) complex, which has a key role in the regulation of the glycolytic flux (30). Noteworthy is the fact that skeletal muscle PDH is affected already during mild sepsis, whereas hepatic PDH is depressed maximally only during severe sepsis (31). Although data on cardiac PDH are currently not available, it seems most likely that, as in skeletal muscle, it is reduced. Because the blood insulin levels are normal (or even increased) and the insulin receptor appears not to be impaired (28), the hyperglycemia has to be caused by postreceptor defects. The reduced pyruvate oxidation of skeletal muscle results in an increased release of pyruvate and lactate, which are primarily used in the liver for gluconeogenesis (28). The increased lipolysis during the trauma-sepsis syndrome arises most probably from high blood levels of catecholamines, cortisol, and glucagon (32). Tumor necrosis factor alpha (TNF$_\alpha$) contributes to the increased triglyceride levels via inhibition of endothelial lipoprotein lipase (33). Taken together, the metabolic status of the body during the trauma-sepsis syndrome mimicks, in various aspects, a state typically observed during severe starvation or insulin-dependent diabetes mellitus; it is aggravated, however, by the specific action of various cytokines.

CARDIAC METABOLISM DURING THE TRAUMA-SEPSIS SYNDROME

The general catabolic effects of trauma-sepsis would also be expected to affect heart muscle in an unfavorable manner. Of particular importance would be a reduction in PDH activity, which would reduce glucose oxidation and result in an increased fatty acid oxidation. Additional citrate would be formed, which is transformed into malonyl-coenzyme A (CoA) in the cytoplasm. By this mechanism, the carnitine palmitoyl transferase-1 activity is reduced and the mitochondrial long-chain fatty acid uptake is adjusted to the functional demands (Fig. 2). The metabolic regulation of the septic heart appears, however, to be more complex, because the uptake of fatty acids and glucose has been found to be markedly diminished, whereas the lactate uptake is increased (34). Furthermore, about 35% to 55% of oxygen uptake could not be accounted for by exogenous substrates (34). Because the relationship between myocardial oxygen consumption and myocardial work is not altered, a normal myocardial oxidative phosphorylation can be inferred (34). One could assume, then, that, in septic shock, the heart depends to a great extent on endogenous energy sources and that perhaps the depletion of energy reserves might underlie the progressive cardiac depression that occurs (34). However, the currently available data suggest normal (35) or even elevated (36) adenosine triphosphate (ATP) levels in the septic heart, demonstrating that energy depletion represents a late process. As regards the endogenous substrate reserves that could be utilized by the heart, one has to take into account the fact that glycogen stores are depleted much earlier than lipid stores, and the heart would thus be expected to depend

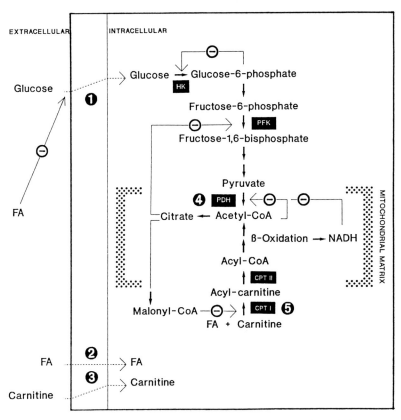

FIG. 2. Currently suspected major abnormalities in cardiac metabolism during the trauma-sepsis syndrome. **Point 1.** Impaired glucose uptake. **Point 2.** Impaired fatty acid uptake. **Point 3.** Impaired carnitine uptake. **Point 4.** Reduced PDH activity. **Point 5.** Reduced CPT-1 activity. (Note: This list is not considered to be complete. In particular, additional substrates typical of the trauma-sepsis syndrome, such as glutamine, have not been taken into account.) *HK*, hexokinase; *PFK*, phosphofructokinase; *PDH*, pyruvate dehydrogenase complex; *CPT*, carnitine palmitoyl transferase; *FA*, nonesterified free fatty acids; *CoA*, coenzyme A; *NADH*, nicotinamide-adenine dinucleotide.

primarily on fatty acid oxidation. Thus, the energy status of the heart muscle would be altered in a manner similar to that observed in severe diabetes mellitus. Because there is increasing evidence that glucose oxidation and the formation of glycolytic ATP are essential for the maintenance of various subcellular processes (37), the metabolic status of heart muscle during sepsis is unfavorable. Little is known about the mechanisms that result in the deranged cardiac metabolism (see Fig. 2). Thus, the question arises why both fatty acid uptake and glucose uptake are reduced in septic shock. The finding that TNF$_\alpha$ inhibits endothelial lipoprotein lipase (33) only partially accounts for the reduced fatty acid uptake. With respect to glucose utilization, various inconsistencies remain. One of the missing links is the activity of glucose transporters as it relates to the PDH activity. Particularly intriguing is the finding of an increased lactate utilization in conjunction with a possibly reduced PDH activity.

Taken together, it appears that a major problem of heart muscle during the trauma-sepsis syndrome relates to the imbalance of substrate utilization. Currently, the importance of substrate utilization is best documented for diabetic cardiomyopathy (38), wherein glucose oxidation is greatly depressed and the mechanical performance is impaired (39). Although it is not clear to what extent glucose utilization is impaired in the septic heart, it is not unexpected that the heart fails to maintain a high cardiac output during the trauma-sepsis syndrome.

A further aspect of the deranged cardiac metabolism relates to the recent findings that subcellular organelles are affected by a shift in cardiac fuel utilization (40–44). For example, myosin heavy chain expression is shifted in the diabetic heart, favoring myosin V3 of a low myofibrillar adenosine triphosphatase (ATPase) activity. Furthermore, the rate of sarcoplasmic reticulum Ca^{2+} uptake is reduced. Although such studies have not been conducted for the heart during the trauma-sepsis syndrome, it appears most likely that functionally comparable alterations occur in subcellular organelles. This contention would be supported by the finding that myofibrillar ATPase was reduced in the hearts of rabbits infected with *Streptococcus viridans* (45,46). Furthermore, sarcolemmal Na^+,K^+-ATPase and sarcolemmal Ca^{2+}-binding were reduced (45,46). The finding that heart rate and body temperature were increased (46) indicates that a generalized sepsis occurred and that the changes in heart muscle might not arise solely from the observed endocarditis. In this respect, is should also be mentioned that the function of subcellular organelles is critically influenced by thyroid hormones. In the trauma-sepsis syndrome, low serum triiodothyronine (T_3) and FT_3 concentrations have been observed (47). A reduced thyroid influence is expected to slow down myocardial performance, producing, for example, a reduced expression of the sarcoplasmic reticulum Ca^{2+}-pump ATPase and the Ca^{2+}-release channel (48). Thus, such a slow-type heart would not be well adapted for the high heart rates required in the trauma-sepsis syndrome.

PROTEIN SYNTHESIS INHIBITING TOXINS
AND THE TRAUMA-SEPSIS SYNDROME

Although during the trauma-sepsis syndrome, the protein catabolism is enhanced, the situation is aggravated in septic states in which protein synthesis is inhibited by toxins. The best characterized example is Pseudomonas exotoxin A, which inhibits protein synthesis via adenosine diphosphate (ADP) ribosylation of elongation factor 2 (10). Because proteolysis is already enhanced, inhibition of protein synthesis represents an additional detrimental factor for heart muscle. To discern the various direct and indirect actions of cytokines, they can be examined in cultured heart muscle cells. In analogy to the contractility of intact hearts, the pulsation amplitude and the beating rate can be determined (49,50). As shown in Table 2, the cytokines differ greatly with respect to the concentration required for inducing a depressed mechanical activity. The cultured heart muscle cells also provide the opportunity of deciding whether a certain toxin has direct effects or whether it acts via the release of sepsis mediators (see Table 1). In the case of exotoxin A, the protein synthesis of cultured neonatal heart muscle cells was inhibited half-maximally by 10 ng/mL during a 24-hour incubation period (2). The consequences of protein synthesis inhibition have been studied in great detail with respect to the β-adrenoceptor/G protein/adenylyl cyclase axis (1,2,19,51; and Müller U, Pfeifer A, Rupp H, Hübner G, and Werdan K, *unpublished data*). As demonstrated in Figure 3, 1 ng/mL exotoxin A, which inhibits global protein synthesis by 20%, had no effect on the number of β_1-adrenoceptors within 2 to 3 days of culture, and it did not interfere with the β_1-adrenoceptor–dependent and β_1-adrenoceptor–independent stimulation of adenylyl cyclase. Also, the norepinephrine-induced downregulation of β_1-adrenoceptors that occurs independently of protein synthesis ("homologous desensitization") was not affected by exotoxin A (see Fig. 3). However, when heart muscle cells were cultured in the presence of norepinephrine and exotoxin A, the forskolin-stimulated adenylyl cyclase activity was not reduced ("heterologous desensitization") (see Fig. 3). The loss of heterologous desensitization arises from the inhibition of the $G_{i\alpha2}$ and $G_{i\alpha3}$ synthesis, which is increased owing to high norepinephrine levels (19,51).

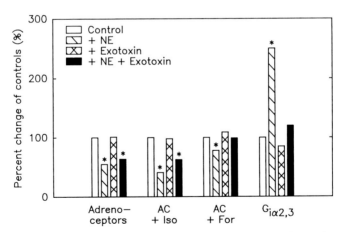

FIG. 3. Influence of *Pseudomonas* exotoxin A on the β_1-adrenoceptor/G protein/adenylyl cyclase axis. Neonatal rat heart muscle cells were cultured for 2 to 3 days in a synthetic medium (control) with the following additions: 1 μM of norepinephrine *(+NE)*, 1 ng/mL of exotoxin A *(+Exotoxin)*, 1 μM of norepinephrine and 1 ng/mL of exotoxin A *(+NE+Exotoxin)*. The following parameters were determined: β_1-adrenoceptor number, 100 μM isoproterenol-stimulated adenylyl cyclase activity *(AC+Iso)*, 100 μM forskolin-stimulated adenylyl cyclase activity *(AC +For)*, and the inhibitory $G_{i\alpha2,3}$ protein synthesis *($G_{i\alpha2,3}$)*. The statistical comparisons *(p<0.05)* refer to heart muscle cells cultured under control conditions. (Data adapted from Werdan et al., refs. 1 and 7; Reithmann et al., refs. 11 and 51; and Müller, Pfeifer, Rupp, Hübner, and Werdan, *unpublished data*.)

Thus, although exotoxin A does not prevent the desensitization secondary to β_1-adrenoceptor downregulation, it does reduce the extent of desensitization arising from the concomitant increase in $G_{i\alpha 2,3}$ proteins. Because of this loss of heterologous desensitization, isoproterenol-stimulated adenylyl cyclase is reduced by only about 35% (homologous desensitization) and not by about 60% (homologous plus heterologous desensitization). Thus, the response of the heart muscle cells to the high catecholamine challenge during the trauma-sepsis syndrome cannot be reduced very efficiently.

The inhibition of protein synthesis affects the β_1-adrenoceptor recovery at a time when blood catecholamine levels become normalized. Thus, in the absence of exotoxin A, β_1-adrenoceptors of the myocyte have been found to recover within 24 hours following the wash-out of norepinephrine. However, in the presence of exotoxin A, synthesis of β_1-adrenoceptors has not been observed, and the heart muscle cells have been found to remain refractory toward catecholamines (19,51). Noteworthy is the fact that this effect occurred even though global protein synthesis was inhibited by only 20%. Thus, it appears that exotoxin A interferes specifically with the synthesis of components involved in adrenergic signal transduction. Further evidence for the specific effects of exotoxin A is provided by studies involving myosin heavy chain expression. The expected increase in the proportion of V1 resulting from isoproterenol (50) was completely prevented by exotoxin A again at concentrations that only partially inhibit protein synthesis (Müller, Pfeifer, Rupp, Hübner, and Werdan, *unpublished data*). The important consequence is that specific derangements in the protein phenotype occur at rather low exotoxin titers, which would not be expected taking into account the effects on global protein synthesis. It should also be noted that the protein synthesis inhibition occurs in the intact organism under conditions favoring protein degradation.

NOVEL THERAPEUTIC REGIMENS DESIGNED TO TREAT THE DERANGED FUEL UTILIZATION

Because glucose intolerance provides a sensitive index for the mortality rate of patients with the trauma-sepsis syndrome (52), one could speculate that improved glucose utilization might prove to be beneficial to these patients. In view of the increasing evidence that signals derived from the glycolytic flux (39–44) affect gene transcription/protein translation, improved glucose utilization might be helpful in normalizing protein synthesis. Among various possibilities for increasing glucose utilization, it appears that an attractive approach could involve the activation of PDH or the inhibition of carnitine palmitoyl transferase-1 (53–55). Carnitine palmitoyl transferase-1 inhibition has been found to increase glucose utilization in insulin-dependent diabetes (56) and to normalize both the myosin heavy chain expression as well as the sarcoplasmic reticulum Ca^{2+}-stimulated ATPase activity (*unpublished data*). Clearly, further experimental work is required to assess the potentially beneficial actions of drugs that normalize fuel utilization in the trauma-sepsis syndrome. In view of the fact that currently available pharmacologic regimens do not efficiently reduce mortality from the trauma-sepsis syndrome, alternative avenues of treatment are needed.

SUMMARY

It is now well known that heart function is impaired in trauma-sepsis syndrome; however, the mechanisms for this are poorly understood. It is becoming evident that the detrimental effects of trauma-sepsis on heart function are mediated through the release of sepsis mediators from the macrophage-monocytes and granulocytes, as well as through neuroendocrine imbalance. A shift occurs in myocardial metabolism, particularly with respect to substrate utilization in trauma-sepsis. In addition, myocardial protein synthesis is inhibited and protein degradation is enhanced. Improvement of glucose utilization, either by the activation of pyruvate dehydrogenase or by inhibition of carnitine palmitoyl transferase, has been suggested to produce beneficial effects on the trauma-sepsis heart dysfunction.

REFERENCES

1. Werdan K, Müller U, Reithmann C, Pfeifer A, Hallström S, Koidl B, Schlag G. Mechanisms in acute septic cardiomyopathy: evidence from isolated myocytes. *Basic Res Cardiol* 1991;86:411–421.
2. Werdan K, Müller U, Reithmann C. "Negative inotropic cascade" in cardiomyocytes triggered by substances relevant to sepsis. In: Schlag G, ed. *Pathophysiology of shock, sepsis and organ failure*. Berlin-Heidelberg-New York: Springer-Verlag [*in press*].
3. Boekstegers P, Werdan K. Muscle tissue oxygen partial pressure in patients with severe infection, sepsis and cardiogenic shock. In: Ehrly AM, Fleckenstein W, Landgraf H, eds. *Clinical oxygen measurement III. Tissue oxygen pressure and transcutaneous oxygen pressure*. Berlin: Blackwell Wissenschaft; 1992:63–72.
4. Parratt JR. Alterations in vascular reactivity in sepsis. In: Vincent JL, ed. *Update in intensive care and emergency medicine*. Berlin-Heidelberg-New York: Springer; 1989:299–308.
5. Cunnion RE, Schaer GL, Parker MM, Natanson C, Parrillo JE. The coronary circulation in human septic shock. *Circulation* 1986;73:637–644.
6. Suffredini AF, Fromm RE, Parker MM, Brenner M, Kovacs JA, Wesley RA, Parrillo JE. The cardiovascular response of normal humans to the administration of endotoxin. *N Engl J Med* 1989;321:280–287.
7. Werdan K, Melnitzki SM, Pilz G, Kapsner T. The cultured rat heart cell: a model to study direct cardiotoxic effects of Pseudomonas endo- and exotoxins. In: Schlag G, Redl H, eds. *Second Vienna shock forum*. New York: Alan R. Liss, Inc.; 1989:247–251.
8. Snell RJ, Parrillo JE. Cardiovascular dysfunction in septic shock. *Chest* 1991;99:1000–1009.
9. Cross AS, Sadoff JC, Iglewski BH, Sokol PA. Evidence for the role of toxin A in the pathogenesis of infection with Pseudomonas aeruginosa in humans. *J Infect Dis* 1980;142:538–546.
10. Saelinger CB. Use of exotoxin A to inhibit protein synthesis. *Methods Enzymol* 1988;165:226–230.
11. Reithmann C, Gierschik P, Müller U, Werdan K, Jakobs KH. Pseudomonas exotoxin A prevents β-adrenoceptor-induced upregulation of G_i protein α-subunits and adenylyl cyclase desensitization in rat heart muscle cells. *Mol Pharmacol* 1990;37:631–638.
12. Thompson A, Halbert SP, Smith U. The toxicity of streptolysin O for beating mammalian heart cells in tissue culture. *J Exp Med* 1970;132:745–763.
13. Bhakdi S, Tranum-Jensen J. Damage to mammalian cells by proteins that form transmembrane pores. *Rev Physiol Biochem Pharmacol* 1987;107:147–223.
14. Bhakdi S, Mannhardt U, Muhly M, Hugo F, Ronneberger H, Hungerer KD. Human hyperimmune

globulin protects against the cytotoxic action of staphylococcal alpha-toxin in vitro and in vivo. *Infect Immun* 1989;57:3214–3220.

15. Bauriedel G, Bohn I, Werdan K. Direkte Wirkung von Staphylokokken-Toxin (α-Toxin) auf Kontraktions- und Ionenflußverhalten kultivierter Herzmuskelzellen. *Z Kardiol* 1986;75[Suppl 1]:57.

16. Yarom R, Hasin Y, Raz S, Yagen B. T-2 toxin effect on cultured myocardial cells. *Toxicol Lett* 1986;31:1–8.

17. Hegewisch S, Weh JH, Hossfeld DK. TNF-induced cardiomyopathy. *Lancet* 1990;I:294–295.

18. Hollenberg SM, Cunnion RE, Lawrence M, Kelly JL, Parrillo JE. Tumor necrosis factor depressed myocardial cell function: results using an in vitro assay of myocyte performance. *Clin Res* 1989; 37:528A.

19. Reithmann C, Gierschik P, Werdan K, Jakobs KH. Tumor necrosis factor α upregulates G_i and G_s proteins and adenylate cyclase responsiveness in rat cardiomyocytes. *Eur J Pharmacol (Mol Pharmacol Section)* 1991;206:53–60.

20. Schuchter LM, Hendricks CB, Holland KH, Shelton BK, Huchins GM, Baughman KL, Ettinger DS. Eosinophilic myocarditis associated with high-dose interleukin-2 therapy. *Am J Med* 1990;88: 439–440.

21. Sonnenblick M, Rosenmann D, Rosin A. Reversible cardiomyopathy induced by interferon. *Br Med J* 1990;300:1174–1175.

22. Wang YC, Herskowitz A, Gu LB, Kanter K, Lattouf O, Sell KW, Ahmed-Ansari A. Influence of cytokines and immunosuppressive drugs in major histocompatibility complex class I/II expression by human cardiac myocytes in vitro. *Hum Immunol* 1991;31:123–133.

23. Del Balzo U, Polley MJ, Levi R. Cardiac anaphylaxis: complement activation as an amplification system. *Circ Res* 1989;65:847–857.

24. Berger HJ, Taratuska A, Smith TW, Halperin JA. Activated complement directly modifies the performance of isolated heart muscle cells from guinea pig and rat. *Am J Physiol [in press]*.

25. Crespo MS, Fernandez-Gallardo S. Pharmacological modulation of PAF: a therapeutic approach to endotoxin shock. *J Lipid Mediators* 1991;4:127–144.

26. Massey CV, Kohout TA, Gaa ST, Lederer WJ, Rogers TB. Molecular and cellular actions of platelet-activating factor in rat heart cells. *J Clin Invest* 1991;88:2106–2116.

27. Wahler GM, Coyle DE, Sperelakis N. Effects of platelet-activating factor on single potassium channel currents in guinea pig ventricular myocytes. *Mol Cell Biochem* 1990;93:69–76.

28. Kispert P, Caldwell MD. Metabolic changes in sepsis and multiple organ failure. In: *Multiple organ failure. Pathophysiology and basic concepts of therapy*. New York: Thieme Medical Publishers; 1990:104–125.

29. Baracos V, Rodemann HP, Dinarello CA, Goldberg AL. Stimulation of muscle protein degradation and prostaglandin E_2 release by leukocytic pyrogen (interleukin-1). *N Engl J Med* 1983;308:553–558.

30. Weiss RG, Chacko VP, Gerstenblith G. Fatty acid regulation of glucose metabolism in the intact beating rat heart assessed by carbon-13 NMR spectroscopy: the critical role of pyruvate dehydrogenase. *J Mol Cell Cardiol* 1989;21:469–478.

31. Vary TC, Siegel JH, Nakatani T, Sato T, Aoyama H. Effect of sepsis on activity of pyruvate dehydrogenase complex in skeletal muscle and liver. *Am J Physiol* 1986;250:E634–E640.

32. Stoner HB, Little RA, Frayn KN, Elebute AE, Tresadern J, Gross E. The effect of sepsis on the oxidation of carbohydrate and fat. *Br J Surg* 1983;70:32–35.

33. Scholl RA, Lang CH, Bagby GJ. Hypertriglyceridemia and its relation to tissue lipoprotein lipase activity in endotoxemic, Escherichia coli bacteremic, and polymicrobial septic rats. *J Surg Res* 1984;37:394–401.

34. Dhainaut JF, Huyghebaert MF, Monsallier JF, Lefevre G, Dall'Ava-Santucci J, Brunet F, Villemant D, Carli A, Raichvarg D. Coronary hemodynamics and myocardial metabolism of lactate, free fatty acids, glucose, and ketones in patients with septic shock. *Circulation* 1987;75:533–541.

35. McDonaugh KH, Lang CH, Spitzer JJ. The effect of hyperdynamic sepsis on myocardial performance. *Circ Shock* 1985;15:247–259.

36. Pasque MK, Murphy CE, Van Trigt P, Pellom GL, Currie WD, Wechsler AS. Myocardial adenosine triphosphate levels during early sepsis. *Arch Surg* 1983;118:1437–1440.

37. Sethi R, Rupp H, Naimark BJ, Barwinsky J, Beamish RE, Dhalla NS. Characteristics and mechanisms of tachyphylaxis of cardiac contractile response to insulin. *Int J Cardiol [in press]*.

38. Nagano M, Dhalla NS. *The diabetic heart*. New York: Raven Press, 1991.

39. Dhalla NS, Elimban V, Rupp H. Paradoxical role of lipid metabolism in heart function and dysfunction. *Mol Cell Biochem* 1992;116:3–9.

40. Rupp H, Elimban V, Dhalla NS. Sucrose feeding prevents changes in myosin isoenzymes and sarcoplasmic reticulum Ca^{2+}-pump ATPase in pressure-loaded rat heart. *Biochem Biophys Res Commun* 1988;156:917–923.
41. Rupp H, Elimban V, Dhalla NS. Diabetes-like action of intermittent fasting on sarcoplasmic reticulum Ca^{2+}-pump ATPase and myosin isoenzymes can be prevented by sucrose. *Biochem Biophys Res Commun* 1989;164:319–325.
42. Rupp H, Wahl R, Hansen M. Influence of diet and carnitine palmitoyltransferase I inhibition on myosin and sarcoplasmic reticulum. *J Appl Physiol* 1992;72:352–360.
43. Rupp H, Elimban V, Dhalla NS. Modification of subcellular organelles in pressure overloaded heart by etomoxir, a carnitine palmitoyltransferase I inhibitor. *FASEB J* 1992;6:2349–2353.
44. Rupp H, Jacob R. Metabolically-modulated growth and phenotype of the rat heart. *Eur Heart J* 1992;13[Suppl D]:56–61.
45. Tomlinson CW, Lee SL, Dhalla NS. Abnormalities in heart membranes and myofibrils during bacterial infective cardiomyopathy in the rabbit. *Circ Res* 1976;39:82–92.
46. Dhalla NS, Ziegelhoffer A, Singal PK, Panagia V, Dhillon KS. Subcellular changes during cardiac hypertrophy and heart failure due to bacterial endocarditis. *Basic Res Cardiol* 1980;75:81–91.
47. Dennhardt R, Gramm HJ, Meinhold K, Voigt K. Patterns of endocrine secretion during sepsis. In: Schlag G, Redl H, eds., *Second Vienna shock forum*. New York: Alan R Liss, Inc.; 1989:751–756.
48. Arai M, Otsu K, MacLennan DH, Alpert NR, Periasamy M. Effect of thyroid hormone on the expression of mRNA encoding sarcoplasmic reticulum proteins. *Circ Res* 1991;69:266–276.
49. Werdan K, Erdmann E. Preparation and culture of embryonic and neonatal heart muscle cells: modification of transport activity. *Methods Enzymol* 1989;173:634–662.
50. Rupp H, Berger HF, Pfeifer A, Werdan K. Effect of positive inotropic agents on myosin isozyme population and mechanical activity of cultured rat heart myocytes. *Circ Res* 1991;68:1164–1173.
51. Reithmann C, Gierschik P, Werdan K, Jakobs KH. Role of inhibitory G protein α-subunits in adenylyl cyclase desensitization. *Mol Cell Endocrinol* 1991;82:C215–C221.
52. Dahn M. Bouwman D, Kirkpatrick JR. The sepsis-glucose intolerance riddle: a hormonal explanation. *Surgery* 1979;86:423–426.
53. Wolf HPO. Aryl-substituted 2-oxirane carboxylic acids: a new group of antidiabetic drugs. In: Bailey CJ, Flatt PR, eds. *New antidiabetic drugs*. London: Smith-Gordon; 1990:217–229.
54. Steiner KE, Lien EL. Hypoglycaemic agents which do not release insulin. *Prog Med Chem* 1987; 24:209–248.
55. Sherratt HSA. Inhibition of gluconeogenesis by non-hormonal hypoglycaemic compounds. In: Hue L, Van de Werve G, eds. *Short-term regulation of liver metabolism*. Amsterdam: Elsevier/North-Holland Biomedical Press; 1981:199–227.
56. Rösen P, Schmitz FJ, Reinauer H. Improvement of myocardial function and metabolism in diabetic rats by the carnitine palmitoyltransferase inhibitor etomoxir. In: Nagano M, Mochizuki S, Dhalla NS, eds. *Cardiovascular disease in diabetes*. Boston: Kluwer Academic Publishers; 1992:361–372.

The Cardiomyopathic Heart, edited by Makoto Nagano, Nobuakira Takeda, and Naranjan S. Dhalla. Raven Press, Ltd., New York © 1994.

27

A Novel Animal Model of Alcoholic Cardiomyopathy

Fumiaki Masani, Ken-ichi Watanabe, *Zhang Shaosong, *Tohru Izumi, and *Akira Shibata

*Division of Cardiology, Niigata Kuwana Hospital and *First Department of Internal Medicine, Niigata University School of Medicine, Niigata 951, Japan*

INTRODUCTION

Alcoholic cardiomyopathy, a condition marked by a dilated heart and compromised pump function, has been thought to be closely related to long-term consumption of large amounts of alcohol. Present studies indicate that the alcohol itself is one of the important factors involved in worsening the congestive cardiomyopathy (1–4). However, the pathophysiology of this alcoholic cardiomyopathy has not yet been elucidated. The main reason why a pathophysiologic study has been delayed is the lack of a good animal model for investigating this cardiac muscle disease. Up until now, no investigator has succeeded in provoking dilated heart in any experimental animals forced to ingest a large amount of ethanol for long periods of time. Frequently, the ethanol concentration in these studies reached an extraordinarily high level so that the animals did not take it spontaneously for a period of time (5). Nonetheless, the results gathered from previous trials suggest that alcohol consumption might be involved in initiating the cardiac muscle disease. It has also been emphasized for many years that the histologic findings associated with this cardiomyopathy include sclerosis and stenosis of myocardial arterioles (6,7). When we examined the myocardial samples obtained by biopsy from patients with alcoholic cardiomyopathy, degenerative endothelium of the myocardial arterioles and capillaries were remarkable in the fine structure (8). Furthermore, our data, obtained by thallium-201 myocardial scintigraphy, supported the view that this disease might be associated with small vessel lesions in the myocardium (9). Thus, in this study, we attempted to experimentally provoke dilated heart and compromised pump function in rats via chronic alcoholic consumption and to induce myocardial ischemia by allylamine administration.

MATERIAL AND METHODS

Fifty-two male Wister rats (5.5 weeks old, Charles River Laboratories, Japan) were used. The rats were divided into four groups: Group A (13 rats) received a 0.1% aqueous solution of allylamine, Group E (13 rats) received a 15% aqueous solution of ethanol, Group AE (13 rats) received an aqueous solution containing 0.1% allylamine and 15% ethanol, and Group C (13 rats) received pure water. In each group, treatment was begun at 5.5 weeks of age. All animals were housed in a room where the temperature and humidity were automatically controlled. They were allowed free access to drinks and a solid diet containing other nutrients, vitamins, and minerals in amounts suitable for normal growth of rats.

At 10 months of age, the animals were anesthetized with intraperitoneal pentobarbital and were sacrificed. The heart of each rat was fixed in 10% formalin and embedded in paraffin by the conventional methods for light microscopy. The heart was sliced horizontally into three parts: at the atrioventricular valve annulus, at the papillary muscle, and at the apex. The sections were then stained with hematoxylin-eosin and Masson-Goldner stain. The transverse diameter (the minimum span of myocardial cells) was measured sequentially, and a median value was determined to allow comparison with that of the others.

RESULTS

After 9 months of treatment, the body weight and the heart weight of the rats in Group A were significantly lower than those in Group C (control group), whereas these parameters in Group E and Group AE did not differ significantly from those in Group C (Table 1).

During the observation period, neither animals in Group E nor Group C died. However, four animals in Group A and three animals in Group E died unexpectedly without showing any apparent abnormalities. Of these seven rats, two in Group A and one in Group AE could be examined by histopathological means. All of these three rats were found to have extensive myocardial infarction in the ventricular

TABLE 1. *Body weight, heart weight, and heart weight/body weight ratio*

	Body weight (g)	Heart weight (g)	Heart weight/body weight ratio (%)
Group A (n = 9)	634 ± 60	1.97 ± 0.19	0.31 ± 0.01
Group E (n = 13)	878 ± 61	2.49 ± 0.23	0.28 ± 0.01
Group AE[a] (n = 9)	886 ± 54	2.74 ± 0.42	0.31 ± 0.03
Group C (n = 13)	879 ± 48	2.64 ± 0.15	0.30 ± 0.01

[a]Data from the rat that developed heart failure after 5 months of treatment is excluded from Group AE.

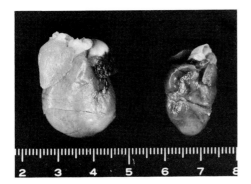

FIG. 1. Formalin-fixed heart of a control rat (*left*) and a rat that developed heart failure (*right*) after 9 months of treatment with allylamine and ethanol combined.

walls. Of the rats except those 7 that died, two in Group AE showed symptomatic heart failure in the fifth and ninth month after treatment, respectively. In both animals, initial signs of heart failure included slow movements, fluffy hair, and piloerection. About ten days after these signs were observed, the animals were noted to have marked facial edema and tended to remain crouching. At autopsy, both animals were found to have massive hydrothorax and ascites. The liver and spleen were very enlarged and the lungs were remarkably congested. The hearts from these animals were much larger than those of the controls. The diseased hearts were dilated in a spherical form (Fig. 1). In both rats, thrombi within the atrium were transparently visible through the right atrial wall. On macroscopic examination, the heart surface was pale-whitish. No myocardial infarction was detectable in a global view. The ventricular lumen was enlarged in both the right and left ventricles. The dilatation was more dominant in the left ventricle. The left ventricular wall was found to have thinned remarkably, whereas the thickness of the right ventricle was comparable to that in the controls (Fig. 2). The diameters of myocardial cells, both in the left ventricular free wall and the ventricular septum, were slightly larger in the two rats with congestive heart failure (median of 12.8 μm) than in the controls (11.5 μm). In addition, the number of myofibrils was reduced in the sarcoplasma in the

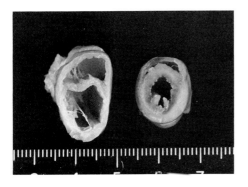

FIG. 2. Transverse section of the hearts shown in Figure 1 at the papillary muscle level. The heart of the rat with heart failure (*right*) shows dilatation of the right and left ventricles and marked thinning of the left ventricular wall.

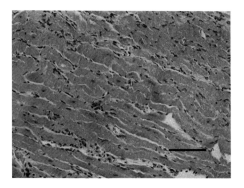

FIG. 3. Light microscopy study of the myocardium of the ventricular septum in a rat that developed heart failure after 5 months of combined treatment with allylamine and ethanol. A slight reduction in the density of myofibrils, as well as myocardial cell hypertrophy, is seen. The arrangement of myocardial cells is normal. (H&E). Scale bar = 50 μm.

two rats with congestive heart failure so that the muscle striation were obscure in some cardiocytes. However, the myofibrils maintained their normal arrangement (Fig. 3).

The interstitium in these two rats showed neither inflammatory cell infiltrates nor an increase in fat cells. Fibrosis was relatively marked in the subendocardium, predominantly in the apex of the heart. Neither extensive nor transmural fibrosis was present. Only several small fibrotic loci were scattered in the myocardium (Fig. 4a,b). Neither of these two animals showed arteriolar obstruction or serious stenosis of vessels. However, hyperplastic smooth muscle was seen in the tunica media, and the endothelium in the arterioles was found to have proliferated. Consequently, the infarcted myocardium was not detectable, even upon detailed investigation. Meanwhile, the surviving rats in Group AE, as well as in Groups A, E, and C did not exhibit cardiac dilatation. Light microscopy studies in these survivors showed more extensive myocardial infarction in comparison with that observed in the congestive

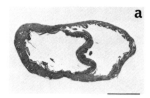

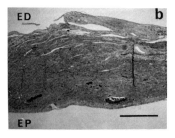

FIG. 4. a: Transverse section of the heart of a rat that developed heart failure after 5 months of combined treatment with allylamine and ethanol. (Masson-Goldner stain.) Scale bar = 5 mm. **b:** Magnification of the heart section shown in 4a. Fibrosis has not spread beyond the subendocardial region. *ED,* endocardium; EP, epicardium. scale bar = 50 μm.

rats. Even transmural infarction was seen in some of these rats. In Groups E and C, no histologic abnormalities were observed.

DISCUSSION

In this study, heart failure developed only in the rats treated with a combination of allylamine and ethanol. Rats treated with allylamine or ethanol alone showed neither a dilated heart nor compromised pump failure. These results suggest that the combined use of allylamine and ethanol are essential to induce this cardiac muscle disease experimentally. The hearts of rats in which heart failure developed showed no evidence of extensive myocardial infarction. Thus, the heart failure in these rats was not caused by an obvious ischemic lesion, such as extensive infarction. The histopathologic features are consistent with the findings in alcoholic cardiomyopathy. The body weight, heart weight, and the ratio of these two values among rats treated with a combination of allylamine and ethanol did not differ from those of ethanol-treated rats or from those of rats receiving pure water or other treatment. Therefore, it is likely that malnutrition did not contribute to the disease in rats treated with a combination of ethanol and allylamine. Allylamine is an unsaturated primary amine. Because this compound has high cardiovascular toxicity, it has been used to produce an experimental model of myocardial ischemia for many years. Extensive myocardial necrosis and infarction, which have been found to develop following allylamine treatment, are primarily attributable to the ischemic changes caused by impaired small coronary arteries (10). The arteriolar impairment is attributable to several factors, including edema and degeneration of the endothelium, hyperplasia of the tunica intima, and necrosis and smooth muscle hyperplasia of the tunica media (11–14). Also in the present study, not only rats treated with allylamine alone but also rats treated with a combination of allylamine and ethanol developed arteriolar hypertrophy in the tunica media, as well as marked myocardial infarction. These results suggest that allylamine induces myocardial ischemia.

It is well known that massive alcohol ingestion can easily cause hypertension (15,16). In addition, the heavy drinker is also likely to have an unbalanced daily uptake of nutrients. Considering these factors, it can be speculated that arteriosclerosis is likely to occur in heavy drinkers. Until now, it has been unclear whether the stenotic lesion of myocardial arterioles, observed in patients with alcoholic cardiomyopathy, is an outcome of long-term and massive alcohol ingestion or a cause of this alcohol-related cardiac muscle disease. The present results support the premise that the arteriolar lesions, which may induce myocardial ischemia, are at least partially responsible for triggering this disease. Even in this context, it has been reported that myocardial contractility was not reduced in patients with severe ischemic heart disease who ingested large amounts of ethanol (17). Therefore, the question has also remained unresolved how to induce the cardiac muscle disease in the presence of chronic alcohol ingestion and myocardial ischemia.

The incidence of sudden death that was thought to be attributable to an acute ischemic event was lower in the group treated with a combination of allylamine and ethanol than in the group treated with allylamine alone. Furthermore, rats with heart failure exhibited no extensive myocardial infarction. Thus, it is likely that the ethanol intake does not accelerate the myocardial ischemia caused by allylamine. The heart failure observed in these rats may be a result of ethanol's effect in modulating the allylamine-induced ischemia. It may not be an outcome of a combination or synergistic effect of ethanol and allylamine in impairing myocardial function. Further studies are required to clarify the underlying mechanism for the initiation of heart failure after treatment with both allylamine and ethanol. Nonetheless, the rats with heart failure that we established experimentally are the first in which the heart failure was caused by long-term alcohol ingestion. This animal model should prove very useful in investigating alcoholic cardiomyopathy in humans.

SUMMARY

To study whether myocardial ischemia can be an important trigger in the development of alcoholic cardiomyopathy, male Wistar rats were forced to ingest a large amount of alcohol for a long time. The induction of extensive myocardial ischemia was proven by the case control study involving allylamine administration to the experimental animals. Apparent chronic heart failure occurred in 2 of the 13 rats, both of which were forced to take an aqueous solution containing both 0.1% allylamine and 15% ethanol. Of these two, one rat developed chronic heart failure within 5 months of treatment, whereas the other developed the condition within 9 months. The control rats, which were treated with allylamine only, ethanol only or pure water only, showed no sign of heart failure. The hearts of rats with congestive heart failure demonstrated remarkably dilated ventricles. Despite this dilatation, histologic examination did not reveal any signs of myocardial infarction or interstitial fibrosis. No histologic changes were noted in the groups receiving ethanol only and pure water only. Some of the allylamine-treated rats showed characteristics of an obvious arteriolar wall thickening and myocardial infarction around the vessels. From these data, it was concluded that the combined use of allylamine and ethanol may produce a dilated heart and pump failure in this experimental animal.

ACKNOWLEDGMENT

The authors gratefully acknowledge Drs. Makoto Kodama and Haruo Hanawa for their assistance. This study was supported by the research fund of the Niigata Medical Association.

REFERENCES

1. Fuster V, Gersh BJ, Giuliani ER, Tajik AJ, Brandenburg RO, Frye RL. The natural history of idiopathic dilated cardiomyopathy. *Am J Cardiol* 1981;47:525–531.
2. Johnson RA, Palacios I. Dilated cardiomyopathy of the adult. *N Engl J Med* 1982;307:1051–1058.
3. Wang R, Mallon J, Alterman AI, McLellan AT. Alcohol and dilated cardiomyopathy: incidence and correlation with clinical outcome. *J Substance Abuse Treat* 1987;4:209–213.
4. Urbano-Marquez A, Estruch R, Navarro-Lopez F, Grau JM, Mont L, Rubin E. The effects of alcoholism on skeletal and cardiac muscle. *N Engl J Med* 1989;320:409–415.
5. Segel LD. The development of alcohol-induced cardiac dysfunction in the rat. *Alcohol Alcoholism* 1988;23:391–401.
6. Factor SM. Intramyocardial small-vessel disease in chronic alcoholism. *Am Heart J* 1976;92:561–575.
7. Burch GE, Giles, TD. The small coronary arteries in alcoholic cardiomyopathy. 1977;94:471–478.
8. Masani F, Kodama M, Yokoyama A, Koike T, Hatano T, Tsuda T, Izumi T, Shibata A. A comparative study on alcoholic cardiomyopathy: left ventricular wall motion and endomyocardial biopsies after total abstinence. *Jpn Circ J* 1988;52[Suppl]:832.
9. Masani F, Sasagawa Y, Kodama M, Kato H, Cyou S, Hatano T, Tsuda T, Izumi T, Shibata A. Comparison of effects of abstinence on alcoholic cardiomyopathy and findings of 201 T1 myocardial scintigraphy. *Jpn Circ J* 1990;54[Suppl]:73.
10. Rubin E. Alcoholic myopathy in heart and skeletal muscle. *N Engl J Med* 1979;301:28–33.
11. Boor PJ, Hysmith RM. Allylamine cardiovascular toxicity. *Toxicology* 1987;44:129–145.
12. Waters LL. Changes in the coronary arteries of the dog following injections of allylamine. *Am Heart J* 1948;35:212–218.
13. Lalich JJ, Paik WCW. Myocardial fibrosis and smooth muscle cell hyperplasia in coronary arteries of allylamine-fed rats. *Am J Pathol* 1972;66:225–230.
14. Boor PJ, Nelson TJ, Chieco P. Allylamine cardiotoxicity: histopathology and histochemistry. *Am J Pathol* 1980;100:739–751.
15. Boor PJ, Ferrans VJ. Ultrastructural alterations in allylamine cardiovascular toxicity: late myocardial and vascular lesions. *Am J Pathol* 1985;121:39–54.
16. Criqui MH, Wallace RB, Mishkel M, Barret-Connor E, Heiss G. Alcohol consumption and blood pressure: the lipid research clinics prevalence study. Hypertension 1981;3:557–565.
17. Klatsky AL, Friedman GD, Armstrong MA. The relationship between alcoholic beverage use and other traits to blood pressure: a new Kaiser Permanente study. *Circulation* 1986;73:628–636.
18. Kelbek H, Heslet L, Skagen K, Munck O, Christensen NJ, Godtfredsen J. Cardiac function after alcohol ingestion in patients with ischemic heart disease and cardiomyopathy: a controlled study. *Alcohol Alcoholism* 1988;23:17–21.

The Cardiomyopathic Heart, edited by Makoto
Nagano, Nobuakira Takeda, and Naranjan S.
Dhalla. Raven Press, Ltd., New York © 1994.

28

Doxorubicin-Induced Cardiomyopathy: A Model of Congestive Heart Failure

Natasa Siveski-Iliskovic, Thomas P. Thomas, Nalini Kaul,
*Jan Slezak, and Pawan K. Singal

*Division of Cardiovascular Sciences, St. Boniface General Hospital Research Centre and
Department of Physiology, Faculty of Medicine, University of Manitoba,
Winnipeg, Canada R2H 2A6; and *Institute for Heart Research,
Slovak Academy of Sciences, 84233 Bratislava, Czech and Slovak Federative Republic*

BACKGROUND AND INTRODUCTION

Features of Doxorubicin

Doxorubicin (Adriamycin) is a member of the anthracyclines class of cytostatic antibiotics and is composed of a tetracycline group attached by a glycoside bond to an amino sugar (Fig. 1). A quinone ring, present in the doxorubicin structure, can undergo cyclic oxidation reduction, which can lead to the formation of free radicals

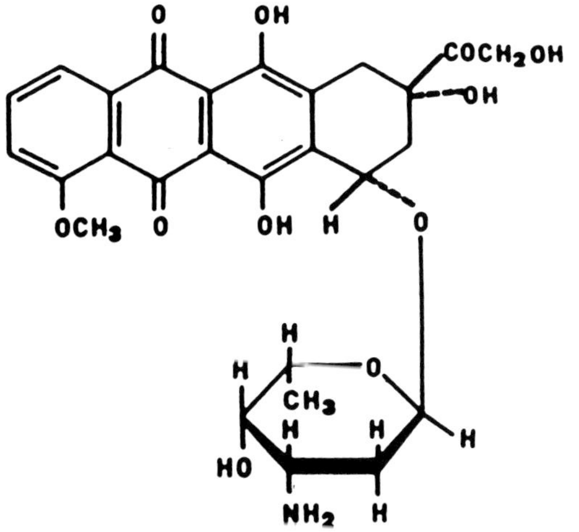

FIG. 1. Structure of the doxorubicin molecule.

277

(1). Doxorubicin is a very potent chemotherapeutic agent, effective against soft and solid human malignant lesions. It is obtained by aerobic fermentation or by chemical synthesis. The molecular structure of doxorubicin confers lipophilicity, and the drug readily permeates the cell membrane (2,3). Within minutes of its administration, the drug is cleared from the plasma and is found in the nucleus, where it intercalates between the base pairs of nucleic acids and exerts an antimitotic effect (1,4). It has a relatively long tissue half-life.

Cardiovascular Side Effects of Doxorubicin

The usefulness of doxorubicin is limited by the fact that repetitive administration in patients is associated with the development of cardiovascular abnormalities leading to cardiomyopathy and heart failure. These cardiovascular side effects may be acute as well as chronic.

Acute cardiovascular effects develop within minutes or hours after intravenous administration of the drug. Major acute effects are tachycardia and various arrhythmias, but these are clinically manageable. Worsening of pre-ejection period (PEP)/left ventricular ejection time (LVET) ratios in patients receiving doxorubicin therapy has also been found to be transient, with values returning to normal within 1 month after discontinuation of therapy (5). A number of studies have also suggested the possibility of an acute left ventricular dysfunction that normally does not become apparent because of the cardiac reserve present (6). However, all of these early changes are transient and reversible and are not of major consequence (1,5).

The chronic cardiovascular effects of doxorubicin, on the other hand, are life-threatening. These effects develop after several weeks or months of treatment, in some cases, even after the therapy has been completed. The worst complication is cardiomyopathy, which often leads to congestive heart failure (5,7,8). The most frequent symptoms of congestive heart failure include tachycardia, shortness of breath, neck vein distention, gallop rhythms, hepatomegaly, cardiomegaly, and pleural effusions (5). Some of the electrocardiographic abnormalities accompanying this condition may include ST-T wave changes, sinus tachycardia, premature ventricular contractions, low voltage of QRS complex, atrial flutter, and fibrillations (5). Increased serum enzyme levels—serum glutamic-oxaloacetic transaminase (SGOT), lactic dehydrogenase (LDH), and creatine phosphokinase (CPK)—have also been reported to accompany heart failure in these patients.

Unique Features of Doxorubicin-Induced Heart Failure

Doxorubicin cardiotoxicity and congestive heart failure in patients are dose-dependent. In a retrospective study of patients receiving doxorubicin, the incidence of heart failure was found to increase from 0% at doses of less than 450 mg/m^2 to 35% at a total cumulative dose exceeding 601 mg/m^2 (5). Characteristically, doxorubicin-induced congestive heart failure is refractory to treatments routinely used to improve cardiac function in patients with heart failure. Heart biopsies have revealed two structural features that are typical of doxorubicin-induced cardiomyopathy. These include loss of myofibrils and dilation of the sarcotubular membranes (5,7). These and other features of doxorubicin-induced cardiomyopathy can be produced in a variety of animals by subchronic treatment with the drug (9–15).

Mechanisms Underlying Doxorubicin-Induced Heart Failure

With respect to mechanisms, experimental data support the involvement of free radicals. Doxorubicin can initiate oxidation chain reactions by the transfer of electrons from endogenous compounds, such as nicotinamide-adenine dinucleotide phosphate (NADPH), to oxygen through quinone-semiquinone reactions. This results in the formation of superoxide radicals that can lead to the formation of hydroxy radicals and hydrogen peroxide. These, in turn, can oxidize unsaturated fatty acids in the biomembranes as well as in other cell constituents, including S-H groups in proteins (1,7). This oxidative stress injury has been suggested as one of the possible mechanisms for the myocardial cell injury caused by doxorubicin (1, 16–19).

EXPERIMENTAL MODEL OF CONGESTIVE HEART FAILURE

Procedure and General Observations

We have established a simple procedure for inducing congestive heart failure in rats. For this, doxorubicin is administered intraperitoneally to rats (250 ± 20 g of body weight) in six equal doses of 2.5 mg/kg each (total cumulative dose of 15 mg/kg) on Monday, Wednesday, and Friday over a 2-week period. After the first or second injection, animals lose their appetites and also start to lose weight. They become slow and inactive and experience a loss of fur. After treatment is discontinued, their appetite improves and the rats start gaining weight. This gain in body weight, however, is dependent on the age as well as the weight of the animal. Animals 1 month of age (175 ± 25 g of body weight) stop gaining weight, but do not lose weight, for the duration of the drug treatment. By contrast, 6-month-old animals (450 ± 25 g of body weight) show about a 22% loss in body weight during the doxorubicin treatment period (13). Younger animals (1 month old) show a recovery in body weight that parallels that of the control group during the posttreatment period. However, 6-month-old animals show only a partial recovery in body weight. Loss of weight with drug treatment (7.5 mg/g of body weight) is dramatic in 9-month-old and older animals, and there is no weight gain in these rats during the posttreatment period.

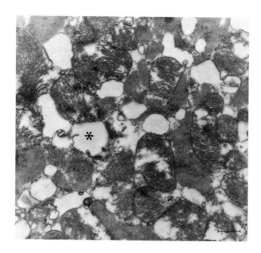

FIG. 2. Ultrastructural changes in the rat heart secondary to treatment with doxorubicin. Animals were treated with doxorubicin (15 mg/kg), as described in the text, and hearts were examined 3 weeks after the last treatment. Dilation of the tubular membrane system (*), mitochondrial damage, and myofibril loss were noted. Scale bar = 1 μM.

Morphologic Changes

Myofibrillar loss and cytoplasmic vacuolization, considered to be characteristic features of the doxorubicin-induced cardiomyopathy, invariably become apparent 3 weeks after treatment (Fig. 2) at the dose described earlier, and these changes progress significantly 6 weeks after treatment. The affected cells are generally distributed in all layers of the myocardium. From a structural viewpoint, cardiomyopathy is clearly established in the experimental model within 3 to 6 weeks. These and other ultrastructural changes, including mitochondrial swelling and degeneration, nucleolar changes, myofibrillar separation and homogenization, separation of the intercalated discs, and cellular and interstitial edema, have also been described in other animal models (9,21). Early changes are limited to the mitochondria and nucleoli, with little myofibrillar destruction, vacuolization, or swelling (21). In addition, in older animals (9 to 12 months of age), extensive collagen deposition is seen, as evidenced by the appearance of white patches of collagen in the heart. The myocardial cell damage caused by doxorubicin, as well as the associated accumulation of lipid peroxides, is dependent on both the amount of drug given and the age of the animal (Table 1).

Hemodynamic Changes

Hemodynamically, one can see in this model a gradually developing heart failure (22). Three weeks after treatment, left ventricular end diastolic pressure (LVEDP) increases, whereas left ventricular systolic pressure (LVSP) is maintained. However, 6 weeks after treatment, LVSP also becomes depressed (22). It has been proposed that a shift to the right on the Frank-Starling curve and other adjustments are able to maintain the aortic pressure during the 3-week posttreatment period (22).

TABLE 1. *Age- and dose-dependent[a] differences in myocardial cell damage and lipid peroxidation induced by doxorubicin in rat hearts*

Age of animals (months)	MDA (% increase)	Histology score
1	0	+
6	100	+ +
9[b]	76	+ +
12[b]	80	+ +

Based on data from Weinberg and Singal, ref. 13, and Deally and Singal, ref. 20.

[a]In younger animals (1 and 6 months of age), the cumulative dose of doxorubicin was 15 mg/kg, whereas in older animals, the dose was 7.5 mg/kg.

[b]Among other changes in these animals (see text), there was marked collagen deposition in the hearts.

However, a chronic increase in LVEDP as early as 3 weeks after treatment probably does cause an increase in back pressure in the lungs, right heart, and major veins, resulting in the congestion of dependent tissues. About this time, some animals start accumulating fluid in the abdominal cavity owing to the heart failure.

Features of Doxorubicin-Induced Heart Failure in Rats

The development of congestive heart failure in this rat model is progressive and is frequently manifested by measurable quantities of fluid retained in the abdominal cavity. It has been shown that it is a degenerative phenomenon, the outcome of which depends on the total cumulative dose administered, as well as on the age of the animal. The incidence of mortality, as well as of ascites, increases with age (Table 2). In fact, in 9-month-old and older animals, the cumulative dose of the drug that is administered is generally reduced to 50% (7.5 mg/kg) in order to obtain a comparable injury, because at a higher dose (15 mg/kg), 100% mortality is experienced.

A characteristic feature of doxorubicin-induced congestive heart failure in patients is its refractoriness to therapeutic interventions (5), which is also noted in the heart failure model in the present study. The in vivo response to epinephrine (10^{-5}

TABLE 2. *Age- and dose-dependent differences in doxorubicin-induced ascites and mortality in rats*

Age (months)	15 mg/kg		7.5 mg/kg	
	Ascites (%)	Mortality (%)	Ascites (%)	Mortality (%)
1–1.5	11	18	–	–
6	100	30	–	–
9	100	100	81	22
12	100	100	77	20

Based on data from Weinberg and Singal, ref. 13, and Deally and Singal, ref. 20.

TABLE 3. *In vitro response to epinephrine (10^{-5} M) in papillary muscles from hearts of control and doxorubicin-treated rats at different ages*

	Doxorubicin (15 mg/kg)		Doxorubicin (7.5 mg/kg)	
	1 Month of age	6 Months of age	9 Months of age	12 Months of age
Controls	+ 54.5 ± 4.1	17.8 ± 2.7	28.0 ± 4.0	27.2 ± 5.2
Doxorubicin-treated rats	+ 27.7[a] ± 9.8	8.7[a] ± 1.9	3.8[a] ± 2.4	− 2.9[a] ± 3.3

Based on data from Weinberg and Singal, ref. 13, and Deally and Singal, ref. 20.
[a]Significantly different ($p < 0.05$) from controls.

M) is reduced by 50% in rats weighing 300 ± 25 g (22). Furthermore, the duration of this blunted positive response to epinephrine is also reduced in doxorubicin-treated animals (22). Reduced responsiveness to epinephrine has also been noted in isolated in vitro papillary muscle preparations (13,20). Papillary muscles from doxorubicin-treated animals were also less responsive to other inotropic interventions, such as high and low calcium and frequency response. This modulation of the inotropic response is also an age-dependent phenomenon (Table 3). In younger animals (1 month to 6 months of age), the responsiveness is reduced by almost 50%, whereas in older animals (9 months and 12 months of age) that were treated with doxorubicin, there was no positive response to epinephrine (Table 3).

SUMMARY

Cardiotoxicity is the main limitation in anticancer treatment with doxorubicin. The present animal model is relatively inexpensive and can be established within weeks for a quick evaluation of drug effects. The induction of cardiomyopathy is highly reproducible and seems to be time- as well as dose-related. It is also possible to obtain different heart failure stages in this animal model. Thus, this rat model may be the closest to an "ideal animal model" for producing congestive heart failure. It provides a useful tool, not only in the study of doxorubicin-induced cardiotoxicity, but also in examining the natural history of congestive heart failure.

ACKNOWLEDGMENTS

Studies reported in this paper were supported by grants from the Manitoba Heart and Stroke Foundation. At the time of this study, Dr. Slezak was a visiting Professor of the Canadian Heart and Stroke Foundation. Dr. Kaul was supported by a Postdoctoral Fellowship from the Faculty of Medicine. Dr. Siveski-Iliskovic was supported by the St. Boniface General Hospital Research Center.

REFERENCES

1. Singal PK, Deally CMR, Weinberg LE. Subcellular effects of adriamycin in the heart: a concise review. *J Mol Cell Cardiol* 1987;19:817–828.
2. Skovsgaard T, Nissen NI. Membrane transport of anthracyclines. *Pharmacol Ther* 1982;18:293–311.
3. Benjamin RS. Clinical pharmacology of adriamycin (NSC-123127). *Cancer Chemother Rep* 1975;6(3):183–185.
4. Bachur NR. Adriamycin (NSC-123127) pharmacology. *Cancer Chemother Rep* 1975;6(3):153–158.
5. Lefrak EA, Pitha J, Rosenheim S, Gottlieb J. A clinicopathologic analysis of adriamycin cardiotoxicity. *Cancer* 1973;32:302–314.
6. Singal PK. Adriamycin does have a potentially depressant effect on left ventricular contractility. *Int J Cardiol* 1985;7:447–449.
7. Ferrans VJ. Anthracycline cardiotoxicity. In: Spitzer JJ, ed. *Myocardial injury*. New York: Plenum Press; 1983:519–532.
8. Von Hoff DD, Layard MW, Basa P, Von Hoff AL, Rozenweiz M, Muzio M. Risk factors for doxorubicin-induced congestive heart failure. *Ann Int Med* 1979;91:710–717.
9. Myers CE, McGuire WP, Liss RH, Ifrim I, Grotzinger K, Young RC. Adriamycin: The role of lipid peroxidation in cardiac toxicity and tumor response. *Science* 1977;19:165–167.
10. Jaenke RS. Anthracycline antibiotic-induced cardiomyopathy in rabbits. *Lab Invest* 1974;30:292–304.
11. Ditchey RV, LeWinter MM, Higgins CB. Acute effects of doxorubicin (adriamycin) on left ventricular function in dogs. *Int J Cardiol* 1984;6:341–350.
12. Kehoe R, Singer DH, Trapain A, Billingham M, Levandowski R, Elson T. Adriamycin-induced cardiac dysrhythmias in an experimental dog model. *Cancer Treat Rep* 1978;62(6):963–978.
13. Weinberg LE, Singal PK. Refractory heart failure and age-related differences in adriamycin-induced myocardial changes in rats. *Can J Physiol Pharmacol* 1987;65:1957–1965.
14. Mettler FP, Young DM, Ward JM. Adriamycin-induced cardiotoxicity (cardiomyopathy and congestive heart failure) in rats. *Cancer Res* 1977;37:2705–2713.
15. Czarnecki A, Hinek A, Soltysiak-Pawluczuk D. Adriamycin-induced cardiomyopathy. A rat model. *Pol J Pharmacol Pharm* 1986;38:171–177.
16. Lee V, Randhawa AK, Singal PK. Adriamycin-induced myocardial dysfunction *in vitro* is mediated by free radicals. *Am J Physiol* 1991;261 [Heart Circ Phys 30]:H989–H995.
17. Thornalley PJ, Dodd NJF. Free radical production from normal and adriamycin treated rat cardiac sarcosomes. *Biochem Pharmacol* 1985;34:669–674.
18. Singal PK, Pierce GN. Adriamycin stimulates low-affinity Ca^{2+} binding and lipid peroxidation but depresses myocardial function. *Am J Physiol* 1986;250 [Heart Circ Physiol 19]: H419–H425.
19. Porta EA, Joun NS, Matsumara L, Nakasone B, Sablan H. Acute adriamycin cardiotoxicity in rats. *Res Commun Chem Pathol Pharm* 1983;41:125–137.
20. Deally CMR, Singal PK. Susceptibility to adriamycin-induced cardiotoxicity increases only up to certain age. *J Appl Cardiol* 1990;5:223–238.
21. Jensen RA, Acton EM, Peters JH. Doxorubicin cardiotoxicity in the rat: comparison of electrocardiogram, transmembrane potential and structural effects. *J Cardiovasc Pharmacol* 1984;6:186–200.
22. Tong J, Ganguly PK, Singal PK. Myocardial adrenergic changes at two stages of heart failure due to adriamycin treatment in rats. *Am J Physiol* 1991;260:H909–H916.

The Cardiomyopathic Heart, edited by Makoto
Nagano, Nobuakira Takeda, and Naranjan S.
Dhalla. Raven Press, Ltd., New York © 1994.

29

Cellular and Molecular Basis for the Immunopathologic Characteristics of the Myocardial Cell Damage Caused by Acute Viral Myocarditis, with Special Reference to Dilated Cardiomyopathy

*†‡Yoshinori Seko, †Yoichi Shinkai, †Hideo Yagita,
†Ko Okumura, and *Yoshio Yazaki

*Third Department of Internal Medicine, Faculty of Medicine, University of Tokyo;
†Department of Immunology, School of Medicine, Juntendo University; and
‡The Institute for Adult Diseases, Asahi Life Foundation, Tokyo 125, Japan

INTRODUCTION

Viral myocarditis can not only produce congestive heart failure as an acute inflammatory disorder, but it has also been strongly implicated in the pathogenesis of idiopathic dilated cardiomyopathy. The pathogenesis of the myocardial cell damage involved is of great clinical significance and remains to be clarified. Many studies (1–3) have been conducted in this field using murine models of viral myocarditis; these studies have shown that cell-mediated cytotoxicity plays an important role. Using a murine model of myocarditis caused by coxsackievirus B3 (CVB3), we have analyzed the phenotypes of the infiltrating cells in the hearts of the animal models and have examined the expression of major histocompatibility complex (MHC) antigens and intercellular adhesion molecule-1 (ICAM-1), as well as the virus genomes in myocardial tissue of acute viral myocarditis. Using Northern blot analysis, we have found that, just after virus inoculation on day 0, virus genomes appear in the heart and replicate, peaking on day 6; they then almost disappear from the heart after day 10. On or around day 5, massive cell infiltration, mainly involving natural killer (NK) cells, occurs in the heart (4). Almost simultaneously, both MHC class I antigen and ICAM-1 are strongly expressed in myocardial cells (5,6). A little later, T-helper (Th) cells, and then cytotoxic T lymphocytes (CTLs), infiltrate the heart sequentially. Our data strongly suggest that, in any early phase of acute myocarditis, NK cells mainly kill virus-infected cardiac myocytes. In a later

285

phase, when virus genomes have almost disappeared from the heart, CTLs recognize virus-derived antigens expressed on the cardiac myocytes with MHC class I antigen and may cause further myocardial cell damage. Both NK cells and CTLs, playing a major part in cell-mediated cytotoxicity, are thought to kill virus-infected cells or tumor cells with the effector molecules contained in their cytoplasmic granules, one of which is named pore-forming protein, or perforin. From the results of in vitro studies, a granule exocytosis model for lymphocyte-mediated target cell killing has been proposed. In response to surface contact between a killer cell and a target cell, cytoplasmic granules of the killer cell rapidly reorient toward the target cell. With the increase in intracellular calcium levels, granule exocytosis occurs. Many perforin monomer molecules are released, and are inserted into the target cell membrane; they then polymerize and assemble to form transmembrane pores, which in turn cause colloid osmotic injury to the target cell (7). Until recently, however, there was no evidence for the role of perforin in cell-mediated cytotoxicity primed in vivo (8–10). Recent studies (11,12) have demonstrated that perforin plays a critical role in cytolysis and can be a good marker for killer cells.

EXPRESSION OF PERFORIN IN INFILTRATING CELLS IN HEARTS AFFECTED BY ACUTE MYOCARDITIS

To determine whether cell-mediated cytotoxicity really occurs in this model of acute viral myocarditis, we examined the expression of perforin in the infiltrating cells using immunoperoxidase and immunoelectron microscopy. C3H/He mice were killed on day 7 after virus inoculation, when myocardial inflammation reached a maximal level. Cryostat sections were prepared from the freshly frozen heart ventricles. After fixation, they were blocked with rabbit serum and incubated with rat anti-mouse perforin monoclonal antibody (mAb), then incubated with biotinylated rabbit anti-rat IgG antibody. After incubation with avidin-biotinylated peroxidase complex, they were reacted with diaminobenzidine tetrahydrochloride with H_2O_2. For immunoelectron microscopy, the reaction was carried out first with 1% dimethylsulfoxide for preincubation, then with H_2O_2. The sections were treated with osmium tetroxide, and were embedded in resin. Then, ultrathin sections were prepared and examined with an electron microscope.

Figures 1 and 2 show immunoperoxidase staining of the ventricular tissues of CVB3-infected mice (day 7) with anti-mouse perforin mAb for light and electron microscopy, respectively. Some of the infiltrating cells were clearly stained in their peripheral cytoplasm, indicating the expression of perforin in their cytoplasmic granules (see Fig. 1, *arrows*). There was apparent heterogeneity in the expression of perforin among different infiltrating cells. The proportion of perforin-positive cells as a fraction of total cells was 13% to 15% on day 5 after virus inoculation, when massive cell infiltration began to appear. This was followed by a gradual decrease. To clarify the mechanism of perforin-mediated cardiac myocyte injury, we investi-

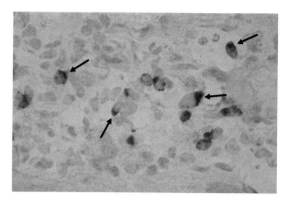

FIG. 1. Immunoperoxidase staining of the infiltrating cells for perforin in the hearts of mice killed on day 7 after CVB3 infection. Note the clear expression of perforin in the cytoplasm of some of the infiltrating cells (*arrows*). There was apparent heterogeneity in the expression of perforin among the infiltrating cells. (×400.)

gated the release of perforin molecules from the infiltrating killer cells using immunoelectron microscopy. Figure 2A (*arrows*) shows the expression of perforin at the peripheral cytoplasm or the surface of the infiltrating cells close to a cardiac myocyte. These cells expressed perforin at the side toward the surface of the cardiac myocyte. It appears that these infiltrating cells began to secrete perforin to the cardiac myocyte. Higher magnification revealed that a large number of perforin molecules were released from the surface of an infiltrating cell and directly reached the surface of a cardiac myocyte (Fig. 2B, *arrowheads*). It is clear that perforin molecules were secreted from the infiltrating cells and passed through a short distance (about 1 μm) of extracellular space, as shown in Fig. 2B, then reached the surface of a cardiac myocyte. Thus, it is strongly suggested that perforin attacks target cells by passing through an extracellular space, with subsequent insertion and polymerization in planar lipid bilayers of the target cell membrane.

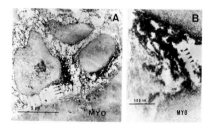

FIG. 2. Electron photomicrographs of the infiltrating cells, stained for perforin with immunoperoxidase, in the hearts of mice killed on day 7 after CVB3 infection. **A**: Note the expression of perforin in infiltrating cells on the side toward the surface of a cardiac myocyte (*MYo*) close by them (*arrows*). **B**: Higher magnification revealed that a large number of perforin molecules were released into the extracellular space between an infiltrating cell and a cardiac myocyte (*MYo*) and directly reached the surface of the cardiac myocyte (*arrowheads*). (Reproduced from Seko et al. (18) by copyright permission of John Wiley & Sons, Ltd.)

DEMONSTRATION OF PERFORIN PORES ON THE MEMBRANE OF CARDIAC MYOCYTES IN ACUTE MYOCARDITIS

Next, to confirm that perforin-mediated cardiac myocyte injury really occurred, we examined the ultrastructural circular lesions formed by perforin molecules on the membrane of cardiac myocytes. Heart ventricles of mice killed on day 7 after virus inoculation were fixed in 2% glutaraldehyde in PBS, and postfixed in 2% osmium tetroxide in PBS. Then, they were dehydrated in ethanol and embedded in resin. Ultrathin sections were prepared, and these were stained with uranyl acetate and lead citrate. To visualize the ultrastructure of the membrane of cardiac myocytes, the ultrathin sections were treated with 0.0125% trypsin in PBS for 2 hours at 37°C, after which they were examined with an electron microscope.

Figure 3 shows the electron micrographs of the membrane of cardiac myocytes in the ventricular tissues of CVB3-infected mice (day 7). As shown in Fig. 3A (*arrows*), there were several circular lesions with the morphologic characteristics of perforin pores formerly reported. Higher magnification revealed that these ring-like lesions formed pores with internal diameters of 15 to 20 nm, a feature that was almost uniform among the lesions (Fig. 3B, *arrows*). The pores formed by the membrane attack complex of complement have morphologic characteristics similar to those of perforin pores with internal diameters of about 10 nm (7). Because the pores formed by perforin are significantly larger than those formed by complement, we can distinguish these two kinds of lesions on the target membrane by electron microscopy. To exclude the possibility that these ring-like lesions were not formed by perforin but were merely artifacts, we also examined the ultrastructure of the membrane of cardiac myocytes of mice without CVB3 infection. There were no such ring-like lesions on the membrane of normal cardiac myocytes.

These data provide direct evidence that, in an early phase of acute myocarditis when virus genomes replicate in the heart, NK cells directly damage the virus-infected cardiac myocytes by the release of perforin. We have also found, by in situ hybridization, that these infiltrating NK cells strongly express cytokines, such as interferon-γ and tumor necrosis factor α (data not shown). Therefore, the infiltrating NK cells may induce MHC class I antigen and ICAM-1 on cardiac myocytes

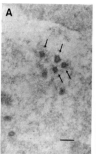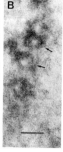

FIG. 3. Electron photomicrographs of the myocardial cell membranes in the hearts of mice killed on day 7 after CVB3 infection. **A**: There were several uniform, ring-like lesions on the membrane of a cardiac myocyte (*arrows*). Scale bar = 100 nm. **B**: Higher magnification revealed that the internal diameter of these ring-like lesions was 15 to 20 nm (*arrows*). Scale bar = 50 nm. (Reproduced from Seko et al. (18) by copyright permission of John Wiley & Sons, Ltd.)

around them, and may facilitate further myocardial cell damage by CTLs, which infiltrate the heart in a later phase.

EXPRESSION OF T-CELL RECEPTOR Vβ GENES IN INFILTRATING CELLS IN HEART AFFECTED BY ACUTE MYOCARDITIS

To clarify the immunologic mechanisms that may cause persistent damage to cardiac myocytes and that may lead to dilated cardiomyopathy, we investigated the pathophysiologic characteristics of the T-cell–mediated autoimmune process in a later phase, when virus genomes had almost disappeared.

In general, foreign antigens, such as viruses, are digested and degraded into peptide fragments in target cell cytoplasm and are then presented on the surface of the target cell membrane by MHC antigens. T cells recognize processed antigens specifically in conjunction with MHC molecules through their T-cell receptors (TCRs), consisting mostly of α and β chain heterodimers. The TCR α chain consists of variable, joining, and constant regions, whereas the β chain consists of variable, diverse, joining, and constant regions. These are designated as Vβ, Dβ, Jβ, and Cβ, respectively. The antigen specificity of the TCRs is defined by V domains encoded by variable, diverse, and joining gene elements that rearrange and join during T-cell differentiation. Recent studies in autoimmune diseases (13–15), allograft rejection (16), and malignant tumors (17) have shown that T cells involved in the local immune response use a limited range of TCR genes, indicating that these T cells interact with a specific antigen and play an important role in the pathologic process. In acute viral myocarditis, to determine the extent of TCR gene usage by the infiltrating cells, and to assess the characteristics of the virus-derived antigen expressed on the cardiac myocytes, we analyzed the expression of TCR Vβ genes in infiltrating cells in the heart using polymerase chain reaction (PCR). Table 1 shows the nucleotide sequences of the primers used for the detection of Vβ messenger RNAs (mRNAs). Twenty different Vβ-specific oligonucleotides, representing the major TCR Vβ subfamilies, were used for the 5′-primers, and a Cβ sequence was used for the 3′-primer. Mice were killed on day 12 after virus inoculation, and heart ventricles and spleen were removed and freshly frozen. Total cytoplasmic RNA was extracted from each sample and was reverse-transcribed with the 3′-Cβ primer. Then, the resulting complementary DNA (cDNA) was amplified by means of each Vβ primer and Cβ primer. After amplification for 30 cycles, we identified the PCR products by Southern blot hybridization using a cDNA probe of Cβ. We also examined the expression of TCR Vβ genes in peripheral blood lymphocytes (PBLs) from a mouse as a positive control.

Figure 4 shows the results of Southern blot hybridization of the PCR products from PBLs, spleen lymphocytes (*Spleen*), and infiltrating cells in the hearts (*Heart*) of mice with acute viral myocarditis. There was almost uniform expression of each Vβ segment except Vβ13, which is known to be only slightly expressed in this strain of mouse, in the PBLs. This result also indicates that all Vβ primers work

TABLE 1. *Sequences of primers used for polymerase chain reaction*

Primer	$5' \rightarrow 3'$ Sequence
Vβ1	TTCGAAATGAGACGGTGCCC
Vβ2	AGAGGTCAAATCTCTTCCCG
Vβ3	CTTCAGCAAATAGACATGAC
Vβ4	TGGACAATCAGACTGCCTCA
vβ5.1	GAGATAAAGGAAACCTGCCC
Vβ5.2	GAGACAAAGGATTCCTACCC
Vβ6	CGACAGGATTCAGGGAAAGG
Vβ7	ATACAGGGTCTCACGGAAGA
Vβ8.1	CATATGTCGCTGACAGCACG
Vβ8.2	CATATGGTGCTGGCAGCACT
Vβ8.3	CATATGGTGCTGGCAACCTT
Vβ9	ACAGGGAAGCTGACACTTTT
Vβ10	AATCAAGTCTGTAGAGCCGG
Vβ11	GGAGTCCCTGACTTACTTTC
Vβ12	AAGATGGTGGGGCTTTCAAG
Vβ13	TCTATAACAGTTGCCCTCGG
Vβ14	CCTCCAGCAACTCTTCTACT
Vβ15	CGCCTCAAAAGGCATTTGAA
Vβ16	CAGCAGATGGAGTTTCTGGT
Vβ17a	ACAGACTTGGTCAAGAAGAG
Cβ	AGGATCTCATAGAGGATGGT

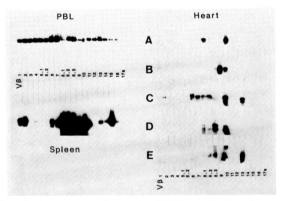

FIG. 4. Detection of polymerase chain reaction (PCR)-amplified products by Southern blot hybridization using a cDNA probe of T-cell receptor Cβ on peripheral blood lymphocytes (*PBL*), spleen lymphocytes (*Spleen*), and infiltrating cells in the hearts (*Heart*) of mice on day 12 after CVB3 infection. There was almost uniform expression of each Vβ gene in the PBLs, whereas heterogeneous expression among the Vβ genes was found in the spleen. Note that only a few Vβ genes were expressed in the infiltrating cells in the hearts of five mice (*A to E*) with acute myocarditis.

effectively. There was heterogeneous expression among the Vβ genes in the spleen lymphocytes. Some of the Vβ genes were not expressed. By contrast, only few Vβ genes were expressed in the infiltrating cells in the hearts of five mice killed on day 12 after virus inoculation. In particular, Vβ10 was expressed in all five hearts. Vβ8.3 and Vβ13 were expressed in two of the five hearts. The restricted usage of TCR Vβ genes in the infiltrating cells strongly suggests that a specific antigen in the heart of viral myocarditis is targeted. Next, to investigate whether the infiltrating T cells really express a restricted repertoire of TCR Vβ gene products, especially Vβ10, we stained with immunoperoxidase the serial sections of the hearts of mice with myocarditis on day 12 for TCR αβ chain and that of Vβ10, respectively. Comparing the rate of the infiltrating cells that were positive for TCR αβ chain and those positive for Vβ10, we were able to confirm that the infiltrating T cells predominantly expressed Vβ10 gene products (data not shown). Studies of murine experimental allergic encephalomyelitis (13,14) have demonstrated that the myelin basic protein-specific T-cell clones predominantly used TCR Vβ8, and that in vivo administration of anti-Vβ8 antibody significantly suppressed the induction of this autoimmune disease. In viral myocarditis, our data also offer a possible in vivo antibody therapy specific for the TCR Vβ gene products against T-cell–mediated myocardial cell damage in a later phase.

Furthermore, to investigate the mechanism by which these T cells cause damage to cardiac myocytes expressing a virus-derived antigen on their surfaces, we examined the expression of perforin in infiltrating CTLs. We double-stained the heart samples of mice with myocarditis on day 12 for CD8 (Lyt 2) and perforin. We found that perforin was also clearly expressed in CD8-positive CTLs (data not shown).

SUMMARY

Cell-mediated autoimmunity has been strongly implicated in the pathogenesis of the myocardial cell damage involved in viral myocarditis, but the underlying mechanism has not been clarified. Our data have revealed that, after virus infection, NK cells infiltrate the heart in an early phase, directly killing virus-infected cardiac myocytes by the release of perforin. They also induce MHC class I antigen and ICAM-1 on cardiac myocytes around them by releasing cytokines, such as interferon-γ and tumor necrosis factor-α. In a later phase, when virus genomes almost disappear from the heart, Th cells, and then CTLs, infiltrate the heart. These cells recognize a virus-derived antigen presented on the membrane of cardiac myocytes in conjunction with MHC antigen specifically through their TCRs mainly consisting of Vβ10 gene products, and they may cause persistent damage to the cardiac myocytes by the release of perforin. The restricted usage of TCR genes in the infiltrating cells strongly suggests that a specific antigen in the heart of mice with myocarditis is targeted. Considering the immunopathology involved in dilated cardiomyopathy as the consequence of viral myocarditis, we hypothesize that persistent expression of MHC antigen and ICAM-1 on cardiac myocytes enables them to be antigen-present-ing cells for cellular immunity which may cause chronic inflammation. This process may lead to chronic destruction of the contractile elements of cardiac muscles and replacement with fibrous tissues, and may finally lead to dilated cardiomyopathy. The cellular and molecular basis for both target cells and immune effector cells for cell-mediated cytotoxicity revealed in this study may explain, at least in part, the pathogenesis of acute viral myocarditis and dilated cardiomyopathy.

REFERENCES

1. Woodruff JF, Woodruff JJ. Involvement of T lymphocytes in the pathogenesis of coxsackievirus B3 heart disease. *J Immunol* 1974;113:1726–1734.
2. Woodruff JF. Viral myocarditis: a review. *Am J Pathol* 1980;101:427–484.
3. Guthrie M, Lodge PA, Huber SA. Cardiac injury in myocarditis induced by coxsackievirus group B, type 3 in Balb/c mice is mediated by Lyt 2$^+$ cytolytic lymphocytes. *Cell Immunol* 1984;88:558–567.
4. Seko Y, Shinkai Y, Kawasaki A, et al. Expression of perforin in infiltrating cells in murine hearts with acute myocarditis caused by coxsackievirus B3. *Circulation* 1991;84:788–795.
5. Seko Y, Tsuchimochi H, Nakamura T, et al. Expression of major histocompatibility complex class I antigen in murine ventricular myocytes infected with coxsackievirus B3. *Circ Res* 1990;67:360–367.
6. Seko Y, Yamazaki T, Shinkai Y, et al. Cellular and molecular bases for the immunopathology of the myocardial cell damage involved in acute viral myocarditis with special references to dilated cardiomyopathy. *Jpn Circ J* 1992;56:1062–1072.
7. Young JDE. Killing of target cells by lymphocytes: a mechanistic view. *Physiol Rev* 1989;69:250–314.
8. Dennert G, Anderson CG, Prochazka G. High activity of N$^\alpha$-benzyloxycarbonyl-L-lysine thiobenzyl ester serine esterase and cytolytic perforin in cloned cell lines is not demonstrable in in vivo-induced cytotoxic effector cells. *Proc Natl Acad Sci USA* 1987;84:5004–5008.
9. Young JDE, Clark WR, Liu CC, Cohn ZA. A calcium- and perforin-independent pathway of killing mediated by murine cytotoxic lymphocytes. *J Exp Med* 1987;166:1894–1899.
10. Berke G, Rosen D. Highly lytic in vivo primed cytotoxic T lymphocytes devoid of lytic granules and BLT-esterase activity acquire these constituents in the presence of T cell growth factor upon blast transformation in vitro. *J Immunol* 1988;141:1429–1436.
11. Young LHY, Klavinskis LS, Oldstone MBA, Young JDE. In vivo expression of perforin by CD8$^+$ lymphocytes during an acute viral infection. *J Exp Med* 1989;169:2159–2171.
12. Young LHY, Peterson LB, Wicker LS, Persechini PM, Young JDE. In vivo expression of perforin by CD8$^+$ lymphocytes in autoimmune disease: studies on spontaneous and adoptively transferred diabetes in nonobese diabetic mice. *J Immunol* 1989;143:3994–3999.
13. Acha-Orbea H, Mitchell DJ, Timmermann L, et al. Limited heterogeneity of T cell receptors from lymphocytes mediating autoimmune encephalomyelitis allows specific immune intervention. *Cell* 1988;54:263–273.
14. Urban JL, Kumar V, Kono DH, et al. Restricted use of T cell receptor V genes in murine autoimmune encephalomyelitis raises possibility for antibody therapy. *Cell* 1988;54:577–592.
15. Paliard X, West SG, Lafferty JA, et al. Evidence for the effects of a superantigen in rheumatoid arthritis. *Science* 1991;253:325–329.
16. Miceli MC, Finn OJ. T cell receptor β-chain selection in human allograft rejection. *J Immunol* 1989;142:81–86.
17. Nitta T, Oksenberg JR, Rao NA, Steinman L. Predominant expression of T cell receptor Vα7 in tumor-infiltrating lymphocytes of uveal melanoma. *Science* 1990;249:672–674.
18. Seko Y, Shinkai Y, Kawasaki A, et al. Evidence of perforin-mediated cardiac myocyte injury in acute murine myocarditis caused by coxsackie virus B3. *J Pathol* 1993;170:53–58.

The Cardiomyopathic Heart, edited by Makoto
Nagano, Nobuakira Takeda, and Naranjan S.
Dhalla. Raven Press, Ltd., New York © 1994.

30

Morphologic Aspects of Experimental Autoimmune Myocarditis

T. Izumi, M. Kodama, H. Hanawa, S. Zhang, M. Saeki, and
A. Shibata

*First Department of Internal Medicine, Niigata University School of Medicine,
Niigata 951, Japan*

INTRODUCTION

Foot spots of autoimmune disorders in the heart have been already indicated in patients with myocarditis and dilated cardiomyopathy (1,2). Through these clinical studies, some cardiac proteins have been suggested as possible self-antigens, which may provoke the muscle cell damage through an autoimmunologic mechanism. These cardiac proteins include myosin, actin (3), adenosine diphosphate (ADP)/ adenosine triphosphate (ATP) carrier protein (4), SRA protein (5), laminin (6), and others. Recently, our interest has been focused on the ability of cardiac myosin to induce myocarditis (7–9).

MYOCARDITIS PROVOKED BY CARDIAC MYOSIN

The myosin fraction was isolated from human hearts according to the method of Murakami and colleagues (10). This cardiac myosin fraction was injected into 6-week-old Lewis rats at a dosage of 5 mg/kg of body weight; booster immunization was administered 1 week later (11). The rats that were immunized with cardiac myosin were sacrificed on the 21st day after the first immunization. Autopsy results revealed massive pericardial effusion, yellow-whitish discolored hearts, and liver congestion. Histologic examination revealed diseased cardiac tissue, with evidence of serious cell infiltrates and extensive myocardial necrosis (Fig. 1). In some, the inflammatory lesions penetrated the whole cardiac wall from the epicardium to the endocardium. In most of the rats, the myocarditis predominantly affected the right ventricle rather than the left.

Some of the rats in which this experimental autoimmune myocarditis was induced had a lethal clinical course. Most of the animals studied were found to be immo-

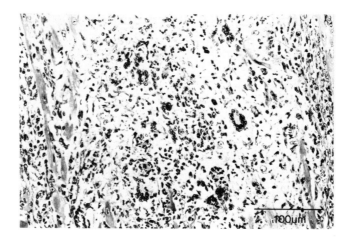

FIG. 1. On the histologic level, the cardiac tissue was found to be diseased, as evidenced by cell infiltrates and extensive myocardial necrosis. In the areas of the myocardium that sustained extensive damage, multinucleated giant cells were seen.

bilized in the corner of the cage on the 16th day after the first immunization, and displayed ruffled fur and quick breathing. Of these, some rats died of symptomatic heart failure. After 42 days, the rats had clinically recovered from the disease. This myocarditis has already been found to be transferable into healthy syngeneic rats using T lymphocyte, but has not been transferable using immunoglobulin (12).

INFILTRATES INTO THE MYOCARDIUM

Immunohistologic examination revealed that 70% of the infiltrates were positive for the monoclonal cell surface antibody, OX42 (Serotec, UK), a representative macrophage marker. Ultrastructurally, the macrophages were approximately 10 μm in diameter, with an oval or irregularly shaped nucleus and abundant phagocytotic vacuoles containing highly dense materials (Fig. 2). Using acid phosphatase staining, the distribution of macrophages was investigated. The macrophages were located not only in the center of inflammatory lesions, but also in the interstitial space, free from the myocardial necrosis. In the infiltrates, the macrophages were clustered, but in the interstitium, they were scattered among the myofibers. Most of the macrophages in the inflammatory lesions were negative for ED2 (Serotec, UK), a specific antibody for the tissue-fixed macrophage. The cells in these lesions must have been free macrophages that had immigrated from the blood. By contrast, the macrophages in the interstitium were positive for ED2, and thus were of the tissue-fixed type.

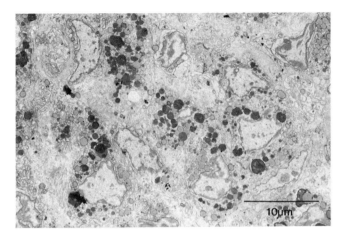

FIG. 2. Ultrastructural examination revealed that the macrophages were approximately 10 μm in diameter, with an oval or irregularly shaped nucleus and abundant phagocytotic vacuoles containing highly dense materials.

CLOSE CONTACT WITH THE CARDIOCYTE

Among the OX42-positive cells, there were also cells that were stained with OX6 (Serotec, UK) that were detectable. These major histocompatibility complex II-positive cells were distributed not only in the interstitium of the cardiac myofiber, but also in the inflammatory lesion on ultrastructural examination, these cells were approximately 10 μml in size, with an irregularly shaped nucleus and a relatively clear cytoplasma compared with the macrophages mentioned earlier. Remarkably, the cell membrane was found to be invaginating in a complicated configuration. Morphologically, these cells were determined to be dendritic cells in the heart. Interestingly, the cells were in close contact to the cardiocyte (Fig. 3).

CD4 T lymphocytes were seen in 20% of the infiltrates. Only a few CD8 T cells were present, and B cells were quite rare. Ultrastructurally, the T cells were also in close contact with the cardiocyte, and in some places, the cells had invaded into the diseased myocyte (Fig. 4).

MULTINUCLEATED GIANT CELL

In the areas of severe inflammation associated with myocardial necrosis, multinucleated giant cells were found in this animal model (see Fig. 1), and this unique figure characterizes the experimental autoimmune myocarditis (13). The giant cells were stained with acid phosphatase for histochemical examination. The surface antigen was positive for OX42. From these data, it was determined that these multi-

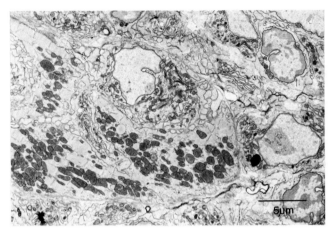

FIG. 3. Large cells with membranes invaginating in a complicated configuration were seen. This dendritic cell was in close contact with the cardiocyte in some places.

nucleated giant cells were derived from the macrophage. On ultrastructural examination, giant cells were confirmed to be constructed through cytofusion with several macrophages (Fig. 5). Between the nuclei, the unit membrane was not present as the boundary of two cells.

CONCLUSION

Morphologic studies have revealed the following:

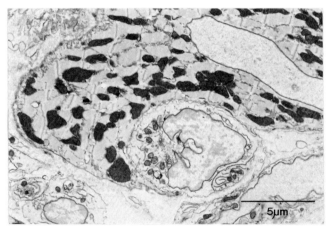

FIG. 4. The T lymphocytes were in close contact with the cardiocyte, and its invasion into the diseased myocyte was documented.

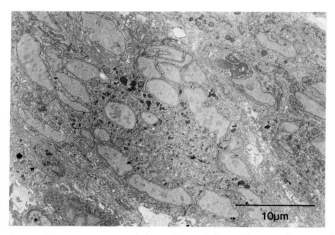

FIG. 5. The giant cells were constructed through cytofusion with several macrophages. Between the nuclei, the unit membrane was not present as the boundary of two cells.

(a) The rat model of experimental autoimmune myocarditis is characterized by cell infiltrates, myocardial necrosis, and the occurrence of multinucleated giant cells.

(b) With respect to the cellular effector of the myocarditis, three kinds of cells—namely, macrophages, dendritic cells, and T lymphocytes—were implicated.

(c) Close contacts with the cardiocyte were seen in both dendritic cells and T lymphocytes.

(d) Multinucleated giant cells among the areas affected by myocardial necrosis were remarkable, as these cells were found to represent cytofusion of several macrophages.

SUMMARY

Recently, our interest has been focused on whether cardiac myosin can cause myocarditis. The myosin, isolated from human hearts, is injected into Lewis rats at a dosage of 5 mg/kg of body weight. Most of the immunized rats showed symptomatic heart failure, and some of them died from the condition. This myocarditis was transferable into healthy syngeneic rats using T lymphocytes, but not with the IgG fraction of the sera. Histologic examination revealed that inflammatory cells had infiltrated into the cardiac wall, causing extensive muscle necrosis. Of the infiltrates, 70% were composed of macrophage, 20% were CD4 cells, a few were CD8 T cells, and B cells were quite rare. This lethal autoimmune myocarditis was characterized by the occurrence of giant cells, which have been proven to be derived from macrophages. Ultrastructurally, the occurrence of dendritic cells was remarkable, and both the dendritic cells and T lymphocytes were in close contact with the cardiocyte.

ACKNOWLEDGMENTS

We sincerely thank Dr. Y. Matsumoto (Niigata University) for his immunologic advice, and Drs. A. Fujiwara, S. Motoda (Denkaseiken Co.), E. Okazaki (Niigata Shimin Hospital) and H. Tsunoda (Niigata Cancer Center) for preparation of human cardiac myosin. This investigation was supported in part by a grant for scientific research (No. 03670444) from the Ministry of Education, Science, and Culture of Japan.

REFERENCES

1. Maisch B, Trostel-Soeder R, Stechemesser E, Berg PA, Kochsiek K. Diagnostic relevance of humoral and cell-mediated immune reactions in patients with acute viral myocarditis. *Clin Exp Immunol* 1982;48:533–545.
2. Caforio ALP, Bonifacio E, Stewart JT, Neglia D, Parodi O, Bottazzo GF, McKenna W. Novel organ-specific circulating cardiac antibodies in dilated cardiomyopathy. *J Am Coll Cardiol* 1990; 15:1527–1534.
3. Beisel KW. Immunogenetic basis of myocarditis: role of fibrillary antigens. *Springer Semin Immunopathol* 1989;11:31–42.
4. Schulze K, Becker BF, Schultheiss HP. Antibodies to the ADP/ATP carrier, an autoantigen in myocarditis and dilated cardiomyopathy, penetrate into myocardial cells and disturb energy metabolism in vivo. *Circ Res* 1989;64:179–192.
5. Acosta AM, Santos-Buch CA. Autoimmune myocarditis induced by Trypanosoma cruzi. *Circulation* 1985;71:1255–1261.
6. Wolff PG, Kuehl U, Schultheiss HP. Laminin distribution and autoantibodies to laminin in dilated cardiomyopathy and myocarditis. *Am Heart J* 1989;117:1303–1309.
7. Kodama M, Izumi T. Experimental autoimmune myocarditis. *Acta Med Biol* 1991;39:1–10.
8. Izumi T, Kodama M, Fujiwara M. Cardiac muscle cell damage through autoimmune mechanism—can cardiac proteins provoke autoimmune myocarditis? *Jpn Circ J* 1991;55:1138–1143.
9. Izumi T, Kodama M, Shibata A. Experimental giant cell myocarditis induced by cardiac myosin immunization. *Eur Heart J* 1991;12 [Suppl B]: 166–168.
10. Murakami U, Uchida K, Hiratuka K. Cardiac myosin from pig heart ventricle: purification and enzymatic properties. *J Biochem* 1976;80:611–619.
11. Kodama M, Matsumoto Y, Fujiwara M, Masani F, Izumi T, Shibata A. A novel experimental model of giant cell myocarditis induced in rats by immunization with cardiac myosin fraction. *Clin Immunol Immunopathol* 1990;57:250–262.
12. Kodama M, Matsumoto Y, Fujiwara M. In vivo lymphocyte-mediated myocardial injuries demonstrated by adoptive transfer of experimental autoimmune myocarditis. *Circulation* 1992;85:1918–1926.
13. Kodama M, Matsumoto Y, Fujiwara M, et al. Characteristics of giant cells and factors related to the formation of giant cells in myocarditis. *Circ Res* 1991;69:1042–1050.

The Cardiomyopathic Heart, edited by Makoto
Nagano, Nobuakira Takeda, and Naranjan S.
Dhalla. Raven Press, Ltd., New York © 1994.

31

Adoptive Transfer of Experimental Giant Cell Myocarditis into Normal Syngeneic Rats

*†Makoto Kodama, *Haruo Hanawa, *Shaosong Zhang,
*Makihiko Saeki, ‡Sen Koyama, *Hiroyuki Hosono,
*Tohru Izumi, and *Akira Shibata

*First Department of Internal Medicine, Niigata University School of Medicine,
Niigata 951; †Department of Medical Technology, The College of Biomedical Technology
of Niigata University, Niigata 951; and ‡Tachikawa Hospital, Nagaoka 940, Japan

INTRODUCTION

Giant cell myocarditis is a severe and frequently fatal inflammatory heart disease (1). The etiology of the disease remains unknown (2). It is also not known whether giant cell myocarditis is a disease entity that is distinct from viral myocarditis or other etiologically specific myocarditic conditions (3). Recently, antiheart antibodies have been detected in the serum of a patient with this disease (4). There have been several reports that giant cell myocarditis can be effectively treated with immunosuppressants (5,6). Occasionally, giant cell myocarditis is complicated by various immunologic disorders (7–10). Therefore, the autoimmune system is speculated to have a role in the pathogenesis of giant cell myocarditis (11).

Recently, we have reported on a new animal model for autoimmune myocarditis (12). Lewis rats immunized with cardiac myosin in complete Freund's adjuvant developed severe myocarditis characterized by congestive heart failure, enlargement of the heart, and the appearance of multinucleated giant cells. The clinical course and pathologic findings closely resembled those of human giant cell myocarditis (13). Experimental autoimmune myocarditis showed both types of myocarditis—giant cell and non-giant cell—depending on the phase of the disease, the severity of the disease, and the immunoadjuvants used.

Several experimental autoimmune diseases have been established in susceptible animals by immunization with organ-specific antigen in complete Freund's adjuvant (14). Most of those organ-specific autoimmune diseases have been demonstrated to be transferable into syngeneic animals using autoantibodies or T cells (15–21). In order to elucidate the pathogenesis of experimental autoimmune giant cell myocarditis, we examined whether the myocarditis could be transferred into normal Lewis rats using immunoglobulin fractions or lymphocytes from the rats previously immunized with cardiac myosin.

METHODS

Animals

Lewis rats were purchased from Charles River Japan, Inc. (Atsugi, Kanagawa, Japan). They were maintained at the Facilities for Comparative Medicine and Animal Experimentation, Niigata University School of Medicine.

Antigen

Purified cardiac myosin was used as the antigen. Cardiac myosin was prepared from the ventricular muscle of human hearts according to the procedure described previously (12).

Induction of Experimental Myocarditis

Cardiac myosin was dissolved at a concentration of 10 mg/mL in phosphate-buffered saline (PBS) containing 0.3 M of KCl. The antigen solution was mixed with an equal volume of complete Freund's adjuvant supplemented with *Mycobacterium tuberculosis* H37Ra (Difco, Detroit, MI) at a concentration of 11 mg/mL. Lewis rats received an injection of 0.2 mL of antigen-adjuvant emulsion in their footpads. The rats received intravenous injections of 1.0 mL of *Bordetella pertussis* vaccine (2×10^9/mL) (Nacalai Tesque, Kyoto, Japan) on days 1 and 3. The rats were immunized again after 7 days (13).

Humoral Transfer

On day 21, serum was collected from the rats that had been immunized with cardiac myosin. These animals showed severe myocarditis at the time of sacrifice. Saturated ammonium sulfate solutions, adjusted to a pH of 7.0, was added to the serum, and the fraction under 33% saturation was collected. After dialysis against PBS, the immunoglobulin fraction was reconstituted with PBS. The protein concentration of this solution was 3.5 mg/mL. The titer of antibodies against cardiac myosin was measured by enzyme-linked immunosorbent assay (ELISA), and this solution tested positive until a dilution of 1,600:1 was reached. Naive syngeneic rats were intraperitoneally injected with 4.5 mL of this solution. Passive myocarditis was assessed on days 14 and 28.

Cellular Transfer

Spleens and lymph nodes were removed from the rats with overt myocarditis, and a single cell suspension was prepared by passing through a stainless steel mesh screen. After washing three times with RPMI-1640, cells were cultured for 3 days at a density of 2×10^6 cells/mL in RPMI-1640 that had been supplemented with 10% fetal bovine serum. 1% sodium pyruvate, 1% nonessential amino acids (GIBCO Laboratories), 0.4% (vol/vol) of penicillin-streptomycin mixture (Bioproducts, Inc., MD), 5×10^{-5} M of 2-mercaptoethanol, and 1 μg/mL of concanavalin A (Con A) (Sigma Chemical, St. Louis, MO). Viable cultured spleen cells or lymph node cells at doses of 3×10^6, 1×10^7, and 3×10^7 were intravenously injected into syngeneic rats. Recipient rats were killed on day 11 or 14 for histologic examination. The effects of another mitogen on activation of myocarditogenic lymphocytes were investigated using LPS.

Histopathology

All rats were killed using ether anesthesia. Hearts were removed immediately after sacrifice. A part of the ventricular muscle was fixed in 10% formalin and embedded in paraffin. Several transverse sections were cut from paraffin-embedded samples and stained with hematoxylin and eosin.

RESULTS

Induction of Experimental Autoimmune Giant Cell Myocarditis

The rats immunized with cardiac myosin became ill by the third week. Rats were killed and sacrificed on day 21. All the rats immunized with cardiac myosin showed macroscopic evidence of myocarditis at sacrifice. Most of them had a large amount of pericardial effusion. In all of these rats, the heart was markedly enlarged. White discolored patches were observed on the surface of the hearts (Fig. 1). The discolored areas did not correspond to the coronary perfusion territories. Histologic examination revealed extensive myocardial necrosis and cellular infiltrations. The inflammatory lesions were composed of macrophages, lymphocytes, polymorphonuclear neutrophils, and fragments of degenerated myocardial fibers. Frequently, multinucleated giant cells were observed in the lesions (Fig. 2).

Humoral Transfer

Rats injected with immunoglobulin fractions were as active as normal Lewis rats. Pericardial effusion or other macroscopic findings of myocarditis were not detected

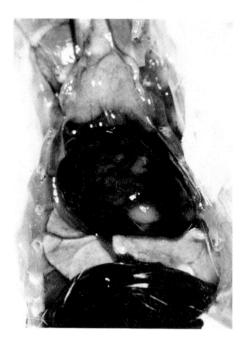

FIG. 1. The findings after thoracotomy in the rats immunized with cardiac myosin. Pericardial effusion and white discoloration of the heart were observed.

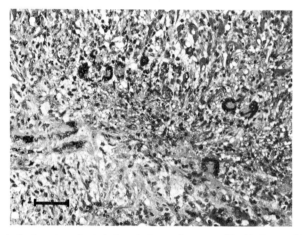

FIG. 2. Histologic findings in actively induced giant cell myocarditis. Various cell infiltrations and extensive myocardial necrosis were observed. Multinucleated giant cells frequently appeared in the lesions. Scale bar = 60 μm.

TABLE 1. *Transfer of autoimmune giant cell myocarditis*

Groups	Day of sacrifice	Total	Diseased	Rate (%)
Immunoglobulin G fraction	14	4	0	0
Immunoglobulin G fraction	28	4	0	0
Concanavalin A: spleen (1×10^7)	14	5	4	80
Concanavalin A: lymph node (3×10^6)	14	7	3	43
Concanavalin A: lymph node (3×10^7)	11	6	6	100
Lipopolysaccharide: lymph node (3×10^7)	14	3	0	0

in the rats injected with humoral factors. Neither inflammatory infiltration nor myocardial necrosis were observed (Table 1).

Cellular Transfer

The activity level and food intake of rats injected with activated lymphocytes from rats previously immunized with cardiac myosin were found to be decreased by the second week. Most of the rats injected with activated T cells had pericardial effusion at sacrifice. The degree of enlargement of the heart and the extent of the discolored areas of the heart in rats injected with activated T cells were similar to that observed in the rats immunized with cardiac myosin (Fig. 3). Histologic studies revealed extensive myocardial necrosis and various kinds of inflammatory infiltra-

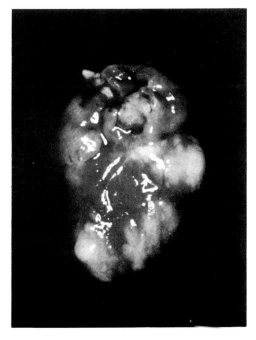

FIG. 3. Macroscopic findings in passively transferred giant cell myocarditis. The heart was enlarged and areas of white discoloration were noted on its surface.

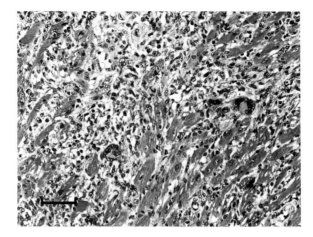

FIG. 4. Histologic findings in the hearts of rats injected with activated lymph node cells. Mononuclear cell infiltration with myocardial necrosis was observed. Multinucleated giant cells were also detected in the lesions. Scale bar = 60 μm.

tions. Multinucleated giant cells were also detected in the lesions (Fig. 4). The histologic findings associated with transferred myocarditis were the same as those for actively induced myocarditis. All of the rats injected with 3×10^7 of Con A-activated lymph node cells developed severe myocarditis on day 11 (see Table 1). Of the five rats injected with 1×10^7 of Con A-activated spleen cells, four showed myocarditis on day 14. However, none of the rats injected with LPS-stimulated lymph node cells developed induced myocarditis.

DISCUSSION

Autoimmune involvement has been postulated in the pathogenesis of myocarditis and dilated cardiomyopathy (22,23). In order to elucidate the precise pathogenesis of autoimmune myocardial injuries, various forms of experimental autoimmune myocarditis have been proposed during the past 30 years (24). The experimental autoimmune myocarditis in rats described in this study has several unique features not established in previous models, including the following:

(a) The clinical course, which was characterized by congestive heart failure
(b) The extremely severe pathologic findings, as evidenced by pericardial effusion and macroscopic evidence of myocarditis
(c) The appearance of multinucleated giant cells in the lesions

(d) The uniformity of effect, as all rats immunized with cardiac myosin developed myocarditis

(e) The distinct susceptibility for this myocarditis among species and strains

What is the effector of myocardial injuries in autoimmune giant cell myocarditis? In several experimental autoimmune diseases, adoptive transfer of the diseases into syngeneic animals has been demonstrated using antibodies or T cells. However, a similar phenomenon has not been precisely demonstrated with regard to myocarditis. In the present study, we have demonstrated that experimental autoimmune giant cell myocarditis is transferable by Con A-activated lymphocytes, not by antibodies. Furthermore, this study showed that LPS-activated lymphocytes—namely, B cells—could not transfer the disease into normal syngeneic rats. Therefore, the effector of experimental giant cell myocarditis in rats appears to be T cells. Recently, this premise was supported by a murine model of myosin-induced autoimmune myocarditis (25).

Previously, we had reported that the onset of actively induced experimental giant cell myocarditis occurred between day 14 and day 16 after the first immunization. In this study, all rats injected with Con A-activated lymph node cells developed severe myocarditis on day 11. Thus, the onset of transferred myocarditis is apparently earlier than that of actively induced myocarditis. Although the precise pathogenesis of this myocarditis has not been analyzed, we propose the following explanation. The first step of this disease is probably an expansion of myocarditogenic T-cell clones in the rats immunized with cardiac myosin. When myocarditogenic T-cell clones expand far enough, they spread in the systemic circulation. The next step seems to be recruitment of effector T cells to the target organs, at which time effector-target interactions may be provoked. In adoptively transferred myocarditis, the initial expansion steps of myocarditogenic T cells is not necessary; thus, the pathogenetic onset of transferred myocarditis occurs earlier than that of actively induced myocarditis.

From the results presented in this study, it is evident that this rat model closely resembles human giant cell myocarditis in terms of clinical course and pathologic findings. Therefore, some human giant cell myocarditis may have the same etiology and pathogenesis as this model. The evidence for autoimmunity is rather obscure in clinical investigation. The elucidation of this evidence may lead to diagnostic information on autoimmune myocarditis—that is, whether cardiac T cells that are reactive to myosin exist in the peripheral blood of affected patients (26). If autoimmune myocarditis can be distinguished from other forms of myocarditis during the patient's life, it would be possible to treat them more effectively (27,28). The pathogenesis of this myocarditis is probably similar to that of experimental allergic encephalomyelitis (29). Accordingly, the relationship between experimental allergic encephalomyelitis and multiple sclerosis may be similar to that between experimental autoimmune myocarditis and some forms of human myocarditis and dilated cardiomyopathy (30,31). Thus, the pathogenesis of this experimental model offers new insights into the clinical study of myocarditis and cardiomyopathy.

SUMMARY

In order to eludicate the pathogenesis of giant cell myocarditis, we examined whether experimental giant cell myocarditis was passively transferable into normal syngeneic animals by humoral or cellular factors. Experimental giant cell myocarditis was elicited in Lewis rats by immunization with cardiac myosin in complete Freund's adjuvant. This myocarditis was characterized by congestive heart failure and the appearance of multinucleated giant cells in the lesions. Adoptive transfer of this disease by humoral factors was examined using immunoglobulin fractions from rats with severe myocarditis. Adoptive transfer by cellular factors was tested using spleen cells and lymph node cells from the rats with actively induced myocarditis. Immunoglobulin fraction could not elicit myocarditis in recipient rats. However, intravenous injection of spleen cells and lymph node cells that had been cultured in medium containing concanavalin A were able to elicit severe myocarditis. Macroscopic and microscopic findings of adoptively transferred myocarditis were the same as those found in actively induced myocarditis. Sufficient doses of viable cells for adoptive transfer were 1×10^7 of spleen cells and 3×10^6 of lymph node cells. The onset of adoptively transferred myocarditis occurred by the 11th day, which is apparently earlier than actively induced myocarditis occurs. Lymphocytes cultured with lipopolysaccharide were not able to transfer the disease into naive syngeneic rats. This study demonstrated direct evidence for in vivo T-cell–mediated myocardial injuries in experimental giant cell myocarditis.

ACKNOWLEDGMENT

This study was supported in part by the Japan Heart Foundation Research Grant for 1991.

REFERENCES

1. Davies MJ, Pomerance A, Teare RD. Idiopathic giant cell myocarditis—a distinctive clinico-pathological entity. *Br Heart J* 1975;37:192–195.
2. Davidoff R, Palacios I, Southern J, Fallon JT, Newell J. Dec GW. Giant cell versus lymphocytic myocarditis. A comparison of their clinical features and long-term outcomes. *Circulation* 1991;83:953–961.
3. Lieberman EB, Hutchins GM, Herskowitz A, Rose NR, Baughman KL. Clinicopathologic description of myocarditis. *J Am Coll Cardiol* 1991;18:1617–1626.
4. Humbert P, Faivre R, Fellman D, Bassand JP, Dupond JL. Giant cell myocarditis: an autoimmune disease? *Am Heart J* 1988;115:485–487.
5. Costanzo-Nordin MR, Silver MA, O'Connell JB, Scanlon PJ, Robinson JA. Giant cell myocarditis: dramatic hemodynamic and histologic improvement with immunosuppressive therapy. *Eur Heart J* 1987;8[Suppl J]:271–274.
6. McFalls EO, Hosenpud JD, McAnulty JH, Kron J, Niles NR. Granulomatous myocarditis. Diagnosis by endomyocardial biopsy and response to corticosteroids in two patients. *Chest* 1986;89:509–511.
7. Hales SA, Theaker JM, Gatter KC. Giant cell myocarditis associated with lymphoma: an immunohistochemical study. *J Clin Pathol* 1987;40:1310–1313.

8. McKeon J, Haagsma B, Nicholas Bett JH, Boyle CM. Fatal giant cell myocarditis after colectomy for ulcerative colitis. *Am Heart J* 1986;111:1208–1209.
9. Burke JS, Medline NM, Katz A. Giant cell myocarditis and myositis. Associated with thymoma and myasthenia gravis. *Arch Pathol* 1969;88:359–366.
10. Kloin JE. Pernicious anemia and giant cell myocarditis. New association. *Am J Med* 1985;78:355–360.
11. Wilson MS, Barth RF, Baker PB, Unverferth DV, Kolibash AJ. Giant cell myocarditis. *Am J Med* 1985;79:647–652.
12. Kodama M, Matsumoto Y, Fujiwara M, Masani F, Izumi T, Shibata A. A novel experimental model of giant cell myocarditis induced in rats by immunization with cardiac myosin fraction. *Clin Immunol Immunopathol* 1990;57:250–262.
13. Kodama M, Matsumoto Y, Fujiwara M, et al. Characteristics of giant cells and factors related to the formation of giant cells in myocarditis. *Circ Res* 1991;69:1042–1050.
14. Matsumoto Y, Fujiwara M. Adoptively transferred experimental allergic encephalomyelitis in chimeric rats: identification of transferred cells in the lesions of the central nervous system. *Immunology* 1988;65:23–29.
15. Panitch HS. Adoptive transfer of experimental allergic encephalomyelitis with activated spleen cells: comparison of in vitro activation by concanavalin A and myelin basic protein. *Cell Immunol* 1980;56:163–171.
16. Mann R, Zakheim B, Clayman M, McCafferty E, Michaud L, Neilson EG. Murine interstitial nephritis. 4. Long-term cultured L3T4$^+$ T cell lines transfer delayed expression of disease as I-A-restricted inducers of the effector T cell repertoire. *J Immunol* 1985;135:286–293.
17. Linington C, Izumo S, Suzuki M, Uyemura K, Meyermann R, Wekerle H. A permanent rat T cell line that mediates experimental allergic neuritis in the Lewis rat in vivo. *J Immunol* 1984;133:1946–1950.
18. Romball CG, Weigle WO. Transfer of experimental autoimmune thyroiditis with T cell clones. *J Immunol* 1987;138:1092–1098.
19. Ogawa M, Mori Y, Mori T, et al. Adoptive transfer of experimental autoimmune hepatitis in mice—cellular interaction between donor and recipient mice. *Clin Exp Immunol* 1988;73:276–282.
20. Holoshitz J, Naparstek Y, Ben-Nun A, Cohen IR. Lines of T lymphocytes induce and vaccinate against autoimmune arthritis. *Science* 1983;219:56–58.
21. Caspi RR, Roberge FG, McAllister CG, et al. T cell lines mediating experimental autoimmune uveoretinitis (EAU) in the rat. *J Immunol* 1986;136:928–933.
22. Caforio AP, Bonifacio E, Stewart JT, et al. Novel organ-specific circulating cardiac autoantibodies in dilated cardiomyopathy. *J Am Coll Cardiol* 1990;15:1527–1534.
23. Neumann DA, Burek CL, Baughman KL, Rose NR, Herskowitz A. Circulating heart-reactive antibodies in patients with myocarditis or cardiomyopathy. *J Am Coll Cardiol* 1990;16:839–846.
24. Kodama M, Izumi T. Experimental autoimmune myocarditis. *Acta Med Biol* 1991;39:1–10.
25. Smith SC, Allen PM. Myosin induced myocarditis is a T cell mediated disease. *J Immunol* 1991;147:2141–2147.
26. Allegretta M, Nicklas JA, Sriram S, Albertini RJ. T cells responsive to myelin basic protein in patients with multiple sclerosis. *Science* 1990;247:718–721.
27. Zhang S, Kodama M, Hanawa H, et al. The effects of cyclosporine and prednisolone on experimental autoimmune myocarditis. *Jpn Circ J* 1990;54:893–894 (abst).
28. Hanawa H, Kodama M, Zhang S, Izumi T, Shibata A. An immunosuppressant compound, FK-506, prevents the progression of autoimmune myocarditis in rats. *Clin Immunol Immunopathol* 1992;62:321–326.
29. Kodama M, Matsumoto Y, Fujiwara M. In vivo lymphocyte-mediated myocardial injuries demonstrated by adoptive transfer of experimental autoimmune myocarditis. *Circulation* 1992;85:1918–1926.
30. Wucherpfennig KW, Ota K, Endo N, et al. Shared human T cell receptor V beta usage to immunodominant regions of myelin basic protein. *Science* 1990;248:1016–1019.
31. Ota K, Matsui M, Milford EL, Mackin GA, Weiner HL, Hafler DA. T-cell recognition of an immunodominant myelin basic protein epitope in multiple sclerosis. *Nature* 1990;346:183–187.

The Cardiomyopathic Heart, edited by Makoto
Nagano, Nobuakira Takeda, and Naranjan S.
Dhalla. Raven Press, Ltd., New York © 1994.

32

Analysis of the Pathogenesis of Coxsackievirus B3 Myocarditis: Comparison of Myocarditic and Amyocarditic Coxsackievirus B3 Strains[1]

Chiharu Kishimoto, *Masahiko Kurokawa, *Hiroshi Ochiai,
Hitoshi Takada, Yuji Hiraoka, Shigetake Sasayama, and
*Kimiyasu Shiraki

*The Second Department of Internal Medicine and *Department of Virology,
Faculty of Medicine, Toyama Medical and Pharmaceutical University,
Toyama 930-01, Japan*

INTRODUCTION

Coxsackievirus B3 (CB3) has been shown to cause severe myocarditis in inbred strains of mice (1). In this murine model, lesions produced in the myocardium, as determined by histologic examination, were found to resemble and reflect those seen in human myocarditis, and were characterized by lymphoid infiltration and necrosis (1). The pathogenesis likely originates from virus-infected cells. Cytotoxic T lymphocytes (CTLs) have been shown to play a major role in the virus-induced myocarditis, especially in its development (1–3). However, the antigens, recognized by CTLs, have not been identified. Recently, we found that there were two variants in CB3 Nancy strain; one of the strains (CB3M) could cause myocarditis in all infected mice, whereas the other (CB3O) failed to do so. Pathologic studies of hearts from CB3M-infected mice showed obvious lymphoid infiltration and myocardial cell necrosis (3,4). However, these phenomena were not observed in the hearts of CB3O-infected mice. Thus, in this study, we analyzed the vital growth and proteins in African green monkey kidney (Vero) cells infected with CB3M and CB3O.

[1]This work was supported in part by research grants of the Japanese Heart Foundation, Education Fellowship of Toyama Medical and Pharmaceutical University, Iwaki Fellowship, Japanese Education of Science and Welfare (Nos. 01570478 and 03670445), and Uchara Memorial Foundation.

MATERIALS AND METHODS

Viruses and Cells

CB3M and CB30 variants (Nancy strain) were obtained from Dr. Creighhead, University of Vermont, Arlington, VT, and Dr. Abelmann, Harvard Medical School, Boston, MA, respectively. Both viruses were propagated in Vero cells. The cultures were frozen and thawed three times, centrifuged at 3,000 rpm for 10 minutes and the culture supernatants were stored at $-80°C$. Vero cells were grown in Eagle's minimal essential medium (MEM) supplemented with 5% heat-inactivated fetal bovine serum (FBS).

Growth Assay

Monolayers of Vero cells in 25-cm^2 flasks were infected with CB3M or CB30 at five plaque-forming units (PFU)/cell for 1 hour. The infected cells were washed three times with phosphate-buffered saline (PBS) and incubated in maintenance medium at 37 °C. At various times after infection, the cultures were frozen and thawed three times, and then supernatants clarified by centrifugation were subjected to plaque assay on Vero cells.

Labeling of Viral Proteins and Immunoprecipitation

Monolayers of cells in 60-mm dishes were infected with CB3M or CB30 at a multiplicity of infection of 5 to 10 PFU/cell. After 1 hour of adsorption, the cells were incubated in maintenance medium (MEM supplemented with 2% FBS). The culture medium was replaced with methionine-free maintenance medium containing [^{35}S] methionine (20 Ci/mL). The labeled cells were lysed in radioimmune precipitation assay (RIPA) buffer and the cell lysates were immunoprecipitated by rabbit anti-CB30 antibody or human immunoglobin.

RESULTS AND DISCUSSION

As shown in Figure 1, no differences were noted between CB3M and CB30 in terms of viral growth assay upon Vero cells. Although no differences in the proteins of total cell lysates or the capsid proteins of virions were noted between CB3M and CB30, there was a difference (27K protein) in gel electrophoretic patterns of immunoprecipitates against rabbit anti-CB30 or human immunoglobulin between CB3M- and CB30-infected Vero cells (Fig. 2). The 27K protein was detected in infected cells late in infection (data not shown).

Newer insights into the immunologic aspects of murine CB3 myocarditis have been gained. The susceptibility of a subject for a viral infection is primarily deter-

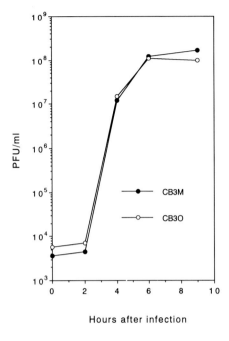

FIG. 1. Growth assay on Vero cells. No differences were noted in viral growth assay between CB3M and CB30 strains. *PFU*, plaque-forming unit.

mined by the age and genetic background of the host (5). Furthermore, the host-virus interaction may not only determine disease susceptibility, but also may control myocardial responses or characteristics of myocardial damage in murine models (5). Unlike B cells, T cells (especially the immature T cell subset) play a role in the development of myocarditis (3,4).

Recently, we obtained an amyocarditic variant of CB3 (CB30); similar antigenic variations were reported in poliovirus type (6) as well as other CB30 (7). Although further research efforts are necessary to characterize the difference between CB3M and CB30, a study designed to analyze the 27K protein is now in progress.

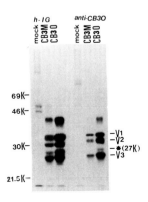

FIG. 2. Gel electrophoretic patterns. Gel electrophoretic analysis of viral proteins immunoprecipitated with anti-CB30 antibody or human immunoglobulin (h-IG). CB3M- or CB30-infected cells were labeled with [^{35}S] methionine for 4 hours beginning 1 hour postinfarction. The labeled cells were lysed and immunoprecipitated.

SUMMARY

Coxsackievirus B3 (CB3) has been shown to cause severe myocarditis in inbred strains of mice. Using this in vivo infection system, we found that there are two types in CB3 Nancy strains. One of the strains (CB3M) could cause myocarditis in infected mice, but another strain (CB30) had no effect. Pathologic studies of hearts from CB3M-infected mice showed obvious lymphoid infiltration and myocardial cell necrosis. However, these phenomena were not observed in CB30-infected mice. These results suggest that the difference in the viral products of CB3M and CB30 is responsible for the pathogenesis of myocarditis in mice. Thus, we compared the viral proteins produced in CB3M- and CB30-infected Vero cells by immunoprecipitation method using rabbit anti-CB30 serum. In cell extract prepared from CB30-infected cells, 27K protein was detectable but in lesser amounts than found in cell extract prepared from CB3M-infected cells. It appears that the 27K viral protein may play an important etiologic role in myocarditis in mice.

REFERENCES

1. Woodruff JF. Viral myocarditis. A review. *Am J Pathol* 1980;101:427–484.
2. Reyes M, Lerner AM. Coxsackievirus myocarditis. With special reference to acute and chronic effects. *Prog Cardiovasc Dis* 1985;27:373–394.
3. Kishimoto C, Abelmann WH. Absence of effects of cyclosporine on myocardial lymphocyte subsets in coxsackievirus B3 myocarditis in the aviremic stage. *Circ Res* 1989;65:934–945.
4. Kishimoto C, Throp KA, Abelmann WH. Immunosuppression with high doses of cyclophosphamide reduces the severity of myocarditis but increases the mortality in murine coxsackievirus B3 myocarditis. *Circulation* 1990;82:982–989.
5. Kishimoto C, Kawai C, Abelmann WH. Immunogenetic aspects of the pathogenesis of experimental viral myocarditis. In: Kawai C, Abelmann WH, eds. *Cardiomyopathy. Pathogenesis of myocarditis and cardiomyopathy*. Tokyo: University of Tokyo Press; 1987;3–7.
6. Nomoto A, Omata T, Toyoda H, Kuge S, Horie H, Kataoka Y, Genba Y, Nakano Y, Imma N. Complete nucleotide sequence of the attenuated poliovirus Sabin 1 strain genome. *Proc Natl Acad Sci USA* 1982;79:5793–5797.
7. Ganutt JC, Trousdale MD, LaBadie DRL, Paque RE, Nealon T. Properties of coxsackievirus B3 variants which are amyocarditic or myocarditic for mice. *J Med Virol* 1979;3:207–220.

The Cardiomyopathic Heart, edited by Makoto
Nagano, Nobuakira Takeda, and Naranjan S.
Dhalla. Raven Press, Ltd., New York © 1994.

33

Mutations of the Mitochondrial DNA in Patients with Hypertrophic Cardiomyopathy

Kazuki Hattori, Toshihiro Obayashi, *Masashi Tanaka,
*Satoru Sugiyama, Takayuki Ito, and *Takayuki Ozawa

*Department of Internal Medicine II and *Department of Biomedical Chemistry,
Faculty of Medicine, University of Nagoya, Tsuruma, Showa-ku, Nagoya 466, Japan*

INTRODUCTION

The pathogenesis of hypertrophic cardiomyopathy (HCM) has attracted much attention because sudden death, probably resulting from ventricular arrhythmias, often occurs in patients with HCM. Accordingly, the diagnosis and treatment of HCM have been investigated extensively. Advances in echocardiography have enabled us to visualize myocardial thickening accurately, and have thus resolved the former problem of definitive diagnosis of HCM (1). However, the etiology of HCM has not been fully elucidated. Accumulating evidence suggests that a genetic defect may be a factor in the genesis of HCM. In some patients with familial HCM, an α/β cardiac myosin heavy chain hybrid gene and a missense mutation in a β myosin heavy chain gene have been reported (2,3), and HCM with an autosomal dominant type of inheritance might be ascribed to this mutation. Nevertheless, HCM with a nonautosomal dominant type of inheritance has also been encountered clinically, and another etiology might be involved in the latter form of HCM.

One important feature of mitochondria is that they have their own DNA, which was first sequenced by Anderson et al. (4). Mitochondrial DNA (mtDNA) encodes 11 subunits of the electron-transfer chain, 2 subunits of adenosine triphosphatase (ATPase), 2 ribosomal RNA (rRNA) and 22 transfer RNA (tRNA) (Fig.1). Recently, mutations in mtDNA as well as in nuclear DNA have been proposed to be contributing factors in various diseases, such as mitochondrial myopathy (5,6). We presumed that such mutations of mtDNA might also have an important role in cardiomyopathy. Another feature of mtDNA is that mtDNA is inherited maternally (7). In this study, we sequenced the total mtDNA from two patients with HCM who did not show autosomal dominant inheritance, and found several point mutations and deletions that might be related to the genesis of HCM.

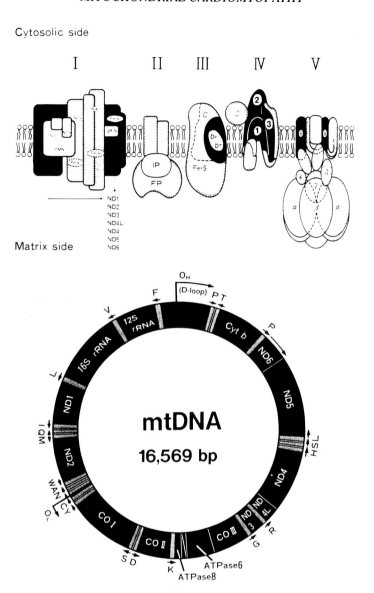

FIG. 1. Schematic representation of the mitochondrial oxidative phosphorylation system (*upper part*) and mitochondrial DNA (*lower part*). The subunits with shadow in the upper part are encoded by mitochondrial DNA; the others are encoded by nuclear DNA.

MATERIALS AND METHODS

Cases

Patient 1

A 43-year-old man with a 20-year history of cardiomegaly was admitted to the hospital because of general malaise and dyspnea on exertion. Chest X-ray studies showed cardiac enlargement and evidence of pulmonary congestion and bilateral pleural effusion. Hemodynamic examination revealed that the left ventricular end diastolic pressure (LVEDP) was 15 mm Hg and the pulmonary artery wedge pressure was 15/4 mm Hg (mean of 9). The cardiac index was 2.5 L/min/m^2. The echocardiogram showed left ventricular enlargement and diffuse hypokinesis in wall motion. The ejection fraction was 20% and the width of the intraventricular septum was 9 mm. Coronary angiography did not reveal abnormalities in the coronary arteries. Microscopic examination of the endomyocardial biopsy samples showed myofiber hypertrophy and marked disarray, which are characteristic of hypertrophic cardiomyopathy, although the hemodynamic features resembled those seen in dilated cardiomyopathy. Two years after the first admission, the patient died of heart and renal failure. His younger sister also had HCM, but no other family member had any known cardiovascular diseases.

Patient 2

A 54-year-old woman was admitted to the hospital because of anorexia and general fatigue. She had been suffering from diabetes mellitus and heart failure for 20 years, and had received insulin injections. Three years before, she had suffered second-degree atrioventricular block, and was fitted with a permanent pacemaker. As she had marked renal dysfunction on admission, she was diagnosed as having diabetic nephropathy. The echocardiogram showed diffuse left ventricular wall thickening and pericardial effusion. The ejection fraction was 66% and the width of the intraventricular septum was 18 mm. She had no neuromuscular symptoms before admission. Microscopic examination of endomyocardial biopsy samples showed myofiber hypertrophy and disarray. She died of sudden cardiac arrest. Her elder sister also has diabetes mellitus, but there was no other family history of heart disease.

DNA Extraction

Total DNA was extracted from 5 mg of biopsy or autopsy specimens of heart muscle, as previously reported (8).

Oligonucleotide Primers

Primers were synthesized with an Applied Biosystems (model 381A) DNA synthesizer (Applied Biosystems Inc., Ramsey, NJ) and then purified on oligonucleotide purification cartridges from Applied Biosystems according to the manufacturer's instructions. The light (L) strand and the heavy (H) strand primers were 20-mer oligonucleotides possessing sequences specific for the L strand and the H strand of mtDNA, respectively. The 5'-end of the L (n) primer corresponded to nucleotide position $(10n + 1)$ and its 3'-end corresponded to nucleotide position $(10n + 20)$. Similarly, the 3'-end of the H (n) primer corresponded to nucleotide position $(10n + 1)$ and its 5'-end corresponded to nucleotide position $(10n + 20)$. The FL primers were 38-mer oligonucleotides possessing both the 18 nucleotides of the M13mp18 forward universal sequence $(-21M13, 5' - $ TGTAAAACGACG-GCCAGT $-3')$ on the 5'-side and a sequence of 20 nucleotides specific for the L strand of mtDNA at the 3'-end.

PCR Amplification

The extracted DNA solution (1 μL) was amplified in 50 μL of reaction mixture containing 200 μM of each deoxyribonucleoside triphosphate (dNTP), 1 μM of each primer, 1.25 units of *Taq* DNA polymerase (Promega, Madison, WI) and polymerase chain reaction (PCR) buffer (50 mM of Tris-HCl with a pH of 8.4, containing 50 mM of KCl, 1.5 mM of $MgCl_2$ and 0.01% gelatin). The reaction was carried out for a total of 30 amplification cycles with the use of a Perkin-Elmer/Cetus Thermal Cycler (Perkin-Elmer/Cetus Corp., Norwalk, CT). The cycle time was as follows: denaturation, 15 sec at 94°C; annealing, 15 sec at 50°C; and primer extension, 80 sec at 72°C. Amplified fragments were separated by electrophoresis on 1% agarose gel and were detected after they had been stained with ethidium bromide.

Asymmetric PCR Amplification for Template Formation of Fluorescence-based Sequencing

Thirty PCR cycles were performed with 1 μL of the first PCR product in a final volume of 50 μL, which included the reagents just mentioned along with 0.5 pmol of FL primer and 50 pmol of H primer, and 20 μM of each dNTP. The amplified single-strand DNA was stored at $-80°C$ for 30 min after the addition of 5 μL of sodium acetate (pH of 7.4) and 120 μL of ethanol, and then centrifuged at $11,000 \times g$ for 10 min. The precipitate was rinsed with 120 μL of 70% ethanol and then centrifuged at $11,000 \times g$ for 5 min, dried in a vacuum chamber for 10 min, and then resuspended in 8 μl of distilled water.

Fluorescence-based Direct Sequencing

The *Taq* sequencing kit was obtained from Applied Biosystems, Osaka, Japan. For sequencing reactions with the Joe dye primer (for adenine; A) and the Fam dye primer (for cytosine; C), the following reagents were mixed to a total volume of 7.75 μL: 1.0 μL of single-strand DNA template, 1.0 μL of each dye primer (dissolved to a concentration of 0.4 pmol/μL), 1.0 μL of $5 \times Taq$ sequencing buffer (50 mM of Tris-HCl with a pH of 8.5, 50 mM of $MgCl_2$, and 250 mM of NaCl), 1.0 μL of each mix of d/ddNTP (deoxynucleoside/dideoxynucleoside triphosphate), 3.5 μL of distilled water, and 1.25 units of *Taq* DNA polymerase. For the sequencing reactions with the Tmra dye primer (for guanine; G) and the Rox dye primer (for thymine; T), the amount of reagents was doubled for a total volume of 15.5 μL. Ten cycles of denaturation at 90°C for 15 sec, and annealing and extension at 70°C for 1 min, were conducted in the thermal cycler. The contents of the four tubes were pooled into a tube containing a mixture of 5 μL of 3-M sodium acetate (pH of 5.2) and 100 μL of ethanol. The mixture was placed at $-20°C$ for 10 min, and then centrifuged at $11,000 \times g$ for 10 min. The pellet was rinsed with 100 μL of 70% ethanol and centrifuged at $11,000 \times g$ for 5 min. The pellet was dried in a vacuum chamber for 10 min and stored at $-20°C$. Just prior to electrophoresis, the pellet was dissolved in a mixture of 5 μL of deionized formamide and 1 μL of 50-mM ethylenediaminetetra-acetic acid (EDTA) (pH of 8.0). The DNA samples were heated at 90°C for 2 min, then immediately cooled on ice and loaded onto 6% polyacrylamide gel. Fluorescence-based automated DNA sequence analysis was carried out using a 373A DNA Sequencer (Applied Biosystems, Inc.) run with the manufacturer's version of 1.0.1 software.

RESULTS

The point mutations in mtDNA of patient 1 are shown in Table 1. Two point mutations that changed amino acids were observed. A transversion from A to T at position 13,258 replaced the conserved serine to cysteine in the ND5 gene. There were 8 silent point mutations. Two point mutations were observed in tRNA genes, which were transitions from G to A at position 5,821 in the cysteine tRNA gene, and from A to G at position 15,951 in the threonine tRNA gene. There was a transition from A to G at position 2,246 in the 16S rRNA gene.

Figure 2 shows the PCR amplification of mtDNA from the heart muscle of patient 1, using primers L853 and H38. Multiple abnormal fragments (3.1kb, 2.4kb, 1.7kb, 1.4kb, 1.0kb), which mean 5.3kb, 6.0kb, 6.7kb, 7.0kb, and 7.4kb deletions of mtDNA, respectively, were detected (lane A). We sequenced the deleted regions of one mutant mtDNA using the direct sequencing method. The crossover sequence of this mutant mtDNA was demonstrated to be a 12-bp directly repeated sequence of 5'-CATCAACAACCG-3', which was located at the boundaries of the deletion be-

TABLE 1. *Point mutations in mtDNA of patient 1*

Number	Region	Std. mut.		Std. mut.		N/C
tRNA genes						
5821	tRNA-Cys	G	A			N
15951	tRNA-Thr	A	G			C
Protein coding genes (replacement of amino acid)						
13258	ND5	A	T	Ser	Cys	C
14180	ND6	T	C	Tyr	Cys	N
Protein coding genes (no replacement of amino acid)						
8020	COII	G	A	Pro		
8450	ATP6	T	C	Leu		
10181	ND3	C	T	Phe		
11185	ND4	C	A	Arg		
13827	ND5	A	G	Gly		
14091	ND5	A	G	Lys		
15217	Cytb	G	A	Gly		
15805	Cytb	A	G	Val		
rRNA genes						
2246	16SrRNA	A	G			

Std., standard mtDNA sequence reported by Anderson et al., ref. 4; Mut., mutation; C, conserved among human, bovine, rat, and mouse; N, nonconserved.

tween the ATPase6 gene and the D-loop region. The deletion spanned 7,436 bp from position 8,649 to position 16,084.

The point mutations in mtDNA of patient 2 are shown in Table 2. Three point mutations that changed amino acids were observed. A transition from T to C at position 3,394 replaced the conserved tyrosine to histidine in the ND1 gene. There were three silent point mutations. One point mutation was observed in the tRNA gene, which was a transition from A to G at position 3,243 in the leucine tRNA gene. This mutation was the same mutation found in patients with myopathy, encephalopathy, lactic acidosis, and stroke-like episodes (MELAS). There was a transversion from C to A at position 964 and a transition from A to G at position 1,041 in the 12S rRNA gene.

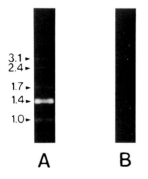

3.1 ►
2.4 ►

1.7 ►
1.4 ►

1.0 ►

A   B

FIG. 2. Ethidium bromide staining of a 1% agarose gel. Detection of deleted mtDNA by PCR amplification using primers L853 and H38. Sizes of amplified fragments are indicated in kb. **Lane A:** Heart mtDNA of patient 1. **Lane B:** Control heart mtDNA. Five kinds of mtDNA deletions were observed in patient 1.

TABLE 2. *Point mutations in mtDNA of patient 2*

Number	Region	Std. mut.		Std. mut.		N/C
tRNA genes						
3243	tRNA-Leu	A	G			C
Protein coding genes (replacement of amino acid)						
3394	ND1	T	C	Tyr His		C
4491	ND2	G	A	Val Ile		N
11963	ND4	G	A	Val Ile		N
Protein coding genes (no replacement of amino acid)						
9242	COIII	A	G	Lys		
10373	ND3	G	A	Glu		
14308	ND6	T	C	Gly		
rRNA genes						
964	12SrRNA	C	A			
1041	12SrRNA	A	G			

DISCUSSION

Mitochondria are unique organelles containing their own DNA, which encode 13 subunits of the ATP-producing system; the other subunits are encoded by nuclear DNA. The rate of mutation in mtDNA is estimated to be much higher than that of nuclear DNA (9). Mitochondria occupy a pivotal position in the cellular energy metabolism, and deterioration (secondary to mtDNA mutation) of various enzymes linked with energy metabolism in mitochondria was shown to be involved in mitochondrial encephalomyopathy (10). We presumed such mutation of mtDNA might also be an important contributor to cardiomyopathy.

We found that multiple deletions, as well as point mutations, existed in the heart mtDNA of patients with HCM. It should be remembered that point mutations in mtDNA are a predisposing factor in the development of mtDNA deletion (9). Accordingly, accumulated point mutations are likely to be linked with the increase in the population of mtDNA with deletion. These mutations of mtDNA would impair ATP production and create a persistent ischemia-like state, which might cause disorganization and an abnormal proliferation of cardiac muscles. Another possibility is that mutations functionally impair a regulatory protein, thereby accelerating the proliferation of cardiac muscles.

The nucleotide sequences of the tRNA gene are highly conserved. Mutations in some tRNA genes might be responsible for the genesis of mitochondrial neuropathy and myopathy; for example, a point mutation in the leucine tRNA gene has been proposed as the cause of MELAS (11), and a mutation in the lysine tRNA gene may be responsible for myoclonic epilepsy with ragged-red fibers (MERRF) (12). Mutations in the tRNA gene may cause an alteration in the secondary structure of the tRNA, which may affect the transport of amino acids to the ribosome and their subsequent translation into protein. Mutations in tRNA genes observed here might be linked with the genesis of HCM. However, there are no common mutations in the mtDNA of patients with HCM. Accordingly, summation of point mutations and deletions might play a key role in the etiology of some types of HCM, and gene analysis of mtDNA would be necessary to make the correct diagnosis of HCM. Although various mechanisms have been proposed concerning the genesis of HCM (13–16), mutations in mtDNA may be a contributory factor in the genesis of HCM with nonautosomal dominant inheritance.

SUMMARY

In order to examine the mechanism of HCM, gene analysis of mitochondrial DNA was performed in two patients who did not show autosomal inheritance. The sequence of total mtDNA from the diseased myocardium revealed several point mutations and deletions. These results suggest that mutations in mtDNA may be involved in the development of HCM.

ACKNOWLEDGMENT

We express our appreciation to Michael Bodman, a language consultant of our department, for reading the previous draft and making suggestions on language and style.

REFERENCES

1. Wynne J, Braunwald E. Hypertrophic cardiomyopathy. In: Braunwald E, ed. *Heart disease, Vol 2*. Philadelphia: WB Saunders; 1992:1404–1415.
2. Tanigawa G, Jarcho JA, Kass S, et al. A molecular basis for familial hypertrophic cardiomyopathy: an α/β cardiac myosin heavy chain hybrid gene. *Cell* 1990;62:991–998.
3. Geisterfer-Lowrance AAT, Kass S, Tanigawa G, et al. A molecular basis for familial hypertrophic cardiomyopathy: a β cardiac myosin heavy chain gene missense mutation. *Cell* 1990;62:999–1006.
4. Anderson S, Bankier AT, Barrell BG, et al. Sequence and organization of the human mitochondrial genome. *Nature* 1981;290:457–465.
5. Wallace DC, Singh G, Lott MT, et al. Mitochondrial DNA mutation associated with Leber's hereditary optic neuropathy. *Science* 1988;242:1427–1430.
6. Yoneda M, Tsuji S, Yamauchi T, et al. Mitochondrial DNA mutations in family with Leber's hereditary optic neuropathy. *Lancet* 1989;1:1076–1077.
7. Ozawa T, Yoneda M, Tanaka M, et al. Maternal inheritance of deleted mitochondrial DNA in a family with mitochondrial myopathy. *Biochem Biophys Res Commun* 1988;154:1240–1247.
8. Hattori K, Tanaka M, Sugiyama S, et al. Age-dependent increase in deleted mitochondrial DNA in the human heart: possible contributory factor to presbycardia. *Am Heart J* 1991;121:1735–1742.
9. Linnane AW, Maruzuki S, Ozawa T, Tanaka M. Mitochondrial DNA mutations as an important contributor to aging and degenerative diseases. *Lancet* 1989;1:642–645.
10. Ozawa T, Tanaka M, Sato W, et al. Mitochondrial DNA mutations as an etiology of human degenerative diseases. In: Kim CH, Ozawa T, eds. *Bioenergetics: molecular biology, biochemistry, and pathology*. New York: Plenum; 1990: 413–427.
11. Ino H, Tanaka M, Ohno K, et al. Mitochondrial leucine tRNA mutations in a mitochondrial encephalomyopathy. *Lancet* 1991;337:234–235.
12. Yoneda M, Tanno Y, Horai S, Ozawa T, Miyatake T, Tsuji S. A common mitochondrial DNA mutation in the tRNA^{Lys} of patients with myoclonus epilepsy associated with ragged-red fibers. *Biochem Int* 1990;21:789–796.

13. Hirzel HO, Tuchschmid CR, Schneider J, Krayenbuehl HP, Schaub MC. Relationship between myosin isoenzyme composition, hemodynamics, and myocardial structure in various forms of human cardiac hypertrophy. *Circ Res* 1985;57:729–740.
14. Komuro I, Kurabayashi M, Takaku F, Yazaki Y. Expression of cellular oncogenes in the myocardium during the developmental stage and pressure-overloaded hypertrophy of the rat heart. *Circ Res* 1988;62:1075–1079.
15. Simpson P. Stimulation of hypertrophy of cultured neonatal rat heart cells through an α_1-adrenergic receptor and induction of beating through an α_1- and β_2-adrenergic receptor interaction. *Circ Res* 1985;56:884–894.
16. Darsee JR, Heymsfield SB, Nutter DO. Hypertrophic cardiomyopathy and human leukocyte antigen linkage. *N Engl J Med* 1979;300:877–882.

The Cardiomyopathic Heart, edited by Makoto
Nagano, Nobuakira Takeda, and Naranjan S.
Dhalla. Raven Press, Ltd., New York © 1994.

34

Pulmonary Hypertension and Right Ventricular Hypertrophy in Rats

Heinz-Gerd Zimmer

Department of Physiology, University of Munich, Munich, Germany

FUNCTIONAL SIGNIFICANCE OF THE RIGHT VENTRICLE

The morphologic, functional, metabolic, and molecular biological changes in experimental cardiac hypertrophy (1,2) have been studied predominantly in the left ventricle (LV). Pharmacologic strategies and the effects of drugs have also been directed to and tested in experimental models of LV hypertrophy. Similar studies specifically designed for the right ventricle (RV) have not been performed on a large scale. In fact, the RV seems to have been neglected to a large extent, both in experimental and clinical cardiology.

From previous experimental studies, it had appeared that the RV may even be dispensable in functional terms. This was concluded from experiments on dogs in which extensive destruction of the entire RV wall by cauterization (3–5) or by ligation of the right coronary artery (6) did not lead to right heart failure. These experimental procedures failed to produce more than a minimal increase in peripheral venous pressure. Furthermore, the force expelling blood into the pulmonary circuit appeared to be derived from sources other than contraction of the external wall of the RV. These forces were thought to be the central venous pressure, the LV via the sinospiral and bulbospiral fibers that envelop the two ventricles (4), the interventricular septum by shortening of the apex–base axis or by bulging into the right ventricle (5), or small regions of the RV muscle that were still functioning (6). These studies may have contributed to the long-lasting underestimation of right heart function, both in physiologic and pathophysiologic conditions.

Additional experimental and clinical studies were needed to put the function of the RV into the correct perspective physiologically. Experiments in which venopulmonary shunts were established to bypass the RV in dogs showed that occlusion of the normal pathway of blood through the RV resulted in a marked reduction in systemic arterial pressure and in elevations of venous pressure (7). Thus, the RV appeared to be an essential pump for the maintenance of normal pressure and flows in the intact circulation. Later experimental studies in dogs in which the RV was impaired by cauterization revealed that damage to the RV produces a syndrome of predominant RV dysfunction (8).

Clinical studies also emphasized the functional importance of the RV. Congenital aplasia of the RV (9) was associated with absence of RV contraction (10). The peak pulse wave in the RV was the right atrial "a" wave. Thus, the main force propelling blood through the lungs was right atrial contraction. Moreover, in patients with diffuse endocardial fibroelastosis and with massive fibrosis of the RV subsequent to RV infarction, pulmonary blood flow was maintained by the contraction of the right atrium, which was greatly hypertrophied. Right heart insufficiency appeared when the right atrium failed to support the pulmonary circulation. Thus, congestive failure coincided with the failure of the right atrium (11).

Catheterization in six patients with RV infarction revealed that the RV was generating very little pressure. In some patients, the pulmonary arterial tracing was nearly identical to that in the right atrium. The hypotension and reduced cardiac output in patients with RV infarction was attributed to inadequate LV filling. RV damage clearly produced evidence of RV failure with increased central venous pressure (12).

The importance of the RV was also supported in people living at high altitudes. The effect of hypoxia on pulmonary arterial blood pressure resulting in constriction of pulmonary vessels had been known since the experimental studies of von Euler and Liljestrand (13). In people native to high altitudes, there was an extensive muscularinization of the peripheral pulmonary arterial branches (14). There was also hypertrophy of the RV in native children living at high altitudes, suggesting that pulmonary hypertension may have been an early feature (15). Moreover, RV hypertrophy secondary to chronic lung or pulmonary embolic disease proved to be the strongest predictor of RV infarction (16).

In view of these experimental and clinical studies, it seemed appropriate to investigate models of RV hypertrophy in a small laboratory animal model. To do this, it was first necessary to establish a method for measuring right heart function in the rat. Based primarily on our own experimental experience, several models of pulmonary hypertension and RV hypertrophy, as well as some pharmacologic interventions in these pathophysiologic conditions, are reviewed in this article.

METHODS FOR MEASURING RIGHT VENTRICULAR FUNCTION

When heart function was to be measured in closed-chest rats, thiobutabarbital sodium (Inactin, Byk Gulden, Konstanz, FRG) was used as an anesthetic at a dosage of 80 mg/kg, administered intraperitoneally. The depth of anesthesia was evaluated by eliciting reflexes in the legs with a forceps. After tracheotomy, a cannula was placed in the trachea through which the animals were breathing spontaneously. RV function was measured with an ultraminiature catheter pressure transducer (model PR-291, Millar Instruments, Inc., Houston, TX). This catheter is curved in such a way as to facilitate the advancement of the catheter tip from the right atrium into the RV (17).

In some animals, catheterization of the pulmonary artery was performed using a similarly tipped catheter manometer with an angle of 120° between tip and shaft (model SPR 392, Millar Instruments). The tip of this catheter has a length of 4 mm and a diameter of 1 mm. The diameter of the shaft is 0.5 mm. The shaft was marked 11 cm distal to the tip. The system has a natural resonant frequency of 35 kHz. This catheter was inserted into the right femoral vein and advanced through the abdominal and thoracic vein to the right atrium, which was reached after a distance of about 10 cm. Location of the catheter in the atrium was confirmed by obtaining atrial pressure signals with an amplitude of less than 10 mm Hg. By carefully rotating the tip, the catheter was placed in the RV and then advanced into the pulmonary artery. The typical change of the shape of the pressure curve illustrated that the catheter had entered the pulmonary artery (18,19). After the measurements had been obtained, the position of the catheter was verified by autopsy.

Heart rate, RV and pulmonary artery pressure, as well as RV dp/dt_{max} were recorded on a Gould Brush 2600 recorder. Cardiac output was measured using the thermodilution method. Total peripheral resistance was calculated on the basis of mean arterial pressure and cardiac output (20).

These methods, which were specifically designed for measurements in rats, do not allow the assessment of coronary blood flow or of regional contractility of the RV. If the need arises to measure these parameters, a larger animal model, such as the dog, must be used. Regional blood flow can be measured with the microsphere technique. To do this, six distinctly radiolabeled microspheres are injected in randomized order into the dog's left atrium within 20 to 30 seconds, while a reference sample of blood is drawn from the abdominal aorta (21). To determine the regional contraction pattern of the RV in dogs, two pairs of miniaturized piezoceramic ultrasonic transducers are implanted in the longitudinal axis of the inflow tract and the outflow tract of the RV free wall (22). Sonomicrometry provides an accurate description of the distance between these two ultrasonic transducers. Myocardial segment length is measured at end diastole and end systole. Maximum and minimum segment length can also be determined. To visualize the dynamics of RV free wall contraction, pressure–length loops can be constructed by computer by plotting phasic changes of segment length against phasic changes of RV pressure during one cardiac cycle (22).

EXPERIMENTAL MODELS OF PULMONARY HYPERTENSION AND RIGHT VENTRICULAR HYPERTROPHY

Acute Models

Norepinephrine

Infusion of norepinephrine (3 μg/kg/min) into the jugular vein of anesthetized female Sprague-Dawley rats had an immediate effect on RV function (17). Heart rate was increased from 392 ± 13 bpm (n = 11) to 495 ± 10 bpm; RV systolic pressure was elevated from 32 ± 1.0 mm Hg to 61 ± 2.6 mm Hg; RV dp/dt$_{max}$ was enhanced from $1,887 \pm 174$ mm Hg/sec to $6,129 \pm 394$ mm Hg/sec, and the pressure-rate product had increased from $12,575 \pm 692$ mm Hg/min to $30,397 \pm 1,547$ mm Hg/min. These acute changes signify an immediate increase in pulmonary vascular resistance by norepinephrine, probably by stimulation of α-adrenergic receptors (23).

Hypoxia

Acute hypoxia, which is known to induce constriction of the pulmonary vessels (13), was induced in female Sprague-Dawley rats by exposing them to a hypoxic gas mixture (13.3% O_2, 0.7% CO_2, and 86% N_2). This mixture was made by mixing carbogen with nitrogen. The proportion of the components was controlled and adjusted by Rotameter metering tubes (Rota Company, Wehr, FRG). The functional parameters of the RV were measured at the end of a 5-minute period of exposure to the hypoxic gas mixture. Heart rate was increased from a control value of 345 ± 10 bpm (n = 6) to 361 ± 9 bpm; RV systolic pressure was elevated from 31 ± 1.1 mm Hg to 55 ± 2.1 mm Hg; RV dp/dt$_{max}$ was enhanced from $2,067 \pm 171$ mm Hg/sec to $2,633 \pm 173$ mm Hg/sec; and the pressure-rate product was increased from $10,561 \pm 406$ mm Hg/min to $19,935 \pm 863$ mm Hg/min (19). This experimental model was used to test the effects of several pharmacologic interventions (see section on pharmacologic interventions).

Pulmonary Microembolism

The lungs of anesthetized dogs were embolized by injection of a single dose of oleic acid (0.01 mL/kg) into the right atrium, followed by repetitive doses (0.5 to 1 g every 3 to 5 minutes, for a total of 0.5 g/kg) of nonsiliconized glass beads (with diameters of 100 μm) suspended and thoroughly mixed in 1 to 2 mL of dextran 50. Embolization was interrupted when mean pulmonary artery pressure had increased by 10 to 15 mm Hg. Thereafter, embolization was continued and terminated when mean pulmonary artery pressure had reached a peak level of about 40 mm Hg. This procedure to induce an acute rise in pulmonary vascular resistance resulted in an increase in RV systolic pressure from 24.0 ± 4.0 mm Hg to 48 ± 9 mm Hg, and an elevation of the mean pulmonary artery pressure from 11 ± 2 mm Hg to 39 ± 4 mm Hg, along with a reduction in mean arterial pressure from 106 ± 15 mm Hg to 85 ± 17 mm Hg. Although stroke volume was diminished, cardiac output was not altered because of a concomitant increase in heart rate (22).

The increase in afterload secondary to pulmonary microembolization caused regionally different changes in local preload and segment shortening in the RV free wall. Sonomicrometry measurements revealed that normalized end diastolic segment length increased significantly in the inflow tract from 10.0 to 10.3 mm, but simultaneously decreased in the outflow tract of the RV from 10.0 to 9.6 mm.

Segment shortening in the inflow tract was not affected, but deteriorated significantly in the outflow tract from 11.6% to 2.7%. Bulging was found at any level of microembolization in the RV outflow tract, but not in the inflow tract. At the same time that lung mechanics and gas exchange had deteriorated, hypercapnia and respiratory acidosis had developed. The results of these studies (22) provide evidence that segment shortening was affected differently by acute pulmonary microembolization in the RV inflow and outflow tracts. The pressure–segment length loops changed from an originally triangular or oval shape to a rectangular shape in both inflow and outflow tracts.

Chronic Models

Hypoxia

Chronic exposure of rats in a hypobaric chamber to a simulated altitude of 6,000 m (345 Torr) for up to 4 weeks resulted in the gradual development of RV hypertrophy secondary to pulmonary hypertension (13). The morphologic substrate indicating pulmonary hypertension was shown to be an increase in the width of the media of small pulmonary arteries from 1.8 to 3.9 μm. With respect to RV hypertrophy, there was an increase in the protein and DNA content of the RV. Most of the DNA-producing cells were shown to be located in the interstitium. The labeling index of these cells increased about sixfold owing to the expansion of the interstitium by proliferation, which was also evident from the presence of frequent mitoses (24). There seemed to be three stages of RV hypertrophy. The first stage was characterized by pure myocyte hypertrophy, with extensive stimulation of protein synthesis that was completely reversible when hypoxia was discontinued. In the second phase, there was an increase in mitochondrial adenosine triphosphatase (ATPase) activity and proliferation of the interstitium, with no further changes in myocardial cells. In the third phase, the myofibrillar content of the cardiomyocytes decreased and the mitochondria exhibited severe alterations (24).

Triiodothyronine

When 3,3′, 5-triiodo-L-thyronine (T_3) was subcutaneously administered in a single daily dose of 0.2 mg/kg for 3 and 16 days, respectively, there was a gradual increase in heart rate, LV systolic pressure, and cardiac output. Also, RV systolic pressure was elevated from 32 ± 1 mm Hg (n = 7) to 41 ± 1 mm Hg (n = 7) and to 49 ± 2 mm Hg (n = 3), respectively (17). After 3 days of daily T_3 administration, the percent increase in RV systolic pressure and RV dp/dt_{max} was greater than that in LV systolic pressure and LV dp/dt_{max}. Also, the increase in the cardiac RNA/DNA ratio and in the heart weight/body weight ratio was more pronounced in the RV (+45% and +22%, respectively) than in the LV (+32% and +10%, respectively) (18). When T_3 treatment was extended to longer periods of time, RV hypertrophy was also predominant (25,26). This can be explained by the fact that the RV has to handle a pressure overload in addition to volume overload. This is also in agreement with the finding that, in chronic hyperthyroidism, the RV shows fibrosis and focal necrosis (27). These typical morphologic signs of pressure overload were not observed in the LV.

Monocrotaline

The administration of monocrotaline is a widely used method for inducing pulmonary hypertension and RV hypertrophy. A single injection of monocrotaline (60 mg/kg) in rats produced thickening of the pulmonary arteries and RV hypertrophy. In addition, there was swelling, focal necrosis, hemorrhage, and hyaline thrombosis of the alveolar walls. Time course studies revealed that the morphologic effects of monocrotaline were primarily related to injury of the alveolar walls, and that hypertrophy of the RV and the pulmonary arterial lesions were probably attributable to pulmonary hypertension (28).

Combined physiologic and morphologic studies showed that, 4 weeks after a single intravenous injection of monocrotaline pyrrole (2 and 4 mg/kg, respectively), a dose-dependent elevation of peak RV pressure occurred, with a concomitant increase in RV end diastolic pressure (RVEDP). The values for the group receiving 4 mg/kg of monocrotaline pyrrole were 4 to 5 times greater than those recorded for the control groups. The RV was markedly dilated and hypertrophied, so that by 4 weeks, the RV weighed almost three times that of the controls. Numerous pulmonary vessels had become partially or completely occluded with fibrin and platelet thrombi as a result of enlargement of the endothelium and hypertrophy of smooth muscle cells in the tunica media. Impairment of pulmonary blood flow had led to tissue hypoxia, which was reflected by an increase in hemoglobin, hematocrit, and erythrocyte count values (29).

In another study, an aqueous solution of monocrotaline hydrochloride, equivalent to a dose of 60 mg/kg, was subcutaneously injected in rats. There was a time-dependent elevation in pulmonary artery pressure and an increase in the medial thickness of small pulmonary blood vessels in relation to postinjection time. RV hypertrophy, which progressed with time, was observed during the second week after monocrotaline injection. There were positive correlations between the elevation in pulmonary artery pressure and the development of RV hypertrophy, between the medial thickness of pulmonary vessels and the weight of the RV, and between the elevation in pulmonary artery pressure and the enlargement of medial thickness of small pulmonary blood vessels as a function of time after monocrotaline injection (30).

Several hours after injection of a large dose of monocrotaline pyrrole, the earliest change noted in rats was an increase in the relative weight of the lungs. No changes were observed in the right heart at this time. It thus appears that toxic effects are primarily exerted at the endothelium of the small pulmonary blood vessels. Therefore, the progressive increase in medial thickness of small pulmonary vessels was responsible for the progressive elevation in pulmonary artery pressure that induced hypertrophy of the RV (30). The volume of cardiac myocytes isolated from the RV of monocrotaline-treated rats was increased owing primarily to an increase in cell cross-sectional area. The cells were only moderately elongated (31). An increase in cross-sectional area is indicative of pressure-induced concentric hypertrophy.

Lung Irradiation

RV hypertrophy can also be created in male Brown-Norway rats by a single bilateral thorax irradiation with x-rays of 300 kV in a dose of 17 Gy. This leads to vascular inflammation with intimal proliferative lesions and fibromuscular hypertrophy. Ultimately, there is fibrous accumulation around pulmonary blood vessels, obliterative intimal and medial thickening, and narrowing of the vessel lumen (32–34). In this experimental model, RV systolic pressure was elevated from 23 ± 3 mm Hg (n = 8) to 62 ± 8 mm Hg (n = 4) after 40 days, and to 81 ± 4 mm Hg (n = 11) after 45 days subsequent to lung irradiation. RV dp/dt_{max} was increased from $1,479 \pm 149$ mm Hg/sec to $2,404 \pm 256$ mm Hg/sec after 40 days and to $3,481 \pm 288$ mm Hg/sec after 45 days. LV systolic pressure and cardiac output were not changed after 40 days, but were decreased after 45 days, indicating impaired filling of the left heart. There was selective hypertrophy of the RV, as evidenced by an 80% increase in the RV weight/heart weight ratio. Also the RNA/DNA ratio was elevated to a similar extent in the RV, whereas it was not altered in the LV (17).

Pulmonary Artery Stenosis

A purely mechanical model of RV hypertrophy in rats is induced by stenosis of the pulmonary artery. After administration of ether anesthesia and subsequent thoracotomy, a band is fixed around the pulmonary artery and a wire 1.7 mm in diameter is placed alongside this vessel. The wire is then removed, leaving the pulmonary artery constricted to an outer diameter equivalent to the diameter of the wire (35). After 2 weeks, RV systolic pressure was increased from 35 ± 2 mm Hg (n = 10) to 61 ± 4 mm Hg (n = 6), with a slight elevation of the RVEDP from 2.3 ± 0.3 mm Hg to 4.7 ± 0.2 mm Hg. There was a selective increase (57%) in the RV weight/body weight ratio. At the cellular level, cardiac myocytes isolated from the RV free wall showed a 58% increase in volume and cross-sectional area (35).

Myocardial Infarction

Large myocardial infarctions in rats, induced by ligation of the descending branch of the left coronary artery, are characterized by a marked elevation in LV end diastolic pressure (LVEDP) from 3.4 ± 0.8 mm Hg (n = 20) to 32 ± 2 mm Hg (n = 14), whereas LV systolic pressure was surprisingly well maintained at 115 ± 3 mm Hg. In these animals, RV systolic pressure was increased from a control value in sham-operated animals of 37 ± 1 mm Hg (n = 19) to 79 ± 2 mm Hg (n = 15). The RV weight/body weight ratio was increased by 90%. Cardiac myocytes isolated from the RV of rats with large myocardial infarction had a 107% and 73% increase in cell volume and cross-sectional area, respectively. This finding clearly indicated pressure-induced concentric hypertrophy of the RV, which must have developed as a consequence of pulmonary hypertension. Histologic studies revealed that there was a marked thickening of the media of small pulmonary arteries, with obstruction of the lumen. This was interpreted to be the morphologic manifestation of an increase in pulmonary vascular resistance (36). Compared to the extent of RV hypertrophy, the 23% increase in septum weight of these infarcted animals was quite moderate. Thus, large myocardial infarctions in rats are characterized by pulmonary hypertension and predominantly pressure-induced RV hypertrophy.

PHARMACOLOGIC INTERVENTIONS IN PULMONARY HYPERTENSION AND RIGHT VENTRICULAR HYPERTROPHY

Calcium Antagonists in Hypoxia-Induced Pulmonary Hypertension

Rats were exposed to two successive 5-minute periods of hypoxia (see the previous section relating to hypoxia in experimental models), separated by a normoxic interval of 60 minutes' duration during which the animals received an intravenous infusion of 0.9% NaCl or of several drugs. Hypoxia caused a marked rise in RV systolic pressure and a moderate increase in RV dp/dt_{max}. The functional response to the second hypoxic period did not differ from the first one when only 0.9% NaCl was infused. All of the calcium antagonists tested reduced the increase in hypoxic pressure in a dose-dependent manner and ultimately abolished it. Nisoldipin was the most effective substance, followed by nifedipine, nitrendipine, and verapamil. By contrast, the α-adrenergic antagonist prazosin and the β-adrenergic blocker propranolol did not influence the hypoxic pressure response. The angiotensin-converting enzyme (ACE) inhibitor captopril and nitroglycerin attenuated the increase in RV systolic pressure to some extent. Thus, when compared with other drugs, calcium antagonists—in particular, nisoldipine—were by far the most effective substances that antagonized the hypoxia-induced increase in RV systolic pressure (19).

Angiotensin-Converting Enzyme Inhibition in Pressure-Induced Right Ventricular Hypertrophy

The influence of the ACE inhibitor ramipril (1 mg/kg orally in a single daily dose) on RV hypertrophy was studied in female Sprague-Dawley rats in which the pulmonary artery had been banded to an outer diameter of 1.7 mm by the method described earlier. After 2 weeks, LV and RV hemodynamic parameters were measured in the anesthetized animals. Moreover, regional heart weights were determined, and myocytes obtained from three different regions of the heart (LV, RV, and septum) were subjected to morphometric analysis. Ramipril slightly reduced LV systolic pressure and LV dp/dt$_{max}$ as compared to banded animals that did not receive treatment. The increase in RV systolic pressure and in the weight gain of the RV free wall were not affected. However, the increase in cell volume of isolated cardiac myocytes was less pronounced in this group ($+27\%$ as compared to $+58\%$ in untreated animals). Thus, ACE inhibition with ramipril appeared to attenuate the cellular hypertrophy in this experimental model without affecting the weight increase of the RV (35). In a model of pressure-induced LV hypertrophy, ramipril had no effect at all on the development of cardiac hypertrophy, both at the macroscopic and the cellular level (37). Thus, ACE inhibition is not effective in preventing the development of cardiac hypertrophy when the pressure imposed on the heart is held constant.

SUMMARY

The function of the RV has been appreciated only recently in experimental studies. This has become possible through the application of methods previously applied to the LV and by miniaturization of catheter-tipped manometers. From all of these investigations, it appears that the RV plays an important role in maintaining circulation in a variety of pathophysiologic conditions, including pulmonary hypertension. Several problems remain to be resolved in this interesting area of active research. For instance, the exact mechanism underlying the hypoxia-induced constriction of pulmonary vessels, as compared to that produced by dilatation in the systemic circulation, has not yet been established. Furthermore, the role of possible growth factors in the thickening of the tunica media of small pulmonary vessels that occurs in chronic hypoxia, monocrotaline treatment, and myocardial infarction remain to be elucidated. Finally, the effect of chronic administration of catecholamines (such as norepinephrine, which induces LV hypertrophy [38]) on the function, morphology, and metabolism of the RV remains to be studied. This is of particular importance as patients with end-stage heart failure are treated with sympathomimetic agents with the understanding that their effects are directed primarily to the LV.

REFERENCES

1. Zimmer H-G. Correlation between haemodynamic and metabolic changes in three models of experimental cardiac hypertrophy. *Eur Heart J* 1984;5 [Suppl F]:171–179.
2. Lompre A-M, Mercadier J-J, Schwartz K. Changes in gene expression during cardiac growth. *Int Rev Cytol* 1991;124:137–186.
3. Starr I, Jeffers WA, Meade RH. The absence of conspicuous increments of venous pressure after severe damage to the right ventricle of the dog, with a discussion of the relation between clinical congestive failure and heart disease. *Am Heart J* 1943;26:291–301.

4. Bakos ACP. The question of the function of the right ventricular myocardium: an experimental study. *Circulation* 1950;1:724–732.
5. Kagan A. Dynamic responses of the right ventricle following extensive damage by cauterization. *Circulation* 1952;5:816–823.
6. Donald DE, Essex HE. Pressure studies after inactivation of the major portion of the canine right ventricle. *Am J Physiol* 1954;176:155–161.
7. Rose JC, Cosimano SJ, Hufnagel CA, Massullo EA. The effect of exclusion of the right ventricle from the circulation in dogs. *J Clin Invest* 1955;34:1625–1631.
8. Guiha NH, Limas CJ, Cohn JN. Predominant right ventricular dysfunction after right ventricular destruction in the dog. *Am J Cardiol* 1974;33:254–258.
9. Uhl HSM. A previously undescribed congenital malformation of the heart: almost total absence of the myocardium of the right ventricle. *Bull Johns Hopkins Hosp* 1952;91:197–209.
10. Cumming GR, Bowman JM, Whytehead L. Congenital aplasia of the myocardium of the right ventricle (Uhl's anomaly). *Am Heart J* 1965;70:671–676.
11. Dalla-Volta S, Battaglia G, Zerbini E. "Auricularization" of right ventricular pressure curve. *Am Heart J* 1961;61:25–33.
12. Cohn JN, Guiha NH, Broder MI, Limas CJ. Right ventricular infarction. Clinical and hemodynamic features. *Am J Cardiol* 1974;33:209–214.
13. von Euler US, Liljestrand G. Observations on the pulmonary arterial blood pressure in the cat. *Acta Physiol Scand* 1947;12:301–320.
14. Arias-Stella J, Saldana M. The terminal portion of the pulmonary arterial tree in people native to high altitudes. *Circulation* 1963;28:915–925.
15. Arias-Stella J, Recavarren S. Right ventricular hypertrophy in native children living at high altitude. *Am J Pathol* 1962;41:55–64.
16. Forman MB, Wilson BH, Sheller JR, Kopelman HA, Vaughn WK, Virmani R, Friesinger GC. Right ventricular hypertrophy is an important determinant of right ventricular infarction complicating acute inferior left ventricular infarction. *J Am Coll Cardiol* 1987;10:1180–1187.
17. Zimmer H-G, Zierhut W, Seesko RC, Varekamp AE. Right heart catheterization in rats with pulmonary hypertension and right ventricular hypertrophy. *Basic Res Cardiol* 1988;83:48–57.
18. Zierhut W, Zimmer H-G. Differential effects of triiodothyronine on rat left and right ventricular function and the influence of metoprolol. *J Mol Cell Cardiol* 1989;21:617–624.
19. Zierhut W, Zimmer H-G. Effect of calcium antagonists and other drugs on the hypoxia-induced increase in rat right ventricular pressure. *J Cardiovasc Pharmacol* 1989;14:311–318.
20. Zimmer H-G, Zierhut W, Marschner G. Combination of ribose with calcium antagonist and β-blocker treatment in closed-chest rats. *J Mol Cell Cardiol* 1987;19:635–639.
21. Zwissler B, Schosser R, Schwickert C, Spengler P, Weiss M, Iber V, Messmer K. Perfusion of the interventricular septum during ventilation with positive end-expiratory pressure. *Crit Care Med* 1991;19:1414–1424.
22. Zwissler B, Forst H, Messmer K. Acute pulmonary microembolism induces different regional changes in preload and contraction pattern in canine right ventricle. *Cardiovasc Res* 1990;24:285–295.
23. Porcelli RJ, Bergofsky EH. Adrenergic receptors in pulmonary vasoconstrictor responses to gaseous and humoral agents. *J Appl Physiol* 1973;34:483–488.
24. Schneider M, Wiese S, Kunkel B, Hauk H, Pfeiffer B. Development and regression of right heart ventricular hypertrophy: biochemical and morphological aspects. *Z Kardiol* 1987;76[Suppl 3]:1–8.
25. Van Liere EJ, Sizemore DA, Hunnel J. Size of cardiac ventricles in experimental hyperthyroidism in the rat. *Proc Soc Exp Biol Med* 1969;132:663–665.
26. Gerdes AM, Moore JA, Hines JM. Regional changes in myocyte size and number in propranolol-treated hyperthyroid rats. *Lab Invest* 1987;57:708–713.
27. Gerdes AM, Moore JA, Bishop SP. Failure of propranolol to prevent chronic hyperthyroid induced cardiac hypertrophy and multifocal cellular necrosis in the rat. *Can J Cardiol* 1985;1:340–345.
28. Hayashi Y, Hussa JF, Lalich JJ. Cor pulmonale in rats. *Lab Invest* 1967;16:875–881.
29. Chesney CF, Allen JR, Hsu IC. Right ventricular hypertrophy in monocrotaline pyrrole treated rats. *Exp Mol Pathol* 1974;20:257–268.
30. Ghodsi F, Will JA. Changes in pulmonary structure and function induced by monocrotaline intoxication. *Am J Physiol* 1981;240:H149–H155.
31. Werchan PM, Summer WR, Gerdes AM, McDonough KH. Right ventricular performance after monocrotaline-induced pulmonary hypertension. *Am J Physiol* 1989;256:H1328–H1336.

32. Gross NJ. The pathogenesis of radiation-induced lung damage. *Lung* 1981;159:115–125.
33. Maisin JR. The ultrastructure of the lung of mice exposed to a supra-lethal dose of ionizing radiation on the thorax. *Radiat Res* 1970;44:545–564.
34. Slauson DO, Hahn FF, Chiffelle TL. The pulmonary vascular pathology of experimental radiation pneumonitis. *Am J Pathol* 1977;88:635–648.
35. Zierhut W, Zimmer H-G, Gerdes AM. Influence of ramipril on right ventricular hypertrophy induced by pulmonary artery stenosis in rats. *J Cardiovasc Pharmacol* 1990;16:480–486.
36. Zimmer H-G, Gerdes AM, Lortet S, Mall G. Changes in heart function and cardiac cell size in rats with chronic myocardial infarction. *J Mol Cell Cardiol* 1990;22:1231–1243.
37. Zierhut W, Zimmer H-G, Gerdes AM. Effect of angiotensin converting enzyme inhibition on pressure-induced left ventricular hypertrophy in rats. *Circ Res* 1991;69:609–617.
38. Zierhut W, Zimmer H-G. Significance of myocardial α- and β-adrenoceptors in catecholamine-induced cardiac hypertrophy. *Circ Res* 1989;65:1417–1425.

The Cardiomyopathic Heart, edited by Makoto
Nagano, Nobuakira Takeda, and Naranjan S.
Dhalla. Raven Press, Ltd., New York © 1994.

35

Effects of Monocrotaline-Induced Pulmonary Hypertension on Right Ventricular Hemodynamic, Biochemical, and Histologic Changes

Yoshiyuki Hirota, Makoto Nagai, Tadanari Ohkubo, and
Makoto Nagano

*Department of Internal Medicine, Aoto Hospital, Jikei University School of Medicine,
Aoto 6-41-2, Katsushika-ku, Tokyo 125, Japan*

INTRODUCTION

Monocrotaline (MCT) is a pyrrolizidine alkaloid extracted from the leaves and seeds of *Crotalaria spectabilis* (1). It is a thoroughly studied substance, and is known to cause characteristic pulmonary vascular lesions, including medial hyperplasia, hypertrophy of pulmonary arterial muscle, muscularization of pulmonary arterioles, and capillary endothelial cell changes. In addition, MCT induces pulmonary hypertension, cardiomegaly with right heart dilatation, and cor pulmonale (2–5). We studied the effect of MCT-induced pulmonary hypertension on the right heart of rats by examining right ventricular hemodynamic, biochemical, and histologic changes. Also, in an effort to learn more about the participation of serotonin in pulmonary hypertension, we evaluated the effect of DV-7028 (DV), a selective 5-hydroxytryptamine$_2$ (5-HT$_2$) receptor antagonist (6), in this experimental model.

MATERIALS AND METHODS

Male Sprague-Dawley rats that weighed 150 to 180 g and that were 7 weeks old received a single 40 mg/kg dose of a 2% MCT solution (7) by subcutaneous injection. Pathologic changes in the right heart were monitored over time (1, 2, and 4 weeks after MCT injection) and compared with those in an untreated control group. The time-course changes occurring after MCT administration were assessed at 1, 2, 4, and 6 weeks after MCT injection (n = 6 in each group).

In addition, the effect of treatment with 20 mg/kg/day of DV-7028 (Daiichi Pharmaceutical Co., Tokyo, Japan), provided continuously in the drinking water, was assessed. The animals were divided into the following five groups (n = 8 in each group): (a) controls, no treatment; (b) PDVC, DV administration only, starting on day 3; (c) MCT, MCT alone; (d) MCT + DV, DV administration starting at the time of MCT injection; and (e) MCT + PDV, DV administration starting 3 days before MCT injection. The following parameters were examined:

(a) *Index of right ventricular hypertrophy.* The ratio of the weight of the right ventricle to that of the left ventricle and interventricular septum was derived in accordance with the method of Fulton et al. (8). The result was used as the index of right ventricular hypertrophy.

(b) *Hemodynamic analysis.* Electrocardiographic studies were conducted using 12 leads, as previously described (9). In addition, right ventricular systolic pressure and dP/dt_{max} were measured. Zimmer's catheter was inserted through the right external jugular vein into the right ventricle for pressure monitoring (10).

(c) *Biochemical analysis of the right ventricle.* The right ventricle was frozen in liquid nitrogen and stored at $-80°C$ for determination of the myosin isoenzyme and hydroxyproline. The analysis of myosin isozyme and hydroxyproline was done with the same homogenate. The extraction and separation of myosin isoenzyme were carried out as described previously (11,12). The isomeric pattern was determined by laser-densitometry after application of Boezy's stain (13). Hydroxyproline content, an indicator for collagen, was also assessed. The hydrolysis of the tissue (50 mg/mL) in 6N HCl was carried out at 120°C for 16 hours. The measurement of hydroxyproline was carried out according to the method of Stegemann and Stalder (14). The resulting values were expressed in terms of the protein concentration (Lowry's method) of the tissue.

(d) *Histologic analysis.* Transverse sections that had been cut serially from the apex to the basal portion of the heart, as well as sections of maximal diameter, were prepared for light microscopic examination. Hematoxylin and eosin and Masson's stains were applied.

Statistical Analysis of the Data

Equality of variances was checked by Bartlett's test. Multiple comparisons were carried out by Duncan's multiple range test. All values were expressed as mean $\pm$ SD. Statistical significance was assumed at $p < 0.05$.

RESULTS

Right Ventricular Hypertrophy

As shown in Figure 1, the group receiving MCT exhibited a marked increase in the index for right ventricular hypertrophy 2 weeks after MCT administration in

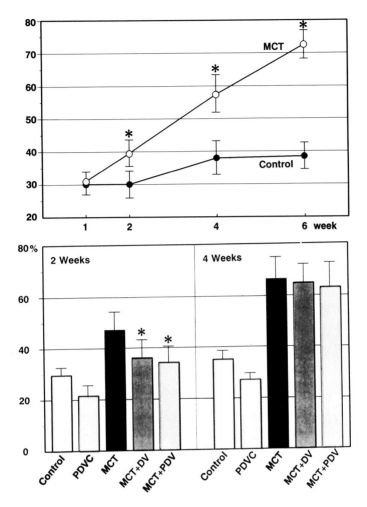

FIG. 1. Changes in the right ventricular index (see description in the text). The upper panel shows the time course of the index, whereas the lower panel illustrates the effect of DV-7028 (DV). *MCT*, monocrotaline; *PDVC*, DV-7028 administration only, starting on day 3; *MCT + DV*, DV administration at the time of MCT injection; *MCT + PDV*, DV administration starting 3 days before MCT injection; *control*, no treatment.

comparison with the control group. The degree of increase rose over time to 74% at 6 weeks. Two weeks after MCT administration, the degree of right ventricular hypertrophy was significantly lowered by treatment with DV. However, this effect was not observed at 4 weeks post-MCT treatment.

Hemodynamic Analysis

ECG Changes

No ECG changes were seen in the control group over time. However, in the group receiving MCT, ECG findings indicated right ventricular hypertrophy (right axis deviation, an increase in the P wave amplitude, and a high R wave and strain pattern from the right thoracic leads) 4 weeks after MCT administration. These features were most striking 6 weeks after MCT administration. By contrast, rats treated with DV exhibited a lesser degree of right ventricular hypertrophy, as evidenced by the observed ECG changes.

Right Ventricular Pressure

Figure 2 shows the temporal change in right ventricular systolic pressure and the effect of DV on this parameter. In the control group, no elevation was seen with the passage of time, whereas a significant elevation in right ventricular systolic pressure was observed in the MCT-treated group 2 weeks after MCT administration (13.3 ± 3.4 mm Hg versus 25.4 ± 2.2 mm Hg). Furthermore, DV decreased right ventricular systolic pressure 2 weeks after MCT administration (MCT + DV: 18.1 ± 2.9 mm Hg; MCT + PDV: 19.1 ± 2.2 mm Hg). However, this effect was not observed 4 weeks post-MCT administration.

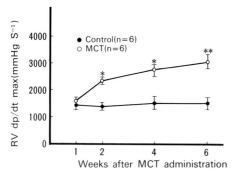

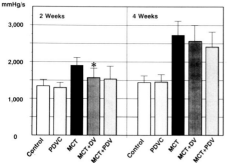

FIG. 2. Changes in the right ventricular (RV) systolic pressure. The upper panel shows the time course of systolic pressure, whereas the lower panel shows the effect of DV-7028. *MCT*, monocrotaline; *PDVC*, DV-7028 administration only, starting on day 3; *MCT + DV*, DV administration at the time of MCT injection; *MCT + PDV*, DV administration starting 3 days before MCT injection; *control*, no treatment.

Right Ventricular dP/dt$_{max}$

Among control animals, no elevation in right ventricular dP/dt$_{max}$ was detected. By contrast, a significant elevation was observed in the group receiving MCT 2 weeks after MCT administration ($1,340 \pm 166$ mm Hg/sec versus $2,310 \pm 144$ mm Hg/sec). DV decreased right ventricular dP/dt$_{max}$ at 2 weeks, but not at 4 weeks, after MCT administration (MCT + DV: $1,920 \pm 123$ mm Hg/sec; MCT + PDV: $1,870 \pm 173$ mm Hg/sec).

Biochemical Analysis

Myosin V3

The myosin isoenzyme profiles in the right ventricle and the effect of DV on the myosin V3 content are depicted in Figure 3. In the MCT-treated group, the myosin isoenzyme pattern showed a tendency to shift from V1 predominance to V3 predominance 4 weeks after MCT administration. When DV was started at the time of MCT injection (MCT + DV group), it reduced the myosin V3 at 4 weeks postadministration. However, when DV was started 3 days prior to MCT injection (MCT + PDV group), this reduction did not occur.

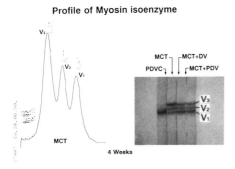

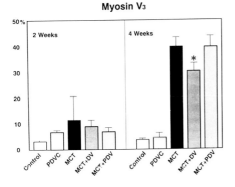

FIG. 3. The upper panel shows the myosin isoenzyme profile in the right ventricle at 4 weeks after MCT administration. The lower panel shows the effect of DV-7028 on the right ventricular V3 content. *MCT,* monocrotaline; *PDVC,* DV-7028 administration only, starting on day 3; *MCT + DV,* DV administration at the time of MCT injection; *MCT + PDV,* DV administration starting 3 days before MCT injection; *control,* no treatment.

Hydroxyproline Content

Figure 4 presents the change over time in the hydroxyproline content of the right and left ventricles and the effect of DV on its concentration in the right ventricle. The controls showed no significant changes in this regard, whereas a marked increase was seen in the right ventricles of the MCT-treated group 2 weeks after administration (1.72 ± 0.18 μg/mg versus 3.64 ± 0.09 μg/mg of protein). However, no further increase occurred thereafter. Similarly, the left ventricular muscle showed an increase in hydroxyproline content 2 weeks after MCT administration (0.42 ± 0.07 μg/mg versus 1.21 ± 0.08 μg/mg of protein), but no additional increase occurred thereafter. DV reduced right ventricular hydroxyproline content 4 weeks after MCT administration.

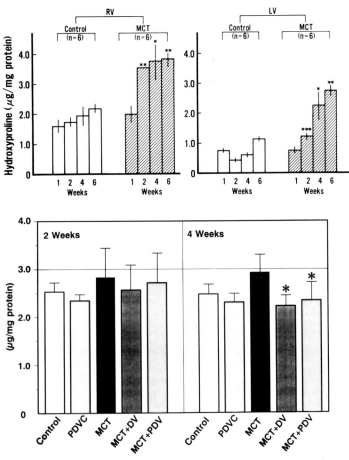

FIG. 4. Changes in the ventricular hydroxyproline concentration. The upper panel represents the time course of hydroxyproline concentration in the right and left ventricles. The lower panel shows the effect of DV-7028 on the right ventricle. *MCT*, monocrotaline; *PDVC*, DV-7028 administration only, starting on day 3; *MCT+DV*, DV administration at the time of MCT injection; *MCT+PDV*, DV administration starting 3 days before MCT injection; *control*, no treatment.

Histological Analysis

Very little change was seen over time in the control specimens. By contrast, a disturbance in the arrangement of the right ventricular myocyte and development of perivascular fibrosis were observed 2 weeks after MCT administration. Only slight hypertrophy of the cardiac muscle cells was noted, but the right ventricle was markedly dilated. Four weeks after MCT administration, severe hyperplasia of the right ventricular myocyte was noted, and nuclear irregularity, widespread hypertrophy and degenerative necrosis of cardiac muscle cells, further perivascular fibrosis, and replacement fibrosis were prominent. Photomicrographs representative of these changes are presented in Figure 5. In animals treated with DV, these fibrotic changes were not prevented or retarded.

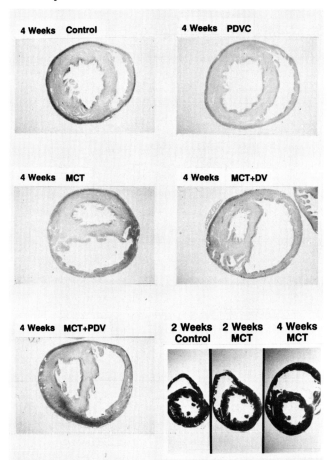

FIG. 5. Hematoxylin-eosin–stained photomicrographs. Each shows the maximum diameter of horizontal sections. The right ventricle was markedly dilated 2 weeks after MCT administration. DV-7028 appeared to have no effect on this process. *MCT*, monocrotaline; *PDVC*, DV-7028 administration only, starting on day 3; *MCT + DV*, DV administration at the time of MCT injection; *MCT + PDV*, DV administration starting 3 days before MCT injection; *control*, no treatment.

DISCUSSION

The characteristic MCT-induced pulmonary vascular lesions are not attributable to MCT itself, but to an active metabolite, monocrotaline pyrrole, which is produced in the liver (15–17). Although the mechanism by which this metabolite produces pulmonary hypertension is unknown, it reportedly causes pulmonary endothelial injury and pulmonary edema (18,19) and, after some weeks, chronic structural changes. Pulmonary endothelial injury, such as degeneration and deciduation, leads to thrombus formation, reduction of the pulmonary vascular bed, and loss of synthesis and release of humoral factors. In addition, 5-HT, histamine, and prostanoids are released from platelets and inflammatory cells (20–22). Therefore, it has been suggested that 5-HT could be involved in the development of pulmonary hypertension.

To investigate the role of 5-HT in the cardiopulmonary response to MCT, the effect of a new 5-HT$_2$ receptor antagonist, DV-7028, was examined in MCT-treated rats. According to the hemodynamic, biochemical, and histologic data compiled, DV-7028 significantly reduced right ventricular hypertrophy for up to 2 weeks after MCT administration. However, this effect did not persist 4 weeks after treatment. Moreover, in similar experiments using Ketanserine (23) (another 5-HT$_2$ receptor antagonist), cotreatment with this agent failed to alter the right ventricular hypertrophic response to MCT. It is likely that DV-7028 and Ketanserine possess different receptor binding affinities. The fact that DV-7028 has no apparent influence on MCT-induced changes at 4 weeks suggests that MCT's potency is greater than that of DV-7028.

SUMMARY

Hemodynamic, biochemical, and histologic changes in the right ventricle were assessed in rats with MCT-induced pulmonary hypertension. A single dose of MCT (40 mg/kg) was injected into male Sprague-Dawley rats weighing 150 to 180 g to induce pulmonary hypertension. This study had two components: one part was concerned with the time-course changes after MCT administration, whereas the other part examined the effect of treatment with 5-HT$_2$ receptor antagonist. The time-course changes were measured at 1, 2, 4, and 6 weeks after MCT injection. 5-HT$_2$ receptor antagonist (20 mg/kg/day, DV-7028) was added to the drinking water and the animals were observed 2 and 4 weeks after MCT administration. The inspected parameters were index of right ventricular hypertrophy, electrocardiographic (ECG) changes, right ventricular systolic pressure, myosin isoenzyme, hydroxyproline content, and light microscopic findings.

ECG studies disclosed right ventricular hypertrophy 4 weeks after the MCT injection, whereas the right ventricular peak pressure and dP/dt$_{max}$ were increased 2 weeks after injection. The myosin isoenzyme pattern shifted toward V3 in hypertrophied right ventricles beginning at 4 weeks after MCT injection. The right ventricular hydroxyproline content increased 2 weeks after MCT administration. Microscopic study revealed marked dilatation and fibrosis of the right ventricle 2 weeks after MCT administration. These results demonstrate that MCT-induced pulmonary hypertension produced right ventricular hypertrophy associated with definite hemodynamic, biochemical, and histologic alterations of the myocardium. The treatment of animals with DV-7028 suppressed the myocardial effects of MCT-induced pulmonary hypertension.

REFERENCES

1. Neal WN, Rusoff LL, Ahmann CF. The isolation and some properties of an alkaloid from Crotalaria spectabilis Roth. *J Am Chem Soc* 1935;57:2560.
2. Kay JM, Harris P, Heath D. Pulmonary hypertension produced in rats by ingestion of Crotalaria spectabilis seeds. Thorax 1968;22:176–79.
3. Lalich JJ, Merkow L. Pulmonary arteritis produced in rats by feeding Crotalaria spectabilis. *Lab Invest* 1961;10:744–50.
4. Hayashi Y, Hussa JF, Lalich JJ. Cor pulmonale in rats. *Lab Invest* 1967;16:875–81.
5. Stotzer H, Herbst M, Reichl R, Kollmer H. Zur pathogeneses der experimentellen pulmonalen hypertonie. *Virchows Arch [A]* 1972;356:331–42.
6. Morishima Y, Tanaka T, Watanabe K, Igarashi T, Yasuoka M, Shibano T. Prevention by DV-7028, a selective 5-HT receptor antagonist, of the formation of coronary thrombi in dogs. *Cardiovasc Res* 1991;25:727–30.
7. Kajihara H, Takanishi A, Kato Y. A method of monocrotaline induced cor pulmonale (right ventricular hypertrophy) in rat (in Japanese). *Methods of cardiac metabolism*. Tokyo: Ishiyaku; 1988;135–138.
8. Fulton RM, Hutchinson EC, Morgam JA. Ventricular weight in cardiac hypertrophy. *Br Heart J* 1952;14:413–20.
9. Takeda A, Nagai M, Takeda N, Kawai S, Okada R, Nagano M. Morphological and biochemical abnormalities in new cardiomyopathic syrian hamster (in Japanese). *Cardiac Struct Metab* 1988; 11:617–29.
10. Zimmer HG, Zierhut W, Seesko RC, Varekamp AE. Right heart catheterization in rats with pulmonary hypertension and right ventricular hypertrophy. *Basic Res Cardiol* 1988;83:48–57.
11. Martin AF, Pagani ED, Solaro RJ. Thyroxine-induced redistribution of isoenzyme of rabbit ventricular myosin. *Circ Res* 1982;50:117–24.
12. Hoh JFY, Megrath PA, Hale PT. Electrophoretic analysis of multiple forms of rat cardiac myosin: effects of hypophysectomy and thyroxine replacement. *J Mol Cell Cardiol* 1977;10:1053–76.
13. Blakesley RW, Boezi JA. A new staining technique for proteins in polyacrylamide gels using Coomassie Brilliant Blue G250. *Anal Biochem* 1977;82:580–582.
14. Stegemann H, Stalder K. Determination of hydroxyproline. *Clin Chim Acta* 1967;18:267–73.
15. Mattocks AR. Toxicity of pyrrolizidine alkaloids. *Nature* 1968;217:723.
16. Plestina R, Stoner HB. Pulmonary edema in rats given monocrotaline pyrrole. *J Pathol* 1972; 106:235.
17. Plestina R, Stoner HB, Glenys J, Butler WH, Mattocks AR. Vascular changes in the lungs of rats after intravenous injection of pyrrole carbamates. *J Pathol* 1977;121:9–18.
18. Sugita T, Hyers TM, Dauber IM, Wagner WW, McMurtry IF, Reeves JT. Lung vessel leak precedes right ventricular hypertrophy in monocrotaline-treated rats. *J Appl Physiol* (*Resp Environ Exercise Physiol*) 1983;54:371.
19. Valdivia E, Sonnad J, Hayashi Y, Lalich JJ. Experimental interstitial pulmonary edema. *Angiology* 1967;18:378.
20. Hilliker KS, Roth RA. Increased vascular responsiveness in lungs of rats with pulmonary hypertension induced by monocrotaline pyrrole. *Am Rev Respir Dis* 1985;131:46–50.

21. Takeoka O, Angevine DM, Lalich JJ. Stimulation of mast cells in rats fed various chemicals. *Am J Pathol* 1962;40:545–54.
22. Scott E, Vaage J, Wiberg T. Lack of release of prostaglandins from isolated perfused lungs during pulmonary hypertension and edema. *Br J Pharmacol* 1979;65:197–204.
23. Ganey E, Hilliker SK, Hadley B, Roth A. Monocrotaline pyrrole-induced cardiopulmonary toxicity is not altered by Metergoline or Ketanserine. *J Pharmacol Exp* 1986;237:226–31.

The Cardiomyopathic Heart, edited by Makoto
Nagano, Nobuakira Takeda, and Naranjan S.
Dhalla. Raven Press, Ltd., New York © 1994.

36

Age-Dependent Differences in Cardiac Growth Response to Workload

Jan Slezak, *Ladislav Zlatos, †Arvinder Randhawa, and
†Pawan K. Singal

*Institute for Heart Research, Slovak Academy of Sciences; *Institute of
Pathophysiology, Medical Faculty, Comenius University, Bratislava, Czech and Slovak
Federative Republic; and †St. Boniface General Hospital Research Centre,
Faculty of Medicine, University of Manitoba, Winnipeg, Canada, R2H 2A6*

INTRODUCTION

Myocardial hypertrophy is the main adaptive response designed to sustain a chronic increase in workload. The cardiac growth response (i.e., cell hyperplasia and/or hypertrophy) may depend on the age at which the load is imposed (1). In embryonic stages, the spontaneous mitotic activity of cardiomyocytes of mammals is intensive, and this rapidly decreases after birth (1–4). In humans as well as other primates, hyperplasia may end in the prenatal period (5). However, in most experimental animals, the mitotic activity of cardiac muscle cells is present even after birth and generally ceases within the first few weeks of postnatal life (1,4,6–8). Thus, the exact stages of involvement of cell hyperplasia, cell hypertrophy, and increased collagen in hypertrophied response remain to be defined.

Although the mechanism of regulation and the cause of cessation of mitotic activity of cardiomyocytes have not yet been elucidated completely, participation of several cellular and extracellular factors has been suggested (6,9). In this regard, cardiomyocyte mitotic activity is inhibited by an increase in contractile proteins (10), DNA-synthesis repressors (11), intracellular pO_2 (12), intracellular NAD^+ (13), and intracellular cyclic adenosine monophosphate (cAMP) (14). Maturation of myocytes, as well as interaction between neighboring myocytes, is also known to influence mitotic activity (6,9). The total number of cardiac muscle cells can be enhanced if the rate of the heart growth during the early postnatal period is accelerated by various physiological or pathologic factors (Table 1). However, only the undifferentiated myocytes have the ability to respond to these factors by increased proliferation (15).

Currently, several experimental models exist in which these factors (see Table 1)

TABLE 1. *Stimuli for the mitotic activity in cardiomyocytes in the early postnatal period*

Physiological Stimuli
    Increased food intake
    Increased heart workload owing to physical training
Pathologic Stimuli
    Increased heart workload owing to pathologic state of the organism
    Low pO_2 in cardiomyocytes
    Inhibition of the postnatal maturation of myocardial sympathetic innervation

can be modified in a systematic fashion. These models differ not only in the degree but also in the rate of hypertrophic growth. Mitotic activity during the perinatal period can be influenced by increased food intake (16); increased physical training (17–19); increased pressure overload (20–22); sideropenic anemia and/or anemic hypoxia (23); chronic hypotensive or normotensive hypoxemic hypoxia (24–26); exogenous thyroid hormone intake (27,28); and chronic sympathectomy of the newborn heart (17–19,29).

In the present study involving newborn puppies and young guinea pigs, we have tried to determine the age at which increases in cellular hypertrophy and connective tissue become the principal adaptive responses to chronically increased pressure overload.

MATERIAL AND METHODS

Pressure overload was induced in puppies and young guinea pigs by narrowing of the aorta.

Puppies

Newborn puppies were operated on the second day after birth. A constricting spiral, made of tantalum wire, was placed around the abdominal aorta and the inner diameter of the metal spiral was adjusted so as to reduce the lumen of the aorta by 60% to 70% (29). For each puppy with the aortic constriction, an age-matched puppy of the same litter, same sex, and approximately the same body weight was used as a control. The animals sacrificed at the age of 7 to 42 days were divided into four groups as follows: *Group A*, controls (1 to 3 weeks of age); *Group B*, 1 to 3-week-old puppies with aortic constriction; *Group C*, controls (4 to 6 weeks of age); and *Group D*, 4 to 6-week-old puppies with aortic constriction. For the recording of blood pressure, animals were anesthetized (pentobarbital, 30 mg/kg, administered intraperitoneally), the aorta was cannulated with a polyethylene catheter, and the pressure was recorded. Following this assessment, the chest was opened and the beating heart was removed, placed in ice-cold saline solution, and rinsed of blood. After dissection of extraneous tissue and great vessels, the free wall of the right ventricle was separated from the left ventricle and septum (30). Myocardial tissue samples for biochemical and ultrastructural examination were taken from the free walls of ventricles, midway between the apex and the base.

Water content in the myocardium was determined in tissue samples weighing 250 to 300 mg by drying the samples to a constant weight in an oven set at 105°C. Hydroxyproline (31), RNA, and DNA levels were determined (32). For ultrastructural studies, 1-mm^3 pieces of the left and right ventricles were immersion-fixed in 2.5% glutaraldehyde in 0.1 phosphate buffer (pH of 7.4) for 3 hours, rinsed in the same buffer overnight, and postfixed for 1 hour in 1% OsO_4 in 0.1 phosphate buffer (pH of 7.4). The samples were then dehydrated in graded ethanol series and propylene oxide, and embedded in Epon 812. Thin sections were prepared using a diamond knife; these were then stained with uranyl acetate and lead citrate and studied using a Tesla 500 electron microscope.

Guinea Pigs

Male guinea pigs (25 ± 3 days old) were anesthetized with methohexital sodium (35 mg/kg, administered intraperitoneally). A mildly constricting band was then placed around the ascending aorta using 3-0 silk (33). For hemodynamic measurements, a catheter with a miniature pressure transducer tip was inserted through the right carotid artery into the aorta and left ventricle. Left ventricular systolic pressure (LVSP), left ventricular end diastolic pressure (LVEDP), and aortic systolic and diastolic pressures were recorded on a precalibrated multichannel dynograph. Hydroxyproline content was estimated by spectrophotometric analysis (34). Histologic processing was also done for morphologic and collagen studies (33).

Student's T-test (unpaired) was used for statistical evaluation of the results. Statistical significance was accepted at the 0.05 level. The results are presented as means $\pm$ S.E.

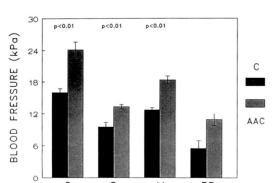

FIG. 1. Mean blood pressure in 1- to 3-week-old puppies with abdominal aortic constriction (*AAC*). *C*, control; *S*, systolic; *D*, diastolic; *M*, mean; *PP*, pulse pressure.

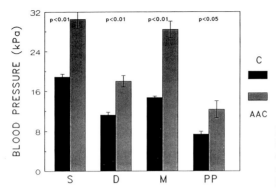

FIG. 2. Mean blood pressure in 4- to 6-week-old puppies with abdominal aortic constriction (*AAC*). *C*, control; *S*, systolic; *D*, diastolic; *M*, mean; *PP*, pulse pressure.

RESULTS

Puppies

In group B, mean blood pressure in the ascending aorta was increased by about 5.52 kPa (41.5 torr), or 42%, over that in the control group A (Fig. 1). In group D, the blood pressure was increased by about 8.35 kPa (62.8 torr), or 57%, compared to that in the control group C (Fig. 2). The mean values of pressure gradient across the constriction in groups B and D are shown in Figure 3.

In group B, the heart weight increased by about 30% and the weight of the left ventricle plus septum was increased by about 40% (Table 2). There was only a slight increase in the weight of the right ventricle. The ratio of the left ventricle plus septum weight to the right ventricle weight in this group was significantly increased ($p<0.01$) as compared to that in group A. When the duration of the increased workload on the hearts of the newborn puppies was prolonged for another 3 weeks, increased hypertrophy of the heart was observed (see Table 2). In group D, the weight of the heart increased by 60%, and the weight of the left ventricle plus septum increased by 72% as compared to that in control group C. This increase in

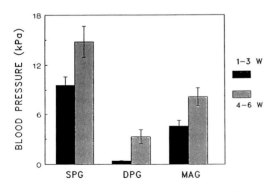

FIG. 3. Blood pressure gradients in puppies 1 to 3 weeks of age (*1–3 W*) and 4 to 6 weeks of age (*4–6 W*) with abdominal aortic constriction. *SPG*, systolic pressure gradient; *DPG*, diastolic pressure gradient; *MAG*, mean aortic pressure gradient.

TABLE 2. *Body weight, total heart weight, and ventricular weight in 1- to 3-week-old and 4- to 6-week-old control puppies (K) and puppies with constriction of the abdominal aorta (S)* ($\bar{x} \pm s_{\bar{x}}$)

Age	Group	Body weight (g)	Heart weight (g)	LV ÷ septum weight (g)	RV weight (g)
1–3 weeks	K (n = 11)	663.63 ± 70.82	4.089 ± 0.428	2.594 ± 0.282	0.916 ± 0.103
	S (n = 11)	639.09 ± 72.96	5.369 ± 0.967	3.655 ± 0.663	1.014 ± 0.174
4–6 weeks	K (n = 9)	1,542.22 ± 121.28	7.896 ± 0.747*	5.452 ± 0.488*	1.502 ± 0.144
	S (n = 9)	1,376.11 ± 100.97	12.611 ± 1.113*	9.377 ± 0.835*	1.938 ± 0.186

*$p < 0.01$.
LV, left ventricle; RV, right ventricle.

left ventricular weight was accompanied by a significant increase ($p < 0.01$) in the wall thickness, as well as in the ratio of left to right ventricle wall thickness ($p < 0.01$). It is noteworthy that, in this older group, there was also a significant increase ($p < 0.01$) in the weight of the right ventricle (see Table 2). However, the ratio of the left ventricular plus septum weight to the right ventricular weight in group D was significantly increased ($p < 0.01$) when compared to that in control group C.

The water content of the right and left ventricles did not differ among groups A through D (Table 3). The hydroxyproline concentration, in the ventricular myocardium as well as the total content, was also recorded (Table 4). Hydroxyproline concentration in the left ventricle of groups B and D was reduced, whereas the total content remained unchanged between groups. There were no changes in the right ventricle with respect to hydroxyproline concentration or content.

RNA concentration in the ventricular myocardium of groups B and D were the same as in the age-matched control groups A and C. However, the total RNA

TABLE 3. *The water content of the ventricular myocardium (expressed as a percentage of the weight) in 1- to 3-week-old and 4- to 6-week-old control puppies (K) and puppies with abdominal aortic constriction (S)*

Age	Group	H_2O percentage of wet weight	
		LV	RV
1–3 weeks	K (n = 11)	81.97 ± 0.13	82.06 ± 0.17
	S (n = 11)	82.07 ± 0.12	81.94 ± 0.18
4–6 weeks	K (n = 9)	80.52 ± 0.24	81.02 ± 0.29
	S (n − 9)	80.19 ± 0.21	80.79 ± 0.24

TABLE 4. *Hydroxyproline concentration (mmol/kg of wet weight) and total content (mg) in the ventricular myocardium of 1- to 3-week-old and 4- to 6-week-old control puppies (K) and puppies with abdominal aortic constriction (S) ($\bar{x} \pm s_{\bar{x}}$)*

Age	Group	Hydroxyproline concentration (mmol/kg) LV	RV	Hydroxyproline content (mg) LV	RV
1–3 weeks	K (n = 7)	7.474* ± 0.450**	10.218* ± 0.601	1.79* ± 0.32	1.36* ± 0.29
	S (n = 7)	5.408 ± 0.608**	9.627 ± 0.936	1.78 ± 0.29	1.32 ± 0.29
4–6 weeks	K (n = 9)	7.471* ± 0.378**	11.993* ± 0.599	3.74* ± 0.23	2.39* ± 0.12
	S (n = 9)	5.699 ± 0.563**	11.255 ± 0.837	3.89 ± 0.24	2.32 ± 0.10

*$p<0.01$; **$p<0.02$.

content in the left and right ventricles of groups B and D increased with an increase in their weights (Table 5).

In group B, the 40% increase in the left ventricular weight was associated with about a 30% increase in the total DNA content (Table 6). In group D, the weight of the left ventricle increased by about 72%, whereas the total DNA content increased by only 44%. The DNA concentration in the ventricular myocardium of puppies in group B was the same as that in the age-matched control group A, whereas in group D, DNA concentration was decreased. The concentration of DNA in the myocardium may also be expressed as the ratio of ventricular wet weight to ventricular DNA content, and this ratio provides information about the myocardial cell size. When the value of this ratio is small, it reflects the prevalence of small cells; likewise, when the value of this ratio is large, it reflects the presence of larger cells. In group B, this ratio was nearly the same as in group A (Table 7), whereas in group D, this ratio was significantly increased ($p<0.01$).

TABLE 5. *RNA concentration (mmol of phosphorus per kg of wet weight) and total content control puppies (K) and puppies with*

Age	Group	RNA concentration (mmol P/kg) LV	RV
1–3 weeks	K (n = 10)	10.41* ± 0.46	9.51* ± 0.55
	S (n = 10)	10.38 ± 0.39	9.70 ± 0.30
4–6 weeks	K (n = 9)	6.95* ± 0.24	6.81[a] ± 0.22
	S (n = 9)	7.03 ± 0.46	7.41 ± 0.50

*$p<0.01$.

The myocardial ultrastructure of groups A and C (Figs. 4 and 5) and groups B and D (Figs. 6 and 7) was also examined. There were signs of increased proteosynthesis, myofibrillogenesis, mitochondriogenesis, and proliferation of the sarcoplasmic reticulum in groups B and D. These differences were more pronounced between groups C and D. Proteosynthesis was indicated by the increased number of ribosomes and polyribosomes, the increase of the free myofilaments or their bundles within the sarcoplasm, and the increased abundance of granulated sarcotubular reticulum of myocyte. Myofibrillogenesis was apparent near the Z-band of preexisting myofibrils (see Fig. 7), as well as near the intercalated disks. In group B, muscle cells exhibiting an ultrastructure similar to that of the embryonic myocytes were also seen (Fig. 8). By contrast, groups A, C, and D did not show any immature myocytes.

Guinea Pigs

Data on heart hypertrophy, hemodynamics, and collagen content for guinea pigs are presented in Table 8. At 10 weeks post surgery, there was a 53% increase in ventricular weight of the guinea pigs that underwent aortic constriction as compared to controls. Left ventricle wall thickness was increased by about 31% in the hypertrophic group. Both systolic and diastolic blood pressures were increased significantly in the hypertrophic group as compared to controls. Left ventricular systolic pressure in the hypertrophic group was increased by 78%, whereas there was no significant change in LVEDP. Both the hydroxyproline content and the collagen content of the left ventricle were significantly increased after 10 weeks of aortic constriction. Histologic studies revealed no mitotic figures in any of the sections from the hypertrophied heart. There was significant deposition of collagen around the blood vessels in hypertrophic hearts. Focal areas of collagen deposition in the interstitium were also seen in hypertrophic heart sections, whereas very little collagen was seen in the sections from control hearts. A study of the ratios of dry

(mg of phosphorus) in the ventricular myocardium of 1- to 3-week-old and 4- to 6-week-old abdominal aortic constriction (S) ($\bar{x} \pm s_{\bar{x}}$)

RNA content (mg P)			
LV		RV	
absolute	% increase	absolute	% increase
0.55 ± 0.06		0.26 ± 0.02	
	41.81		11.54
0.78 ± 0.13		0.29 ± 0.05	
0.80 ± 0.08		0.32 ± 0.04	
	83.75		40.63
1.47 ± 0.20		0.45 ± 0.06	

TABLE 6. *DNA concentration (mmol of phosphorus per kg of wet weight) and total content control puppies (K) and puppies with*

Age	Group	DNA concentration (mmol P/kg)	
		LV	RV
1–3 weeks	K (n = 9)	8.97 ± 0.23	9.62 ± 0.35
	S (n = 9)	8.27 ± 0.52	8.90 ± 0.69
4–6 weeks	K (n = 9)	8.28 ± 0.35*	8.59 ± 0.29
	S (n = 9)	6.71 ± 0.41*	8.15 ± 0.54

*$p < 0.02$

weight to wet weight in the heart, liver, and lungs revealed no indication of tissue edema.

DISCUSSION

The constriction of the ascending aorta (20,33) or the abdominal aorta (35,36) is one of the most widely used experimental approaches to imposing increased work-load on the heart. Animal models with pressure overload have been used in the study of adaptive biochemical, functional, and morphologic changes occurring in the myocardium in response to an increased workload in the early postnatal period. However, in most of these studies, the cardiac work overload was imposed at the end of the third week of postnatal life or later. For the study of mitotic activity in these models, this timing is associated with a distinct disadvantage, as the proliferation of myocardial muscle cells is markedly reduced, or almost completely ceased

TABLE 7. *Mean values for the ratio of ventricular wet weight to ventricular DNA content (mg/mg) in 1- to 3-week-old and 4- to 6-week-old control puppies (K) and puppies with abdominal aortic constriction (S) ($\bar{x} \pm s_{\bar{x}}$)*

Age	Group	Wet weight/DNA (mg/mg)	
		LV	RV
1–3 weeks	K (n = 9)	3646.66 ± 95.43	3422.88 ± 125.51
	S (n = 9)	4073.33 ± 327.80	3938.22 ± 391.21
4–6 weeks	K (n = 9)	3889.89 ± 198.26*	3836.33 ± 132.27
	S (n = 9)	4958.22 ± 275.48*	4137.00 ± 277.64

*$p < 0.01$

(mg of phosphorus) in the ventricular myocardium of 1- to 3-week-old and 4- to 6-week-old abdominal aortic constriction (S) ($\bar{x} \pm s_{\bar{x}}$)

DNA content (mg P)			
LV		RV	
absolute	% increase	absolute	% increase
0.48 ± 0.05		0.27 ± 0.03	
	29.16		0.00
0.62 ± 0.08		0.27 ± 0.04	
0.93 ± 0.07		0.39 ± 0.03	
	44.08		20.51
1.34 ± 0.12		0.47 ± 0.04	

by that time (37). In our puppy model, the aortic constriction was produced as early as the second day after birth, and the lumen of the aorta was reduced by 60% to 70%. During the rapid growth of the neonatal period, the aorta rapidly increases in size while the metal spiral around the aorta maintains the same diameter. Thus, the degree of the aortic constriction increases with age. The workload of the left ventricle in the present study was found to be increased as early as the first week of life, as demonstrated by blood pressure measurements in the ascending aorta and by the values of the blood pressure gradients across aortic constriction.

In terms of DNA concentration as well as total DNA content, the interpretation of these data is generally complicated by the heterogeneous cell composition of the myocardium (muscle cells, fibroblasts, and vascular endothelial cells). It may be

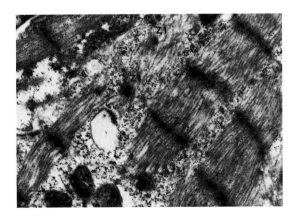

FIG. 4. Electron micrograph of the left ventricular muscle cell from an 8-day-old control puppy. The sarcoplasm of the cell contains few myofibrils and little mitochondria. The myofibrils are only partially developed. The sarcomeres reveal relatively wide Z bands, and their M line and H zone are absent. In some places, Z-band–like material (Zl) and numerous unaligned myofilaments are seen. Z, Z band. Scale bar = 1 μm.

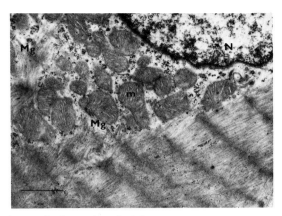

FIG. 5. Electron micrograph of a portion of a left ventricular myocyte from a 20-day-old control puppy. In the perinuclear area, there are numerous mitochondria (*m*), and myofibrillogenesis (*Mg*) is seen within the sarcoplasm. *N*, nucleus. Scale bar = 1 μm.

further complicated by the potential multiplication of DNA with or without subsequent division of the nuclei (polyploidy and polynucleation), as well as by enhanced synthesis of mitochondrial DNA. Mitochondrial DNA accounts for less than 1% of the total DNA content in the myocardium and is considerably stable (38,39). Thus, a change in mitochondrial DNA may represent only a minor component in the increase in total DNA content that occurred in response to aortic banding in our study. The data on the ventricular water content showed that the increase in the

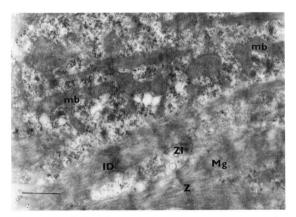

FIG. 6. Electron micrograph of the left ventricular myocyte from a 14-day-old puppy with abdominal aortic constriction. Loose bundles of myofilaments and signs of intensive myofibrillogenesis (*Mg*), as well as signs of mitochondrial multiplication, can be seen in the sarcoplasm of the cell. *ID*, intercalated disk; *Z*, Z band; *Zl*, Z-band–like material; *mb*, dividing mitochondrion. Scale bar = 1 μm.

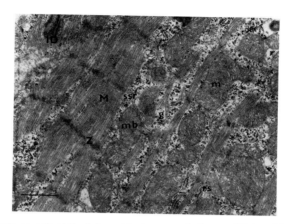

FIG. 7. Electron micrograph of the left ventricular myocyte from a 35-day-old puppy with abdominal aortic constriction. Myofibrils with the typical internal structure of mature sarcomeres, along with myofibrils with undifferentiated sarcomeres and loose myofilaments, are seen within the sarcoplasm. *ID*, intercalated disk; *Z*, Z band; *M*, M line; *g*, glycogen; *ssr*, smooth sarcoplasmic reticulum; *rs*, granular sarcoplasmic reticulum; *m*, mitochondrion; *mb*, dividing mitochondrion. Scale bar = 1 μm.

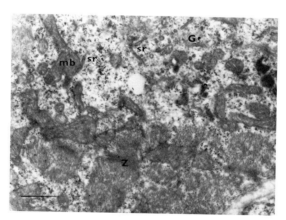

FIG. 8. Electron micrograph of the left ventricular muscle cell from a 20-day-old puppy with abdominal aortic constriction. The cell has the appearance of an embryonic cardiac muscle cell. The sarcoplasm contains only a small amount of chaotically oriented free myofilaments and protofibrils. Numerous small mitochondria are also present. Both smooth and rough endoplasmic reticulum (*sr*) are abundant. *G*, golgi complex; *Z*, Z band; *mb*, dividing mitochondrion. Scale bar = 1 μm.

TABLE 8. *Data on heart hypertrophy and hemodynamic function in guinea pigs after 10 weeks of aortic constriction*

Parameter	Control	Banded
Body weight (BW) (g)	727 ± 32	716 ± 22
Ventricular weight (VW) (g)	1.6 ± 0.2	2.5 ± 0.2*
(VW/BW) × 10³	2.2 ± 0.1	3.5 ± 0.1*
LV wall thickness (mm)	4.5 ± 0.1	5.9 ± 0.4*
Aortic pressure (mm Hg)		
Systolic	73.4 ± 3.1	97.0 ± 1.2*
Diastolic	58.2 ± 2.2	75.9 ± 3.0*
LV pressure (mm Hg)		
Systolic	76.5 ± 2.8	136.5 ± 2.2*
Diastolic	5.2 ± 1.4	6.2 ± 0.7
Hydroxyproline content (mg/g, wet weight)	5.3 ± 0.8	8.5 ± 0.5*
Collagen content (mg/g, wet weight)	40.3 ± 1.0	64.6 ± 1.0*

Data is mean ± S.E. of 6 to 7 experiments.
*$p < 0.05$ from control value.

heart weight of both age groups of puppies with constriction of the aorta was not attributable to the accumulation of tissue fluid. Increased heart weight, as well as the changes in the content and concentration of DNA, may, therefore, predominantly reflect alterations in the volume or the total number of different cell types, such as myocytes, fibroblasts, and endothelial cells in the myocardium.

Myocyte and nonmyocyte cell growth may occur independent of each other, both during normal development and during hypertrophy (40,41). The degree of connective tissue response during hypertrophy is dependent on the type of stimulus used, as well as upon the age (42). The biochemical measurement of hydroxyproline has been shown to be both specific and reproducible, and thus serves as a quantitative index of tissue collagen (43). Our study of the changes in ventricular hydroxyproline concentration and total content revealed that a chronic increase in cardiac workload in the newborn puppy does not cause proliferation of myocardial connective tissue cells. On the other hand, in guinea pigs, there was an increase in hydroxyproline content of more than 60% without any morphologic evidence of mitotic activity.

Among the three major cell types comprising the myocardium of newborn animals, vascular endothelial cells represent the smallest portion (44). In the puppies studied, during the first 8 weeks of postnatal life, approximately 85% of cell nuclei were classified as muscle cell nuclei and only 15 percent were classified as nonmuscle cell nuclei. A similar cell distribution has been reported in puppies with aortic stenosis (20). This ratio is exactly opposite to the distribution of cell types previously reported for the adult heart (45). Increased proliferation of blood vessels occurs during the development of hypertrophy in newborn animals (46–49). In view of the mentioned ratio of muscle cells to nonmuscle cells, this can account for the observed 30% and 44% increase in total DNA content in the left ventricular myocardium of the 1- to 3-week-old puppies and of the 4- to 6-week-old puppies with aortic constriction.

The fact that there was an increase in total DNA content in group B, but no change in DNA concentration in the left ventricular myocardium, indicates that the increase in DNA content and the increase in the number of myocardial muscle cells may be proportional. Myocardial muscle cell volume must not have changed substantially, as the ratio of left ventricular wet weight to ventricular DNA content (expressed in mg/mg) was the same as in the age-matched control animals. Therefore, it can be concluded that the increased muscular mass of myocardium in the puppies with aortic constriction within the first 3 weeks of postnatal life is mainly attributable to the increase in muscle cell number (i.e., owing to hyperplasia). By contrast, in the adaptation period that follows, it is mainly the enlargement of the muscle cells (i.e., cellular hypertrophy) that may be responsible for the increased myocardial muscle mass. This assumption is supported by the fact that, in the older group of puppies with aortic constriction (Group D), the DNA concentration of the left ventricle was significantly decreased and the ratio of left ventricular wet weight to ventricular DNA content was significantly increased in comparison to the control group.

The results of our electron microscopic study are in agreement with the biochemical findings. Seldom are there dividing muscle cells in growing myocardium of newborn animals. However, some authors regard the occurrence of electron-lucent myocytes, the sarcoplasm of which contains loose bundles of chaotically distributed myofilaments or a small amount of irregularly arranged myofibrils, as structural proof for the presence of cardiac muscle cell mitosis (4,20,50). These cells resemble embryonic muscle cells. Immature cardiomyocytes of this kind were apparent only in the myocardium of the younger group (Group B) of puppies with aortic constriction. We suggest that these embryonic myocytes may represent newly formed cells. However, direct evidence can be obtained only by further analysis with radiolabeled thymidine.

From our data on puppies as well as from our studies in guinea pigs, we have concluded that cardiac growth in response to pressure overload up to the first 3 weeks of postnatal life is primarily attributable to cell hyperplasia. Thereafter, up to 6 weeks of age, cardiac growth occurs mainly by cellular hypertrophy. Only in later stages (i.e., after 6 weeks) does an increase in collagen contribute toward an increase in heart weight. Hence, the growth response of the postnatal heart to increased workload is met through different cellular processes depending on the postnatal age.

SUMMARY

Banding of the abdominal aorta in newborn puppies resulted in a 30% and 60% increase in heart weight at 3 weeks and 6 weeks of age, respectively. Studies of the changes in water and hydroxyproline content showed that the increase in heart weight was primarily attributable to an increase in cardiac muscle mass. Studies of the changes in the DNA concentration, as well as total DNA content, indicated that this increase in muscle mass, occurring within the first 3 weeks of life, was mainly attributable to an increase in the cell number. Some muscle cells in these hearts exhibited an ultrastructure similar to that of embryonic myocytes. Thereafter and up to 6 weeks of age, cell hypertrophy appeared to be the primary contributor to increased muscle mass. The ultrastructural characteristics of cardiomyocytes in the latter group of puppies included increased proteosynthesis, sarcomerogenesis, myofibrillogenesis, and mitochondriogenesis. Addition of new myofilaments occurred at the level of intercalated disks and Z-bands of the preexisting myofibrils. On the other hand, in young guinea pigs (25 ± 3 days), hypertrophy at 10 weeks was accompanied by an increase in collagen, and animals showed increased peak LVSP with no change in LVEDP. No mitotic figures were seen in any of the sections from hypertrophic hearts of guinea pigs. It is suggested that the cardiac growth response during heart hypertrophy secondary to an increased cardiac workload may depend on the age at which the load is imposed.

ACKNOWLEDGMENTS

Dr. J. Slezak was a Visiting Scientist supported by the Heart and Stroke Foundation of Canada. Ms. A. Randhawa was supported by a studentship from the Manitoba Health Research Council. A portion of the research was supported by a grant from the Medical Research Council of Canada.

REFERENCES

1. Zak R. Development and proliferative capacity of cardiac muscle cells. *Circ Res* 1974;34–35[Suppl II]:17–26.
2. Hay DA, Low FN. The fine structure of progressive stages of myocardial mitosis in chick embryos. *Am J Anat* 1972;134:175–203.
3. Chacko S. DNA synthesis, mitosis and differentiation in cardiac myogenesis. *Dev Biol* 1973;35:1–18.
4. Rumyantsev PP. *Kardiomiocity v processsach reprodukcii, differencirovki i regeneracii.* Leningrad: Nauka: 1982;288.
5. Goss RJ. Hypertrophy versus hyperplasia. *Science* 1966;153:1615–1620.
6. Manasek FJ. Mitosis in developing cardiac muscle. *J Cell Biol* 1968;37:191–196.
7. Claycomb WC. Cardiac muscle hypertrophy. Differentiation and growth of the heart cell during development. *Biochem J* 1977;168:599–601.
8. Rakusan K. Postnatal development of the heart. In: Bournei GH, ed. *Hearts and heart-like organs*, Vol. 1. New York: Academic Press; 1980:415.
9. Nag CA, Cheng M. DNA synthesis in heart cells. Comparative studies of monolayer and aggregate cultures. *Cell Mol Biol* 1983;29:451–459.
10. Rumyantsev PP, Snigirevskaya E. The ultrastructure of differentiating cells of the heart muscle in the state of mitotic division. *Acta Morphol Acad Sci Hung* 1968;16:271–283.
11. Hurrelbrink LE, Claycomb WC. Chalone and DNA replication in differentiating cardiac muscle. *J Cell Biol* 1978;79:326.
12. Hollenberg M, Honbo N, Samorodin AJ. Effect of hypoxia on cardiac growth in neonatal rat. *Am J Physiol* 1976;231:1445–1450.
13. Ghani QP, Hollenberg M. Poly (adenosine diphosphate ribose) metabolism and regulation of myocardial cell growth by oxygen. *Biochem J* 1978;170:387–394.
14. Claycomb WC. Poly (adenosine diphosphate ribose) polymerase activity and nicotinamide adenine dinucleotide in differentiating cardiac muscle. *Biochem J* 1976;154:387–393.

15. Walker BE. The origin of myoblasts and the problem of differentiation. *Exp Cell Res* 1962;30:80–92.
16. Dowell RT. Nutritional modification of rat heart postnatal development. *Am J Physiol* 1984;246: H332–H338.
17. Zlatos L, Holzerova J, Kvaszova E, Danihel L. The adaptation mechanism of the myocardium to increased work load in newborn rats with chemical sympathectomy. *Acta Facult Med Univ Brunensia* 1985;92:137–143. In: Vasku J, Dostal M, eds. *New trends in pathological physiology.* Brno: J.E. Purkyne University, Medical Faculty, 1985:599.
18. Slezak J, Zlatos L. Effect of chemical sympathectomy on the ultrastructure of the healthy and of the overloaded myocardium of rats in the early postnatal period. *Bratisl Lek Listy* 1986;86:577–592.
19. Zlatos L, Holzerova J, Slezak J, Kvaszova E, Danihel L. The effect of chemical sympathectomy on the myocardium of the rat during physiological growth and increased work load in the early postnatal period. *Folia Fac Med Univ Comenianae Bratislava* 1989;27:9–75.
20. Bishop SP. Effect of aortic stenosis on myocardial cell growth, hyperplasia and ultrastructure in neonatal dogs. In: Dhalla NS, ed. *Recent advances in studies on cardiac structure and metabolism. Myocardial metabolism*, Vol 3. Munchen: Urban und Schwarzenberg; 1974:878.
21. Zlatos L, Holzerova J, Sapakova E, Kvaszova E. Simple surgical method for producing a model of an experimentally enlarged heart in newborn puppies. *Bratisl Lek Listy* 1977;68:576–582.
22. Campbell SE, Rakusan K, Gerdes AM. Change in cardiac myocyte size distribution in aortic-constricted neonatal rats. *Basic Res Cardiol* 1989;84:247–258.
23. Rakusan K, Poupa O. Differences in capillary supply of hypertrophied and hyperplastics hearts. *Cardiologia* 1966;49:293–298.
24. Peitschmann M, Bartels H. Cellular hyperplasia and hypertrophy, capillary proliferation and myoglobin concentration in the heart of newborn and adult rats at high altitude. *Respir Physiol* 1985; 59:347–360.
25. Mortola JP, Xu L, Lauzon A-M. Body growth, lung and heart weight, and DNA content in newborn rats exposed to different levels of chronic hypoxia. *Can J Physiol Pharmacol* 1990;68:1590–1594.
26. Penney DG. Carbon monoxide induced cardiac hypertrophy. In: Zak R, ed. *Growth of the heart in health and disease.* New York: Raven Press; 1984:337–362.
27. Gerdes AM, Kriseman J, Bishop SP. Changes in myocardial cell size and number during the development and reversal of hyperthyroidism in neonatal rats. *Lab Invest* 1983;48:598–602.
28. Wachtlova M, Ostadal B, Mares V. Thyroxine-induced cardiomegaly in rats of different age. *Physiol Bohemoslov* 1985;34:385–394.
29. Kugler JD, Gillette PC, Graham SP, Garson A Jr., Goldstein MA, Thompson HK Jr. Effect of chemical sympathectomy on myocardial cell division in the newborn rat. *Pediatr Res* 1980;14:881–884.
30. Fulton RM, Hutchinson EC, Jones AM. Ventricular weight in cardiac hypertrophy. *Br Heart J* 1952;14:413–420.
31. Prockop DJ, Undenfriend S. A specific method for the analysis of hydroxyproline in tissue and urine. *Analyt Biochem* 1960;1:228–239.
32. Canev RG, Markov GG. K voprosu o kolicestvennom spektrofotometriceskom opredelenii nukleovej kisloty. *Biochimija* 1960;25:151–159.
33. Randhawa AK, Singal PK. Pressure overload induced cardiac hypertrophy with and without dilation. *J Am Coll Cardiol* 1992;20:1569–1575.
34. Chiariello M, Ambrosio G, Cappelli, Bigazzi M, Perrone-Filardi P, Brigante F, Sifola C. A biochemical method for the quantitation of myocardial scarring after experimental coronary artery occlusion. *J Mol Cell Cardiol* 1986;18:283–290.
35. Dowell RT, McManus RT III. Pressure-induced cardiac enlargement in neonatal and adult rats. Left ventricular functional characteristics and evidence of cardiac muscle cell proliferation in the neonate. *Circ Res* 1978;42:303–310.
36. Gupta M, Singal PK. Higher antioxidative capacity during a chronic stable heart hypertrophy. *Circ Res* 1989;64:398–406.
37. Rakusan K, Korecky B. Regression of cardiomegaly induced in newborn rats. *Can J Cardiol* 1985; 1:217–222.
38. Rabinowitz M, Swift H. Mitochondrial nucleic acids and their relation to the biogenesis of mitochondria. *Physiol Rev* 1970;50:376–427.
39. Rabinowitz M, Zak R. Biochemical and cellular changes in cardiac hypertrophy. *Ann Rev Med* 1972;23:245–262.
40. Ruskoaho HJ, Savolainen E-R. Effects of long-term verapamil treatment on blood pressure, cardiac

hypertrophy and collagen metabolism in spontaneously hypertensive rats. *Cardiovasc Res* 1985; 19:355–362.
41. Weber KT, Brilla ChG. Pathological hypertrophy and cardiac interstitium. Fibrosis and renin-angiotensin-aldosterone system. *Circulation* 1991;83:1849–1865.
42. Bishop SP, Melsen LR. Myocardial necrosis, fibrosis, and DNA synthesis in experimental cardiac hypertrophy induced by sudden pressure overload. *Clin Res* 1976;39:238–245.
43. Buccino RA, Harris E, Spain JF Jr, Sonnenblick EH. Response of myocardial connective tissue to development of experimental hypertrophy. *Am J Physiol* 1969;216:425–428.
44. Hollenberg M, Honbo N, Samorodin AJ. Cardiac cellular response to altered nutrition in the neonatal rat. *Am J Physiol* 1977;233:H356–H360.
45. Grove D, Zak R, Nair KG, Aschenbrenner V. Biochemical correlates of cardiac hypertrophy. IV. Observations on the cellular organization of growth during myocardial hypertrophy in the rat. *Circ Res* 1969;25:473–485.
46. Poupa O, Korecky B, Krofta K, Rakusan K, Prochazka J. The effect of anaemia during the early postnatal development on vascularization of the myocardium and its resistance to anoxia. *Physiol Bohemoslov* 1964;13:281–287.
47. Tomanek RJ, Searls JC, Lachenbruch PA. Quantitative changes in the capillary bed during developing, peak and stabilized cardiac hypertrophy in the spontaneously hypertensive rat. *Circ Res* 1982; 51:295–304.
48. Rakusan K, Turek Z. A new look into the microscope: proliferation and regression of myocardial capillaries. *Can J Cardiol* 1986;2:94–97.
49. Rakusan K, Campbell SE. Spatial relationship between cardiac mast cells and coronary capillaries in neonatal rats with cardiomegaly. *Can J Physiol* 1991;69:1750–1753.
50. Rumyantsev PP. Ultrastructure reorganization DNA synthesis and mitotic division of myocytes in atria of rat with left ventricle infarction. An electron microscopic and autoradiographic study. *Virchow's Arch [Cell Pathol]* 1974;15:357–378.

The Cardiomyopathic Heart, edited by Makoto
Nagano, Nobuakira Takeda, and Naranjan S.
Dhalla. Raven Press, Ltd., New York © 1994.

37

Parallel Changes in the β-Adrenoceptor/ Adenylyl Cyclase System between the Failing Human Heart and the Noradrenaline-Treated Guinea Pig

Sian E. Harding, Lesley A. Brown, Federica del Monte,
Peter O'Gara, Dylan G. Wynne, and Philip A. Poole-Wilson

*Department of Cardiac Medicine, National Heart and Lung Institute,
London SW3 6LY, UK*

INTRODUCTION

The reduction in sensitivity of failing human myocardium to β-adrenoceptor agonists is now well documented (1). There is certainly a loss in cell surface β-receptor number on the order of 30% to 60% (2,3). Because there is little spare receptor capacity in human myocardium (3,4), this accounts for some of the reduction in the maximum inotropic effects of β-agonists in isolated muscle strips from failing human heart (3). There are also lesions distal to the receptor, with decreases in both the activity of adenylyl cyclase and the basal level of cyclic adenosine monophosphate (cAMP) (5,6). Noradrenaline concentrations are increased in the plasma of patients with heart failure and are reduced in the myocardial tissue (5). This is taken as evidence of increased activation of the sympathetic nervous system, probably as a reflex response to the impaired cardiac output. Plasma noradrenaline can be a good indicator of prognosis in patients with heart failure (7). It has been proposed that the reduction in β-adrenoceptor sensitivity represents an agonist-induced desensitization secondary to overexposure to noradrenaline (3,8).

To investigate this hypothesis, we developed an animal model whereby we exposed guinea pigs to chronically increased plasma noradrenaline levels. We then examined the responses of the myocardium to β-adrenoceptor agonists, as well as to agents that act on the distal adenylyl cyclase pathway. These include forskolin (which activates the catalytic subunit of adenylyl cyclase directly), phosphodiesterase inhibitors (which prevent the breakdown of cAMP), lipophilic analogs of cAMP (dibutyryl cAMP and chlorophenylthio-cAMP) and pertussis toxin, which inactivates the inhibitory guanine nucleotide binding protein (G_i).

The myocardial preparation that we chose was the single cardiac myocyte, obtained from the atria or ventricle of human (9–12) or animal (13–15) hearts. Single cells were isolated enzymatically from small pieces of tissue, then superfused and electrically stimulated, and their contraction was studied using a video/edge detection system. Concentration-response curves to β-adrenoceptor agonists and other pharmacologic agents were constructed. Myocytes were useful for these studies, both because of the range of techniques that they permitted and also because of the avoidance of some significant artifacts. For this particular study, we were concerned about the possibility of noradrenaline release from nerve endings within intact muscle strips. In a previous investigation, we had found evidence of tonic release of noradrenaline in electrically stimulated guinea pig papillary muscle (16). It is possible that continued exposure to high noradrenaline levels in the animal model could change either the degree of loading of the nerve stores, or the sensitivity of the presynaptic receptor system, thus altering the contribution of noradrenaline release in intact myocardial strips. Similarly, as failing human myocardium is depleted of noradrenaline compared to normal tissue (5), noradrenaline release within electrically stimulated muscle strips could produce artifactual differences between results in failing and nonfailing hearts.

Much of our previous work has been directed toward investigating the suitability of the isolated myocyte as a tool for studying β-adrenoceptor desensitization in the heart. We have shown that β-adrenoceptor responses in normal cells are reproducible, and that the enzyme treatment itself does not reduce tissue sensitivity to catecholamines (17,18). We have directly compared the extent of functional β-adrenoceptor densensitization in an animal model, the isoprenaline (isoproterenol)-treated rabbit. Rabbits were infused with isoprenaline for 7 days using osmotic minipumps, and contractile responses of myocytes or papillary muscles from the hearts were compared. Concentration-response curves to isoprenaline in vitro were right-shifted and depressed by a similar extent, compared with controls, in the two preparations (18). This indicates that no significant resensitization had occurred during the period of cell preparation.

We can also detect β-adrenoceptor desensitization in single atrial or ventricular muscle cells from failing human heart (9,12). Our results with myocytes from human tissue are in broad agreement with those in the literature (5). β-adrenoceptor subsensitivity correlates with heart failure severity, as defined by the New York Heart Association (NYHA) classification system, which is based on symptoms of the patient, left ventricular ejection fraction, and the left ventricular end diastolic pressure (LVEDP) (9,12,19,20). The effect is not confined to a single etiology of disease (12), although there are some variations with etiology. The age of the patient was also found to affect the contraction amplitude of the ventricular myocytes and the degree of β-adrenoceptor desensitisation (12). With these preliminary data on human and animal myocytes showing reproducible β-adrenoceptor desensitization, we felt justified in performing more detailed comparisons between the noradrenaline-treated guinea pig and the failing human heart.

METHODS

Human ventricular myocardium was obtained at the time of transplant, or during routine cardiac surgery. Informed consent was obtained prior to the operation. Tissue was transported in cold cardioplegic solution; the average transit time to the laboratory was 1 hour. Guinea pigs underwent subcutaneous implantation of osmotic mini-pumps (Alzet) as previously described (21).

Human ventricle (1–2 g) was cut into chunks approximately 1 mm^3 using a razor array. These chunks were then incubated at 35°C, with shaking, in 25 to 50 mL of a low-calcium (LC) medium containing nitrilotriacetic acid (NTA) as a calcium buffer. The composition of the LC medium, expressed in the millimoles, was NaCl, 120; KC1, 5.4; MgSO$_4$, 5; pyruvate, 5; glucose, 20; taurine, 20; HEPES, 10; and NTA, 5; this was bubbled with 100% O$_2$. The pH was adjusted to 6.95, and the measured free [Ca^{2+}] was 1 to 3 μM. The medium was changed three times at 3-minute intervals (twelve minutes total). The chunks were then drained and transferred to LC medium without NTA, with the addition of 50 μM of calcium, and containing 4 U/mL of Sigma type XXIV protease (pronase) at the same temperature for 45 min. The solution was shaken gently in an atmosphere of 100% O$_2$ throughout the preparation. Two further 45-minute digests were then carried out using collagenase (Boehringer) at 400 IU/mL. The cell suspension was filtered through 300 μM gauze to remove undigested tissue, and the myocytes were pelleted by gentle centrifugation. The pellets were then washed and resuspended in preoxygenated LC medium without NTA. Rod-shaped myocytes were obtained from both collagenase digests. The proportion of rod-shaped cells was variable, occasionally as high as 70%, but usually much lower.

For preparation of myocytes from guinea pig ventricle, the heart was perfused by the Langendorff method. There was an initial period of stabilization (approximately 5 minutes) with Krebs-Henseleit (KH) solution, which contained the following (expressed in millimoles): NaCl, 119; KCI, 4.2; MgSO$_4$, 0.94; KH$_2$PO$_4$, 1.2; NaHCO$_3$, 25; glucose, 11.5. Moreover, the solution contained 1 mM of Ca^{2+} and was equilibrated with 95% O$_2$/5% CO$_2$. Following this, the perfusate was quickly changed to LC solution without NTA (final Ca^{2+} of 12 to 14 μM) for 5 minutes at 37°C. The heart was then perfused with pronase, 4 U/mL, prepared as described earlier for 2 minutes, followed by 10 minutes' perfusion with collagenase (0.3 mg/mL, Worthington) and hyaluronidase (0.6 mg/mL, Sigma). The ventricles were chopped and shaken in the collagenase mixture for two additional 5-minute periods, and the cells were separated as before.

The contraction amplitude of single ventricular myocytes superfused at 32°C with KH solution (1.3 mM of Ca^{2+}) and electrically stimulated with biphasic pulses (0.2 Hz, human; 0.5 Hz, guinea pig) was monitored using a video/length detection system (17). Myocytes were chosen for study on the basis of a number of criteria: (a) morphologic appearance (rod-shaped, with no large blebs or areas of hypercontracture); (b) a sarcomere length of greater than 1.60 μm; (c) no spontaneous contractions when unstimulated in 1.3 mM of Ca^{2+}; (d) steady contraction amplitude and diastolic length at basal stimulation rates; and (e) response to and complete recovery from challenge with maximally activating Ca^{2+} concentrations (10 to 25 mM). Following the exposure to high Ca^{2+}, sequential concentration-response curves to agonists were constructed. A maximum was judged to be reached either when there was no further increase in amplitude with increasing dose, or when signs of toxicity were observed (arrhythmias, sharp decreases in diastolic length). Only if signs of toxicity were reversible on washout of agonist were the data included in the analysis; this is to exclude cells which spontaneously developed arrhythmias and rounded up. Controls were performed to compensate for any change in sensitivity of the preparation with time.

Myocytes were incubated with pertussis toxin immediately after digestion as previously described (21). The success of the procedure was determined by the response of each cell to 10 μM of adenosine, following stimulation with a submaximal concentration of isoprenaline. A reversal of the isoprenaline-induced increase in contraction amplitude with adenosine showed the integrity of the G_i pathway. When this response was lost, the functional inactivation of G_i was deemed complete.

Concentrations for half-maximal effect (EC_{50}s) were calculated using an iterative nonlinear curve fitting program on an IBM-compatible computer. Significances were assessed on grouped data using the Student's T-test, and one-way analysis of variance (ANOVA) was performed with the program Minitab.

MATERIALS

Salts were from BDH, and were AnalaR grade except for KC1, taurine, and glucose, which were AristaR grade. BDH AnalaR water was used for the low-Ca^{2+} solutions, and double-distilled deionized water (MilliQ system) was used for the remainder. Isoprenaline-HC1, isobutylmethylxanthine (IBMX), forskolin, adenosine, dibutyryl cAMP, and chlorophenylthio-cAMP were obtained from Sigma. Pertussis toxin was obtained from Porton. Smith Kline & French (SK&F) 94120 and SK&F 94836 were the kind gifts of Dr. Brian Warrington, SB, Welwyn.

RESULTS AND DISCUSSION

Parallels Between Human and Guinea Pig Myocytes

The Maximum Response to Increasing Ca^{2+} Is Unchanged

The maximum contraction amplitude obtained by increasing extracellular Ca^{2+} was $10.0 \pm 0.38\%$ cell shortening (mean ± SEM) in ventricular myocytes from 34 patients in moderate (NYHA class III) or severe (NYHA class IV) failure (results pooled from up to 8 cells per patient). This compares with $9.31 \pm 0.68\%$ in cells from six nonfailing hearts. ANOVA showed that between-cell variation in the same patient was minimal compared to the variation between patients ($p<0.001$) (12). Similarly, myocytes from the left ventricle of noradrenaline-treated guinea pigs had a maximum amplitude of $10.8\pm0.8\%$ shortening ($n=14$), compared with $10.4\pm0.8\%$ ($n=12$) in sham-operated controls.

Concentration-Response Curves to Isoprenaline Are Right-Shifted and Depressed

Figure 1 compares concentration-response curves to isoprenaline in human and guinea pig myocytes (left ventricle). Change in contraction amplitude with each dose of isoprenaline was normalized to that produced by high Ca^{2+} in the same cell. In cells from both failing human hearts and hearts from noradrenaline-treated guinea pigs, the curves were shifted to the right by more than an order of magnitude, and the maximum response was significantly reduced. The change was progressive; when the data from the human ventricle were divided into three grades of failure, the mild-moderate group data lay between the nonfailing and severe data. Similarly, treatment of guinea pigs with a lower dose of noradrenaline (600 µg/kg/hr instead of

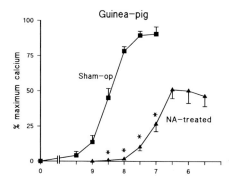

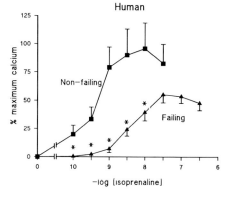

FIG. 1. Increase in contraction amplitude of single ventricular myocytes from guinea pig (**A**) or human (**B**) hearts with increasing isoprenaline concentration (expressed relative to the maximum change with high Ca^{2+} in the same cell). Myocytes were isolated from the hearts of sham-operated (*sham-op*; $n=13$ cells) and noradrenaline (NA)-treated ($n=19$) guinea pigs, and from patients without heart failure ($n=14$) and those with moderate to end-stage failure (NYHA class III–IV, $n=32$). *, $p\leq0.05$ compared to control tissue.

900 µg/kg/hr) produced a shift in the EC_{50} for isoprenaline from 4.8 ± 0.63 nM ($n = 11$) to 167 ± 42 nM (5) ($p < 0.001$), but only a slight depression in maximum response. The progressive nature of the change has been noted previously in our study on rats implanted with noradrenaline-containing mini-pumps (13).

In both human ventricular and atrial myocytes, the shift and depression occurred in concert, so that a significant correlation between decreasing maximum response and increasing EC_{50} was seen (9,12). Such a pattern of desensitization can be attributable to loss of sarcolemmal β-adrenoceptors in a tissue when there is a lack of spare receptors. This is certainly the case for human ventricle, in which the absence of spare β-adrenoceptors has been documented, but it is not known whether the same is true for the guinea pig. The observation that a shift in the EC_{50} can precede the depression of maximum response (see above) tends to suggest that there are some spare receptors, at least initially, in guinea pig myocytes. An alternative explanation for this pattern of desensitization is that there is a change in the distal adenylyl cyclase pathway, in addition to receptor loss. The results discussed below would support this latter interpretation.

Desensitization is Less Pronounced in the Right Than the Left Ventricle

Figure 2a shows the effect of isoprenaline in myocytes from the right and left ventricles of noradrenaline-treated guinea pigs. There is a significant difference between the two in the degree of depression of the maximum response. Similar results have been seen with noradrenaline-treated rats (13). Our human data (12) were complicated by the different patient populations contributing to the data in the left and right ventricle groups. However, it was more difficult to demonstrate a relationship between severity of failure and degree of desensitization in the right ventricle, despite numbers being greater in that group. Direct comparison between cells from the right and left ventricles of patients with ischemic heart disease showed a tendency for myocytes from the left ventricle to have a more pronounced depression of the isoprenaline/calcium ratio (Fig. 2b).

It was thought that this might represent a contribution of the effect of hypertrophy to the apparent β-adrenoceptor desensitization, but preliminary results do not support this hypothesis. The right/left differences were apparent in a group of noradrenaline-treated guinea pigs, in which there was neither an increase in heart weight/body weight ratio nor an increase in myocyte area (data not shown).

Responses to Both Forskolin and cAMP Analogs Are Depressed

Figure 3 shows maximum responses to forskolin and cAMP analogues in ventricular myocytes from human and guinea pig hearts. In humans, the division is the same as for Figure 1, with nonfailing hearts compared to hearts with moderate or severe failure. There is no evidence, in either species, that forskolin or the cAMP analog can yield maximum responses in desensitized myocytes that are any greater

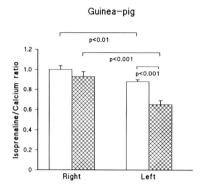

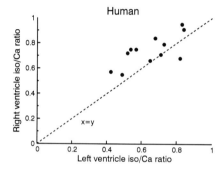

FIG. 2. a: Comparison of the isoprenaline/calcium ratio in right and left ventricle myocytes from sham-operated (n = 12, open bars) and noradrenaline-treated (n = 14, hatched bars) guinea pigs. **b**: Comparison of the isoprenaline (iso)/calcium ratio in right and left ventricle myocytes from 12 patients with ischemic heart disease.

than those yielded by increasing isoprenaline. The concentration-response curves to forskolin are not significantly right-shifted in human cells (22), whereas the EC_{50} is only slightly increased in noradrenaline-treated guinea pig myocytes (from 107 ± 40 nM to 280 ± 64 nM, n = 5 for both; $p < 0.02$). This suggests that the depression of maximum responses to agents that raise cAMP is attributable to a postreceptor lesion, but that the shift in the isoprenaline concentration-response curves is a separate phenomenon, particularly in human cells. It is likely that the increase in EC_{50} for isoprenaline is related to the well-documented loss in cell surface β-adrenoceptors.

The loss of effect of the cAMP analog suggests that the depression of maximum response in these cells is independent of the production of cAMP. Some change in the excitation-contraction coupling system results in the inability of cAMP to exert a maximum effect. This could result from changes in protein kinase A activation, or in the proteins that this enzyme phosphorylates. It could also be related to the arrhythmogenic effect of the catecholamines. The concentration-response curves for isoprenaline, forskolin, and dibutyryl cAMP are often limited by the appearance of arrhythmias, even in desensitized cells. Changes in the myocyte following noradrenaline exposure could result in the appearance of arrhythmias at a lower inotropic level (22).

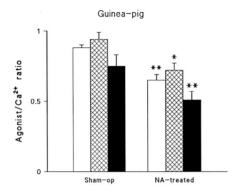

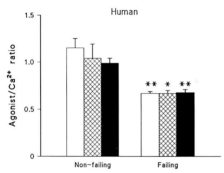

FIG. 3. Maximum responses to isoprenaline (open bars), forskolin (hatched bars), and dibutyryl cAMP (solid bars) in myocytes from the hearts of sham-operated (sham-op; n = 7–12) and noradrenaline (NA)-treated (n = 5–14) guinea pigs (**A**) and from nonfailing (n = 3–5) or failing (n = 11–32) human hearts (**B**). (Ratio to maximum calcium in the same cell; significantly less than control tissue, *$p < 0.02$, **$p < 0.01$)

Phosphodiesterase Inhibitors Potentiate the Effects of Isoprenaline on Desensitized Cells without Fully Restoring Maximum Response Levels

Another pharmacologic approach to the question of whether increasing intracellular cAMP can reverse β-adrenoceptor desensitization is the use of phosphodiesterase inhibitors. By preventing cAMP breakdown, these agents potentiate the response to β-adrenoceptor stimulation. We have used the nonspecific phosphodiesterase inhibitor IBMX, as well as SK&F 94120 and SK&F 94836, which are more specific type III inhibitors. Threshold inotropic concentrations of these agents shift the concentration-response curves to isoprenaline to the right approximately tenfold. The maximum response to isoprenaline is enhanced, but remains significantly below that in control cells. This is true for myocytes from both failing human heart and hearts from noradrenaline-treated guinea pigs (23). The maximum response of myocytes from normal hearts to isoprenaline is unaffected by the presence of phosphodiesterase inhibitors.

These results are in accord with those obtained using cAMP analogs, and confirm that there is a defect in both the response to cAMP and its production by β-adrenoceptor stimulation.

Inactivation of G_i with Pertussis Toxin Reverses β-Adrenoceptor Desensitization

The efficacy of the treatment with pertussis toxin was verified by challenge of each cell with adenosine (see Methods section). Desensitized myocytes in which the treatment had inactivated G_i display an enhanced response to isoprenaline (21). Figure 4a, b shows the maximum isoprenaline/calcium ratio in pertussis-treated cells compared with those incubated at 35°C in the absence of toxin. In myocytes from both failing human hearts and hearts from noradrenaline-treated guinea pig, pertussis toxin increases the maximum response to isoprenaline and shifts the concentration-response curve to the left (21). No such potentiation of maximum response is seen in control myocytes from either species, although the EC_{50} is reduced (21,24). This is clear evidence for the involvement of G_i in the β-adrenoceptor

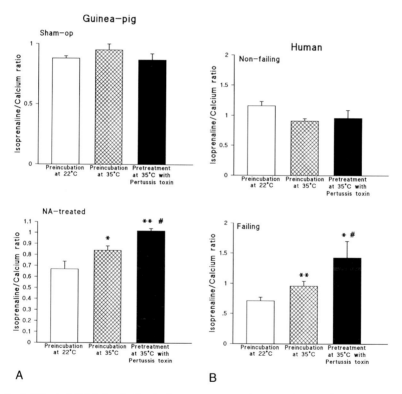

FIG. 4. **A**: Effect of 35° C-incubation in the presence or absence of pertussis toxin on the iso-prenaline/calcium ratio in myocytes from sham-operated (n = 6) and noradrenaline (NA) treated (n = 6) guinea pigs. (Significantly different from 22°C control, $*p<0.02$, $**p<0.01$; significantly different from 35°C control, $\#p<0.05$.) **B**: Effect of 35°C incubation in the presence or absence of pertussis toxin on the isoprenaline/calcium ratio in myocytes from nonfailing (n = 3–6) or failing (n = 5–7) human hearts. (Significantly different from 22°C control, $*p<0.05$, $**p<0.01$; significantly different from 35°C control, $\#p<0.05$.)

desensitization that occurs in both the human disease and the animal model, and supports the biochemical data which suggest that levels of this protein are increased in human heart failure (25,26).

Incubation of Desensitized Myocytes at 35°C Reverses β-Adrenoceptor Desensitization

Freshly isolated myocytes are usually kept at room temperature (22°C) after preparation in our laboratory. No significant resensitization has been seen during the period in which we work on the cells, which can be as long as 12 hours. However, the 3- to 6-hour incubation at 35°C, which serves as a control for the pertussis toxin treatment, causes a significant increase in maximum isoprenaline response (Fig. 4a, b) (21). There is no accompanying shift in the position of the concentration-response curves. The effect is specific for the desensitized myocytes; there is no change in maximum response with changes in temperature in control cells. We have speculated that the removal of the cells from the noradrenaline-rich environment in vivo allows some reversal of the β-adrenoceptor desensitization in both humans and guinea pigs (21).

Conclusions

The similarity between the responses of myocytes from failing human hearts and those from the noradrenaline-treated guinea pig is impressive. We have not yet found a characteristic of the β-adrenoceptor/adenylyl cyclase system in cells from failing hearts that cannot be reproduced in the animal model. This is supporting evidence that the increased noradrenaline level in cardiac patients is the cause of the observed β-adrenoceptor subsensitivity. The results correlate well with our previous observations, which suggested that the duration and severity of the disease, rather than its etiology, largely determine the degree of desensitization. However, other researchers have found some relation between etiology and β-adrenoceptor subsensitivity, with tissue from patients with idiopathic dilated cardiomyopathy having a greater reduction in β-adrenoceptor number, but less depression of functional response to isoprenaline, than that from patients with ischemic heart disease at the time of transplant (5). It may be that the large numbers of patients used for that study were necessary to observe differences between idiopathic and ischemic disease. Alternatively, the difference could lie in factors other than the myocyte, and this could account for our failure to obtain the same results.

The difference between ventricles in terms of extent of β-adrenoceptor desensitization has been noticed before in human and animal studies (5,27). This could be advanced as an argument against the hypothesis that increased sympathetic drive is solely responsible for the changes in heart failure. However, the present study suggests that there is an intrinsic difference between the ventricles in their response to noradrenaline exposure. This may reflect differences in the uptake of transmitter into neuronal and extraneuronal storage sites, or in some postsynaptic coupling mechanism. Our preliminary experiments appear to eliminate hypertrophy as the compounding factor. We had thought that cells from the left ventricle might be tonically desensitized even in normal hearts, but the results with pertussis toxin, which had no effect on the maximum response in left ventricular myocytes from untreated guinea pig hearts, suggest that this is not the case.

The lesion seems to be reversible within a short time, either by incubation at 35°C or with pertussis toxin. This observation itself eliminates the possibility that changes in cell geometry or structure can play a role. Further experiments are necessary to determine whether the recovery at 35°C requires resynthesis of proteins within the cell.

The reversal of β-adrenoceptor desensitization following pertussis toxin treatment is the first evidence that the increased levels of G_i observed in the failing human heart might have functional importance. However, the hypothesis has been that increased G_i exerts its effect by suppressing β-adrenoceptor–stimulated cAMP production. According to this theory, pertussis toxin reverses desensitization by increasing isoprenaline-stimulated cAMP production. This is hard to reconcile with our observations that the effect of cAMP, as well as its production, is decreased. We suggest that there is an additional effect of G_i, which decreases β-adrenoceptor responses independent of cAMP synthesis. One theory is that an increase in G_i potentiates the arrhythmogenic effect of cAMP-producing agents, possibly by acting on sarcolemmal membrane channels in the same way that G_s acts on the L-type Ca^{2+} channel. It is interesting that noradrenaline-induced β-adrenoceptor desensitization in the rat is not accompanied by such pronounced reduction in the responses to forskolin or dibutyryl cAMP. The action potential characteristics of guinea pig and human myocytes are similar, but those of the rat are markedly different. The arrhythmogenic effects of agents that increase cAMP levels may depend on the nature of the currents making up the action potential.

In an attempt to clarify the mechanism of action of G_i, we have investigated the effect of pertussis toxin treatment on the postreceptor defect in myocytes from noradrenaline-treated guinea pigs. Preliminary data show that the reduction in the response to a cAMP analog can be reversed by pertussis toxin (28) (Fig. 5). This confirms that increased G_i may contribute to the lesion in the maximum effect of cAMP. In future studies, we hope to repeat this experiment on myocytes isolated from failing human heart.

SUMMARY

Reduced sensitivity to β-adrenoceptor stimulation is characteristic of failing human myocardium. It has been suggested that this is a consequence of exposure to the increased noradrenaline levels observed in these patients. We have developed an animal model for catecholamine-induced cardiomyopathy by infusing guinea pigs with noradrenaline (900 μg/kg/hr for 7 days) using osmotic mini-pumps. Compari-

Guinea–pig

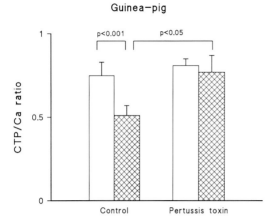

FIG. 5. Effect of pertussis toxin treatment on the maximum response of myocytes to chlorophenylthio (CPT)-cAMP in control (n = 7) and noradrenaline-treated (n = 5–9) guinea pigs.

sons have been made between myocytes isolated from this animal model and those from failing human hearts, and many parallel changes have been observed. In both cases, contractile responses to β-adrenoceptor agonists were reduced, with concentration-response curves to isoprenaline being both right-shifted and depressed. Right/left ventricle differences were observed in both the noradrenaline-treated guinea pigs and in human tissue. Responses to agents acting distal to the β-adrenoceptor were also affected, with maximum responses to forskolin and cAMP analogs being significantly reduced. Simultaneous application of phosphodiesterase inhibitors potentiated the response to low doses of isoprenaline but did not fully restore the maximum to control levels. Incubation of desensitized myocytes, from either human or animal hearts, at 35°C for 2 to 6 hours restored responses to isoprenaline (isoproterenol) close to control levels. Treatment with pertussis toxin at 35°C increased β-adrenoceptor function in desensitized human or guinea pig cells to a greater extent than incubation at 35°C alone. These parallels between the catecholamine cardiomyopathy model and human heart failure support the hypothesis that increased noradrenaline is the common etiologic factor, possibly exerting an effect on the inhibitory guanine nucleotide binding protein (G_i).

ACKNOWLEDGMENTS

We are grateful for the continuing advice and support of Dr. John Pepper and Professor Sir Magdi Yacoub. This work was supported by grants from the Medical Research Council and British Heart Foundation.

REFERENCES

1. Brodde OE. Beta 1- and beta 2-adrenoceptors in the human heart: properties, function, and alterations in chronic heart failure. *Pharmacol Rev* 1991;43:203–242.

2. Bohm M, Beuckelmann D, Brown L, Feiler G, Lorenz B, Nabuaer M, Kemkes B, et al. Reduction of beta-adrenoceptor density and evaluation of positive inotropic responses in isolated diseased human myocardium. *Eur Heart J* 1988;9:844–852.
3. Bristow MR, Ginsburg R, Minobe W, Cubicciotti RS, Sageman WS, Lurie K, Billingham ME, et al. Decreased catecholamine sensitivity and beta-adrenergic receptor density in failing human hearts. *N Engl J Med* 1982;307:205–211.
4. Schwinger RH, Bohm M, Erdmann E. Evidence against spare or uncoupled beta-adrenoceptors in the human heart. *Am Heart J* 1990;119:899–904.
5. Bristow MR, Anderson FL, Port JD, Skerl L, Hershberger RE, Larrabee P, O'Connell JB, et al. Differences in beta-adrenergic neuroeffector mechanisms in ischemic versus dilated cardiomyopathy. *Circulation* 1991;84:1024–1039.
6. Feldman MD, Copelas BS, Gwathmey JK, Phillips P, Warren SE, Schoen FJ, Grossman W, et al. Deficient production of cyclic AMP: pharmacologic evidence of an important cause of contractile dysfunction in patients with end-stage failure. *Circulation* 1987;2:331–339.
7. Cohn JN, Levine TB, Olivari MT, Garberg V, Lura D, Francis GS, Simon AB, et al. Plasma norepinephrine as a guide to prognosis in patients with chronic congestive heart failure. *N Engl J Med* 1984;311:819–823.
8. Thomas JA, Marks BH. Plasma norepinephrine in congestive heart failure. *Am J Cardiol* 1978;41: 233–243.
9. Harding SE, Jones SM, O'Gara P, Vescovo G, Poole-Wilson PA. Reduced beta-agonist sensitivity in single atrial cells from failing human hearts. *Am J Physiol* 1990;259:H1009–H1014.
10. Harding SE, MacLeod KT, Jones SM, Vescovo G, Poole-Wilson PA. Contractile responses of myocytes isolated from patients with cardiomyopathy. *Eur Heart J* 1991;12 [Suppl D]:44–48.
11. Harding SE, Gurden JM, Poole-Wilson PA. A comparison of contractile function between papillary muscles and isolated myocytes from the same human hearts. *Cardioscience* 1991;2:141–146.
12. Harding SE, Jones SM, O'Gara P, del Monte F, Vescovo G, Poole-Wilson PA. Isolated ventricular myocytes from failing and non-failing human heart: the relation of age and clinical status of patients to isoproterenol response. *J Mol Cell Cardiol* 1992;24:549–564.
13. Jones SM, Hunt NA, del Monte F, Harding SE. Contraction of cardiac myocytes from noradrenaline-treated rats in response to isoprenaline, forskolin and dibutyryl cAMP. *Eur J Pharmacol* 1990; 191:129–140.
14. Jones SM, Kirby MS, Harding SE, Vescovo G, Wanless RB, Dalla Libera L, Poole-Wilson PA. Adriamycin cardiomyopathy in the rabbit: alterations in contractile proteins and myocyte function. *Cardiovasc Res* 1990;24:834–842.
15. Vescovo G, Jones SM, Harding SE, Poole-Wilson PA. Isoproterenol sensitivity of isolated cardiac myocytes from rats with monocrotaline-induced right-sided hypertrophy and heart failure. *J Mol Cell Cardiol* 1989;21:1047–1061.
16. Hopwood AM, Harding SE, Harris P. An antiadrenergic effect of adenosine on guinea-pig but not rabbit ventricles. *Eur J Pharmacol* 1987;137:67–75.
17. Harding SE, Vescovo G, Kirby M, Jones SM, Gurden J, Poole-Wilson PA. Contractile responses of isolated rat and rabbit myocytes to isoproterenol and calcium. *J Mol Cell Cardiol* 1988;20:635–647.
18. Jones SM, Gurden J, Harding SE, Poole-Wilson PA. Beta-adrenoceptor desensitisation in papillary muscles and myocytes from the hearts of isoprenaline-treated rabbits. *J Mol Cell Cardiol* 1989;21 [Suppl II]:199 (abst).
19. Harding SE, Hunt NA, Jones SM, O'Gara P, Poole-Wilson PA. Correlation between contractile response to isoprenaline in human left ventricular myocytes and indicators of heart failure. *J Mol Cell Cardiol* 1990;22[suppl III]:s94 (abst).
20. Harding SE, Jones SM, O'Gara P, Vescovo G, Poole-Wilson PA. Decreased response to isoproterenol in single ventricular myocytes from failing human hearts: variation with etiology of disease. *Eur Heart J* 1990;11:404 (abst).
21. Brown LA, Harding SE. The effect of pertussis toxin on β-adrenoceptor responses in isolated cardiac myocytes from noradrenaline-treated guinea-pigs and patients with cardiac failure. *Br J Pharmacol* 1992;106:115–122.
22. Harding SE, Jones SM, Vescovo G, del Monte F, Poole-Wilson PA. Reduced response to forskolin and cyclic AMP analogues in myocytes from failing human ventricle [*submitted*].
23. Wynne DG, Poole-Wilson PA, Harding SE. Partial restoration of β-adrenoceptor function by phosphodiesterase inhibitors in myocytes from noradrenaline-treated guinea-pig and failing human hearts [*submitted*].
24. Brown LA, Humphrey SM, Harding SE. The antiadrenergic effect of adenosine and its blockade by

pertussis toxin. A comparative study in myocytes isolated from guinea-pig, rat and failing human hearts. *Br J Pharmacol* 1990;101:484–488.

25. Feldman AM, Cates AE, Veazey WB, Hershberger RE, Bristow MR, Baughman KL, Baumgartner WA, et al. Increase of the 40,000-mol wt pertussis toxin substrate (G protein) in the failing human heart. *J Clin Invest* 1988;82:189–197.

26. Neumann J, Schmitz W, Scholz H, von Meyernick L, Doring V, Kalmar P. Increase in myocardial Gi-proteins in heart failure. *Lancet* 1988;2:936–937.

27. Fan T, Liang CS, Kawashima S, Banerjee SP. Alterations in cardiac beta-adrenoceptor responsiveness and adenylate cyclase system by congestive heart failure in dogs. *Eur J Pharmacol* 1987; 140:123–132.

28. Harding SE, Brown LA, Vescovo G, del Monte F, Poole-Wilson PA. Reduced response to cAMP analogues in myocytes from noradrenaline treated guinea-pig and failing human heart: reversal by pertussis toxin. *J Mol Cell Cardiol* 1992;24(SI):S86 (abst).

The Cardiomyopathic Heart, edited by Makoto
Nagano, Nobuakira Takeda, and Naranjan S.
Dhalla. Raven Press, Ltd., New York © 1994.

38

Ontogenetic Development of Cardiotoxicity for Catecholamines

Bohuslav Ošťádal, Zdeněk Rychter, and Ivana Ošťádalová

Institute of Physiology, Academy of Sciences of the Czech Republic, Vídeňská 1083, 142 20 Prague 4, Czech Republic

INTRODUCTION

Catecholamines are involved in the regulation of a wide variety of vital functions, including heart rate, myocardial contractility, smooth muscle tone, blood pressure and metabolism of fat and carbohydrates. Low concentrations of circulating catecholamines are thus considered to be beneficial in the regulation of heart function. Excessive release or administration of catecholamines exceeding physiologic doses may, however, deplete the energy reserve of cardiac muscle cells, and this may lead to marked biochemical and structural changes associated with cellular necrosis. The cardiotoxic properties of catecholamines have been recognized since 1905 when the occurrence of cardiac lesions after epinephrine administration was reported by Ziegler (1). However, only after the discovery of Rona and colleagues (2)—that severe myocardial necrosis could be consistently produced in rats with synthetic β-mimetic catecholamine (isoproterenol [IPRO])—did an avenue for systemic examination of catecholamine-induced myocardial lesions (3) emerge.

CARDIOTOXICITY OF CATECHOLAMINES IN ADULTS

Catecholamine-induced cardiac changes are localized predominantly in the subendocardium (2). Moreover, it has been demonstrated that IPRO is a more potent cardiotoxic agent than the naturally occurring catecholamines epinephrine and norepinephrine. This striking difference in the action of these hormones is related to their diverse effects on coronary circulation (4). However, it should be recognized that the pathogenesis of catecholamine-induced myocardial lesions is multifactorial; the major hypotheses (3,5) include a relative hypoxia, coronary microcirculatory effects, altered membrane permeability, myofilament overstimulation, high-energy phosphate deficiency, catecholamine oxidation products, and calcium overload.

	n	cardiac necrosis %
POIKILOTHERMS		
Fish (tench)	99	3
Amphibians (frog)	43	0
Reptiles (turtle)	32	30
HOMOIOTHERMS		
Birds (pigeon)	12	100
Mammals (rat)	30	100

FIG. 1. Cardiotoxicity of isoproterenol in different species of adult warm-blooded and cold-blooded animals. (Data from Oštádal et al., refs. 12 and 14.)

Since the discovery of Rona and associates (2), IPRO-induced cardiac lesions have been demonstrated in a number of adult homeotherms, such as dogs (6), hamsters (7), rabbits (8), cats (9), monkeys (10), mice (11), pigeons (12), and hens (13). Similar changes were described also in some poikilotherms, such as tench (12) and turtles (14). The frog's heart was resistant to the necrotizing effect of IPRO (12). The sensitivity of homeotherms was, however, significantly higher compared to that of poikilothermic animals (Fig. 1). In this regard, it is interesting to note that, in poikilothermic animals, the IPRO-induced necrotic changes are localized predominantly in the inner spongious musculature, which has no vascular supply but which has higher activities of enzymes connected with aerobic oxidation (15).

Whereas abundant data are available concerning the cardiotoxicity of catecholamines in adult animals, much less is known about the toxic effect of these substances on the developing heart. The interest in this topic was stimulated in recent years by an increasing clinical use of catecholamines during early phases of ontogenetic development, particularly during pregnancy (as a tocolytic therapy or treatment for intrapartum fetal distress) or as a treatment of heart pump failure in pediatric cardiology. In this brief overview, we summarize some of our data dealing with the cardiotoxicity of β-mimetic catecholamines during ontogenetic development in both avian and mammalian hearts.

CARDIOTOXICITY OF β-MIMETIC CATECHOLAMINES DURING CHICK EMBRYONIC LIFE

Intra-amniotic administration of IPRO induces serious disturbances in the embryonic cardiovascular system (16,17). The type of change depends upon the time at which the β-adrenergic agonist was administered. From the second to the sixth embryonic day, malformations of the heart and large vessels can be observed. Starting from the fifth embryonic day, cardiomegaly occurred, partly as a result of the increased water content within the myocardium. The slight increase in cardiac dry weight was caused, as in adult hearts, by the combination of the direct proteosynthetic effect of catecholamines and the increased workload induced by their β-stimulating effect. From the seventh to the fifteenth embryonic day, IPRO has been found to exert a negative influence on the coronary vessels. A block in the development of coronary vascularization, always associated with the persistence of an evolutionary older type of blood supply (diffusion from the ventricular cavity), occurs in the nonvascularized portions of the ventricular muscle. Electron microscopic findings (18) are characterized by cellular edema with increased lucidity of sarcoplasm, prominent sarcoplasmic organelles, and swollen mitochondria. Cytoplasmic accumulation of glycogen, seen also in control embryos, was more prominent in the IPRO-treated hearts. Hypercontractions and necrosis of myofibrils, characteristic of catecholamine-induced cardiac lesions in adults, were, however, rather exceptional in embryonic hearts.

A more detailed analysis of the IPRO-induced cardiovascular malformations is presented in Figure 2. The large defects in the interventricular septum were observed on the second embryonic day, the incumbent and transposed aorta occurred on the third and fourth embryonic day, persistent truncus arteriosus was observed on the fourth to fifth embryonic day, and the aortic arch anomalies were observed on the fifth and sixth embryonic day.

Myocardial β-adrenergic stimulation is ordinarily accompanied by an increase in cyclic adenosine monophosphate (cAMP) levels. The IPRO-induced increase in cAMP levels at a period of high cardiotoxicity (i.e., on the seventh embryonic day) was significantly higher as compared with the fifteenth embryonic day, which is characterized by a considerably lower sensitivity to high doses of IPRO (19) (Fig. 3). These observations indicate that cAMP accumulation in the chick embryonic heart in response to IPRO may not only be associated with IPRO-induced modulation of contractile activity (20), but also with its cardiotoxic effect. It should be noted that direct cardiotoxic effects of cAMP analogs have already been demonstrated in adult animals (21,22). The experiments with dibutyryl cAMP in chick embryos, however, yielded results that were not entirely consistent with this hy-

	Embryonic day			
	2	3	4	5	6
Aortic arch anomalies				▭
Persistent truncus art.				▭	
Transposed aorta		▭		
Incumbent aorta		▭		
Defect of i.v. septum	▭▭▭			

FIG. 2. Isoproterenol-induced cardiovascular malformations in the chick embryonic heart. (Data from Rychter and Oštádal, ref. 17.) *art*, arteriosus; *i.v.*, interventricular.

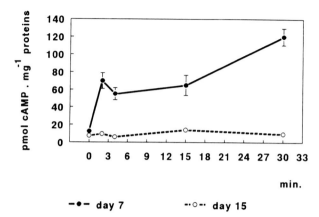

FIG. 3. cAMP levels in the chick embryonic heart after intraamniotic administration of iso-proterenol during periods of high cardiotoxicity (seventh embryonic day, closed circles) and low cardiotoxicity (15th embryonic day, open circles). (Adapted from Ošťádal et al., ref. 19.)

pothesis (23). It was found that cAMP increased the mortality of chick embryos and induced myocardial lesions; in comparison with IPRO, however, the effect of cAMP was significantly less pronounced.

It may be assumed that the cardiotoxicity of catecholamines changes significantly during chick embryonic development. It increased from the second to the twelfth embryonic day and then gradually decreased. Starting from the sixteenth embryonic day, the heart seemed to be resistant to the toxic effect of these drugs. The lack of toxic effect in the last week of embryonic life correlates with the period of the lowest cardiac sensitivity to pharmacologic doses of catecholamines (24).

The mechanism by which sympathomimetic amines cause embryonic cardio-vascular disturbances has not yet been elucidated. Cardiotoxic effects were dose-dependent (17,25) and the order of potency was as follows: the effects of iso-proterenol were greater than those of epinephrine, which were greater than those of norepinephrine (25). The prior administration of either propranolol or the β_1-adrenergic antagonist practolol reduced the incidence of IPRO-induced cardio-vascular malformations as early as the second to the fifth embryonic day (25,26). Because butoxamine, which is more potent in antagonizing the B_2-adrenoreceptors, was less effective in reducing cardiovascular effects, it was suggested that IPRO-induced aortic arch anomalies in chick embryos may be attributable to stimulation of β_1-adrenoreceptors (26). We have observed (17), however, that not all anomalies induced by IPRO up to the sixth embryonic day can be blocked by propranolol, and that all morphogenetic effects of catecholamines are not mediated by a receptor system during this early developmental period. At a later developmental stage (embryonic day 10), propranolol completely prevented the cardiotoxic effect of iso-proterenol (27), an effect similar to that which occurs in adult hearts. Fleckenstein (28) postulated that catecholamine-induced cardiac damage in adult animals was primarily caused by intracellular calcium overloading. This concept was supported

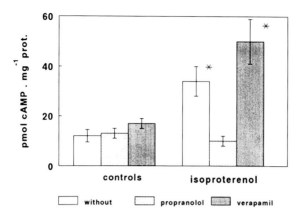

FIG. 4. Different effect of propranolol (1 mg/kg^{-1}) and verapamil (1 mg/kg^{-1}) on the cAMP level in the embryonic heart in control and isoproterenol (10 mg/kg^{-1})-treated chick embryos. *prot.*, protein. (Data from Ošťádal et al., ref. 27.)

by the observation that the cardiotoxic effect of IPRO in adult rats was significantly reduced by the administration of calcium antagonists. We tried, therefore, to repeat this experiment in the chick embryonic heart. Whereas propranolol completely prevented the cardiotoxic effect of IPRO, verapamil (in doses up to 10 mg/kg^{-1}) was ineffective in protecting the immature heart (27) (Fig. 4). Moreover, higher doses of verapamil dramatically increased the mortality of experimental embryos. The inability of the calcium antagonist to protect the embryonic heart may, at least in part, be attributable to the absence or limited number of functional, operative slow calcium channels in the embryonic period. It should be mentioned, however, that calcium overload has not yet been demonstrated in the embryonic myocardium. This possibility is supported by experiments in which [85]Sr was used as a calcium homologue (29–31). IPRO increased [85]Sr uptake in adult rats with hearts having necrotic lesions, but no significant elevation in uptake was observed in the chick embryonic myocardium. It seems, therefore, that IPRO-induced (non-necrotic) changes in the chick embryonic heart are not necessarily attributable to intracellular calcium overload.

ONTOGENETIC DEVELOPMENT OF CARDIOTOXICITY FOR CATECHOLAMINES IN MAMMALS

There are many discrepancies in the literature dealing with responsiveness of the developing mammalian heart to catecholamines (32,33). The situation seems to be even more complex with respect to the possible age-related changes in cardiotoxicity. The information on this aspect of research is insufficient, even though catecholamines are used in clinical practice, both during pregnancy and just after birth. It should be noted that β-sympathomimetic drugs are known to cross the placental barrier and reach the fetus, and their concentration in the fetal blood is nearly equal to that in the mother (34).

The acute administration of high doses of IPRO to rats during prenatal ontogeny does not cause any necrotic changes in the myocardium. The administration of this drug, however, retards the growth of the animals and increases the dry weight of the heart (35). From birth up to the end of the fourth postnatal week, the rat heart has been shown to be resistant to the toxic effect of isoproterenol. The first microscopic changes have been observed on the 30th day of postnatal life, and the incidence of such changes has been found to increase with the age of the animal (Fig. 5).

These results are supported by recent experiments involving [85]Sr (29,31). In 14-day-old animals that were resistant to the necrogenic action of IPRO, the uptake of [85]Sr was not increased, whereas in 30- to 120-day-old hearts, the [85]Sr uptake was significantly increased by IPRO (see Fig. 5). The exact mechanisms for the early postnatal subsensitivity to necrogenic doses of catecholamines are poorly understood.

Unfortunately, no adequate studies have been conducted on possible catecholamine toxicity in the human cardiovascular system. Serious maternal complications of tocolytic therapy, including pulmonary edema, metabolic acidosis, myocardial ischemia, cardiac arrhythmias, and maternal death, have been reviewed by Benedetti (36). The effects of tocolytic therapy in children have included arrhythmias, cardiac insufficiency, cardiomegaly, dyspnea, muscular hypotony, and increased cretine kinase levels (37). Nevertheless, these data are not convincing, and the crucial question of cardiotoxicity of catecholamines during early stages of human development warrants further experimental and clinical investigation.

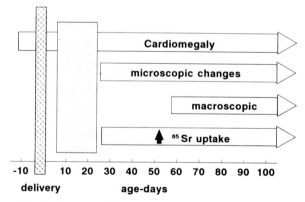

FIG. 5. Ontogenetic development of isoproterenol-induced cardiotoxicity in rats. The hatched area refers to the period of low sensitivity to the toxic effect of isoproterenol. (Adapted from Ošťádal et al., ref. 33, and based on data from Ošťádalová and Ošťádal, ref. 31, and Ošťádal, ref. 35.)

SUMMARY

It seems likely that, despite possible interspecies differences, developmental changes in the cardiotoxicity for catecholamines may exist in all homeotherms, depending on the degree of maturation of systems involved in β-adrenergic interactions. All the existing data draw attention to the possible negative consequences of the clinical use of β-sympathomimetic agents during early phases of cardiac development.

REFERENCES

1. Ziegler K. Über die Wirkung intravenöser adrenalin Injektion auf das Gefässystems und ihre Beziehungen zur Arteriosklerose. *Beitr Pathol Anat u.z. allg Path* 1905;38:229–254.
2. Rona G, Chappel CI, Balasz T, Gaudry R. An infarct-like myocardial lesion and other toxic manifestations produced by isoproterenol in the rat. *Arch Pathol* 1959;67:443–455.
3. Dhalla NS, Yates JC, Naimark B, Dhalla KS, Beamish RE, Oštádal B. Cardiotoxicity of catecholamines and related agents. In: Acosta D, ed. *Cardiovascular toxicology.* New York: Raven Press; 1992:239–282.
4. Boutet M, Hüttner I, Rona G. Aspect microcirculatoire des lesions myocardiques provoquee's par l'infusion de catecholamines. Etude ultrastructural a l'aide de traceurs de diffusion. I. Isoproterenol. *Pathol Biol (Paris)* 1973;21:811–825.
5. Rona G. Catecholamine cardiotoxicity. *J Mol Cell Cardiol* 1985;17:291–306.
6. Rona G, Zsoter T, Chappel C, Gaudry R. Myocardial lesions, circulatory and electrographic changes produced by isoproterenol in the dog. *Rev Can Biol* 1959b;18:83–94.
7. Handforth CP. Myocardial infarction and necrotizing arteritis in hamsters, produced by isoproterenol (Isuprel). *Med Serv J Can* 1962;18:506–512.
8. Amelin AZ, Anshelevich JV, Melzobar MJ. Eksperimentalnyje izmenenija miokarda pri vozdějstvii izadrinom (isopropylnoradrenalinom). *Arkh Pathol* 1963;25:25–30.
9. Rosenblum I, Wohl A, Stein AA. Studies in cardiac necrosis. I. Production of cardiac lesions with sympathomimetic amines. *Toxicol Appl Pharmacol* 1965;7:1–8.
10. Maruffo CA. Fine structural study of myocardial changes induced by isoproterenol in Rhesus monkeys (Macaca mulatta). *Am J Pathol* 1967;50:27–37.
11. Zbinden G, Moe RA. Pharmacological studies on heart muscle lesions induced by isoproterenol. *Ann NY Acad Sci* 1969;156:294–308.
12. Oštádal B, Rychterová V. Effect of necrogenic doses of isoproterenol on the heart of the tench (Tinca tinca—Osteoichthyes), the frog (Rana temporaria—Anura) and the pigeon (Columba livia—Aves). *Physiol Bohemoslov* 1971;20:541–547.
13. Oštádal B, Rychter Z, Rychterová V. Comparison of the different sensitivity of the chick and rat heart to isoproterenol during the prenatal and postnatal development. *Acta Univ Carol Med Praha* 1973;56:183–187.
14. Oštádal B, Rychterova V, Poupa O. Isoproterenol-induced acute experimental cardiac necrosis in the turtle (Testudo horsfieldi). *Am Heart J* 1968;76:645–649.
15. Bass A, Oštádal B, Pelouch V, Vitek V. Differences in weight parameters, myosin-ATPase activity and the enzyme pattern of energy supplying metabolism between the compact and spongious cardiac musculature of carp (Cyprinus carpio) and turtle (Testudo horsfieldi). *Pflügers Arch* 1973;343:65–67.
16. Oštádal B, Rychter Z, Rychterová V. The action of isoproterenol on the chick embryo heart. *J Mol Cell Cardiol* 1976;8:533–544.
17. Rychter Z, Oštádal B. The relationship between the dose of beta mimetic catecholamine and the type of induced cardiovascular anomalies in early chick embryo. *Verh Anat Ges* 1986;80:275–276.
18. Dušek J, Oštádal B. Ultrastructure of isoproterenol-induced myocardial damage in chick embryos. *Physiol Bohemoslov* 1985;34:297–302.
19. Oštádal B, Krause EG, Beyerdorfer I, Pelouch V, Wollenberger A. Effect of intraamnial administra-

tion of the cardiotoxic dose of isoproterenol on cyclic AMP levels in the chick embryo heart. *J Mol Cell Cardiol* 1979;11:1183–1187.

20. Polson JB, Golberg ND, Shideman FE. Norepinephrine and isoproterenol induced changes in cardiac contractility and cyclic adenosine 3′, 5′-monophosphate levels during early development of the embryonic chick. *J Pharmacol Exp Ther* 1977;200:630–637.
21. Dhalla NS, Chernecki S, Gandhi SS, McNamara D, Naimark A. Cardiac and metabolic effect of dibutyryl cyclic AMP in the intact dog heart and the isolated perfused rat heart. *Rec Adv Studies Cardiac Struct Metab* 1973;3:233–250.
22. Lee JC, Downing SE. Cyclic AMP and the pathogenesis of myocardial injury. *Res Commun Chem Pathol Pharmacol* 1980;27:305–318.
23. Janatová T, Ošťádal B, Dušek J. The effect of intraamnial administration of isoprenaline and dibutyryl cAMP on the chick embryonic heart. *Physiol Bohemoslov* 1981;30:432.
24. Higgins D. The ontogeny of the response of the avian embryo heart to autonomic neurotransmitter and to neurotransmitter-like drugs. *Pharmacol Ther* 1983;22:53–77.
25. Hodach RJ, Hodach AE, Fallon JF, Folts JD, Bruyere HJ, Gilbert EF. The role of beta adrenergic activity in the production of cardiac and aortic arch anomalies in chick embryos. *Teratology* 1975; 12:33–46.
26. Gilbert EF, Bruyere HJ, Ishikawa S, Cheung MO, Hodach RJ. The effect of practolol and butoxamine on aortic arch malformations in beta adrenoreceptor stimulated chick embryos. *Teratology* 1977;15:317–324.
27. Ošťádal B, Janatová T, Krause EG, Pelouch V, Dušek J. Different effect of propranolol and verapamil on isoprenaline-induced changes in the chick embryonic heart. *Physiol Bohemoslov* 1987; 36:301–311.
28. Fleckenstein A. Specific inhibitors and promoters of calcium action in the excitation-contraction coupling of heart muscle and their role in the prevention or production of myocardial lesions. In: Harris P, Opie LH, eds. *Calcium and the heart*. London: Academic Press; 1971:135–188.
29. Ošťádalová I, Ošťádal B. Effect of isoprenaline on [85]Sr accumulation in the myocardium of the adult rat. *Physiol Bohemoslov* 1988;37:351–353.
30. Ošťádalová I, Ošťádal B. [85]Sr uptake by the chick embryonic heart. Effect of high doses of isoproterenol. *Can J Physiol Pharmacol* 1992;70:959–962.
31. Ošťádalová I, Ošťádal B. Ontogenetic differences in isoproterenol-induced [85]Sr uptake in the myocardium. In Nagano M, Takeda N, Dhalla NS, eds. *The Cardiomyopathic Heart*. New York: Raven Press, 1993.
32. Driscoll DJ. Use of inotropic and chronotropic agents in neonates. *Clin Perinatol* 1987;14:931–948.
33. Ošťádal B, Beamish RE, Barwinsky J, Dhalla NS. Ontogenetic development of cardiac sensitivity to catecholamines. *J Appl Cardiol* 1989;4:467–486.
34. Caritis SN, Shei Lin L, Toig G, Wonk LK. Pharmacodynamics of ritodrine in pregnant women during pre-term labor. *Am J Obstet Gynecol* 1983;147:752–759.
35. Ošťádal B. Phylogenetic and ontogenetic development of the terminal vascular bed in the heart muscle and its effect on the development of experimental cardiac necrosis. *Proceedings of the Second Annual Meeting of the Inter. Study Gr. for Res. in Cardiac Metabolism*. Milano: Istituto Lombardo, Fond. Baselli; 1970:111–132.
36. Benedetti TJ. Life-threatening complications of beta mimetic therapy for pre-term labor inhibition. *Clin Perinatol* 1986;13:843–852.
37. Wischnik A, Hotzinger B, Wischnik B, Schroll A, Trenkwalder V, Weidenback A. Zum Einfluss des Betablockers Metropolol auf das Zyklische 3,5 Adenosine-Monophosphat in verschiedenen Gewebsarten unter Langzeittokolyse mit Fenoterol. *Arzneimittel-forsch* 1984;34:684–687.

The Cardiomyopathic Heart, edited by Makoto
Nagano, Nobuakira Takeda, and Naranjan S.
Dhalla. Raven Press, Ltd., New York © 1994.

39

Isoproterenol-Induced Changes in Metabolic Regulations in the Canine Heart: Protective Effect of K^+,Mg^{2+}-Aspartate

Attila Ziegelhoeffer, Jan Slezák, Tatiana Ravingerová, and
Narcisa Tribulová

*Institute for Heart Research, Slovak Academy of Sciences, Dubravska cesta 9,
842 33 Bratislava, Czech Republic*

INTRODUCTION

The synthetic catecholamine derivative isoproterenol (ISO), with its β-adrenergic stimulatory effect, has been widely used, not only as a drug but also in experimental cardiology studies related to metabolic regulations in the myocardium (Fig. 1), calcium overload in the heart, infarction, and cardiomyopathy (1–7). ISO-induced, infarction-like cardiac lesions were first described by Rona et al. (8). Since then, the suggested mechanism for their genesis has been the subject of several reviews (9–11). It is generally concluded that (a) hypoxia secondary to the constriction of coronary arteries and/or to the interaction between hemodynamic and biochemical effects of the ISO results in a shift of the electrolyte composition in cardiac tissue; and (b) enhancement in transmembrane Ca^{2+} influx is followed by excessive activation of Ca^{2+}-dependent adenosine triphosphatase (ATPase) systems in the cardiac cells. A dramatic increase in Ca^{2+} concentration in the cardiomyocytes results in functional deterioration of the mitochondria. The latter significantly contributes to the already persisting intracellular energy deficiency induced by Ca^{2+}-dependent stimulation of the high-energy phosphate breakdown (3,10,12).

Besides these generally accepted mechanisms, an intracellular concentration of free calcium over a threshold level is also thought to interfere with several processes that depend on maintenance of Mg^{2+}, Na^+, and K^+ homeostasis, as well as with the intracellular and transsarcolemmal shuttle of cations in cardiac tissue. It was demonstrated that substances preventing excessive intracellular Ca^{2+} accumulation may protect the heart against ISO-caused alterations (3–5,10). It was also shown that K^+,Mg^{2+}-(D,L)-aspartate (K,Mg-ASP) may be beneficial in mitigating the cardiotoxic effect of high doses of ISO (12–14). The present study represents an

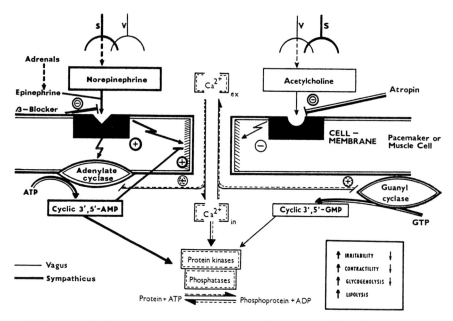

FIG. 1. Hypothetical sequence of reactions in neurohumoral regulation of heart function.

update on the effects of high doses of ISO on the dog myocardium and their prevention by K,Mg-ASP with respect to the metabolic, membrane, and ultrastructural characteristics.

MATERIALS AND METHODS

Experimental Protocol

Male mongrel dogs, 3 to 6 years of age and weighing 8 to 12 kg, were used in the experiments. Animals received an intraperitoneal injection of isoproterenol (7.5 mg/kg) in saline; the controls (group I) received saline only. Dogs in groups II and IV were anesthetized with pentobarbital (30 mg/kg of body weight, SPOFA) and were cardiectomized 2 or 24 hours after administration of the drug. In groups III and V, K,Mg-ASP (4.2 mmol in 50 mL of 10% glucose) was administered intravenously along with the ISO; the animals in these groups also underwent cardiectomy 2 or 24 hours after treatment. Tissue specimens for morphologic examination were taken at 5 minutes and at 2, 4, 6, and 24 hours after ISO treatment.

Determination of Metabolites

Tissue samples for determination of creatine phosphate (CP); adenosine triphosphate (ATP); the total of adenine nucleotides (ADNs), including ATP, adenosine diphosphate (ADP), and adenosine monophosphate (AMP); lactate; pyruvate; and glycogen were taken from the left ventricle (apex) by means of the freeze-clamp technique. The products of intermediary metabolism just enumerated were determined enzymatically (13,15), utilizing the principle of the Warburg's optical test.

Isolation of Subcellular Membrane Fractions

Sarcolemma. Isolated hearts were quickly cooled down and washed free of blood. After removal of fat as well as the epicardial and endocardial membranes, the tissue of the left ventricle (apex) was minced with scissors. Further steps applied in isolation and characterization of the sarcolemmal membrane preparation by a modification of the hypotonic shock method were described recently (16).

Sarcoplasma Reticulum. The initial treatment of the myocardial tissue samples taken from the left ventricle was similar to that described in preparation of sarcolemma. Further procedures applied in preparation of a membrane fraction enriched in sarcoplasma reticulum were described earlier (17).

Mitochondria and Myofibrils. Initial treatment of the tissue samples from left ventricular myocardium was the same as in the case of sarcolemma and sarcoplasma reticulum. Mitochondrial preparation was isolated according to the technique described by Lindenmayer et al. (18). The myofibrils were isolated by the method used previously (17).

Estimation of ATPase Activities. The specific activities of the sarcolemma, sarcoplasma reticulum, myofibril, and mitochondrial ATPase were estimated by measuring the amount of phosphate liberated from ATP splitting. In all cases, the reaction was allowed to proceed for 10 minutes at 37°C in 1 mL of medium with special composition for each ATPase; it was started by the addition of ATP and terminated by 1 mL of ice-cold trichloroacetic acid. Further details with respect to the specific composition of the respective reaction media, as well as the calculation of the enzyme activities, are described elsewhere (16,17).

Estimation of Calcium Binding and Uptake by Subcellular Organelles. Calcium binding and uptake were studied employing ^{45}Ca and the Millipore filtration method. This method has also been used in studies on sarcoplasma reticulum and mitochondria (12,13).

Electron Microscopy and Histochemistry. Blocks of tissue from the middle layer of the apical part of the heart, measuring approximately 0.5 to 1 mm^3, were fixed for electron microscopy in 3% glutaraldehyde in 0.1 mol/L^{-1} of phosphate buffer (pH of 7.4) for 3 hours and were subsequently washed in 0.15 mol L^{-1} of phosphate buffer. Finally, the tissue samples were fixed in 1% phosphate-buffered OsO$_4$ for 1 hour. Dehydration of the samples was carried out gradually using alcohols, and the tissue was finally embedded in Epon 812. At the same time, other pieces of tissue were frozen in liquid nitrogen-cooled hexan for cryostat sectioning for histochemistry. Further technical details are available elsewhere (14).

Drugs and Chemicals. K,Mg-ASP (Tromcardin) was kindly provided by Trommsdorff, Ltd. Aachen, BRD. Tris-ATP, (D,L)-isoproterenol, ouabain, imidazole, oligomycin, sodium azide, as well as all substances used for electron microscopy, were purchased from Sigma, Ltd. $^{45}CaCl_2$ was obtained from Amersham, Ltd. All other reagents were obtained from Lachema (CSFR) and were of analytical grade as well.

RESULTS AND DISCUSSION

The data shown in Figure 2A indicate about a 50% decrease in the ATP content and approximately an 80% loss in the creatine phosphate content in myocardial tissue (as compared to controls) 2 hours after ISO administration (group II). In contrast to the results in group III, to which K,Mg-ASP was administered simultaneously with ISO, the high-energy phosphate compounds remained significantly preserved ($p < 0.01$). The protective effect of K,Mg-ASP became markedly evident 24 hours after ISO administration (group V) in comparison with group IV, which received no K,Mg-ASP.

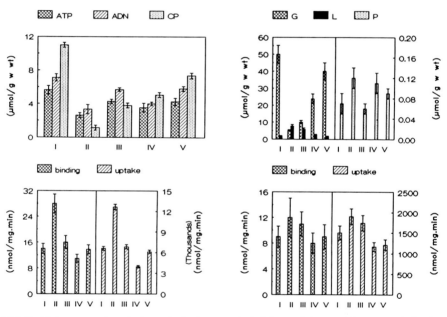

FIG. 2. High-energy phosphate content, glycogenolysis intermediates, and Ca accumulation in sarcoplasmic reticulum and mitochondria from the dog heart in controls (group I), in groups II and IV 2 and 24 hours after administration of ISO, and in groups III and V 2 and 24 hours after administration of ISO plus K,Mg-ASP. **A:** Changes in ATP, total adenine nucleotides (ADN) and creatine phosphate (CP) levels. Values are means ± S.E. of 5 to 10 experiments expressed in μmol/g of wet weight **B:** Changes in glycogen (G), lactate (L), and pyruvate (P) levels. Values are means ± S.E. expressed in μmol/g wet weight. **C:** Ca accumulation in the sarcoplasmic reticulum of the heart in the absence or presence of oxalate. Values are means ± S.E. of 6 experiments expressed in nmol/mg/min. **D:** Calcium accumulation in heart mitochondria. Values are means ± S.E. of 6 experiments expressed in nmol/mg/min.

An 85% and 47% decrease in glycogen content, a 363% and 40% increase in lactate content, and a 70% and 60% increase in pyruvate content were observed in cardiac tissue (as compared to controls) at 2 hours and 24 hours, respectively, after administration of a single dose of ISO (see Fig. 2B). When K,Mg-ASP was simultaneously administered to animals with ISO, a marked protective influence was observed.

Our results concerning the influence of ISO on the intermediary and energy metabolism of the dog myocardium confirmed our expectations (derived from studying the findings of other investigators) (3–5,9,10). These also seem to prove that the anaerobiosis, and particularly, the energy deficiency observed, results from Ca^{2+} overload of the myocardial cells. Until now, it has not been clear how potent K,Mg-ASP may be in antagonizing the ISO-induced massive increase in Ca^{2+} influx into cardiomyocytes. In any case, K,Mg-ASP appears to contribute to the maintenance of the intracellular cation homeostasis. Consequently, in addition to protection of glycogen and energy metabolism of the heart, the beneficial effect of K,Mg-ASP is also reflected in the considerable protection, afforded by the subcellular Ca^{2+} sequestration systems localized in sarcoplasmic reticulum and mitochondria, against functional deterioration caused by excess calcium (see Fig. 2C).

The capacity of sarcoplasmic reticulum, isolated from dog hearts 2 and 24 hours after ISO administration, with and without simultaneous application of K,Mg-ASP, to accumulate Ca^{2+} in the absence (binding) and presence of oxalate (uptake) was found to be doubled 2 hours after ISO application. On the other hand, both of these parameters were decreased below control values 24 hours after ISO administration. The in vivo administration of K,Mg-ASP in millimolar concentrations at the onset of the experiment almost entirely prevented the ISO-induced alterations in Ca^{2+} accumulation ($p<0.05$).

Both Ca^{2+} binding (in the absence of Pi and succinate) and Ca^{2+} uptake (in the presence of 4 mmol/L^{-1} of Pi and 5 mmol/L^{-1} of succinate) were also studied in mitochondria obtained from controls, ISO-treated hearts, as well as hearts treated with both ISO and K,Mg-ASP. The results, shown in Fig. 2D, indicate that Ca^{2+} binding was not changed significantly ($p>0.05$), but that Ca^{2+} uptake was significantly higher ($p<0.05$) 2 hours after ISO administration in the group that did not receive K,Mg-ASP. However, 24 hours after administration of ISO or ISO and K,Mg-ASP, calcium uptake was found to be significantly lower than in controls ($p<0.05$).

Based on the results presented here, and taking into consideration the essential role of the cellular membrane systems in the regulation of heart function (19), as well as other information about the crucial role of membrane defects in the development of genetic cardiomyopathies (20,21), we may assume that there does exist a real biochemical basis for the heart failure. Although this premise has recently been argued by Opie (22), the existence of a biochemical basis for heart failure would not exclude the involvement of other factors, such as O_2 imbalance.

The changes induced by administration of ISO or ISO and K,Mg-ASP in the (Mg^{2+},Ca^{2+})-ATPase activity of the isolated sarcoplasmic reticulum are reported

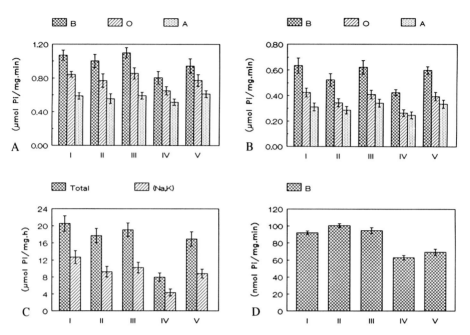

FIG. 3. Changes in ATPase activity in the dog myocardium in controls (group I), in groups II and IV 2 and 24 hours after administration of ISO, and in groups III and V 2 and 24 hours after administration of ISO plus K,Mg-ASP. **A**: (Mg,Ca)-ATPase activity of dog heart sarcoplasmic reticulum. Results are means ± S.E. of 5 experiments expressed in μmol Pi/mg/min. **B**: Mg-ATPase activity of dog heart mitochondria. Results are means ± S.E. of 5 experiments expressed in μmol Pi/mg/min. **C**: Total and (Na,K)-ATPase activity of dog heart sarcolemma. Results are means ± S.E. expressed in μmol Pi/mg/hr. **D**: Myofibrillar ATPase activity of dog heart. Values are means ± S.E. of 5 to 10 experiments expressed in nmol Pi/mg/min. *B*, basic activity; *O*, influenced by oligomycin; *A*, influenced by sodium azide.

in Figure 3A. The activity of this enzyme, suggested to be involved in Ca^{2+} transport into the vesicles of the sarcoplasmic reticulum, was found to be depressed considerably ($p < 0.05$) 24 hours after administration of ISO only; this depression could be fully prevented by treatment with K,Mg-ASP. Contrary to the findings obtained in vitro (17), no specific influence of K,Mg-ASP on the (Mg^{2+}, Ca^{2+})-ATPase of sarcoplasmic reticulum was observed 2 hours after administration of the substance to ISO-untreated animals in vivo (data not shown). The unchanged sensitivity of the (Mg^{2+}, Ca^{2+})-ATPase to oligomycin and sodium azide, found in all sarcoplasmic reticulum preparations, serves as a proof of an unaltered quality of the isolated subcellular fractions investigated.

These findings practically exclude the possibility that a catecholamine-induced lipid peroxidation may be involved in the ISO-induced damage of sarcoplasmic reticulum function in the heart (23). Because the essential SH groups located in the ATP-binding site of the Ca^{2+} pump can be seen to represent the first target for free radicals (24), our findings indicate that the enzymatic part of the Ca^{2+} pump may not be involved in the ISO-induced depression of Ca^{2+} accumulation by cardiac sarcoplasmic reticulum.

ATP hydrolyzing activity of the mitochondrial fraction was also determined; the results are reported in Figure 3B. Similar to the (Mg^{2+},Ca^{2+})-ATPase of cardiac sarcoplasmic reticulum, no marked change in ATPase activity of the mitochondria was found in any group except for one, 24 hours after ISO administration, when the latter ATPase activity was decreased significantly ($p<0.01$). The interpretation offered for findings in the sarcoplasmic reticulum seems to be valid also for the mitochondria, because the mitochondria would represent a particularly suitable target for spontaneously formed peroxides. Because K,Mg-ASP cannot be considered as a potent free radical scavenger, its protective action against the ISO-induced myocardial damage may be ascribed to its ability to maintain cation homeostasis in cardiac cells.

Two hours after administration of ISO, the activity of Ca^{2+}-dependent ATPase of cardiac myofibrils was found to be stimulated significantly ($p<0.01$) (see Fig. 3D). However, in the presence of K,Mg-ASP, activation of the Ca^{2+}-dependent myofibrillar ATPase did not differ from that in controls. Conversely, 24 hours after ISO administration, the ATPase activity of cardiac myofibrils was severely depressed ($p<0.001$). This cardiotoxic effect of ISO could not be antagonized by K,Mg-ASP.

Particularly interesting effects of ISO have been observed when investigating the specific activity of (Na,K)-ATPase in cardiac sarcolemma (see Fig. 3C). Although the activity of the enzyme was found to be slightly decreased 2 hours after treatment of animals with ISO, a significant ($p<0.001$) depression in sarcolemmal (Na,K)-ATPase activity was observed only 24 hours after administration of the drug. ISO-induced changes in the total Mg^{2+}- plus (Na,K)-ATPase activity of sarcolemma, as well as in the 5'-nucleotidase and succinic dehydrogenase activities of sarcolemma (data not shown), followed those of the (Na,K)-ATPase. Paralleling the decrease in sarcolemmal enzyme activities, the yield of the membrane fraction enriched in sarcolemma in ISO-treated hearts was found to be increased. Further, using the marker enzymes of sarcoplasmic reticulum and mitochondria as measures of purity, no increase in contamination of the sarcolemma with the former organelles was observed (25). Investigation of specific properties of (Na,K)-ATPase revealed an alteration in the pH optimum, a changed Km value, and increased sensitivity to $HgCL_2$, without any change in content of the protein-bound sulfhydryl groups (25). In particular, the latter finding indicates the deteriorating effect of high doses of ISO on the sarcolemma; a mechanism not involving the action of free radicals.

The molecular mechanisms underlying the protective effect of K,Mg-ASP on the (Na,K)-ATPase of cardiac sarcolemma (clearly manifested 2 and 24 hours after ISO administration) were also investigated in vitro (17,26). Contrary to the results from in vivo studies, the latter experiments demonstrated an expressed inhibition (allosteric type) of (Na,K)-ATPase by K,Mg-ASP. The basic inhibitory constituent of the compound proved to be the aspartic moiety. Unfortunately, these findings do not contribute directly to an explanation of the protective effect of K,Mg-ASP against the ISO-induced damage to the heart. The reason is that the inhibition of the heart sarcolemma (Na,K)-ATPase in its ouabain-binding site by K,Mg-ASP (which may lead to a positive inotropic effect) could hardly be expected to be responsible for elimination of the ISO-induced effect on the enzyme.

The morphologic changes associated with the ISO-induced myocardial changes are in good agreement with the biochemical changes discussed earlier. First marked ISO-induced changes could be observed in electron microscope as early as 5 minutes after administration of the drug; increased number of lipid droplets, lightly stained with OsO_4 (Fig. 4A). The most striking changes, however, were observed 4 to 6 hours after ISO injection: a great amount of lipid droplets; mitochondria with decreased density of matrix and focal loss of cristae (Fig. 4B). In other areas the prominent features were focal destruction of I-band material, loss of actin filaments, irregular and wide Z-bands and spots of Z-band-like material (Fig. 5A). The amount of glycogen was mostly unchanged. Intercalated discs and sarcoplasmic reticulum did not show any significant alterations. Nuclei were edematous (Fig. 5B). In some places sarcomeres were contracted while in others they were relaxed.

Further morphological changes that occurred later than 6 hours after ISO-application were reported elsewhere (14). They comprised a diminished amount of gly-

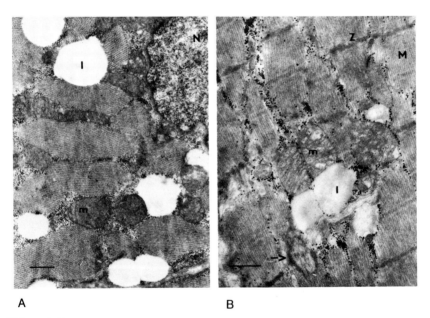

A   B

FIG. 4. A: Electron micrograph of the myocardium 5 minutes after ISO administration. Note the marked increase in the number of lipid droplets (*l*), the decreased density of the mitochondrial matrix (*m*), and the nucleus (*N*) with its even distribution of chromatin. Scale bar = 1 μm. **B**: Electron micrograph 4 to 6 hours after ISO injection. The mitochondria (*m*) reveal decreased density of matrix and focal loss of cristae. Z-band irregularities (*arrow*) are also seen. *Z*, Z band; *M*, M line; *l*, lipid droplet. Scale bar = 1 μm.

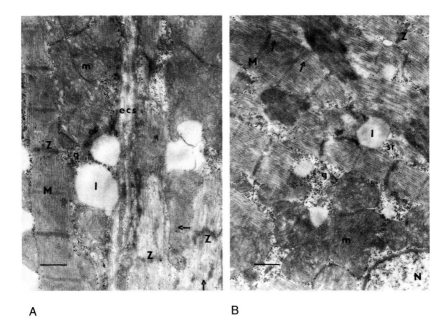

A   B

FIG. 5. A: Ultrastructure of cardiac tissue 2 to 6 hours after ISO injection. Arrows point to areas of local loss of actin filaments. Irregularities of Z bands (*Z*) are seen. Glycogen (*g*) levels are not significantly diminished. *I*, lipid droplet; *m*, mitochondrion; *M*, M line; *ecs*, extracellular space. Scale bar = 1 μm. **B**: Ultrastructure of cardiac tissue 2 to 6 hours after ISO injection. Three areas of electron-dense Z-band–like material are present. One of them is indicated by arrows. An edematous nucleus (*N*) is seen in the lower right corner. *m*, mitochondrion; *sr*, sarcoplasmic reticulum; *Z*, wide and irregular Z bands; *M*, M line. Scale bar = 1 μm.

cogen granules, widened intercalated discs, nuclei with marked swelling and margination of chromatin, and an increased number of free ribosomes, as well as rough endoplasmic reticulum in the perinuclear areas. The changes after 24 hours were much more pronounced. In the neighborhood of severely damaged areas characterized by loss of myofibrils and severely injured mitochondria (in addition to already described changes), relatively well-preserved areas were observed (14). Administration of K,Mg-ASP alone induced only minor and not specific changes in the ultrastructure of the myocardium (14). When K,Mg-ASP was administered simultaneously with ISO, after 24 hours most of the myocardial cells did not differ from normal, except for a higher amount of lipid droplets (Fig. 6A and B). With other changes, like fusion of mitochondria, sausagelike wide cristae of mitochondria resembled those due to enhanced metabolic activity.

The findings concerning the effect of high doses of ISO on the heart, particularly those demonstrating changes typical for the lack of oxygen and for Ca^{2+} overload, were similar to those reported by others (8,9,27). All morphologic changes demonstrated result from severely altered metabolism and function of the subcellular (particularly, the membrane) systems in myocardial cells, discussed earlier. In conclu-

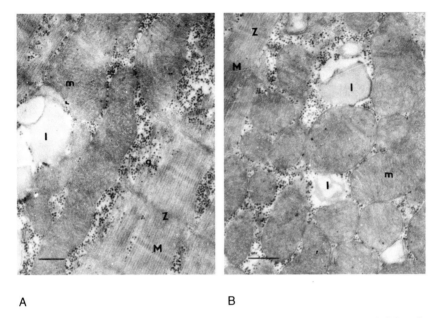

A   B

FIG. 6. Electromicrographs of the myocardium 24 hours after simultaneous administration of ISO and K,Mg-ASP. Almost normal ultrastructure, except for an increased amount of lipid droplets, is seen. **A,** In more than three sarcomeres, long mitochondrion and sausage-like, wide, and dense cristae are seen. There is a normal amount of glycogen present. *M,* M line; *Z,* Z band; *g,* glycogen; *l,* lipid droplet; *m,* mitochondrion. Scale bar = 1 μm. **B:** Normal amount of glycogen is present. *Z,* Z band; *M,* M line; *l,* lipid droplets; *m,* mitochondrion. Scale bar = 1 μm.

sion, the biochemical and morphologic data presented can be regarded as evidence for the existence of a real biochemical foundation for the development of cardio-myopathies secondary to high levels of circulating catecholamines.

SUMMARY

Isoproterenol is known to induce a dose-dependent increase in transmembrane calcium influx with subsequent activation of glycolysis, energy consumption by Ca^{2+}-dependent intracellular systems, and cardiac lesions. Substances preventing excessive intracellular Ca^{2+} accumulation may antagonize the isoproterenol-caused myocardial alterations. Two hours after administration of a single dose of isoproterenol (7.5 mg/kg^{-1} of body weight, intramuscularly [IM]) in male mongrel dogs, high energy phosphate stores and glycogen levels were reduced, whereas lactate and pyruvate levels, the lactate/pyruvate ratio, and myofibrillar adenosine triphosphatase (ATPase) activity, as well as Ca^{2+} accumulation by the sarcoplasmic reticulum and mitochondria, were elevated ($p<0.01$). After 24 hours, a partial recovery (except for myofibrillar ATPase activity and Ca^{2+} uptake by the sarcoplasmic reticulum, which were decreased below control values) was observed. K^+, Mg^{2+}-aspartate (4.2 mmol/L^{-1}), administered simultaneously with isoproterenol, completely prevented the changes in myofibrillar ATPase activity and Ca^{2+} uptake by the sarcoplasmic reticulum and partially affected other parameters 2 hours after administration. After 24 hours, all parameters investigated were close to control levels. Biochemical findings were in agreement with the morphologic changes, thus supporting the view that maintenance of cation homeostasis may prevent the development of isoproterenol-induced cardiac lesions.

REFERENCES

1. Nayler WG. Calcium exchange in cardiac muscle: a basic mechanism of drug action. *Am Heart J* 1967;73:379–394.
2. Fedelešová M, Ziegelhoeffer A. Enhanced calcium accumulation related to increased protein phosphorylation in cardiac sarcoplasmic reticulum induced by cyclic 3',5'-AMP or isoproterenol. *Experientia* 1975;31:518–520.
3. Fleckenstein A. *Calcium antagonism in heart and smooth muscle. Experimental facts and therapeutic prospects.* New York: John Wiley & Sons; 1983.
4. Fleckenstein A, Frey M, Fleckenstein-Gruen G. Myocardial and vascular damage by intracellular calcium overload. Preventive actions of calcium antagonists. In: Godfraind T, Vanhoutte PM, Govoni S, Paoletti R, eds. *Calcium entry blockers and tissue protection.* New York: Raven Press; 1985:91–105.
5. Stoclet JC, Lugnier C, Follenius A, Scheftel JM, Gérard D. Calmodulin and calcium regulation: effect of antagonists. In: Godfraind T, Vanhoutte PM, Govoni S, Paoletti R, eds. *Calcium entry blockers and tissue protection.* New York: Raven Press; 1985:31–40.
6. Ošťádal B, Rychter Z, Ošťádalová I. Ontogenetic development of cardiotoxicity for catecholamines. *J Mol Cell Cardiol* 1992;24 [Suppl II]:0–8, 43.
7. Sugiyama S, Hattori K, Hanaki Y, Akiyama N, Kato T, Ozawa T. Involvement of the autonomic nervous system in the genesis of cardiomyopathy in rats. *J Mol Cell Cardiol* 1992;24 [Suppl II]:0–9,43.
8. Rona G, Chappel CI, Balazs T, Gaudry R. An infarct-like myocardial lesion and other toxic manifestations produced by isoproterenol in rat. *Arch Pathol* 1959;67:443–455.
9. Rona G, Boutet M, Huettner I, Peters H. Pathogenesis of isoproterenol-induced myocardial alterations: functional and morphological correlates. In: Dhalla NS, ed. *Recent advances in studies on cardiac structure and metabolism. Vol. 3. Myocardial metabolism.* Baltimore: University Park Press; 1973:507–525.
10. Fleckenstein A. Specific inhibitors and promoters of calcium action in the excitation-contraction coupling of the heart muscle and their role in the prevention or production of myocardial lesions. In: Harris P, Opie LH, eds. *Calcium and the heart.* London/New York: Academic Press; 1991:135–188.
11. Urbánek E, Vašku J, Bednařík B, Praslička M, Pospíšil M. Electrolyte changes in myocardial injury. In: Fleckenstein A, Rona G, eds. *Recent advances in studies on cardiac structure and metabolism. Vol. 6. Pathophysiology and morphology of myocardial cell alterations.* Baltimore: University Park Press; 1975:59–73.
12. Fedelešová M, Ziegelhoeffer A, Luknárová O, Kostolanský Š. Prevention by K^+, Mg^{2+}-aspartate of isoproterenol-induced metabolic changes in the myocardium. In: Fleckenstein A, Rona G, eds. *Recent advances in studies on cardiac structure and metabolism. Vol. 6. Pathophysiology and morphology of myocardial cell alterations.* Baltimore: University Park Press; 1975:43–58.
13. Fedelešová M, Ziegelhoeffer A, Luknárová O, Kostolanský Š. K^+, Mg^{2+}-aspartate (K,Mg-ASP)-mediated prevention of isoproterenol (ISO)-induced metabolic changes in the myocardium. *Arzneimittelforsch (Drug Res)* 1975;25:760–765.
14. Slezák J, Tribulová N. Morphological changes after simultaneous administration of isoproterenol (ISO) and $K^+, Mg^{2\pm}$ aspartate (K,Mg-ASP) as a physiological Ca^{2+}-antagonist. *Arzneimittelforsch (Drug Res)* 1975;25:908–923.

15. Slezák J, Tribulová N, Gabauer I, Ziegelhoeffer A, Holec V. Diminution of "reperfusion injury" in reperfused ischemic myocardium by phenothiazines. A quantitative morphological study. *Gen Physiol Biophys* 1987;6:304–312.
16. Džurba A, Ziegelhoeffer A, Breier A, Vrbjar N, Szekeres L. Increased activity of sarcolemmal (Na^+K^+)-ATPase is involved in the late cardioprotective action of 7-oxo-prostacyclin. *Cardioscience* 1991;2:105–108.
17. Fedelešová M, Ziegelhoeffer A, Luknárová O, DŽurba S, Kostolanský Š. Influence of K^+,Mg^{2+}-(D,L)-aspartate on various ATPase activities of the dog heart. *Arzneimittelforsch (Drug Res)* 1973; 23:1048–1053.
18. Lindenmayer GK, Sordahl LA, Schwartz A. Reevaluation of oxidative phosphorylation in cardiac mitochondria from normal animals and animals in heart failure. *Circ Res* 1968;23:439–449.
19. Dhalla NS, Ziegelhoeffer A, Harrow JAC. Regulatory role of membrane systems in heart function. *Can J Physiol Pharmacol* 1977;55;1211–1232.
20. Dhalla NS. Sequence of membrane defects during the development of genetic cardiomyopathy in hamsters. *J Mol Cell Cardiol* 1992;24 [Suppl II]:0–12, 44.
21. Tsuruya Y, Ikeda U, Yamamoto K, Seino Y, Oguchi A, Shimada K. Decreased Na,K-ATPase gene expression in cardiomyopathic hamster hearts. *J Mol Cell Cardiol* 1992;24 [Suppl II]:0–24,48.
22. Opie L. Is there a biochemical basis for heart failure? *J Mol Cell Cardiol* 1992;24 [Suppl I]: S04–1, 18.
23. Singal PK, Beamish RE, Dhalla NS. Potential oxidative pathways of catecholamines in the formation of lipid peroxides and genesis of heart disease. In: Spitzer GG, ed. *Myocardial injury.* New York: Plenum Publishing; 1983:391–401.
24. Huang W-H, Wang Y, Askari A. $(Na^+ + K^+)$-ATPase: inactivation and degradation induced by oxygen radicals. *Int J Biochem* 1992;24:621–625.
25. Fedelešová M, Džurba A, Ziegelhoeffer A. Effect of isoproterenol on the activity of Na^+,K^+-adenosine triphosphatase from dog hearts. *Biochem Pharmacol* 1974;23:2887–2893.
26. Fedelešová M, Džurba A, Ziegelhoeffer A. Studies on the mechanism of dog heart $(Na^+ + K^+)$-ATPase inhibition by D,L-aspartic acid and its K^+ and Mg^{2+} salts. *Biochem Pharmacol* 1975;24: 1847–1850.
27. Borgers M. Morphological assessment of tissue protection. In: Godfraind T, Vanhoutte PM, Govoni S, Paoletti R, eds. *Calcium entry blockers and tissue protection.* New York: Raven Press; 1985: 173–181.

The Cardiomyopathic Heart, edited by Makoto
Nagano, Nobuakira Takeda, and Naranjan S.
Dhalla. Raven Press, Ltd., New York © 1994.

40

Ontogenetic Differences in Isoproterenol-Induced ^{85}Sr Uptake in the Myocardium

Ivana Ošťádalová and Bohuslav Ošťádal

*Institute of Physiology, Academy of Sciences of the Czech Republic, Vídeňská 1083,
142 20 Prague 4, Czech Republic*

INTRODUCTION

Administration of large doses of the β-mimetic synthetic catecholamine isoproterenol (IPRO) to adult experimental animals produces necrotic lesions in their
myocardium (1). The administration of the same drug to chick embryos, however,
induces different nonnecrotic cardiovascular disturbances (2,3). The type of change
was shown to depend upon the time at which the β agonist was administered during
embryogenesis. Defects of the interventricular septum occurred on the second embryonic day, malformations of the large vessels were observed on the third to sixth
embryonic day, cardiomegaly was noted on the 10th to 17th embryonic day, and a
block in the development of coronary vascularization, associated with the persistence of an evolutionarily older type of blood supply (diffusion from the ventricular
cavity), occurred on the 7th to 14th embryonic day. Myocardial cellular edema was
the most prominent ultrastructural feature (4). The degree of cardiotoxicity increased from the 2nd to the 12th embryonic day, then gradually decreased; starting
from the 16th embryonic day, chick heart seemed to be resistant to the toxic effect
of IPRO (3).

According to Fleckenstein (5), the main pathogenetic mechanism of the cardiac
damage in adults is an excess of intracellular calcium, followed by depletion of
high-energy phosphates and injury to the mitochondria. The development of IPRO-
induced cardiac lesions can be quantified by the measurement of ^{45}Ca uptake into
the myocardial cells (5,6). The pathogenesis of IPRO-induced disturbances of the
embryonic heart is, however, poorly understood (7). One of the possible mechanisms could be an excess of intracellular calcium, as occurs in adult myocardium.
Strontium, as a homologous element of calcium, is interchangeable with it in the
process of the excitation-contraction coupling in the myocardium (8–10). Therefore, we were interested in whether (a) the two elements would also display similarity in their response to the administration of IPRO in rats during postnatal on-

togeny and (b) whether the intraamniotic administration of IPRO to chick embryos would increase cardiac accumulation of the homologue element of calcium (i.e., strontium). The reason for the use of strontium is its methodological advantage. ^{45}Ca is a source of β radiation, so biological samples must be modified before they can actually be measured. By contrast ^{85}Sr is measurable as a gamma emitter; therefore, samples need no modification and work with them is quicker and simpler.

EFFECT OF IPRO ON ^{85}SR ACCUMULATION IN THE MYOCARDIUM OF THE RAT DURING POSTNATAL ONTOGENY

Experiments were performed on 14-, 30-, 60- and 120-day-old male laboratory rats (Wistar strain). The experimental males were given IPRO (1 mg/kg), whereas the controls received the same volume of distilled water. Two hours later, ^{85}SrCl$_2$ was administered subcutaneously to 60- and 120-day-old control and experimental rats in a dose of 0.56 MBq (15 μCi)/kg and to all 14- and 30-day-old animals in a dose of 3.73 MBq (100 μCi)/kg (specific activity 57 MBq/mg Sr). After an additional 3 hours, the animals were decapitated. Blood and heart samples were weighed and their ^{85}Sr content was measured with an automatic gamma system (Searle Nuclear Chicago model 1185). ^{85}Sr incorporation into the tissues was expressed as a percentage of the administered dose.

In 14-day-old animals, which were resistant to the necrogenic action of IPRO, the content as well as the concentration of ^{85}Sr was not increased, whereas in 30- to 120-day-old hearts, these values were significantly increased by IPRO (Figs. 1 and 2). Similar developmental changes were noted in the heart/blood ratio (Fig. 3).

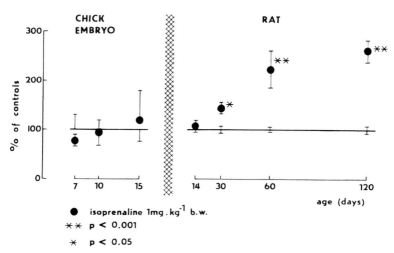

FIG. 1. Effect of isoproterenol on myocardial ^{85}Sr content in the chick embryonic heart (*left*) and rat heart (*right*). Values (means ± SEM) are expressed as a percentage of the administered dose. *b.w.*, body weight.

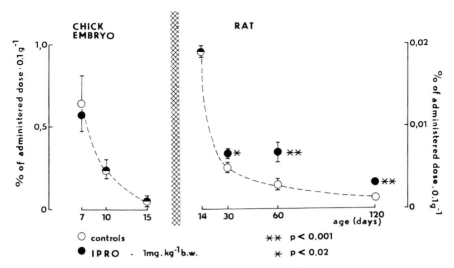

FIG. 2. Effect of isoproterenol on myocardial concentration of ^{85}Sr in the chick embryonic heart (*left*) and rat heart (*right*). Values (means ± SEM) are expressed as a percentage of the administered dose.

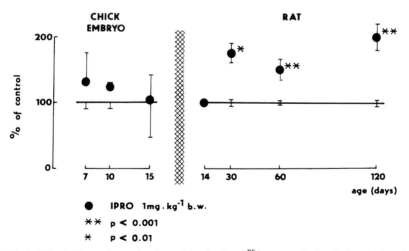

FIG. 3. Effect of isoproterenol on heart/blood ratio of ^{85}Sr concentration in the chick embryonic heart (*left*) and rat heart (*right*). Values (means ± SEM) are expressed as a percentage of controls.

The IPRO-induced increase observed in [85]Sr accumulation in the myocardium of adult rats is comparable to the repeatedly described changes in radioactive calcium uptake (6,11,12). It can be assumed that IPRO-stimulated uptake of strontium by the myocardial cells is affected by voltage-dependent calcium channels (8). This possibility is supported by the findings of Luchowski and colleagues (13), whose research showed that the transport of strontium across the membranes of smooth muscle cells can be blocked by nitrendipine, a calcium antagonist. It may be assumed that IPRO-induced stimulation of [85]Sr uptake in the rat myocardium is strictly age-dependent, and is connected with the development of necrotic lesions.

EFFECT OF IPRO ON [85]SR ACCUMULATION IN THE CHICK EMBRYONIC HEART

To determine the time course of [85]Sr uptake, 10-day-old embryos of white Leghorn chickens were used. The animals were exposed to [85]SrCl$_2$ administered in a single dose of 0.285 MBq (7.7 µCi) in 100 µL of saline (specific activity, 140 MBq/mg Sr), into the amniotic sac. At various times (1, 2, 3, and 5 hours) after the injection, the embryos were removed, freed of the yolk sac, rinsed, dried, and weighed. After decapitation, the mixed blood was collected on preweighed filter paper. The total hearts were dried and weighed.

For the study of the effect of IPRO, embryos aged 7 days, 10 days (the period of highest cardiotoxicity), and 15 days (the period of lowest cardiotoxicity) (3) were used. IPRO was administered intraamniotically to experimental animals in a single teratogenic dose (3) of 4 mg in 40 µL of saline/egg (i.e., approximately 80 mg/kg); the same volume of saline was administered intraamniotically to control embryos. All embryos were exposed simultaneously to [85]SrCl$_2$ in a single intraamniotic dose of 0.285 MBq in 100 µL of saline. Five hours after this procedure, total heart as well as blood samples were collected, as described earlier. The content of [85]Sr was measured on a Searle Nuclear Chicago 1185 automatic gamma system.

Blood and heart uptake of [85]Sr in 10-day-old embryos increased from 1 to 3 hours after intraamniotic administration of the isotope. No significant changes were observed between the intervals of 3 and 5 hours (Fig. 4). The time interval with the highest [85]Sr uptake in embryonic tissues was the same as in adult rat myocardium.

The concentration of [85]Sr in embryonic tissues decreases with increasing age of the animals (see Fig. 2); this trend was more pronounced in heart as compared with blood. Because the extracellular calcium concentration exceeds the intracellular level by more than three to four orders of magnitude, this finding may be attributable to the decrease in cardiac hydration during embryogenesis (3). In addition, the maturation of systems involved in the calcium (strontium) handling has to be taken into consideration.

As mentioned earlier, toxic doses of IPRO significantly increased the accumulation of [85]Sr in the adult rat heart. By contrast, the administration of IPRO did not influence the content and concentration of [85]Sr in the chick embryonic heart in any

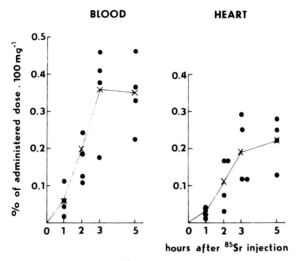

FIG. 4. ^{85}Sr concentration in blood and heart of 10-day-old chick embryos 1, 2, 3, and 5 hours after injection of ^{85}Sr. Individual values, •; means, ×.

of the investigated developmental periods (see Figs. 1 and 2). Consequently, also unchanged was the appropriate heart/blood ratio. These findings are in agreement with the finding that verapamil, a calcium antagonist, was ineffective in preventing the toxic effects of high doses of catecholamines in young chick embryonic hearts (14).

The mechanisms by which sympathomimetic amines produce cardiovascular abnormalities in the chick embryo have not yet been clarified (7). Some of them may be attributable to the hemodynamic changes induced by catecholamine stimulation of β receptors (2,14,15). It should be mentioned, however, that calcium overloading has not yet been demonstrated in the embryonic myocardium. This possibility is supported by our experiments in which ^{85}Sr was used as a calcium homologue. It seems, therefore, that not only type but also mechanisms of IPRO-induced cardiotoxicity depend on the stage of ontogenetic development (Table 1). Our conclusion is that nonnecrotic developmental changes in the chick embryonic myocardium are not necessarily the result of intracellular calcium overload.

TABLE 1. *Cardiotoxicity of isoproterenol; ontogenetic development*

Ontogenetic period	Effect of IPRO	^{85}Sr uptake
- prenatal	malformations	0
- postnatal		
suckling	0	0
weaning	0	0
adolescence	necroses	↑
adulthood	necroses	↑

SUMMARY

The aim of this study was to establish whether the administration of toxic doses of IPRO would increase accumulation of strontium—the homologue element of calcium—in the developing heart. It was shown that IPRO stimulates ^{85}Sr uptake by the rat heart beginning on the 30th day of postnatal life, and that it is connected with the development of cardiac necroses. On the other hand, IPRO did not influence ^{85}Sr uptake in the chick embryonic heart. It may be concluded that IPRO-induced cardiac abnormalities of the chick embryonic heart are not necessarily connected with calcium overload.

REFERENCES

1. Rona G. Catecholamine cardiotoxicity. *J Mol Cell Cardiol* 1985;17:291–306.
2. Hodach RJ, Hodach AE, Fallon JF, Folts JD, Bruyere HJ, Gilbert EF. The role of beta adrenergic activity in the production of cardiac and aortic arch anomalies in chick embryos. *Teratology* 1975;12:33–46.
3. Oštádal B, Rychter Z, Rychterová V. The action of isoproterenol on the chick embryo heart. *J Mol Cell Cardiol* 1976;8:533–544.
4. Dušek J, Oštádal B. Ultrastructure of isoproterenol-induced myocardial damage in chick embryos. *Physiol Bohemoslov* 1985;34:297–302.
5. Fleckenstein A. Specific inhibitors and promotors of calcium actions in the excitation-contraction coupling of heart muscle and their role in the prevention or protection of myocardial lesions. In: Harris P, Opie LH, eds. *Calcium and the heart*. London: Academic Press; 1971:135–188.
6. Mráz M, Faltová E, Šedivý J, Protivová J, Pilný J. Quantitative evaluation of the development of isoprenaline-induced heart lesions. *Physiol Bohemoslov* 1980;29:323–331.
7. Oštádal B, Beamish RE, Barwinsky J, Dhalla NS. Ontogenetic development of cardiac sensitivity to catecholamine. *J Appl Cardiol* 1989;4:467–486.
8. Kohlhardt M, Haastert BP, Krause H. Evidence of nonspecificity of the calcium channel in mammalian myocardial fibre membranes. Substitution of Ca by Sr, Ba or Mg as charge carriers. *Pfügers Arch* 1973;342:125–136.
9. Bass BG, Ciulla EM, Klop P, VanBaal S. Some electrical and mechanical effects of strontium on toad ventricular muscle: comparison to calcium. *J Physiol (Lond)* 1975;252:547–564.
10. Pang DC. Effect of inotropic agents on the calcium binding to isolated cardiac sarcolemma. *Biochim Biophys Acta* 1980;598:528–542.
11. Fleckenstein A. Myokardstoffwechsel und Nekrose. In: Heilmeyer L, and Holtmeier HJ, eds. *Herzinfarkt und Shock*. Stutgart: Georg Thieme; 1968:94–109.
12. Fleckenstein A. *Calcium antagonism in heart and smooth muscle. Experimental facts and therapeutic prospects*. New York: John Wiley and Sons; 1983.
13. Luchowski EM, Yousif F, Triggle DJ, Maurer SC, Sarmiento JG, Janis RA. Effect of metal cations and calmodulin antagonists on cardiac muscle. *J Pharm Exp Ther* 1984;230:607–613.
14. Oštádal B, Janatová T, Krause EG, Pelouch V, Dušek J. Different effect of propranolol and verapamil on isoprenaline-induced changes in the chick embryonic heart. *Physiol Bohemoslov* 1987; 36:301–311.
15. Gilbert EF, Bruyere HJ, Ishikawa S, Cheung MO, Hodach RJ. The effect of practolol and butoxamine on aortic arch malformations in beta adrenoreceptor stimulated chick embryos. *Teratology* 1977;15:317–324.

The Cardiomyopathic Heart, edited by Makoto
Nagano, Nobuakira Takeda, and Naranjan S.
Dhalla. Raven Press, Ltd., New York © 1994.

41

Primary Stress Damage to the Heart

Felix Z. Meerson

Institute of General Pathology and Pathophysiology, Baltijskaya 8.,
Moscow 125315, Russia

INTRODUCTION

Stress and ischemia, and most often their combination, play a main role in the development of major heart diseases. Nevertheless, these two factors are unequal in their place in cardiac pathology. Indeed, genetic defects in the hepatic cholesterol-eliminating systems and the excess cholesterol in food, with its associated atherogenic dyslipidemia and stenosing coronary atherosclerosis, are generally recognized as the key links in the pathogenesis of ischemic heart disease; the role of stress in heart pathology is less definite. On the one hand, an excessively strong and long stress reaction is known to provoke atherosclerosis, spasm, thrombosis, overloading of the heart, and other conditions engendering or aggravating ischemia. On the other hand, there is indeed self-contained, noncoronarogenic, nonischemia-linked, direct stress damage of the heart. What are the exact biochemical, morphologic, and physiological substrates for such damage? Can such damage to the heart evolve because of stress disorders in other organs? Finally, what is the clinical significance of such stress-related heart damage, in particular, for the pathogenesis of noncoronarogenic cardiosclerosis, arrhythmias, and sudden cardiac death?

Diagnoses such as "stress heart" or "stress arrhythmic heart disease" are absent in the accepted nosology. Yet the idea that cardiac stress damage is a reality in many patients and that it need not be associated with ischemic heart disease has been confirmed by a number of clinical studies. First, several cases have been described of stress-induced death caused by ventricular fibrillation in young individuals without coronary atherosclerosis (1,2) but with inherited resistance to stress (3). Second, a peculiar epidemic of sudden cardiac death is known to occur among humans without documented coronary atherosclerosis who experience prior stressful situations (4). Finally, as it has been recently shown by 24-hour monitoring of persons without apparent disease, a high percentage of these people suffer from arrhythmias progressing with age; these arrhythmias are as common as the stress situations in our everyday life (5). An important argument in favor of primary stress damage to the heart and its richly innervated conduction system (6,7) is the presence of persistent arrhythmias, which are often progressive with age, in persons with neurocirculatory dystonia (8,9); these dystonias are often revealed by special stress loads (10,11). On the whole, these data make it possible to discuss the following problems: (a) primary stress damage to the heart; (b) the role of ischemia-unrelated damage in the development of arrhythmias and sudden death of humans, and (c) the differences between clinical findings and therapeutic tactics of ischemic heart disease and stress arrhythmic disease.

STRESS DAMAGE TO THE HEART

Stress reaction has evolved not as an independent phenomenon but as a necessary link with another, broader vital process, adaptation of the organism to the environment (12,13). With respect to the heart, the adaptive importance of stress has been proven in special studies. It was shown that short-term stress, manifesting itself in physiologic phenomena like tachycardia or increased systolic pressure in the ventricles, was accompanied by an enhancement of contractile function and resistance to hypoxia in isolated hearts from stressed animals. On the other hand, long-term stress was accompanied by a decrease in contractile function and resistance to hypoxia of isolated hearts (14). It seems that the study by Miller and Malov (15) was one of the first experimental investigations of stress-induced myocardial injury. The stress situation was created in rats by electric footshocks through the chamber floor. Myocardial damage revealed itself by pronounced leakage of enzymes from isolated hearts of stressed animals and enhanced incorporation of technetium-labeled pyrophosphate routinely used to diagnose myocardial infarction. Upon administration of nembutal, the same "dose" of electric stimulation produced no cardiac damage. Thus, in a sufficiently long and intense stress reaction, we observed not merely an inclusion of a cardiac component into the reaction, but genuine cardiac damage, caused not by such physical factors as electricity, but by pain and impossibility to escape (i.e., by an emotional factor).

In further studying the mechanism of stress damage to the heart, we have demonstrated that its main component is strikingly increased in comparison with the normal multiple effect of stress hormones, such as catecholamines, occurring in the cardiomyocyte membrane lipid bilayer. In this process, the so-called lipid triad develops. This triad consists of the activation of lipid peroxidation (LP), lipases, and phospholipases (16), which results in a disturbed activity of lipid-dependent membrane-bound enzymes in sarcolemma and sarcoplasmic reticulum (SR).

The sarcolemmal Na, K pump is known to play a decisive role in maintaining the transmembrane cation gradient and, therefore, the physiological levels of resting potential (RP), generation and conduction of action potentials, and electric stability of the heart. We have studied the effect of emotionally painful stress (EPS) on Na,K-ATPase activity in the myocardium, as well as the possibility of preventing the observed depression of enzyme activity with β-adrenoblocker (inderal, propranolol) and antioxidant (ionol, butylated hydroxytoluene) (17). The Na, K-

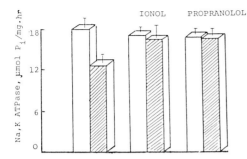

FIG. 1. Prevention of stress-induced myocardial sarcolemmal Na, K-ATPase activity with the antioxidant ionol (butylated hydroxytoluene) and the β-blocker propranolol. *Open blocks*, control; *shaded blocks*, stress.

ATPase activity in the myocardium of rats exposed to EPS was found to decrease by 28%, and this could be prevented by preliminary administration of inderal or ionol (Fig. 1). Moreover, it appeared that the Na, K-ATPase thermal inactivation proceeded much more rapidly in the myocardium of stress-exposed animals than in controls, so that the half-inactivation time was decreased by 50% (Fig. 2). The administration of ionol (50 mg/kg of body weight) prior to stress completely prevented such stress alterations accompanying Na, K-ATPase activity.

Na, K-ATPase activity is known to be localized in sarcolemma. Correspondingly, disorders of its activity are accompanied by sarcolemmal injury. The injury manifests itself first by an enhancement of enzyme leakage into perfusate from isolated hearts of stress-exposed animals (15,18). In addition, a combination of electron microscopic and histochemical techniques has revealed the penetration of lanthanum through sarcolemma into the myocardial cytoplasm of stress-exposed animals as compared to controls (19).

Considering the decisive role of Na, K-ATPase activity in maintaining the RP, we have estimated the effect of stress on the stability of this parameter in cooling and subsequent heating. In an experiment presented in Figure 3, hearts were chilled to 4°C by perfusing them with a cool solution for 1.5 hours; the RP subsequently declined. The temperature of the perfusing solution was then returned to 36°C and the dynamic of RP restoration was monitored. In the control group (curve 1) the

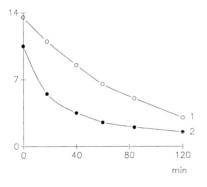

FIG. 2. Heat inactivation of rat cardiac sarcolemmal Na,K-ATPase activity. Enzyme activity at 52°C in controls (*1*) and following emotionally painful stress (2). The abscissa represents time expressed in minutes; the ordinate represents activity (μmol/hr/mg of protein.

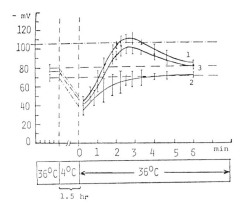

FIG. 3. Effect of cooling and subsequent warming of isolated rat heart on the rest potential (RP) in left ventricular cardiomyocytes. The abscissa represents time before and after cooling (expressed in minutes); the ordinate is the RP expressed in millivolts. *1,* controls; *2,* with stress; *3,* with ionol plus stress.

cooling decreased the RP from -80 to -45 mV. A subsequent rise from 4°C to 36°C resulted in restoration and "overshooting" of the RP to a maximum of -100 ± 5 mV within 2 to 2.5 min. The restoration rate at the point of maximum hyperpolarization was about 0.7 mV/s. In animals subjected to EPS (curve 2), the RP was initially diminished by 10 mV. Upon cooling, it fell to -35 ± 2 mV; in the course of RP restoration, there was no hyperpolarization and the maximum restoration rate did not exceed 0.7 mV/s, (i.e., approximately one third of that in controls.) Thus, even a single 6-hour stress reduces Na,K-ATPase activity, which reduction is accompanied by a profound disturbance in cardiomyocyte capacity for preventing a decrease in an important parameter such as RP, designed to maintain the heart's electrical stability [20].

The other important mechanism providing the rhythmic activity and electric stability of the heart is the SR Ca pump, the function of which is disordered by stress as well. We have studied SR elements isolated from the myocardium 2 hours following 6 hours of EPS [21]. Calcium uptake in the presence of oxalate was monitored by radioactive ^{45}Ca. ATPase activities were measured pH-metrically by the rate of acidification of the medium secondary to ATPase hydrolysis. It appeared that, with EPS, Ca-ATPase activity decreased by almost 30%, whereas the Mg-ATPase level was not affected. The rate of Ca^{2+} accumulation in the presence of oxalate declined by 38%. This significantly attenuated performance of the SR Ca pump appears to be attributable not only to the lowered activity of the calcium transporting enzyme, but also to increased calcium permeability of damaged SR membranes.

It is essential that stress damage to the SR Ca pump be accompanied by an increase in cardiomyocyte Ca pump activity, as proven both by combined histochemical and electron microscopic techniques [14,19] and by the increase in myocardial ^{45}Ca [21]. These disturbances of Ca^{2+} homeostasis have broad negative consequences for myocardial contractile function and electrical stability. For instance, it has been shown that isolated hearts from stress-exposed animals respond to an increase in external Ca^{2+} by a much greater enhancement of stroke volume and to a decrease in external Ca^{2+} by a much greater decline in stroke volume than do hearts from control animals (22). In other words, the dependence of stress-damaged hearts on external Ca^{2+} increases owing to a disturbance in calcium homeostasis (usually maintained by the Ca pump). Atrial myocardium and papillary muscle from such hearts require greater force to be stretched to an optimal length; this phenomenon has been named "stress rigidity of the myocardium" (23). It has been shown that stress potentiates the development of contracture and fibrillation in isolated hearts exposed to high Ca^{2+} concentrations (24). It also appears that stress triggers arrhythmias that develop after the termination of high-frequency stimulation of papillary muscle and in the presence of isoproterenol in the incubation medium (25). Disorders in SR Ca pump function play an important role in the mechanism of such arrhythmias. This trigger mechanism was shown to be involved in many cases of arrhythmia in cardiac hypertrophy (26) and acute myocardial infarction (27).

These injuries of the lipid-dependent membrane Ca and Na,K pumps present an important prerequisite for disturbances of cardiac electrical stability induced by stress in vivo. In our experiments (14), cardiac electrical stability was estimated in rats exposed to 10-hour immobilization stress by measuring the heart fibrillation threshold and the resistance of sinus node automatism upon the inhibitory vagus action. The curves in Figure 4 show that, 2 hours after the end of the stress exposure, the fibrillation threshold fell twofold and remained decreased for at least the next 2 days. The same figure shows that stress substantially enhanced sensitivity of the sinus pacemaker to the negatively chronotropic vagal influence simultaneously. This shift manifested itself by a more pronounced vagal bradycardia than in controls, and remained significant 12 and 24 hours after stress, after which time it regressed. The finding of decreased sinus node resistance to the inhibitory vagal influence is in accord with electron microscopic data that shows that the sinus node is the most vulnerable part of the cardiac conduction system during periods of lengthy stress. The most intense penetration of lanthanum and the most pronounced decrease in the number of mitochondrial crista are observed just in specific cells of

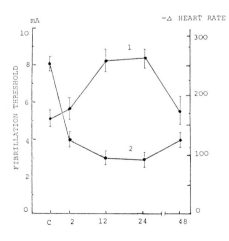

FIG. 4. Dynamics of the fibrillation threshold and the negative chronotropic vagal effect on the heart after stress. The abscissa represents time after the end of stress; *C* denotes the control values. **1, right ordinate**: Reduced heart rate upon vagal stimulation. **2, left ordinate**: Fibrillation threshold expressed in milliamperes.

sinus node (14). It is obvious that the decreased fibrillation threshold induced by the ectopic stimulation of the heart apex, combined with a simultaneous decrease in the resistance of the sinus node to the inhibitory vagal influence, enhances the probability of heterotopic automatism, which cannot be suppressed in a timely manner by the sinus node. In other words, this combination is arrhythmogenic.

On the whole, this complex of alterations—decreased activity of Na,K-ATPase and RP, reduced activity of the SR Ca pump, diminished resistance to adrenergic triggered arrhythmias (25), and, finally, decreased electrical threshold of cardiac fibrillation with a simultaneous decrease in the resistance of automatism of damaged sinus nodes—signifies that, in so-called "stress heart," the damage of membranes and membrane-bound pumps greatly enhances the risk of arrhythmias. This risk increases even more in response to stress-induced disorders of energy systems and focal lesions of the myocardium. The disorders of myocardial energy systems were studied in the conditions of a whole working heart instantly frozen according to the Wollenberger method. These disorders manifested themselves in a decrease in glycogen concentration by one third and in an approximately similar decrease in creatine phosphate (CP) concentration and creatine phosphokinase (CPK) activity, whereas the content of adenosine triphosphate (ATP) and other adenine nucleotides remained at normal levels (28). These shifts, then, can contribute to disturbances of cation pump functioning, as their energy supply is provided by creatine kinase and glycolytic systems to a considerable extent (29,30).

Stress-induced damage of myocardial structures, as revealed by a combination of light and polarization microscopy, has a microfocal character. The damage is manifested in the development of contracture with the merging of the A disks of myofibrils forming anisotropic conglomerates. These hypercalcium contractual alterations undergo regression. Alternatively, they may be subjected to necrobiosis with the formation of cell infiltrates around necrotic muscle fibers which subsequently transform to small foci of poststress noncoronary cardiosclerosis. Such foci increase the physiologic heterogeneity of the myocardium (13). Taking into account the preferential damage to the conducting system that possesses the richest adrenergic innervation (6), one may assume that poststress foci of cardiosclerosis can contribute to the development of phenomena such as partial blockade and ectopic foci of excitation. On the whole, these complex alterations form the basis for the notion of "stress heart," and provide evidence that such a heart is prone to arrhythmias with a high extent of probability.

Indeed, in next stress attack to the heart, when already existing and newly formed microfocal lesions become sources of ectopic impulses (for instance, by the mechanism of triggered arrhythmias associated with the disturbed SR Ca^{2+} transport), these impulses retrogradely propagating may cause extrasystoles. Because ectopic loci of such excitation can be numerous, and because the excitation wave passes zones of decelerated conduction induced by decreased RP, the extrasystoles can also become multiple. By this process, they cannot be suppressed by the sinus pacemaker, not only because of its relative weakness, but also because reduced Na, K-pump activity in peripheral regions of the conducting system is unable to keep up with the normal heart phenomenon called "overdrive suppression." In the presence of this phenomenon, a high frequency of stimulation makes the Na, K-pump increase the sodium extrusion much more than the potassium entry, and thereby restores the necessary degree of polarization or even hyperpolarizes the membranes, preventing the generation of ectopic impulses (31). In principle, the diversity of ectopic focus localization, along with partial blockades, may result not only in arrhythmias, but also in cardiac fibrillation. We have seen that the electrical threshold of fibrillation was reduced after stress.

In order to estimate the actual significance of stress-induced disorders of cardiac electrical stability for cardiologic clinic, one should keep in mind at least three statements. The first one is that, in a severe stressful situation, the β-adrenergic effect of catecholamines is the main arrhythmogenic factor inducing the damage to cardiomyocyte membranes. This effect can occur against the background of increased coronary blood flow, and accordingly, is in no way related to ischemic damage to the heart. The data in Table 1 show that the β-adrenoblocker administered prior to the 6-hour period of immobilization stress prevented the stress-induced decline in the electrical fibrillation threshold, whereas the α-blocker lacked such an effect. Similarly it was shown that practically all of the disorders involving cation pump activity (just described), energetics, and cardiac structure were prevented with β-adrenoblockers (14). Thus, the disorders of cardiac electrical stability that occur after stress are essentially a β-adrenergic injury. In recent years, the studies of whole organism's response to behavioral stress situations are in accord with this premise.

Verrier and Lown (32) studied changes in cardiac susceptibility to fibrillation, and in doing so tried to assess the mechanism through which the adrenergic action on the heart affects cardiac electrical stability. It was found that various stress conditions, such as those evoked by pain, fear, or rage caused by taking away food, significantly enhanced the myocardial blood flow. That is, in the healthy animal, behavioral stress elicits not ischemia, but hyperemia of the myocardium, with a simultaneous reduction in the heart fibrillation threshold. Similar data have been

TABLE 1. *Effect of α- and β-adrenoblockers on the cardiac fibrillation threshold in control animals and in animals subjected to stress*

Conditions	Fibrillation threshold (mA)[a]
Control (n = 12)	6.5 ± 6.3
Propranolol (β-blocker) (n = 10)	11.0 ± 1.50[b]
Prazosin (α-blocker) (n = 10)	6.1 ± 0.54
Stress (n = 10)	2.9 ± 0.26[b]
Propranolol + stress (n = 17)[c]	6.6 ± 0.44
Prazosin + stress (n = 17)[c]	3.1 ± 0.40[b]

[a]The threshold was determined 1 hour after the end of a 6-hour period of immobilization stress.
[b]$p < 0.05$ as compared to controls.
[c]The adrenoblockers were administered at a dose of 1 mg/kg of body weight 30 minutes before stress.

obtained by Vatner and Hintze (33) in continuous measurement of coronary blood flow in monkeys.

When evaluating from this viewpoint the new data on adrenergic damage to the myocardium that is unassociated with ischemia, it should be emphasized that β-adrenergic damage to the heart unassociated with ischemia was discovered and described in detail more than 30 years ago in the excellent studies of Rona and associates (34). These researchers were the first to find that large doses of a synthetic norepinephrine analog, β-agonist isoproterenol, act through the adenylate cyclase of the heart, adipose tissue, and other organs to cause enhanced Ca^{2+} entry into myocardial cells; this, together with an excess of fatty acids, was found to uncouple oxidative phosphorylation in mitochondria and to decrease the cell content of ATP and CP. Simultaneously, excess calcium induces myofibrillar contracture. These mostly microfocal lesions develop at the background of cardiac hypertrophy. At moderate doses of the agonist they may not impair the contractile function, whereas at large doses, they depress it. The outcome, if not lethal, is focal necrobiotic damage to the myocardium with ensuing focal cardiosclerosis. Thus, both new and earlier data provide evidence that β-adrenergic nonischemic damage to the myocardium caused by catecholamines, taking place both in the whole organism and in the isolated heart, is associated with marked impairment of cardiac electrical stability, and is probably involved in the development of arrhythmias.

An important feature of stress damage to the heart is that the consequences of such damage are reversible to a high degree; this is seen, for instance, in the dynamics of restoration of the decreased fibrillation threshold (Fig. 4). Moreover, stress damage may not manifest itself under the action of many sufficiently serious stressful situations on the organism. This optional nature and reversibility of stress damage are attributable, first of all, to the fact that in the process of organism development, a stress-realizing hypophysial-adrenal system is formed not separately but simultaneously with a whole complex of central and local stress-limiting systems. Excitation of stress-limiting systems is coupled with stress reaction to block the latter, limiting its intensity and duration and thereby restricting stress damage. The schema in Figure 5 shows that central stress-limiting systems include GABAergic, opioidergic, serotoninergic, dopaminergic, and other systems, and that local stress-limiting systems include the adenosinergic, prostaglandin (PG) and antioxidant system, as well as others. The role of stress-limiting systems in the protection of the organism is substantiated by at least three facts. First, adaptation to repeated short-term stress results in activation of stress-limiting systems and accumulation of their metabolites (35–42). Another argument in favor of the important role of stress-limiting systems is that adaptation to stress prevents stress injuries: namely, stress-induced anorexia (43), oncogenic effects of stress (44), stress damage to the heart (45), disorders of cardiac contractile function (46), and cardiac electrical stability (47) in experimental myocardial infarction and acute ischemia. Finally, an important factor substantiating the role of stress-limiting systems is that most of the protective effects of adaptation may be reproduced with metabolites of stress-limiting systems or their synthetic analogs. For instance, cardiac arrhythmias induced by

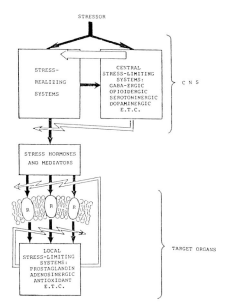

FIG. 5. Central and local stress-limiting systems.

acute ischemia and reperfusion can be abolished or reduced with GABA (48), benzodiazepine receptor activator phenazepam [(17-bromide-5-chlorophenyl)-2, 3-dihydro-H-1,4-benzodiazepine-2-OH] (49), and β-endorphine synthetic analog dalargin (D-Ala^2-Leu^5-Arg^6-enkephalin) (49), antioxidant ionol (50), and hydroxypyridine (51). In other words, the protective effects of stress-limiting systems are sufficiently reproducible with metabolites of stress-limiting systems or their synthetic analogs.

With respect to cardiology, the concept of stress-limiting systems means that in equal stress action, humans with genetically determined potent stress-limiting systems do not respond with cardiac stress damage and arrhythmias, whereas humans with inferior stress-limiting systems develop such disorders.

THE ROLE OF CARDIAC STRESS DAMAGE IN THE DEVELOPMENT OF ARRHYTHMIAS IN HUMANS

Because any normal person experiences multiple, more or less serious stress episodes, we could see that stress induces disturbances of cardiac electrical stability. A reasonable conclusion is that stress and adrenergic effects on the heart may often entail transient and, therefore, nonhazardous arrhythmias. Indeed, this suggestion is favored by the now commonly known fact that, with continuous monitoring, various disturbances of cardiac rhythm and conduction are found no less frequently than the inevitable stress situations of everyday life (5,50–57).

The well known fact that some situations of life can provoke arrhythmias in practically healthy persons who are highly tolerant to physical load is in line with the idea that many arrhythmias may be of stress origin. This premise is supported by, among other things, the very existence of a peculiar disease that had been often called cardiac neurosis (58), a cardiac form of neurocirculatory dystonia (8,9). In recent years, this has been referred to in both the Russian and English literature as idiopathic arrhythmia—that is, an arrhythmia whose cause is unknown (59,60). Of course, this term can cover arrhythmias of toxicoinfectious origin or those resulting from congenital defects.

First, many patients with such "idiopathic" arrhythmias exhibit a pronounced neurotization in the form of hypochondriac, anxiety depressive, cardiophobic, and less frequently, hysteric syndromes, of varying degrees of severity; the extent of the arrhythmia is often proportionate to the severity of the neurotic syndrome, and may disappear as the syndrome is eliminated by successful pharmacotherapy. Second, along with the complete absence of myocardial ischemia and a rather high tolerance to physical loads in such arrhythmias, there often are defects in specific stress-limiting systems. Thus it has been shown (8) that, in 10 patients with neurocirculatory dystonia who had attacks of paroxysmal supraventricular tachycardia, a GABA derivative, phenibut (acting like the known GABA-receptor agonist baclophen), decreased the number of attacks by a factor of 5.5 and prolonged the fitness period to 6 months. In half of 32 patients with ventricular extrasystoles, this activator of the GABAergic system completely abolished or decreased the number of extra-systoles by 75% or more. The antiarrhythmic effect of the drug was accompanied by a positive psychotropic effect. It is known that the GABAergic system can be activated via the benzodiazepine receptors; accordingly, benzodiazepine receptor agonists have also been successfully used as antiarrhythmics. The abolishment of arrhythmias by activation of an important stress-limiting system is an indication of the considerable role of stress in the development of these arrhythmias.

The studies of Smetnev and colleagues (59) demonstrate the involvement of defects in the PG system in arrhythmogenesis. In patients with idiopathic paroxysmal supraventricular rhythm disorders, the attacks of tachycardia develop with enhanced coronary blood flow (i.e., without ischemic manifestations). In patients with ischemic heart disease, similar attacks are not accompanied by adequately enhanced coronary blood flow, and this is why they may in some cases lead to cornonary insufficiency. Further studies have shown that persistence of idiopathic non-ischemic arrhythmias and increasing frequency of supraventricular arrhythmia paroxysms are attended by progressive impairment of the regulatory systems of PG and cyclic nucleotides: decreasing $PGE/PGF_{2\alpha}$ ratio in coronary sinus blood, increasing thromboxan A/PGI_2 ratio, and decreasing cyclic adenosine monophosphate (cAMP)/cyclic guanosine monophosphate (cGMP) in the blood flowing to the heart. Thus, a preexisting or evolving deficiency of the systems limiting the adrenergic effects on the heart may play a substantial role in the development of arrhythmias having no organic basis in the heart, and this can be taken as evidence for the stress origin of such arrhythmias.

The third argument in favor of idiopathic arrhythmias caused by stress is that myocardial needle biopsy in such patients often reveals focal alterations and fibrosis similar to those described in experimental stress damage to animal hearts. Recently, investigators studied 44 patients without ischemic disease or cardiac failure but with complaints of palpitation, heart pains, and faints in whom ventricular arrhythmias or conduction defects were demonstrated. Myocardial biopsy performed on 13 of these patients demonstrated hypertrophy of muscle fibers and focal interstitial fibrosis of both ventricles in 7, and of only the left ventricle in 5. Finally, weighty evidence for the role of stress in idiopathic arrhythmias has been obtained through the clinical use of special psychoemotional or stress loads (SLs). Such techniques have been rather popular in recent years (11). For instance, the inducibility of arrhythmias with SL has been compared in patients with ischemic heart disease and those with neurocirculatory dystonia or idiopathic arrhythmias and pronounced neurasthenic syndrome. According to Rizhinashivili et al. (10), among the whole contingent of cardiology patients with possible cardiac rhythm disorders, the SL test elicited arrhythmias in 18% of cases, whereas in patients with idiopathic arrhythmias and anxiety depressive syndrome, arrhythmias were reported in 42% to 46%. These arrhythmias could be abolished with a benzodiazepine receptor agonist, seduxen, which is known to activate the brain's stress-limiting GABAergic system. Thus, even such moderate, standard clinical stress tests can evoke arrhythmias in a large proportion of people with certain disturbances of cardiac neural regulation.

Together with Khalfen and Lyamina, we compared the adrenergic and cardiac responses to physical loads and SLs in 98 healthy male subjects (mean age of 35) and in 48 male patients of the same age with neurocirculatory dystonia. The latter patients responded to the SL with a 90% increase in noradrenaline excretion in urine (i.e., almost four times as high as that reported in controls.) Atrial or ventricular arrhythmias developed in 25% of cases. The physical load induced arrhythmias with much less frequency, and none of these persons showed electrocardiographic (ECG) alterations characteristic of myocardial ischemia. Thus, the stress action on patients with neurocirculatory dystonia resulted in increased activation of the adrenergic system and, simultaneously, in arrhythmias of nonischemic origin.

Evidence of the existence of arrhythmic stress disease can be obtained from the reports of sudden death in infants and young men without documented coronary atherosclerosis. Such events are often observed in families with a hereditary intolerance to stress. Thus, Green and colleagues (3) reported sudden death in three generations, including a 14-year-old girl who died after being told that her 15-year-old brother had died immediately after a running competition. In a family studied by McRae et al. (61), one son suddenly died at the age of 17 years after being frightened by a friend, another died at the age of 12 years while swimming, and the third also died at the age of 12 years when startled by a spider. Their mother had a history of about 25 syncopal episodes that occurred between the ages of 15 and 25 years, each of which had been preceded by emotional stress causing fear and anger. Her fourth son initially showed no symptoms, but at 11 years of age, was found to have a shortened PR interval and a pronounced U wave. His first syncopal episode occurred at the age of 12.5 years when he got angry during a game of baseball. In the clinic, no rhythm disorders were observed when the patient was left alone and quiet. However, any diagnostic procedure from venipuncture to the administration of anesthesia and catheterization caused great anxiety, resulting in sinus tachycardia, multifocal ventricular extrasystoles, and sometimes, ventricular fibrillation.

In all these cases, cardiac deaths were predetermined by the genetically attenuated resistance of these individuals to stress, likely a result of inferior stress-limiting systems. There have also been other cases reported in which sudden cardiac death resulted from ventricular fibrillation in the absence of documented coronary disease but under the direct action of a stress episode (1,62–65). On the whole, such cases unambiguously prove only the basic possibility of primary stress fibrillation and sudden death, but they provide no clue as to their incidence. Of special interest, therefore, are descriptions of thoroughly examined patients in whom cardiac fibrillation and clinical death with subsequent resuscitation were not attended by any alterations in the coronary arteries.

Cebelin and Hirsh (66) conducted a comparative pathomorphologic examination of 15 persons who had died of sudden cardiac death immediately in response to heavy stress, 15 who had been killed in traffic accidents, and 15 who had died of stenosing coronary artery atherosclerosis. The fatal stress situations included conflicts with parents or neighbors and homicidal assaults. Pathoanatomic examination of these patients revealed groups of cardiomyocytes with contractural injuries and dispersion of myofibrils, as well as interstitial connective tissue that had homogeneous regions alternating with zones of granulation. Such microfocal alterations bear much resemblance to those demonstrated in the myocardium by the author's group in response to EPS or by Rona et al. (34) upon administration of isoproterenol. The authors of the study under consideration (66) justly attributed these lesions to the action of catecholamines and calcium. As already stated, these alterations substantially increase the heterogeneity of the myocardium and may give rise to ectopic loci of recurrent excitation—that is, they may seriously disturb cardiac electrical stability. In essence, these data provide evidence that, in a certain proportion of patients, at the moment of sudden death, the heart had no irreversible organic alterations that could be regarded as the cause of the ischemia disturbing myocardial performance.

Two more groups of similar patients have recently been described in different clinics (67,68). Peculiar "epidemics" of sudden cardiac death were reported among young people without coronary atherosclerosis, such as among Malay and Cambodian immigrants in the United States (4). The overwhelming majority of those who suddenly died had no minimal coronary sclerosis, but differed from others of the same nationality in their relatively poorer prospects of social adaptation (i.e., an element of desolation). These people usually died at night, practically instantly, as apparently healthy young Japanese male patients have been known to die of well-known Pokkuri disease, which has now been shown to result from ventricular fibrillation (69).

In the aggregate, the abovementioned clinical situations (i.e., apparently healthy persons with arrhythmias demonstrated by continuous ECG monitoring, patients with neurocirculatory dystonia, and patients in whom sudden cardiac death occurred in clear absence of coronary atherosclerosis) seem to outline the dynamics of a certain progressive stress disease of the heart. The main factor in its pathogenesis is not an ischemic, coronarogenic cardiac injury, but direct adrenergic damage to the conduction system and contractile myocardium. In evaluating the possible causes for such a disease, one should keep in mind that patients with reduced resistance to stress diseases—that is, those with inferior stress-limiting systems—as well as all other humans, experience numerous stress situations during their lives. Stress damage, which develops every time in this process, may accumulate, resulting in rather voluminous stress lesions of the myocardium and particularly of the conduction system with the most dense adrenergic and cholinergic innervation (6,7).

Of considerable interest in this respect are the results of autopsies performed from 1963 until 1981 on 200 patients with electrocardiographically documented complete atrioventricular (AV) block. The data from this study, summarized by Davies and associates (62), indicate that ischemic disease could be regarded as the cause of impaired conduction in only 17% of the patients with AV block. Even disregarding calcification of the node, congenital cardiomyopathy, and other causes, there were still 38% of the cases in which the underlying process was of unknown etiology (i.e., idiopathic bilateral His bundle-branch fibrosis). Thus, the possible role of adrenergic stress injury in the development of a chronic process leading to this rather frequent finding deserves special study. Another morphologic phenomenon often observed in autopsies of patients dying of sudden cardiac failure—pronounced myocardial hypertrophy—may also be caused by prolonged action of high concentrations of catecholamine (70); along with focal cardiosclerosis, this high catecholamine concentration may be a plausible factor impairing cardiac electrical stability.

COMPARISON OF ISCHEMIC AND STRESS-RELATED DAMAGE TO THE HEART

From the foregoing discussion, it is evident that stress, involving high catecholamine concentrations acting on β-adrenoceptors, damages the myocardial cell membranes, disorders the work of cation pumps, and can result in profound disturbances of cardiac electrical stability directly, without associated ischemia. Accumulating in the course of individual life inevitably repeated stresses, the disorders of cardiac metabolism and structure at the background of stress-limiting system insufficiency, may underlie chronic progressive arrhythmias, as peculiar heart disease. This phenomenon is profoundly different in etiology, pathogenesis, and clinical manifestations from what is usually implied by the term ischemic disease. Indeed, stenosing coronary sclerosis causing myocardial ischemia is now well known to be itself the sequel of genetic defects in or alimentary overloading of the hepatic mechanisms for metabolic elimination of cholesterol. This idea has been supported by the studies of Anichkov (71) on experimental alimentary atherosclerosis and by the works of Brown and Goldstein (72), who reported on a hepatic system of receptors removing low-density lipoproteins from the blood, and convincingly proven by dietary and other measures for preventing coronary disease. As to stress damage to the heart, it is a result of exceedingly long and strong stress reactions. As experiments on animals have shown, it can be more or less completely prevented by adaptation to short-term stress exposures which activate the modulatory stress-limiting systems of the organism (see Fig. 5). Notably, it is the genetic or acquired deficiency of these central and local systems of protection from stress, and not secondary ischemia caused by stress spasm and thrombosis, that is, in many cases, the basis for stress-related arrhythmias, blocks, and cardiopathies.

The set of distinctions between ischemic heart disease and stress-induced arrhythmic heart disease listed in Table 2 support this working hypothesis. The main justification of this concept is not the etiology and the pathogenesis of these two conditions, but also the fact that their prognosis, prophylaxis, and treatment differ in many aspects of clinical importance. When differentiating the etiology, pathogenesis, and clinical finding of these two processes, we should at the same time keep in mind their pronounced mutual potentiation, for which three basic mechanisms can be discerned.

First, stress, by exerting direct noncoronarogenic damage to the conduction system and contractile myocardium, can give rise to multiple zones of depolarization and conduction defects. This stress-induced enhancement of the electric hetero-

TABLE 2. *Differentiation between ischemic heart disease and stress-induced arrhythmic heart disease*

	Ischemic heart disease	Stress-induced arrhythmic heart disease
Etiology	Defects in cholesterol-eliminating systems	Defects in stress-limiting systems
Key pathogenetic link	Stenosing coronary sclerosis leading to myocardial ischemia	Excessive stress reaction leading to stress damage to the heart
Ischemic response to physical load	Marked "ischemic" ECG changes and cardiac pains	Absent
Arrhythmic response to physical load	Rare at peak load	Absent, or occurs after load
Ischemic response to stress load	Occurs in about one third of cases	Absent
Arrhythmic response to stress load	Rarely occurs (about 10% of cases)	Frequent
Arrhythmias at rest	Secondary, ischemia-linked; can be abolished with vasodilators	Primary; without ischemia; vasodilators are poorly effective
Myocardial infarcts	Vast; early	Microfocal; late
Treatment with sedatives, neuroleptics, tranquilizers, or adrenoblockers	Partially effective, restricts secondary stress reaction to ischemia	Quite effective; restricts primary stress reaction
Prophylaxis by adaptation to hypoxia, physical load, etc.	Partially effective	Quite effective

geneity of the heart is aggravated by interruption of intercellular contacts by excess calcium and adds to the depolarization blocks caused by ischemia. As a result, cardiac electrical stability, which we have observed to be only relative even in apparently healthy people, turns out to be deeply impaired and brings on serious arrhythmias, fibrillation, and cardiac arrest. The second and more conventional mechanism is that, under certain conditions, stress can lead to further development of coronary sclerosis, coronary spasm, and coronary thrombosis, thereby worsening the ischemia and leading to acute myocardial infarction which, in turn, is complicated by arrhythmias and cardiac fibrillation. The third mechanism is that the ischemic focus or infarct causes pain and fear, giving rise to a stress reaction which, as we have seen, damages the nonischemic myocardial regions, increases the load on the heart, and may directly aggravate ischemia.

The major issue relating to these three mechanisms is that prevention, restriction, or abolishment of a stress "attack" on the heart can be highly effective in protecting the heart not only from arrhythmias, but also from ischemia that is induced or aggravated by stress. The hypotheses relating to the relationship between stress and ischemic damage do not withdraw the question of real differences between stress heart disease and ischemic heart disease. At the same time, they show that, by protecting the organism from stress-induced arrhythmic disease (by methods that differ from those used for ischemic heart disease), we can simultaneously prevent the stress factor from influencing the pathogenesis of ischemic heart disease.

SUMMARY

Stress-induced electrical instability has been shown to occur as a result of impaired function of the sarcolemmal Na-K pump, as well as the sarcoplasmic reticular Ca pump mechanisms. The actions of stress are mediated by hormones, such as catecholamines, which affect both cardiomyocytes and conducting systems. The central stress-limiting systems have been suggested to involve gamma-aminobutyric acid (GABA), opioids, serotonins, and dopamines, whereas the local stress-limiting systems are considered to include prostaglandins, adenosines, and antioxidants. The stress-induced damage is prevented by antioxidants and β-adrenergic receptor blockers and is known to differ from ischemia-induced alterations. However, under certain conditions, stress can develop coronary sclerosis, coronary spasm, and coronary thrombosis, and thus may enhance the effects of ischemia for the development of myocardial infarction.

REFERENCES

1. Lown B. Sudden cardiac death: biobehavioral perspective. *Circulation* 1987;76 (Suppl, Pt 1): 186.
2. Rozenberg VD, Nepomnyaschikh LM. *Coronarography in pathological morphology.* Novosibirski: 1987 (Russian).
3. Green JR, Korovetz MJ, Shanklin DR, De Vito JJ, Taylor WJ. Sudden unexpected death in three generations. *Arch Intern Med* 1969;124:359.

4. Baron R, Kirscher R. Sudden night-time death among South East Asians. *Lancet* 1983;1:764.
5. Bjerregaard P. Prevalence of cardiac arrhythmias in healthy subjects. In: Chumberlain DA, Kulbertus H, eds. *Cardiac arrhythmias in active population.* Sweden: MoIndad; 1980;24.
6. Kubler W. The conduction and cardiac sympathetic system. *J Am Coll Cardiol* 1985;5(Suppl 6):157B.
7. Bailey JC, Kovach RJ, Rardon DP. Anatomical, biochemical and electrophysiological evidence for parasympathetic innervation of the ventricle. In: Reiser HJ, Horowitz LN, eds. *Mechanisms and treatment of cardiac arrhythmias.* Baltimore, MD: 1985:57.
8. Skibitzky VV. Effect of phenibut and eglonil on the frequency of paroxysms of tachoarrhythmia and cebtra hemodynamics in patients with neurocirculatory dystonia. *Vrach Delo* 1983;8:22 (Russian).
9. Berezin FB, Miroshnikov MN, Rozhanets RV. *The methods of many-sided examination of the personality in clinical medicine and psychohygiene.* Moscow: Nauka, 1976 (Russian).
10. Rizhinashvili ZA, Golitzyn SP, Khramelashvili VV, Smetnev AS. Use of psychoemotional test in patients with different cardiovascular disease. *Kardiologiia* 1981;6:66 (Russian).
11. Lowler KA. Cardiovascular and electrodermal response pattern in heart rate reactive individuals deriving psychological stress. *Psychophysiology* 1980;17:467.
12. Selye H. *The story of the adaptation syndrome.* Montreal: Acta, Inc. Medical Publishers; 1952.
13. Meerson FZ. *Adaptation, stress and prophylaxis.* Berlin: Springer Verlag, 1984.
14. Meerson FZ. *Adaptive protection of the heart: protecting against stress and ischemic damage.* Boca Raton, FL: CRC Press;1991.
15. Miller DG, Malov S. Quantitative determination of stress-induced myocardial damage in rats. *Pharmacol Biochem Behav* 1977;7:139.
16. Meerson FZ, Didenko VV, Belkina LM, Manukhina EB. Lipid peroxidation and antioxidant protection of the heart in stress, ischemia, and arrhythmias. In: Chow ChK, ed. *Cellular antioxidant defense mechanisms,* Vol. 5. Boca Raton, FL: CRC Press;1988:215.
17. Meerson FZ, Medvedev LN, Golubeva LYu, Ustinova EE. Effect of emotional pain stress in the Na, K ATPase activity in the cardiac muscle. *Biull Eksper Biol Med* 1982; No. 8: 61 (Russian).
18. Ustinova EE. Effects of long-term and short-term stress actions on the heart resistance to anoxia. *Biull Eksp Biol Med* 1983;1:21 (Russian).
19. Meerson FZ, Samosudova NV, Glagoleva EV, Shimkovich MV, Belkina LM. Disturbance of myocardial contractile function and ultrastructure of cardiomyocytes after emotional stress. *Arkh Anat Gistol Embriol* 1983;2:43 (Russian).
20. Sudakov KV, Yumatov EA, Ul'yaninsky LS. Systemic mechanisms of emotional stress. In: Furduj FI, Khaidarliu SKh, Shtirtu EI, Nadvodnyuk AI, Mamalyga LM, eds. *Stress development mechanisms.* Kishinev: Shtiintza;1987:52 (Russian).
21. Meerson FZ, Arkhipenko YuV, Rozhitskaya II, Kagan VE. Damage to the sarcoplasmic reticulum Ca-transporting system in emotional pain stress. *Kardiologiia* 1981;4:60 (Russian).
22. Meerson FZ, Shimkovich MV, Khorunzhij VA. Effect of emotional painful stress on heart muscle reactivity to changes in calcium concentration. *Biull Eksp Biol Med* 1980;9:281 (Russian).
23. Meerson FZ. *Pathogenesis and prevention of stress-induced and ischemic damages of the heart.* Moscow: Meditzina,1984 (Russian).
24. Meerson FZ, Abdikaliev NA, Kalvinsh IYA. Antiarrhythmic effect of EDIHYP, a synthetic analogue of acetylcholine and its bioelectric mechanism. In: *Program and Abstracts of the 8th Meeting of the International Society for Heart Research.* Niigata City, Japan: 1990; S45.
25. Meerson FZ, Vovk VI. Effect of adaptation to stress and to intermittent hypoxia on triggering activity of papillary muscle cardiomyocytes of the rat heart. *Biull Eksp Biol Med* 1991;112(11):456 (Russian).
26. Aronson RS. Afterpotentials and triggered activity in hypertrophied myocardium from tars with renal hypertension. *Circ Res* 1981;48:720.
27. El-Sherif W, Gough WB, Zeiler RH, Mehra R. Triggered ventricular rhythms in 1-day-old myocardial infarction in the dog. *Circ Res* 1983;52:566.
28. Golubeva LYU, Meerson FZ. Decreased activity of creatine phosphokinase in heart muscle during stress. *Kardiologiia* 1986;9:108 (Russian).
29. Jacobus WE. Respiratory control and integration of heat high-energy phosphate metabolism by mitochondrial creatine kinase. *Annu Rev Physiol* 1985;47:707.
30. Saks VA, Rosenshtraukh LV, Chazov EI, Smirnov VN. Role of creatine phosphokinase in cellular function and metabolism. *Can J Physiol* 1978;56:691.
31. Vassalle M. The relationship among cardiac pacemakers: overdrive suppression. *Circ Res* 1977; 41:269.

32. Verrier RL, Lown B. Sympathetic-parasympathetic interactions and ventricular electrical stability. In: Schwartz PT, Brown HM, Mallian A, Zanchetti A, eds. *Neural mechanisms in cardiac arrhythmias*. New York: Raven Press;1986:75.
33. Vatner SF, Hintze TH. Mechanism of constriction of large coronary arteries by β-adrenergic receptor blockade. *Circ Res* 1983;53:389.
34. Rona G, Chappel CI, Balazs T, Baudry R. An infarct-like myocardial lesion and other toxic manifestations produced by isoproterenol in the rat. *Arch Pathol* 1959;67:443.
35. Meerson FZ, Pshennikova Mg, Shabunina EV, Sazontova TG, Belkina LM. Stress-limiting systems of the organism and *Meditzinskikh Nauk SSSR* 1987;6:47 (Russian).
36. Meerson FZ, Ustinova EE, Orlova EH. Prevention and elimination of heart arrhythmias by adaptation to intermittent high altitude hypoxia. *Clin Cardiol* 1987;10:783.
37. Meerson FZ, Dmitriev AD, Zayatz VI, Manukhina EB. Prevention of disturbances of heart function in experimental infarction by adaptation to stressful activity: the role of opioid peptides in this phenomenon. In: Smirnov VN, Katz AM, eds. *Myocardial metabolism*. Soviet Medical Reviews, Harwood Academic Publishers; 1987:508.
38. Meerson FZ, Kalvinsh IYa, Abdikaliev NA. Elimination of disturbances of heart electric stability and arrhythmia with synthetic acetylcholine analogue. *Biull Eksp Biol Med* 1991;1:13 (Russian).
39. Meerson FZ, Arkhipenko YuV, Rozhitzkaya II, Didenko VV, Sazontova TG. Opposite effects of adaptations to continuous and intermittent hypoxia on antioxidant enzymes. *Biull Eksp Biol Med* 1992; *[in press]* (Russian).
40. Meerson FZ. Protective effects of adaptation to hypoxia and prospects on the development of adaptive medicine. *CV World Rep* 1990;3:116.
41. Wallace J, Cohen M. Gastric mucosal protection with chronic mild restraint: role of endogenous prostaglandins. *Am J Physiol* 1984;247:6127.
42. Anderson SM, Len JR, Kant GJ. Chronic stress increases the binding of the A_1 adenosine receptor agonist, [^{3}H]cyclohexyladenosine, to rat hypothalamus. *Pharmacol Biochem Behav* 1988;30:169.
43. Stone EA, Platt JE. Brain adrenergic receptors and resistance to stress. *Brain Res* 1982;237:405.
44. Meerson FZ, Sukhikh GT, Katkova LS, Vanko PV. Prevention of depressed activity of natural killers and myocardial contractile function in long-term stress by preliminary adaptation of the organism to short-term stress exposure. *Dokl Akad Nauk SSSR* 1984;274:241 (Russian).
45. Meerson FZ, Dolgikh VT, Smolentzeva VN, Bratchenko ER. Prevention of disturbed metabolism and function of the heart by preliminary adaptation to short-term stress exposure. *Vopr Med Khim* 1985;3:41 (Russian).
46. Meerson FZ, Omitriev AD, Zayatz VI. Prevention of disturbances of cardiac contractile function in experimental myocardial infarction by preliminary adaptation to stress exposure and opioid peptides. *Kardiologiia*, 1984;9:81 (Russian).
47. Meerson FZ, Belkina LM, Dyusenov SS, Saltykova VA, Shabunina EV. Prevention of disturbances of heart electric stability in experimental myocardial infarction by preliminary adaptation to short-term stress exposure and antioxidant ional. *Kardiologiia* 1984;8:91 (Russian).
48. Meerson FZ, Shabunina EV, Belkina LM, Pshennikova MG. Prevention of cardiac fibrillation with a factor causing GABA accumulation in the brain. *Kardiologiia* 1987;5:87 (Russian).
49. Meerson FZ, Pshennikova MG, Belkina LM, Abdikaliev NA, Malyshev IYU. Prevention of ischemic arrhythmias by activation of stress-limiting systems in the organism. *CV World Rep* 1989; 2:205 (Russian).
50. Meerson FZ, Kagan VE, Kozlov YUP, Belkina LM, Arkhipernko YUV. The role of lipid peroxidation in pathogenesis of ischemic damage and the antioxidant protection of the heart. *Basic Res Cardiol* 1982;77:465.
51. Meerson FZ, Abdikaliev NA, Golubeva LYU. Prevention of hypoxic damage to the heart with antioxidant of the oxypyridine class. *Biull Eksp Biol Med* 1981;9:281 (Russian).
52. Brodsky M, Wu D, Denes DP. Arrhythmias documented by 24-hour continuous electrocardiographic monitoring. *Clin J Cardiol* 1977;39:390.
53. Djiane K, Egre A, Bory M. L'enregistrement electrocardiographique continu des 50 sujects normal. In: Puel P, ed. *Troubles des rythme et electroestimulation*. Toulouse; 1977:161.
54. Clarke JM, Hamer G, Shelton JP. The rhythm of the normal human heart. *Lancet* 1976;2:508.
55. Engel UK, Burckhardt D. Haufigkeit und Art von Herzrhythmussforungen Sowie EKG. Veranderungen bei Jungendlichen Herzgesunden Problemden. *Schweiz Med Wochenschr* 1975;105:1467.
56. Von Dietz A, Kirchhoff HW. Die Variationsbreite von Herzrhythmussformgen bei Hergesunden. *Z Kardiol* 1973;62:289.
57. Meerson FZ, Bukina TN. On detection of latent nonischemic arrhythmias in pilot with stress load.

In: Natoradze DA, Gel'man BL, eds. *Problems of clinical medicine in civil aviation*. Moscow: Gosudarstvennyj NII Grazhdanskoj Aviatzii; 1988: 70 (Russian).
58. Karvasarskij BD. *Neuroses*. Moscow: Meditsina; 1980 (Russian).
59. Smetnev AS, Bunin YuA, Firstova MI, Malyshev YuM, Klembovsky AA, Nargizyan AB, Asymbekova EU. The state of myocardial blood flow in patients with various forms of supraventricular cardiac rhythm disturbances. *Kardiologiia* 1985;3:39 (Russian).
60. Lombardi F, Malfatto G, Belloni A, Garimoldi M. Effect of sympathetic activation in ventricular ectopic beats in subjects with and without evidence of organic heart disease. *Eur Heart J* 1987; 8:1965.
61. McRae JR, Wagner GS, Rogers MC, Canen RV. Paroxysmal familial ventricular fibrillation. *J Pediatr* 1974;84:515.
62. Davies MS, Anderson RH, Becker AE. *The conduction of the heart*. London: Butterworth; 1983.
63. Wolf S. Behavioral aspects of cardiac arrhythmia and sudden cardiac death. *Circulation* 1987; 76(Pt 2, I): 1974.
64. Vlay SC. Ventricular tachycardia-fibrillation on the first day of medical school. *Am J Cardiol* 1986;57:483.
65. Wellens HJJ, Vermenlen A, Durrer D. Ventricular fibrillation occurring on arousal from sleep by auditory stimuli. *Circulation* 1972;46:661.
66. Cebelin MS, Hirsh CS. Human stress cardiomyopathy. Myocardial lesions in victims of homicidal assaults without internal injuries. *Hum Pathol* 1980;11:123.
67. McLaran CJ, Gersh BJ, Sugrue DD et al. Out of hospital cardiac arrest in patients without clinically significant coronary artery disease. Comparison of electrophysiological and survival characteristics with those in similar patients who have clinically significant coronary artery disease. *Br Heart J* 1982;58:583.
68. Belhaussen B, Shapira I, Shosbani D, Paredes A, Miller H, Laniado S. Idiopathic ventricular fibrillation: inducibility and beneficial effects of class I antiarrhythmic agents. *Circulation* 1987;75: 809.
69. Hayashi M, Murata M, Saton M. Sudden noctural death in young males from ventricular flutter. *Jpn Heart J* 1985;26:585.
70. Panagia V, Pierce GN, Dhalla KK, Ganguly PK, Beamish RE, Dhalla NS. Adaptive changes in subcellular calcium transport during catecholamine-induced cardiomyopathy. *J Mol Cell Cardiol* 1985;17:411.
71. Anichkov MN. Main results of studies carried out at the Department of Pathological Medicine (USSR AMS) on the problem of atherosclerosis. *Vestn Akad Med Nauk SSSR* 1961;11:29 (Russian).
72. Brown, MS, Goldstein DL. How low-density lipoprotein receptors affect cholesterol metabolism and development of atherosclerosis. *V Mire Nauki* (transl. *Sci Am*) 1985;1:(Russian).

The *Cardiomyopathic Heart*, edited by Makoto
Nagano, Nobuakira Takeda, and Naranjan S.
Dhalla. Raven Press, Ltd., New York © 1994.

42

Dysfunction of Cardiac Sarcoplasmic Reticulum in the Diabetic Dog

Issei Imanaga and Yojiro Kamegawa

*Department of Physiology, School of Medicine, Fukuoka University,
Fukuoka 814-01, Japan*

INTRODUCTION

It has been proposed that cardiomyopathy in the diabetic heart is caused by chronic overload of Ca^{2+} in the cytoplasm (1,2). The continuous increase in cytoplasmic Ca^{2+} concentration in diabetic myocardial cell results from several factors.

The first is an increase in transmembrane Ca^{2+} influx caused by the intracellular accumulation of long-chain acyl carnitine (e.g., palmitoyl carnitine) (3) which acts as a calcium channel activator or like elevated levels of external Ca^{2+} (4,5). The second is an increase in transmembrane Ca^{2+} influx caused by activation of reverse Na^+-Ca^{2+} exchange (Na^+_i-dependent Ca^{2+} influx) as a result of the depression of the sarcolemmal Na^+, K^+-ATPase activity (6–11). The third is a reduction of sarcolemmal Ca^{2+} pump activity caused by the depression of the sarcolemmal Ca^{2+}/Mg^{2+} ATPase activity (12,13). The fourth is a reduction of Ca^{2+} uptake into the sarcoplasmic reticulum (SR) as a result of the depression of the Ca^{2+}-stimulated ATPase activity of the SR membrane (14–17).

The other possibility is an enhancement of spontaneously gradual loss or leakage of Ca^{2+} from the SR into the cytoplasm, which leads to a diminution of Ca^{2+} stored within the SR.

The present studies were performed to determine whether spontaneous leakage of Ca^{2+} from the SR is enhanced in the diabetic heart. The results suggest that it is.

METHODS AND MATERIALS

Tiny cylindric trabecular muscle (0.5 to 1.0 mm in diameter, 5 mm in length) was isolated from the right ventricle of hearts removed from male dogs weighing 5 to 6 kg that had been anesthetized with 50 mg/kg of pentobarbital sodium, administered intravenously. The preparation was fixed in the perfusing chamber (0.4 mL in volume) and superfused with well-oxygenated Tyrode's solution or test solution at a constant flow rate (5 mL/min) and at a constant temperature (at 37°C, or at 20°C in some experiments). Isometric twitch contraction of the muscle was recorded with a force transducer (Nihonkoden, TB612T) that was electrically driven at a frequency of 0.5 Hz.

The first contraction after some rest intervals (e.g., the postrest contraction [PRC]) was taken as an index of the amount of calcium ions (Ca^{2+}) released from the SR and was evaluated by comparing the ratio of the first PRC to the contraction before rest.

To reduce the Na^+ concentration of the solution, Na^+ was substituted with 1-methyl-D-glucamine that had been adjusted with HC1 to a pH of 7.4.

Male dogs weighing 5 to 6 kg were fasted overnight and were made diabetic by a single intravenous injection of streptozotocin (STZ) (Boehringer Mannheim) at a dosage of 50 mg/kg of body weight. The STZ solution was freshly dissolved in 0.1 M of citrate buffer (pH of 4.5) prior to injection.

A glucose tolerance test was done 2 or 3 weeks later, prior to sacrifice of the experimental animal. The diabetic state was assessed by observations that the fasting blood glucose level exceeded 200 mg/dL and the K value of the intravenous glucose tolerance test (IVGTT) was less than 0.95 (18). Tests for urine ketone bodies yielded negative results. Ventricular weight expressed in g/body weight (g), was $6.45 \pm 0.17 \times 10^{-3}$ in the diabetic and $6.08 \pm 0.15 \times 10^{-3}$ in the control heart (mean $\pm$ SEM, *$p < 0.05$), respectively.

RESULTS

Isometric Twitch Contraction

In the diabetic heart, the magnitude of the developed contraction and the maximum rate of development of the contraction were significantly reduced in comparison with controls. Moreover, the time interval to complete relaxation was remarkably longer in the diabetic heart than in the normal heart. Alterations of these parameters are shown in Table 1.

TABLE 1. *Comparison of several parameters of twitch contraction in normal versus diabetic hearts*[a]

	DT (mN/mg tissue)	dT/dt (nN/sec)	TPT (m sec)	TRC (m sec)
Normal heart	1.6 ± 0.1	13.6 ± 0.4	160.4 ± 5.8	230.3 ± 6.1
Diabetic heart	1.0 ± 0.2*	10.8 ± 0.2*	163.8 ± 4.8	283.8 ± 9.4*

[a]The preparation was stimulated at 0.5 Hz. Each value represents the mean and $\pm$ SE.
*$p < 0.001$ compared to normal; statistically significant.
DT, developed contraction; dT/dt, maximum rate of development of the contraction; TPT, time to peak contraction; TRC, time to complete relaxation.

Postrest Contraction

In the rhythmically contracted preparation, the magnitude of the first contraction (PRC) was greater than that of the following second contraction after a rest interval. The magnitude of the PRC was greater or less than that of the contraction before rest, depending on the duration of the rest interval.

The relationship between the PRC and the rest interval is shown in Figures 1 and 2. The magnitude of the PRC was greater at relatively short rest intervals (10 sec to 3 min) and smaller at relatively long rest intervals (5 to 10 min) than that of the

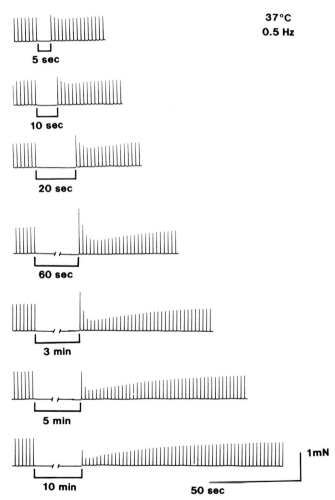

FIG. 1. An example of the postrest contraction of the normal heart at various rest intervals ranging from 5 seconds to 10 minutes. The preparation was driven at 0.5 Hz at a temperature of 37°C.

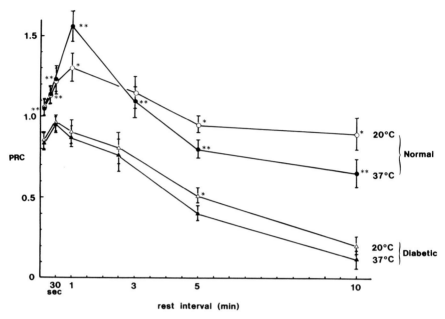

FIG. 2. The relationship between the rest interval and the postrest contraction (PRC) at temperatures of 37°C and 20°C in normal versus diabetic hearts. Each point represents a mean value; each vertical bar is ± SE. *$p<0.001$, compared to the state at the temperature of 37°C; **$p<0.001$, compared to the diabetic heart (statistically significant).

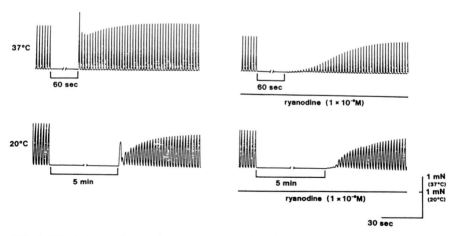

FIG. 3. Effect of ryanodine on the postrest contraction of the normal heart at temperatures of 37°C and 20°C. Ryanodine (1×10^{-6} M) was administered for 20 minutes before cessation of stimulation.

contraction before rest. In the normal heart, the maximum response was obtained at a rest interval of about 60 seconds.

The PRC was completely abolished by treatment with ryanodine (5×10^{-7} M, 30 mins) (Fig. 3) or caffeine (10 mM, ten mins) (data not shown), whereas it was augmented by treatment with ouabain (5×10^{-7} M, 10 mins) or by reduction of external Na^{2+} concentration during a period of rest (Fig. 4).

As the rest interval was prolonged from 5 to 10 minutes, the PRC decreased gradually, a process known as rest decay (19). The rest decay could be prevented by treatment with ouabain ($5 \times 10^{-7} - 1 \times 10^{-6}$, [10 minutes], by reduction of external Na^+ concentration during a period of rest, or by lowering the temperature of the perfusing solution (19°C to 21°C) (see Figs. 2 and 4). By perfusing the solution with the low external Na^+ concentration at 20°C, the rest decay was recovered considerably.

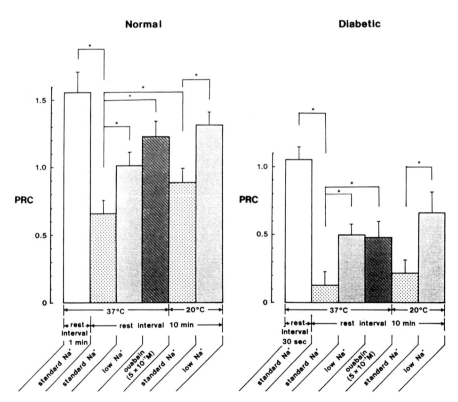

FIG. 4. The effects of reduction of external Na^+ concentration, treatment with ouabain, and lowering of temperature on the postrest contraction (PRC) in normal (*left panel*) and diabetic (*right panel*) hearts. Each column and bar represent the mean ± the SE, respectively. *$p < 0.001$, statistically significant.

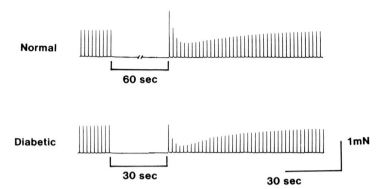

FIG. 5. Original examples of the maximum postrest contraction in the normal (*upper panel*) and the diabetic (*lower panel*) heart.

Comparison of the Postrest Contraction and the Rest Decay in Normal Versus Diabetic Hearts

The maximum response of the postrest potentiation occurred at rest intervals of about 60 seconds in the normal heart and about 30 seconds in the diabetic heart, respectively (Fig. 2). The magnitude of the PRC was significantly smaller in the diabetic than in the normal heart (Figs. 2 and 5). The rest decay at longer rest intervals was greater in terms of rate and magnitude, in the diabetic heart than in the normal heart.

Recovery of the rest decay by reduction of external Na^+ concentration, administration of ouabain (5×10^{-7}, 10 mins), lowering of temperature (20°C) or reduction of external Na^+ concentration during the period of low temperature was considerably impaired in the diabetic heart (see Fig. 4).

DISCUSSION

In the diabetic dog heart, a decrease in the developed contraction and prolongation of the relaxation time of the contraction were observed.

The delay in the relaxation time can be explained by a reduced rate of Ca^{2+} reuptake into the SR, as reduced activity of Ca^{2+}-activated ATPase of the SR membrane (14–17) has been observed in the diabetic heart.

A decrease in the developed contraction is generally attributable to a reduction in Ca^{2+} current through the plasma membrane, a hypofunction of the contractile protein, or a decrease in the amount of Ca^{2+} released from the SR.

Whether Ca^{2+} current (slow inward current) is reduced in the diabetic heart has not yet been confirmed. Rather than Ca^{2+} current may possibly be enhanced because palmitoyl carnitine, one of the metabolites of carnitine that act as Ca^{2+} channel activator (4,5), accumulates in the myocardial cell during diabetes (3). Moreover, it has been observed in a binding experiment of [^{3}H]PN200–110 that the voltage-sensitive Ca^{2+} channel is increased in the diabetic rat heart (20). Therefore, an impairment of the contractile force in the diabetic heart may depend on factors other than transmembrane Ca^{2+} current.

In chronic diabetic hearts, remarkable depression in the activity of myofibrillar Ca^{2+}-stimulated ATPase (21,22), actomyosin Ca^{2+}-stimulated ATPase (23–25), and myosin Ca^{2+} ATPase (23,24,26) has been observed. On the other hand, these enzymatic factors may not contribute substantially to the impaired ability of the preparation to generate contractile force after a short term (2–3 weeks) the diabetic state.

A decrease in the amount of Ca^{2+} released from the SR in the diabetic heart may result from several possibilities. One is inactivation of the Ca^{2+} release channel (e.g., the ryanodine-sensitive channel) of the SR membrane. This possibility has not yet been documented in the diabetic heart, however. Another possible factor is a decrease in the Ca^{2+} content of the SR caused by reduction of Ca^{2+} reuptake into the SR secondary to depression of Ca^{2+}-activated ATPase activity in the SR membrane (14–17). Finally, the spontaneous release (27–30), loss or leakage (31,32) of Ca^{2+} from the SR into cytoplasm may play a role.

In isometrically contracted mammalian cardiac muscle driven at a constant frequency, the magnitude of the first twitch contraction after a rest interval (the PRC) is greater than that of the following second contraction, and greater than that of the contraction before rest after a relatively short rest interval.

Potentiation of the PRC is caused by a large amount of Ca^{2+} being released from the SR, as it can be completely abolished by agents affecting the cardiac SR, including ryanodine (a Ca^{2+} depletor (33), Ca^{2+} release inhibitors (34), or caffeine (also a Ca^{2+} depletor (35,36)). The PRC is potentiated when the amount of Ca^{2+} is stored in the SR during a period of rest. The mechanism of the PRC is thought to be related to a decrease in Ca^{2+} efflux via forward $Na^+ - Ca^{2+}$ exchange (Na^+_o-dependent Ca^{2+} efflux) during a period of rest (37). This premise is supported by evidence that the PRC is potentiated by a reduction in external Na^+ concentration or by administration of ouabain (37; the present study).

As the rest interval is prolonged over 5 minutes, the magnitude of the PRC is gradually decreased (rest decay) (18). The rest decay may be caused by leakage or a spontaneous, gradual loss of Ca^{2+} from the SR (19,31,32).

Observations that the magnitude of the rest decay is mitigated by a reduction in external Na^+ concentration or by the administration ouabain have been reported elsewhere (37) and in the present study. These results suggest a replenishment of the SR with Ca^{2+} during a long period of rest through activation of the reverse $Na^+ - Ca^{2+}$ exchange.

Moreover, the rest decay may be prevented by lowering the temperature of the perfusing solution. In the chemically skinned mammalian cardiac muscle, spontaneous Ca^{2+} release from the SR was found to be increased at physiological temperatures (37°C to 38°C) and suppressed at low temperatures (around 20°C) at which the sensitivity of the contractile system to Ca^{2+} remains unaffected (38).

Additionally, it has been reported that, in sheep cardiac SR, at relatively high concentrations of Ca^{2+}, the Ca^{2+} release channel of the SR remains closed at 23°C, whereas at markedly low temperatures (0°C to 5°C), the probability of an open Ca^{2+} channel of the SR and the amount of Ca^{2+} released from SR are enhanced. (The low temperature results in a so-called "rapid cooling contracture") (39).

Therefore, it is possible that the SR membrane becomes less leaky to Ca^{2+} at low temperatures around 20°C. More Ca^{2+} is preserved in the SR at this temperature range.

Depression of the PRC was previously reported in the diabetic rat (40). In both a previous study (41) and the present one, this property was also observed in the diabetic dog heart. Moreover, the present study has revealed that the rest decay is greater in the diabetic heart than in the normal heart, and that the recovery of the rest decay—through the reduction of external Na^+ concentration, administration of ouabain, or lowering of temperature—is impaired in the diabetic heart. These results suggest that the SR membrane of the diabetic heart has a property of easy leakage of Ca^{2+}, which leads to a gradual loss of Ca^{2+} from the SR.

Almost all Ca^{2+} that is leaked from the SR is extruded outside the cell via the forward $Na^+ - Ca^{2+}$ exchange system, it is then pumped out from the cell by activation of sarcolemmal Ca^{2+}/Mg^{2+} ATPase or it is reaccumulated in the SR by activation of the Ca^{2+}-stimulated ATPase of the SR membrane. However, the activities of these enzymes (12–17) and of sarcolemmal $Na^+ - K^+$ ATPase (6–11) are impaired in the diabetic heart. Therefore, enhanced leakage of Ca^{2+} from the SR in the diabetic heart is responsible not only for a decrease in Ca^{2+} content in the SR, which generates reduced contractile force, but also for an increase in cytoplasmic Ca^{2+} concentration. These changes may result in chronic Ca^{2+} overload in the cytoplasm, which could contribute to the development of diabetic cardiomyopathy.

SUMMARY

Cardiac SR function was studied in the diabetic dog. The magnitude of the PRC, which is a good index of the amount of Ca^{2+} released from the SR, was reduced in the diabetic heart as compared to the normal heart. The rate and magnitude of the rest decay at a relatively long period of rest were increased in the diabetic heart compared to the normal heart. Recovery of the rest decay—through reduction of external Na^+ concentration, treatment with ouabain, or lowering of the temperature of the perfusing solution—was remarkably impaired in the diabetic heart in comparison with the normal heart.

These results suggest that the SR membrane of the diabetic heart allows greater leakage of Ca^{2+}. This may be one of the factors contributing to chronic Ca^{2+} cytoplasmic overload, which, in turn, can result in the development of diabetic cardiomyopathy.

ACKNOWLEDGMENT

A portion of this study was supported by a Research Grant (1988–1990) from the Central Research Institute of Fukuoka University.

REFERENCES

1. Afzal N, Ganguly PK, Dhalla KS, Pierce GN, Singal PK, Dhalla NS. Beneficial effects of verapamil in diabetic cardiomyopathy. *Diabetes* 1988;37:936–942.
2. Dhalla NS, Pierce GN, Innes IR, Beamish RE. Pathogenesis of cardiac dysfunction in diabetes mellitus. *Can J Cardiol* 1985;1:263–281.
3. Pieper GM, Murray WJ. In vivo and in vitro intervention with L-carnitine prevents abnormal energy metabolism in isolated diabetic rat heart: chemical and phosphorus-31 NMR evidence. *Biochem Med Metabol Biol* 1987;38:111–120.
4. Inoue D, Pappano AJ. L-Palmitoylcarnitine and calcium ions act similarly on excitatory ionic currents in avian ventricular muscle. *Circ Res* 1983;52:625–634.
5. Spedding M, Mir AK. Direct activation of Ca^{2+} channels by palmitoyl carnitine, a putative endogenous ligand. *Br J Pharmacol* 1987;92:457–468.
6. Imanaga I, Kamei R, Kuroiwa M, Uehara A. Effect of insulin on diabetic mammalian cardiac muscle. *J Mol Cell Cardiol* 1981;13[Suppl 2]:40 (Abst).
7. Imanaga I, Kamegawa Y. Mechanisms of low sarcolemmal $Na^+ - K^+$ ATPase activity in diabetic myocardium. *J Mol Cell Cardiol* 1990;22[Suppl II]:S38 (Abst).
8. Imanaga I, Kamegawa Y, Kamei R, Kuroiwa M. Cardiac sarcolemmal $Na^+ - K^+$ adenosine triphosphatase (ATPase) activity in diabetic dog. In: Nagano M, Dhalla NS, eds. *The diabetic heart.* New York: Raven Press; 1991:237–247.
9. Ku DD. Decreased sodium pump activity in heart and thoracic aorta of streptozotocin (STZ)-induced diabetic rats. *Pharmacologist* 1980;22:288.
10. Oniji T, Liu MS. Effects of alloxan-diabetes on the sodium-potassium adenosine triphosphatase enzyme system in dog hearts. *Biochem Biophys Res Commun* 1980;96:799–804.
11. Pierce GN, Dhalla NS. Sarcolemmal $Na^+ - K^+$ ATPase activity in diabetic rat heart. *Am J Physiol* 1983;245:C241–C247.
12. Heyliger CE, Prakash A, McNeill JH. Alterations in cardiac sarcolemmal Ca^{2+} pump activity during diabetes mellitus. *Am J Physiol* 1987;252:H540–H544.
13. Makino N, Dhalla KS, Elimban V, Dhalla NS. Sarcolemmal Ca^{2+} transport in streptozotocin-induced diabetic cardiomyopathy in rats. *Am J Physiol* 1987;253:E202–E207.
14. Ganguly PK, Pierce GN, Dhalla KS, Dhalla NS. Defective sarcoplasmic reticular calcium transport in diabetic cardiomyopathy. *Am J Physiol* 1983;244:E528–E535.
15. Lopaschuk GD, Katz S, McNeill JH. The effect of alloxan- and streptozotocin-induced diabetes on calcium transport in rat cardiac sarcoplasmic reticulum. The possible involvement of long chain acylcarnitines. *Can J Physiol Pharmacol* 1983;61:439–448.
16. Lopaschuk GD, Eibschutz B, Katz S, McNeill JH. Depression of calcium transport in sarcoplasmic reticulum from diabetic rats: lack of involvement by specific regulatory mediators. *Gen Pharmacol* 1984;15:1–5.
17. Penpargkul S, Fein FS, Sonnenblick EH, Scheuer J. Depressed cardiac sarcoplasmic reticular function from diabetic rats. *J Mol Cell Cardiol* 1981;13:303–309.
18. Lundbaek K. Intravenous glucose tolerance as a tool in definition and diagnosis of diabetes mellitus. *Br Med J* 1962;1:1507–1513.
19. Allen DG, Jewell BR, Wood EH. Studies of the contractility of mammalian myocardium at low rates of stimulation. *J Physiol* 1976;254:1–17.
20. Kashiwagi A, Nishino T, Ogawa T, et al. Increase in voltage-sensitive calcium channel of cardiac and skeletal muscle in streptozotocin-induced diabetic rats. In Nagano M, Mochizuki S, Dhalla NS, eds. *Cardiovascular disease in diabetes.* Boston: Kluwer Academic Publishers; 1992:173–182.
21. Pierce GN, Dhalla NS. Cardiac myofibrillar ATPase activity in diabetic rats. *J Mol Cell Cardiol* 1981;13:1063–1069.

22. Pierce GN, Dhalla NS. Mechanisms of the defect in cardiac myofibrillar function during diabetes. *Am J Physiol* 1985;248:E170–E175.
23. Dillmann WH. Diabetes mellitus induces changes in cardiac myosin of the rat. *Diabetes* 1980;29: 579–582.
24. Malhotra A, Penpargkul S, Fein FS, Sonnenblick EH, Scheuer J. The effect of streptozotocin-induced diabetes in rats on cardiac contractile proteins. *Circ Res* 1981;49:1243–1250.
25. Malhotra A. Cardiac contractile proteins in diabetic cardiomyopathy. In: Nagano M, Dhalla NS, eds. *The diabetic heart.* New York: Raven Press; 1991:281–290.
26. Garber DW, Neely JR. Decreased myocardial function and myosin ATPase in hearts from diabetic rats. *Am J Physiol* 1983;244:H586–H591.
27. Bose D, Kobayashi T, Bouchard RA, Hryshko LV. Scattered light intensity fluctuation in the canine ventricular myocardium: correlation with inotropic drug effect. *Can J Physiol Pharmacol* 1988;66: 1232–1238.
28. Capogrossi MC, Stern MD, Spurgeon HA, Lakatta EG. Spontaneous Ca^{2+} release from the sarcoplasmic reticulum limits Ca^{2+}-dependent twitch potentiation in individual cardiac myocytes. A mechanism for maximum inotropy in the myocardium. *J Gen Physiol* 1988;91:133–155.
29. Kort AA, Lakatta EG. Spontaneous sarcoplasmic reticulum calcium release in rat and rabbit cardiac muscle: relation to transient and rested-state twitch tension. *Circ Res* 1988;63:969–979.
30. Stern MD, Capogrossi MC, Lakatta EG. Spontaneous calcium release from the sarcoplasmic reticulum in myocardial cells: mechanisms and consequences. *Cell Calcium* 1988;9:247–258.
31. Bers DM, Bridge JHB. Effect of acetylstrophanthidin on twitches, microscopic tension fluctuations and cooling contractures in rabbit ventricle. *J Physiol* 1988;404:53–69.
32. Hryshko LV, Stiffel V, Bers DM. Rapid cooling contractures as an index of sarcoplasmic reticulum calcium content in rabbit ventricular myocytes. *Am J Physiol* 1989;257:H1369–H1377.
33. Hansford RG, Lakatta EG. Ryanodine releases calcium from sarcoplasmic reticulum in calcium-tolerant rat cardiac myocytes. *J Physiol* 1987;390:453–467.
34. Sutko JL, Kenyon JL. Ryanodine modification of cardiac muscle responses to potassium-free solutions: evidence for inhibition of sarcoplasmic reticulum calcium release. *J Gen Physiol* 1983;82: 385–404.
35. Blayney LH, Muir TJ, Henderson A. Action of caffeine on calcium transport by isolated fractions of myofibrils, mitochondria and sarcoplasmic reticulum from rabbit heart. *Circ Res* 1978;43:520–526.
36. Fabiato A, Fabiato F. Contractions induced by a calcium-triggered release of calcium from the sarcoplasmic reticulum of single skinned cardiac cells. *J Physiol* 1975;249:469–495.
37. Sutko J, Bers DM, Reeves JP. Postrest inotropy in rabbit ventricle: Na^+-Ca^{2+} exchange determines sarcoplasmic reticulum Ca^{2+} content. *Am J Physiol* 1986;250:H654–H662.
38. Asayama J, Tatsumi T, Yamahara Y, et al. Spontaneous cyclic Ca^{2+} release from sarcoplasmic reticulum in the absence and presence of free Ca^{2+} sufficient to overload sarcoplasmic reticulum. *Jpn J Appl Physiol* 1992;22:1–7.
39. Sitsapesan R, Montgomery RAP, MacLeod KT, Williams AJ. Sheep cardiac sarcoplasmic reticulum calcium-release channels: modification of conductance and gating by temperature. *J Physiol* 1991; 434:469–488.
40. Bouchard RA, Bose D. Influence of experimental diabetes on sarcoplasmic reticulum function in rat ventricular muscle. *Am J Physiol* 1991;260:H341–H354.
41. Kamegawa Y, Imanaga I. Deteriorative function of sarcoplasmic reticulum in diabetic heart muscle *J Mol Cell Cardiol* 1991;23[Suppl II]:S46 (Abst).

The Cardiomyopathic Heart, edited by Makoto
Nagano, Nobuakira Takeda, and Naranjan S.
Dhalla. Raven Press, Ltd., New York © 1994.

43

Electron Microscopic and Endocrinologic Studies of Hypertrophic Hearts of Infants from Streptozotocin-Induced Diabetic Pregnant Rats

Naoki Ohta, Yutaka Takino, Tutomu Iwasaki, Susumu Imai,
*Tadashi Suzuki, Shoichi Tomono, Shoji Kawazu, and
Kazuhiko Murata

*The Second Department of Internal Medicine, Gunma University School of Medicine, and
*College of Medical Care and Technology, Gunma University 3-39-15, Showa-machi,
Macbashi-city, Gunma 371 Japan*

INTRODUCTION

Miller and Wilson (1) reported that a transient form of cardiac hypertrophy—asymmetric septal hypertrophy (ASH)—occurred in infants born from diabetic mothers. We have previously reported that infants from streptozotocin (STZ)-induced diabetic female rats (IDM) showed ASH with occasional cellular disarray representing cardiac cellular immaturity (2). Recently, insulin-like growth factor I (IGF-I) and insulin have been found to act as growth factors during fetal development. They play an important role in differentiation processes and maturation in a very wide range of cell types (3–5).

In this study, we investigated the morphologic characteristics of the intercellular connections of cardiocytes in fetuses and infants from STZ-induced diabetic pregnant rats (FDM and IDM, respectively) using transmission electron microscopy (TEM) and scanning electron microscopy (SEM). Furthermore, we also measured the serum levels of IGF-I and insulin content in the pancreatic tissue of the FDMs and IDMs and correlated these values with cardiac development in the IDMs.

TABLE 1. *Comparison of various measurements*

		n	Body weight (g)	Heart weight (mg)
Fetuses (21 days	Control	40	5.51 ± 0.29 _*	22.33 ± 3.68
gestational age	DM	22	4.88 ± 0.63	22.6 ± 2.81
Infants (2 days old)	Control	72	5.79 ± 0.80	23.33 ± 3.96 _*
	DM	22	5.95 ± 0.88	26.70 ± 5.16

[a]Values are expressed as means ± SD.
*p<0.05; **p<0.01.
DM, diabetic mother; IVST, interventricular septal thickness; LVFWT, left ventricular free wall thickness.

MATERIALS AND METHODS

Experimental Protocol

Thirty-nine virgin female Wistar rats, weighing approximately 200 g each, received an intraperitoneal injection of STZ (Sigma, 50 mg/kg) and were mated with male rats overnight 1 week after the injection. Fourteen control rats received isotonic saline in the same dose. The female rats were examined on the next day for the presence of sperm. The day when sperm was detected was counted as day 0 of gestation. The offspring of these rats were sacrificed on the 21st day of gestation or on the 2nd day after birth. The hearts were immediately removed and immersed in 3% phosphate-buffered glutaraldehyde solution for a few minutes. The ventricles were incised parallel to the atrioventricular groove, midway between the aortic root and the apex, and were weighed.

Light Microscopic Studies

For light microscopic examination, basal portions of the ventricles were fixed in 3% phosphate-buffered glutaraldehyde solution, postfixed in 1% osmium tetroxide, dehydrated with an ascending series of ethanol, and embedded in epoxy resin. An entire cross section (4 μm thick) was stained with alkaline toluidine blue. Left ventricular free wall thickness (LVFWT) and interventricular septal thickness (IVST) were measured on micrographs of the sections at 60-fold magnification. Wall thickness was measured at the thickest site excluding the papillary muscles and the trabeculae. Then, the ratio of septal to free wall thickness was calculated.

Electron Microscopic Studies

Several small tissue blocks were excised from the remaining apical portion and fixed in 3% phosphate-buffered glutaraldehyde solution for 3 hours at 4°C. For TEM, the specimens were postfixed in 1% osmium tetroxide, dehydrated with an *in rat fetuses and infants*[a]

Heart wt/ body wt ($\times 10^{-3}$)	n	IVST ($\times 10^{-1}$mm)	LVFWT ($\times 10^{-1}$mm)	IVST/LVFWT
4.01 ± 0.48 *	10	6.12 ± 1.44	4.65 ± 0.64	1.31 ± 0.23
4.60 ± 0.44 *	16	6.48 ± 1.81	4.80 ± 1.10	1.36 ± 0.27
4.03 ± 0.36 *	26	6.61 ± 0.82 **	6.08 ± 0.80	1.10 ± 0.11 **
4.49 ± 0.55 *	14	8.17 ± 1.33 **	6.12 ± 0.79	1.34 ± 0.18 **

ascending series of ethanol, and embedded in epoxy resin. Ultrathin sections were stained with uranyl acetate and lead citrate and examined by TEM. For SEM, the specimens were dehydrated with an ascending series of ethanol, dried in a critical point drier, coated with platinum, and examined with a field-emission type of scanning electron microscope.

Cardiac intercellular connections were classified into two types according to their connective patterns established by TEM: (a) end-to-end connections (mature form); and (b) side-to-side connections and side-to-end connections (immature forms). The frequency of these connection types was determined in the control and diabetic mother (DM) groups, and the proportion of end-to-end type connections was calculated.

Endocrinologic Studies

Seventeen additional female Wistar rats weighing 200 g were prepared to comprise a DM (n = 7) and a control (n = 10) group in the same manner as described earlier, and their offspring were studied. After measuring the body weight of the offspring on the 21st day of gestation or on the 2nd day after birth, blood samples were collected and serum levels of glucose were measured by glucose oxidase method. Serum levels of IGF-I were also measured by radioimmunoassay using anti-rat IGF-I antibodies. The heart and pancreas of the animals were removed and weighed. After extracting the insulin from the pancreas by acid-ethanol method, pancreatic insulin content was measured by radioimmunassay applying rat insulin as a standard.

Statistical Analysis

All values were expressed as a mean ± SD. Unpaired Student's *t*-test and chi-square were used in the analysis of data. Statistical significance was defined as $p < 0.05$.

RESULTS

Body weight, heart weight, and heart weight/body weight ratios in FDMs and IDMs are shown in Table 1. On the 21st day of gestation, the fetuses from diabetic pregnant rats were found to have a smaller body weight and a greater heart weight/body weight ratio than did controls. Heart weight and heart weight/body weight ratio of the IDMs were significantly higher than those of controls.

Microscopic Studies

Table 1 presents data relating to IVST, LVFWT, and IVST/LVFWT ratio. The fetuses of both the control and DM groups had ASH, with a similar IVST/LVFWT ratio (control = 1.31 ± 0.23; DM = 1.36 ± 0.27; NS). The IVST and IVST/LVFWT of the IDMs were significantly larger than those of controls, and also showed evidence of ASH (control = 1.10 ± 0.11; DM = 1.34 ± 0.18; $p < 0.01$).

The correlation between heart weight/body weight ratio and IVST/LVFWT ratio in infants is shown in Fig. 1A. In the infants, a positive correlation was observed between the two ($r = 0.506$; $p < 0.01$).

Electron Microscopic Studies

By TEM, side-to-side or side-to-end connections were frequently observed, with almost equal incidences in both FDMs and controls. By SEM, the three-dimensional structure of these connections could be seen. On the second day after birth, the myofibrils of the controls were parallel and the striations were also clearly visible by TEM. The intercellular connections of cardiocytes were almost at the position of the Z band, and end-to-end connections had been formed (Fig. 2A). SEM study revealed that the area of junction was broad, and dense end-to-end connections were conspicuous (Fig. 2B). Intercellular connections in the IDMs frequently showed side-to-side connections by TEM (Fig. 2C). SEM study revealed that the cardiocytes were clearly distributed in parallel, and were linked by side-to-side connections (Fig. 2D).

The proportion of end-to-end intercellular connections in FDMs and IDMs is presented in Figure 3. On the 21st day of gestation, end-to-end connections (mature form) were less common, both in controls and FDMs, than were side-to-side and side-to-end connections (immature forms). On the second day after birth, end-to-end connections were significantly less common in the IDMs (32.9%) than in the controls (46.1%) ($p < 0.01$).

Endocrinologic Studies

Blood glucose and serum IGF-I levels, as well as pancreatic insulin content, in FDMs and IDMs are presented in Fig. 4. On the 21st day of gestation, blood glu-

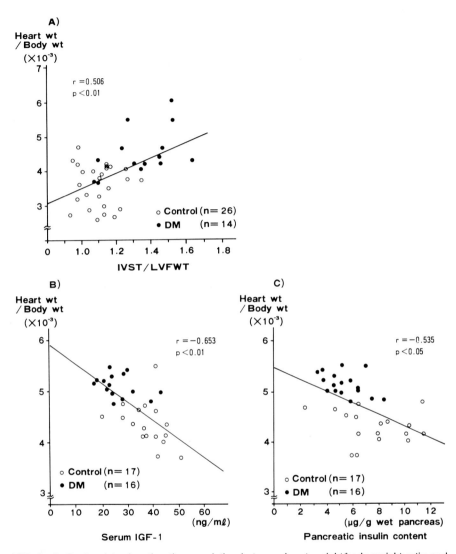

FIG. 1. A: Scatterplots denoting the correlation between heart weight/body weight ratio and IVST/LVFWT of infants on the second day after birth. In the infants, a positive correlation was observed between these two parameters. **B** and **C**: Scatterplots denoting the correlations between the heart weight/body weight ratio and serum IGF-I levels (B) and pancreatic insulin content (C) in 2-day-old infants. In the infants, negative correlations were observed between the heart weight/body weight ratio and both serum IGF-I levels and pancreatic insulin content. *IVST*, interventricular septal thickness; *LVFWT*, left ventricular free wall thickness; *IGF-I*, insulin-like growth factor I; *DM*, diabetic mother.

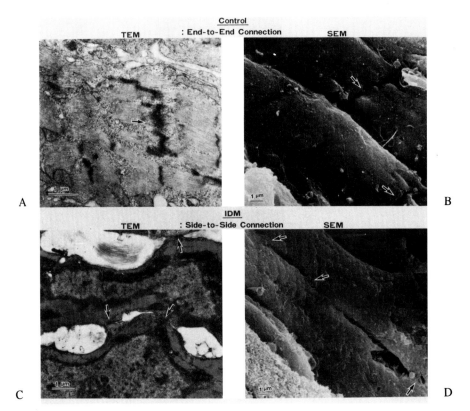

FIG. 2. Electron micrographs of cardiac cell connections (*arrows*) in infants of controls (**A** and **B**) and infants of diabetic mothers (IDMs) (**C** and **D**) on the second day after birth. Scanning electron microscopic (SEM) images (**B** and **D**) correspond to transmission electron microscopic (TEM) images (**A** and **C**), and are useful in visualizing the cellular connections three-dimensionally. Side-to-side or side-to-end connections were observed more frequently in IDMs than in controls.

cose levels in FDMs were significantly higher than those in controls. On the second day after birth, blood glucose levels in IDMs still exceeded those in controls. By contrast, the serum IGF-I levels and pancreatic insulin content in FDMs and IDMs were lower than those in controls.

Correlations between heart weight/body weight ratios and serum IGF-I levels and pancreatic insulin content are shown in Figure 1B, C. On the second day after birth, a negative correlation was observed in the infants between serum IGF-I level and heart weight/body weight ratio ($r = -0.653$; $p<0.01$). A negative correlation was also observed between pancreatic insulin content and heart weight/body weight ratio ($r = -0.535$; $p<0.05$).

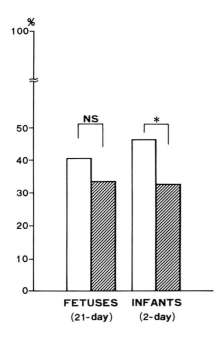

FIG. 3. Percentage of end-to-end types of inter-cellular connections in fetus and infants of diabetic mothers (FDMs and IDMs, respectively). On the 21st day of gestation, end-to-end connections (mature forms) were less common both in controls and in FDM hearts than were immature forms. On the second day after birth, end-to-end connections were significantly less common in IDMs than in controls. Open bars represent the percentage in controls, whereas the crosshatched bars represent the percentage in FDMs and IDMs. $*p<0.01$; *NS*, not significant.

DISCUSSION

Maron and colleagues (6) reported that a disproportionate thickening of the ventricular septum was a common finding in the developing hearts of normal human embryos and during subsequent prenatal and postnatal growth, but that disproportionate septal thickening became progressively less common later. We observed that the hearts of fetuses from both control and diabetic rats showed disproportionate septal thickening. However, on the second day after birth, disproportionate septal thickening disappeared in the infants from the control rats, whereas it persisted in the hearts of IDMs. ASH in the IDMs observed in this study might reflect the immaturity of the hearts of these animals. We also observed a positive correlation between heart weight/body weight ratio and IVST/LVFWT in IDMs, which showed that the heart weight/body weight ratio was relevant to the immaturity of the hearts in these animals.

We investigated the maturity of cardiac cytoarchitecture by determining the proportion of end-to-end type (mature form) intercellular connections. The proportion of end-to-end type connections was similar in both controls and FDMs, and these types of connections were found to be less common than the immature forms. On the second day after birth, the proportion of end-to-end type connections in the controls increased, whereas in the IDMs, it remained. These results suggest that the cardiac cytoarchitecture in IDMs may be immature.

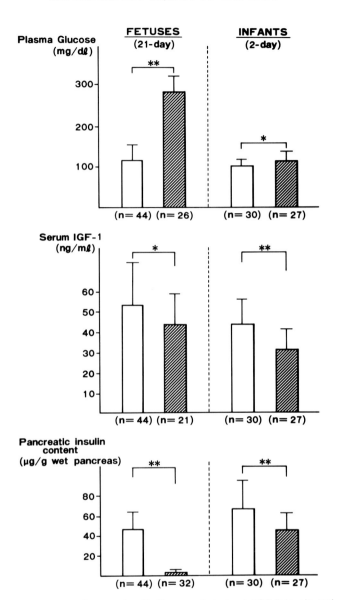

FIG. 4. Plasma glucose and serum insulin-like growth factor I (IGF-I) levels and pancreatic insulin content. Plasma glucose levels were higher in fetuses (FDMs) and infants (IDMs) of diabetic pregnant rats than in controls, whereas pancreatic insulin content and serum IGF-I levels were lower in the offspring of diabetic rats than in controls. Open bars represent mean values of the control; crosshatched bars represent values for FDMs and IDMs. *p<0.05; **p<0.01.

The plasma glucose level in FDMs was significantly higher than that in controls, which factor might explain the significant reduction in pancreatic insulin content in FDMs. On the second day after birth, IDMs showed a similar but less extensive increase in plasma glucose level, as well as a less extensive decrease in pancreatic insulin content compared to controls. The influence of high plasma glucose levels in the DM rat appearted to remain in the offspring even after birth. Serum IGF-I levels and pancreatic insulin content were lower in both the FDMs and the IDMs than in controls. Moreover, there were negative correlations between heart weight/body weight ratios (relevant to the immaturity of the hearts) and serum IGF-I levels and pancreatic insulin content in IDMs. IGF-I and insulin can promote cellular differentiation and maturation (3–5). These results suggest that the insufficient secretion of these hormones during development may result in an immature form of cardiac architecture, as evidenced by the immature form of cellular connections and ASH.

SUMMARY

The persistence of disproportionate septal hypertrophy and immature cardiac intercellular connections even after birth in IDMs suggests that the hearts of IDMs are immature. Moreover, the reduction in pancreatic insulin content and serum IGF-I concentration was presumed to be relevant to the immaturity of the hearts in IDMs.

ACKNOWLEDGMENT

We express our heartfelt thanks for the aid received from Fujisawa Pharmaceutical Co., Ltd. (Osaka) in the radioimmunoassay of rat IGF-I.

REFERENCES

1. Miller HC, Wilson HM. Macrosomia, cardiac hypertrophy, erythroblastosis and hyperplasia of the islets of Langerhans in infants born to diabetic mothers. *J Pediatr* 1943;23:251–266.
2. Takino Y, Iwasaki T, Suzuki T. The cardiomyopathy in infants of streptozotosin-induced diabetic female rats. *Jpn Circ J* 1990;54:1554–1562.
3. Guler HP, Zapf J, Froesch ER. Short-term metabolic effects of recombinant insulin-like growth factor in healthy adults. *N Engl J Med* 1987;317:137–140.
4. De Pablo F, Roth J. Endocrinization of the early embryo: an emerging role for hormones and hormone-like factors. *Trends Biochem Sci* 1990;15:339–342.
5. De Pablo F, Scott LA, Roth J. Insulin and insulin-like growth factor I in early development: peptide receptors and biological events. *Endocr Rev* 1990;11:558–577.
6. Maron BJ, Verter J, Kapur S. Disproportionate ventricular septal thickening in the developing normal human heart. *Circulation* 1978;57:520–526.

The Cardiomyopathic Heart, edited by Makoto
Nagano, Nobuakira Takeda, and Naranjan S.
Dhalla. Raven Press, Ltd., New York © 1994.

44

Involvement of the Parasympathetic Nervous System in Heart Mitochondrial Dysfunction Associated with Hypothyroidism in Rats

Satoru Sugiyama, *Yoshihiro Hanaki, *Kazuki Hattori,
*Naohiko Akiyama, Tomoko Kato, and Takayuki Ozawa

*Departments of Biomedical Chemistry and *Internal Medicine, Faculty of Medicine,
University of Nagoya, Nagoya, Japan*

INTRODUCTION

Cardiovascular function is greatly influenced by hormonal factors, and cardiac failure, associated with endocrine disorders such as hypothyroidism, is often encountered clinically (1). The mechanism of hypothyroid cardiomyopathy has attracted much interest because of its variety of symptoms based on various morphologic and biochemical alterations (2). Because these alterations revert back to normal with replacement of thyroid hormone (3), the lack of thyroid hormone itself has been considered to be responsible for the genesis of this condition. Accordingly, the involvement of thyroid-hormone–regulated contractile components, such as the myosin heavy chains and calcium-dependent adenosine triphosphatase (ATPase), has been studied extensively (4,5).

Morphologic changes in mitochondria also accompany hypothyroid cardiomyopathy (6). Mitochondria play a crucial role in energy metabolism. Recent research has revealed that mitochondrial abnormality is closely related to the development of myopathy. Nevertheless, few reports have been published concerning the correlation between cardiac mitochondrial dysfunction and hypothyroidism. We have indicated that alterations in the autonomic nervous system are involved in the genesis of mitochondrial dysfunction (7,8). It is well known that hormonal changes induce alterations in the autonomic nervous system and vice versa. The present study focuses on whether or not alterations in the autonomic nervous system occur in rats with hypothyroidism, and if so, what the relationship is between alterations in the autonomic nervous system and mitochondrial dysfunction.

METHODS

Experiments were conducted using male specific pathogen free Wistar rats weighing 60 to 70 g at 4 weeks of age. Animals were maintained in our animal facility until the time of the study. The experiments performed conformed to the *Position of the American Heart Association on Research Animal Use*, adopted on November 11, 1984 by the American Heart Association.

Surgical Procedure

Hypothyroidism was achieved by surgical thyroidectomy with simultaneous transplantation of the parathyroid glands in the neck muscles (9). Rats were anesthesized using ethyl ether, and using a stereomicroscope, the parathyroid glands were localized from the neck muscles. Thereafter, surgical thyroidectomy was performed. The success of thyroidectomy was judged by the radioimmunoassay determination of triiodothyronine (T_3) (described below).

Experimental Design

Rats were divided into five groups: Group 1, in which hypothyroidism was achieved by thyroidectomy and experiments were performed 3 weeks after surgery; Group 2, in which a sham operation was performed and experiments were performed 3 weeks after surgery; Group 3, in which hypothyroidism was achieved by thyroidectomy and experiments were performed 6 weeks after surgery; Group 4, in which hypothyroidism was achieved by thyroidectomy and hormonal supplementation was initiated (daily subcutaneous injections of 10 mg/kg of T_3 in a volume of 1 mL/kg dissolved in 4 mM of NaOH in 0.9% NaCl) for a period of 3 weeks beginning 3 weeks and 6 weeks after surgery, after which times the experiments were performed; and Group 5, in which a sham operation was performed and experiments were performed 6 weeks after surgery.

Radioimmunoassay of Triiodothyronine

Blood was collected via the inferior vena cava from sacrificed animals for analysis of T_3 levels. Plasma T_3 levels were measured by radioimmunoassay kits (Dainabot).

Isolation of Heart Mitochondria

Rats underwent cervical dislocation, after which the hearts were removed rapidly and washed in cold saline. The cardiac mitochondrial fraction was prepared by differential centrifugation according to the method of Hatefi and associates (10), and was suspended in 0.25 M of sucrose/10 mM of Tris-HCl (pH of 7.8) buffer. Because of the large amount of protein required for measurement of mitochondrial electron transport activity, segments from three hearts were combined for preparation of the mitochondrial fraction.

Measurement of Electron Transport Activity

The specific activity of nicotinamide adenine dinucleotide (NADH) (reduced form) cytochrome *c* reductase was determined by a modification of the method of Hatefi and Rieske (11). The reaction mixture consisted of 0.06 mL of potassium phosphate (1.0 M, pH of 8.0), 0.1 mL of NaN_3 (0.1 M), 0.06 mL of ethylenediaminetetraacetic acid (EDTA) (1 mM), 5 μL of 1% deoxycholic acid (pH of 8.0), 0.18 mL of 1% ferricytochrome *c*, and 2.6 mL of distilled water. The reaction was initiated by adding 10 μL of mitochondrial suspension and 75 μL of NADH (0.01 M). After 15 seconds, incubation at 30°C, the reaction rate was followed for 1 minute by recording the increase in absorbance of cytochrome *c* at 550 nm. The activity of NADH cytochrome *c* reductase was calculated from the rate of increase in the absorbance.

The specific activity of succinate-cytochrome *c* reductase was determined by the method of Tisdale (12). The reaction mixture consisted of 0.3 mL of potassium phosphate (0.1 M, pH of 7.4), 0.03 mL of NaN_3 (0.1 M), 0.06 mL of EDTA (0.01 M), 0.15 mL of 10% bovine serum albumin (BSA), 0.3 mL of potassium succinate (0.1 M), 0.3 mL of 1% ferricytochrome *c*, and 1.86 mL of distilled water. The reaction was initiated by adding 10 μl of mitochondrial suspension. As with NADH-cytochrome *c* reductase, after 15 seconds incubation at 30°C, the reaction rate was followed for 1 minute by recording the increase in absorbance of cytochrome *c* at 550 nm. The activity of succinate-cytochrome *c* reductase was deduced from the rate of increase in the absorbance.

The specific activity of cytochrome *c* oxidase was determined by a modification of the method of Wharton and Tzagoloff (13). To prepare ferrocytochrome *c*, 1% ferricytochrome *c* was reduced completely by dithionate, and excess dithionate was removed by passing the solution through a column of Sephadex G-25 (fine). Potassium phosphate (2.67 mL, 50 mM; pH of 7.0) and 30 μL of 10% Triton X-100 were added to 100 μL of ferrocytochrome *c* solution. Immediately after the addition of 0.1 mL of mitochondrial suspension, the reaction rate was followed for 10 seconds by recording the decrease in absorbance of cytochrome *c* at 550 nm. The activity of cytochrome *c* oxidase was deduced from the rate of decrease in the absorbance.

Tissue Preparations

The left ventricles were isolated and frozen in liquid nitrogen and stored at −70°C until use. Tissue was prepared according to the modified method described previously (14).

Acetylcholine and Norepinephrine Quantification

Acetycholine was separated from choline by reverse-phase high-performance liquid chromatography (HPLC), and was converted enzymatically into hydrogen peroxide in a postcolumn reaction system with acetylcholinesterase and choline oxidase. Production of hydrogen peroxide was detected by electrochemical detection (ECD). A modification of the method of Potter et al. (15), using an immobilized enzyme column as a postcolumn reactor, was used for the quantification of acetylcholine (14). The norepinephrine assay was conducted by the usual HPLC-ECD method described previously (14).

Morphologic Study

The tissue was cut into 1-mm cubes and fixed with 2% glutaraldehyde in phosphate buffer (0.1 M, pH of 7.4) for 2 hours at 4°C, postfixed with 1% osmium tetraoxide in the same buffer for 1 hour, dehydrated in ethanol, and embedded in Epon 812. Ultrathin sections were cut with a Porter-Blum ultramicrotome (MT-2), stained with uranyl acetate and lead citrate, and examined with a Nihon Denshi electron microscope (JEM 100S).

Statistical Analysis

All results are shown as mean $\pm$ SD, and analysis of variance with Duncan's test was used for statistical analysis of the data. Analysis was performed between Groups 1 and 2, and between Groups 3, 4, and 5. Differences were considered to be significant when probability values (p) were less than 0.05.

RESULTS

Effects of Thyroid Status on T_3 Levels, Heart Weight, and Body Weight

The effect of thyroid status on blood T_3 levels, heart weight, body weight, and heart weight/body weight ratio in each group is shown in Table 1. A significant decrease in T_3 level was observed 3 and 6 weeks after thyroidectomy. Supplementation with thyroid hormone resulted in a lesser decrease. Significant decreases in heart weight/body weight ratio were seen either 3 or 6 weeks after thyroidectomy. Administration of thyroid hormone resulted in a lesser decrease in this parameter. Heart weight/body weight ratios were maintained in rats receiving thyroid hormone replacement therapy.

TABLE 1. *Effects of thyroid status on triiodothyronine (T_3) level, heart weight (HW), body weight (BW), and HW/BW ratio*[a]

	T_3 (ng/ml)	HW (mg)	BW (g)	HW/BW ($\times 10^{-3}$)
Hypothyroid—3 weeks	0.55 ± 0.07**	267 ± 41**	155 ± 9**	1.7 ± 0.2**
Control	1.02 ± 0.11	709 ± 58	215 ± 10	3.3 ± 0.2
Hypothyroid—6 weeks	0.47 ± 0.08**	358 ± 49**	174 ± 17**	2.1 ± 0.3**
Hypothyroid—6 weeks, with T_3 therapy	0.77 ± 0.15*,***	692 ± 58**,***	273 ± 23**,***	2.5 ± 0.1***
Control	0.93 ± 0.06	908 ± 38	333 ± 9	2.7 ± 0.1

[a]Values expressed as means ± SD.
*$p < 0.05$ versus respective control group; **$p < 0.01$ versus respective control group; ***$p < 0.01$ versus hypothyroid—6 weeks group.

Effects of Thyroid Status on Electron Transport Activity

The activities of the electron transport chain in heart mitochondria in each group are shown in Table 2. Although no significant difference was observed in the activity of NADH-cytochrome c reductase 3 weeks after thyroidectomy, a significant decrease was observed 6 weeks after thyroidectomy. Thyroid hormone supplementation prevented this decrease. Similar tendencies were observed in the activity of cytochrome c oxidase. However, there was no significant difference between groups in terms of the activities of succinate-cytochrome c reductase.

TABLE 2. *Effects of thyroid status on electron transport activity*[a]

	NADH cytochrome c reductase	Succinate-cytochrome c reductase	Cytochrome c oxidase
Hypothyroid—3 weeks	396 ± 70	376 ± 49	2293 ± 260
Control	420 ± 54	368 ± 44	2214 ± 174
Hypothyroid—6 weeks	334 ± 72*	358 ± 39	1932 ± 211*
Hypothyroid—6 weeks, with T_3 therapy	442 ± 57**	384 ± 57	2347 ± 254**
Control	439 ± 55	364 ± 43	2333 ± 244

[a]Values expressed in nmol/mg protein/min and as means ± SD.
*$p < 0.05$ versus control group; **$p < 0.05$ versus hypothyroid—6 weeks group.
NADH, nicotinamide adenine dinucleotide, reduced form; T_3, triiodothyronine.

Effects of Thyroid Status on Acetylcholine and Norepinephrine Levels

The acetylcholine and norepinephrine contents of the left ventricle of rats in each group are shown in Figure 1. Although no significant difference was reported in the left ventricular acetylcholine content 3 weeks after thyroidectomy, a significant decrease was seen 6 weeks after thyroidectomy. Supplementation with thyroid hormone resulted in a lesser decrease. Thyroidectomy increased norepinephrine content significantly compared with the norepinephrine level in sham-operated rats. Again, thyroid hormone supplementation prevented this increase.

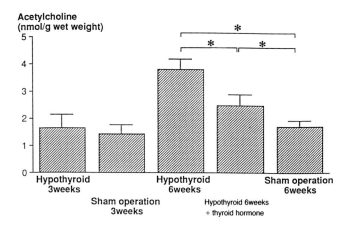

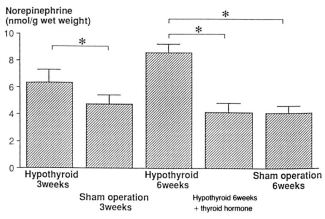

FIG. 1. Effects of thyroid status on acetylcholine (*upper panel*) and norepinephrine (*lower panel*) contents. Acetylcholine contents in the left ventricle increased 6 weeks after thyroidectomy; norepinephrine content increased 3 weeks after surgery. (*$p<0.01$.)

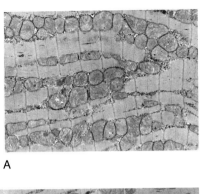

A

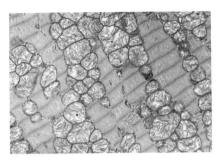

B

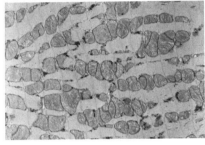

C

FIG. 2. **A:** Typical histologic features of the cardiac tissue from the control group. No significant changes were observed. **B:** Typical histologic features of the cardiac tissue from rats 6 weeks after thyroidectomy. Mitochondrial swelling was observed. **C:** Typical histologic features of the cardiac tissue from thyroidectomized rats treated with triiodothyronine. The alterations seen in Figure 2B were lessened.

Effects of Thyroid Status on Myocardial Structure

Electron microscopic photographs were obtained from sections of cardiac tissue in each group (Fig. 2). In the sham-operated group, no significant changes were observed (Fig. 2A). In rats undergoing thyroidectomy, mitochondrial swelling was observed 6 weeks after surgery (Fig. 2B). However, this swelling decreased with thyroid hormone supplementation (Fig. 2C).

DISCUSSION

Mitochondria and Hypothyroidism

Because mitochondria exclusively produce high-energy phosphates, an impairment in cardiac mitochondrial enzymatic activities can be seen to cause cardiac dysfunction. In the present study, mitochondrial dysfunction was not seen 3 weeks after thyroidectomy. However, decreases in NADH cytochrome c reductase and cytochrome c oxidase activities were observed in rat myocardium 6 weeks after thyroidectomy, although no significant change was seen in succinate-cytochrome c reductase. Administration of thyroid hormone mitigated these decreases significantly. Morphologic results corresponded with biochemical functional analysis. These results suggested that long-term hypothyroidism caused mitochondrial dysfunction, although short-term hypothyroidism did not introduce significant mitochondrial dysfunction.

Hypothyroid myopathy is widely accepted. Abnormalities in ultrastructure and mitochondrial function have been reported (16). However, reports indicate that histologic changes were absent in myopathy in acute hypothyroidism (17). These reports are consistent with our results. Khaleeli and colleagues (16) have suggested that the severity of hypothyroid myopathy is closely related to the chronicity and the severity of the hypothyroidism. In the present study, similar findings involving both structural changes and biochemical abnormalities were revealed. Cardiac dysfunction associated with hypothyroidism may be attributable to mitochondrial dysfunction, as thyroid hormone regulates physiologically mitochondrial biogenesis.

Sympathetic Nervous System and Hypothyroidism

It is well known that a decrease in peripheral adrenergic function, an alteration in responsiveness to catecholamines, and a decrease in the density and responsiveness of β-adrenergic receptors are seen in hypothyroidism (18–20). These changes may be reversed by thyroid hormone replacement (20). In the present study, a significant increase in left ventricular norepinephrine level was observed either 3 weeks or 6 weeks after thyroidectomy. Supplementation with thyroid hormone reduced the increase significantly, suggesting that changes in the sympathetic nervous system were attributable to alterations in the thyroid status. Accordingly, an increase in left ventricular norepinephrine levels was caused by thyroidectomy. Mitochondrial dysfunction was not observed 3 weeks after surgery, despite a left ventricular norepinephrine increase. Accordingly, this increase may not be directly related to mitochondrial dysfunction. Hence, an increase in norepinephrine observed 6 weeks after thyroidectomy also may not be related to mitochondrial dysfunction.

Parasympathetic Nervous System and Hypothyroidism

It is unclear whether or not the parasympathetic nervous system impairment is related to hypothyroidism. In a previous study, we demonstrated that an acetylcholinesterase inhibitor, pyridostigmine, impaired mitochondrial electron transport activity in accordance with elevated acetylcholine levels (7,8). These results suggest that acetylcholine, a transmitter of the parasympathetic nervous system, causes cardiomyopathy. In the present study, a significant increase in left ventricular acetylcholine level was seen 6 weeks after thyroidectomy, although only an insignificant increase was observed 3 weeks after thyroidectomy. The increases in acetylcholine observed in this study were comparable to those seen in rats receiving pyridostigmine (7,8). Supplementation with thyroid hormone lessened these increases. The changes in acetylcholine levels seemed to correlate with the changes in electron transport activities. These results suggest that an increase in acetylcholine level is related to mitochondrial dysfunction caused by hypothyroidism rather than to an increase in norepinephrine. Tsuboi and associates (14) have demonstrated an elevation in acetylcholine in spontaneously hypertensive rats, and streptozotocin-induced diabetic rats have been reported to have an increased acetylcholine content in the left ventricle (21). We have shown that cyclophosphamide causes heart mitochondrial dysfunction associated with autonomic disturbances (22). In hypothyroidism, similar autonomic disturbances may occur.

Clinical Implication

Hypothyroidism appears to influence autonomic nervous system. Mitochondrial dysfunction associated with hypothyroidism may be closely linked to an increase in left ventricular acetylcholine level. It is suggested that an impairment in the parasympathetic nervous system is involved in the genesis of cardiomyopathy.

SUMMARY

The involvement of the autonomic nervous system in the genesis of cardiomyopathy has been suggested. In the present study, the role of acetylcholine, a transmitter of the parasympathetic nervous system, in hypothyroid cardiomyopathy was investigated using surgically thyroidectomized rats. Hearts were isolated 3 or 6 weeks after thyroidectomy. Heart mitochondrial electron transport activities (NADH-cytochrome c reductase, succinate-cytochrome c reductase and cytochrome c oxidase) were measured by enzymatic assay. Acetylcholine and norepinephrine levels of the left ventricles were measured by HPLC. Structural changes in cardiac muscles were observed by electron microscopy of cardiac sections. No significant changes in the electron transport activities were observed 3 weeks after thyroidectomy. However, activities of NADH-cytochrome c reductase and cytochrome c oxidase were significantly reduced 6 weeks after thyroidectomy. A significant increase in acetylcholine level was noted 6 weeks after thyroidectomy, although no significant change was seen 3 weeks after thyroidectomy. By contrast, a significant increase in norepinephrine levels was reported either 3 or 6 weeks after thyroidectomy. Marked mitochondrial changes were observed 6 weeks after thyroidectomy. Administration of T_3 partially prevented these changes. Thus, an increase in acetylcholine associated with mitochondrial dysfunction and pathologic changes was observed in long-term hypothyroid rats. However, changes in norepinephrine levels did not correspond with mitochondrial changes. Accordingly, it was concluded that an impairment of the parasympathetic nervous system might be involved in the genesis of hypothyroid cardiomyopathy.

REFERENCES

1. Tachman ML, Guthrie GP. Hypothyroidism: diversity of presentation. *Endocr Rev* 1984;5:456–65.
2. Nishiki K, Erecinska M, Wilson DF, Cooper S. Evaluation of oxidative phosphorylation in hearts from euthyroid, hypothyroid, and hyperthyroid rats. *Am J Physiol* 1978;235:C212–19.
3. Shenoy MM, Goldman JM. Hypothyroid cardiomyopathy: echocardiographic documentation of reversibility. *Am J Med Sci* 1987;294:1–9.
4. Everett AW, Umeda PK, Sinha AM, Rabinowitz M, Zak R. Expression of myosin heavy chains during thyroid hormone-induced cardiac growth. *Fed Proc* 1986;45:2568–72.
5. Roher D, Dillmann WH. Thyroid hormone markedly increases the mRNA coding for sarcoplasmic reticulum Ca^{2+}-ATPase in the rat heart. *J Biol Chem* 1988;263:6941–4.
6. Skelton CL, Sonnenblick EH. The cardiovascular system. In Werner A, ed. *The Thyroid. A fundamental and clinical text.* Philadelphia: JB Lippincott; 1986:1140–8.
7. Kato T, Sugiyama S, Hanaki Y, et al. Role of acetylcholine in pyridostigmine-induced myocardial injury: Possible involvement of parasympathetic nervous system in the genesis of cardiomyopathy. *Arch Toxicol* 1989;63:137–43.
8. Ito T, Akiyama N, Ogawa T, et al. Changes in myocardial mitochondrial electron transport activity in rats administered with acetylcholinesterase inhibitor. *Biochem Biophys Res Commun* 1989;164:997–1002.
9. Capasso G, Tepper D, Capasso JM, Sonnenblick EH. Effects of hypothyroidism and hypoparathyroidism on rat myocardium: mechanical and electrical alterations. *Am J Med Sci* 1986;291:232–40.
10. Hatefi Y, Jurtsshuk P, Haavik AG. Studies on the electron transport system. XXIII. Respiratory control in beef heart mitochondria. *Arch Biochem Biophys* 1961;94:148–55.
11. Hatefi Y, Rieske JS. The preparation and properties of DPNH-cytochrome c reductase (complex I-III of the respiratory chain). In: Estabrook RW, Pullman ME, eds. *Methods in enzymology*, Vol 10. New York: Academic Press; 1967:225–31.
12. Tisdale HD. Preparation and properties of succinic-cytochrome c reductase (complex II-III). In: Estabrook RW, Pullman ME, eds. *Methods in enzymology*, Vol 10. New York: Academic Press; 1967:213–5.
13. Wharton DC, Tzagoloff A. Cytochrome oxidase from beef heart mitochondria. In: Estabrook RW, Pullman ME, eds. *Methods in enzymology*, Vol 10. New York: Academic Press; 1967:245–50.
14. Tsuboi H, Ohno O, Ogawa K, et al. Acetylcholine and norepinephrine concentration in hearts of spontaneously hypertensive rats: A parasympathetic role in hypertension. *J Hypertens* 1987;5:323–30.
15. Potter PE, Meek JL, Neff NH. Acetylcholine and choline in neuronal tissue measured by HPLC with electrochemical detection. *J Neurochem* 1983;41:188–94.
16. Khaleeli AA, Gohil K, McPhail G, Round JM, Edwards R. Muscle morphology and metabolism in hypothyroid myopathy: effects of treatment. *J Clin Pathol* 1983;36:519–26.
17. Kung AWC, Ma JTC, Yu YL, et al. Myopathy in acute hypothyroidism. *Postgrad Med J* 1987;63:661–63.
18. Kunos G, Mucci L, O'Regan S. The influence of hormonal and neuronal factors on rat heart adrenoceptors. *Br J Pharmacol* 1980;71:371–86.
19. Fox AW, Juberg EN, May M, Johnson RD, Abel PW, Minneman KP. Thyroid status and adrenergic receptor subtypes in rat: comparison of receptor density and responsiveness. *J Pharm Exp Ther* 1985;235:715–23.
20. Chu DTW, Shikama H, Khatra BS, Exton JH. Effects of altered thyroid status on β-adrenergic actions on skeletal muscle glycogen metabolism. *J Biol Chem* 1985;260:9994–10,000.
21. Akiyama N, Okumura K, Watanabe Y, et al. Altered acetylcholine and norepinephrine concentrations in diabetic rat hearts. *Diabetes* 1989;38:231–36.
22. Hanaki Y, Sugiyama S, Akiyama N, Ozawa T. Role of the autonomic nervous system in cyclophosphamide-induced heart mitochondrial dysfunction in rats. *Biochem Int* 1990;21:289–295.

Subject Index

NOTE: Page numbers followed by a *t* indicate tables; page numbers followed by an *f* indicate figures.

Contractile protein abnormalities
  in cardiomyopathic hamster, 31–39
  in Keshan disease, 216*t*, 216–217,
    217*t*
Costameres
  properties of, 250
  vinculin-containing, of cardiomyocytes,
    245–255
Coxsackievirus B3
  myocarditic and amyocarditic strains,
    comparison, 309–312
  myocarditis, 309–312
  immunopathology, 285–292
Creatine kinase
  distribution, in Keshan disease model,
    226, 226*f*, 228*t*
  mitochondrial, in experimental
    cardiomyopathy, 191–192
  myocardial, in Keshan disease, 212,
    212*t*, 214–215, 215*f*
  myofibrillar, in experimental
    cardiomyopathy, 192
  serum, in cardiomyopathic hamster
    and ACE inhibitor treatment, 159,
      159*f*
    and PGE₁ treatment, 161, 161*f*
  serum, in Keshan disease, 223
Creatine phosphate, myocardial
  in canine tissue
    in isoproterenol cardiotoxicity, 386,
      386*f*
    measurement, 384
  in cardiomyopathic hamster, 3, 5*f*
Creatine phosphokinase, serum, in
    cardiomyopathic hamster, 69,
    70*f*
Cyclic adenosine monophosphate
  intracellular, in failing myocardium,
    197–198
  lipophilic analogs to, response to, in
    catecholamine cardiomyopathy
    model and failing human heart,
    361, 366–367, 368*f*, 372
CYP. *See* Iodocyanopindolol
Cytochrome oxidase, in Keshan disease,
    212–213, 213*t*
Cytokines, effects in trauma-sepsis
    syndrome, 258–259, 259*t*,
    262–264, 263*f*

D

DCM. *See* Dilated cardiomyopathy
Dendritic cells, in close contact with
    cardiocytes, in autoimmune
    myocarditis induced by myosin,
    295, 296*f*
Diabetes
  canine model, cardiac sarcoplasmic
    reticular function in, 419–428
  rodent model
    cardiac hypertrophy in infants of
      diabetic mothers in, 429–437
    ventricular myosin isoenzyme pattern
      in, 28
Diabetic dog
  cardiac sarcoplasmic reticular function
    in, 419–428
  trabecular muscle
    isolation, 419–420
    isometric twitch contraction, 420,
      420*t*
    postrest contraction, 420, 421*f*,
      421–424, 422*f*–424*f*
    rest decay, comparison to normal
      muscle, 424–426
Diacylglycerol
  in myopathic hamster heart, 115–123,
    119*f*
  in phosphatidylinositol turnover, 105
Diastolic stiffness, in experimental
    cardiomyopathies, 185–195
Dilated cardiomyopathy, 141
  calcium handling in, 206–207
  force-frequency relationship in,
    197–209
  hamster model of, 57–58
  inotropic interventions and, 197–209
DNA
  extraction, from heart muscle, 315
  in hamster ventricular tissues, 119–120,
    121*f*
  determination of, 117
  mitochondrial
    electron transfer chain subunits
      encoded by, 313, 314*f*
    fluorescence-based direct sequencing,
      317
    mutations, in hypertrophic
      cardiomyopathy, 313–321